Therapeutic Modalities in Rehabilitation

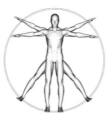

Therapeutic Modalities in Rehabilitation

Fourth Edition

William E. Prentice, PhD, PT, ATC, FNATA

Professor, Coordinator of Sports Medicine Program
Department of Exercise and Sport Science
University of North Carolina at Chapel Hill
Chapel Hill, North Carolina

With Case Studies and Lab Activities Contributed by:

William S. Quillen, PhD, PT, SCS, FACSM

Associate Dean, College of Medicine
Professor and Director, School of Physical
Therapy and Rehabilitation Sciences
University of South Florida
Tampa, Florida

Frank Underwood, PhD, MPT, ECS

Professor, Department of Physical Therapy
University of Evansville
Clinical Electrophysiologist, Rehabilitation Service
Orthopaedic Associates, Inc.
Evansville, Indiana

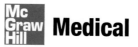

New York   Chicago   San Francisco   Lisbon   London   Madrid   Mexico City
Milan   New Delhi   San Juan   Seoul   Singapore   Sydney   Toronto

Therapeutic Modalities in Rehabilitation, Fourth Edition

Copyright © 2011, 2005 by The McGraw-Hill Companies, Inc. All rights reserved.
Printed in China. Except as permitted under the United States Copyright Act of 1976,
no part of this publication may be reproduced or distributed in any form or by any
means, or stored in a database or retrieval system, without the prior written permission
of the publisher.

Previous editions published as *Therapeutic Modalities for Physical Therapists*, copyright
© 2002 by The McGraw-Hill Companies, Inc., and as *Therapeutic Modalities for Allied
Health Professionals*, copyright © 1998 by The McGraw-Hill Companies, Inc.

3 4 5 6 7 8 9 0 CTP/CTP 14 13 12

ISBN 978-0-07-173769-2
MHID 0-07-173769-3

This book was set in Minion Pro by Thomson Digital.
The editors were Joseph Morita and Peter J. Boyle.
The production supervisor was Phil Galea.
Project management was provided by Pooja Khurana, Thomson Digital.
The interior designer is Eve Siegel.
China Translation & Printing, Ltd., was printer and binder.

Cataloging-in-publication data for this title is on file at the Library of Congress.

McGraw-Hill books are available at special quantity discounts to use as premiums and
sales promotions, or for use in corporate training programs. To contact a representative
please e-mail us at bulksales@mcgraw-hill.com.

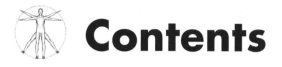

Contents

PART THREE
Thermal Energy Modalities

PART FOUR
Sound Energy Modalities

PART SIX
Mechanical Energy Modalities

Contributors to This and Previous Editions

Bob Blake, PhD, LMT
Assistant Professor
Chair, Chemical Education
Department of Chemistry and Biochemistry
Texas Tech University
Lubbock, Texas

Craig R. Denegar, PhD, PT, ATC, FNATA
Professor and Department Head
in Physical Therapy
Neag School of Education
University of Connecticut
Stoors, Connecticut

Phillip B. Donley, MS, PT, ATC
Director, Chester County Orthopaedic
and Sports
Physical Therapy
West Chester, Pennsylvania

David O. Draper, EdD, ATC
Professor of Sports Medicine/Athletic Training
Department of Exercise Sciences
College of Health and Human Performance
Brigham Young University
Provo, Utah

David Greathouse, PhD, PT, ECS, FAPTA
Adjunct Professor
United States Army- Baylor University
Fort Sam Houston, Texas
Revisions and updates for
Chapter 8, Fourth Edition

John Halle, PhD, PT, ECS
Professor and Associate Dean
School of Physical Therapy
Belmont University
Nashville, Tennessee
Revisions and updates for
Chapter 8, Fourth Edition

Daniel N. Hooker, PhD, PT, SCS, ATC
Associate Director of Sports Medicine
Division of Sports Medicine
Campus Health Service
University of North Carolina
Chapel Hill, North Carolina

Pamela E. Houghton, PhD, BSc PT
Chair, MSc Program
Associate Professor
School of Physical Therapy
University of Western Ontario
London, Ontario
Revisions and updates for
Chapter 3, Fourth Edition

William E. Prentice, PhD, PT, ATC, FNATA
Professor, Coordinator of Sports
Medicine Program
Department of Exercise and Sport Science
University of North Carolina
Chapel Hill, North Carolina

William S. Quillen, PhD, PT, SCS, FACSM
Associate Dean, College of Medicine
Professor and Director, School of Physical
Therapy and Rehabilitation Sciences
University of South Florida
Tampa, Florida

Ethan N. Saliba, PhD, PT, ATC
Head Athletic Trainer, Assistant Athletics
Director for Sports Medicine,
Department of Athletics
Assistant Professor, Department of Kinesiology
Adjunct Assistant Professor, Department of
Physical Medicine and Rehabilitation
University of Virginia
Charlottesville, Virginia

Susan Foreman-Saliba, PhD, MPT, ATC
Assistant Professor, Sports Medicine and
Athletic Training Advisor and Director,
Department of Kinesiology
Assistant Professor, Department of Physical
Medicine and Rehabilitation
Assistant Professor, Department of
Orthopedic Surgery
University of Virginia
Charlottesville, Virginia

Charles Thigpen, PhD, PT, ATC
Clinical Research Scientist
Proaxis Therapy, Innovative
Therapy Resource
Greenville, South Carolina
Revisions and updates for
Chapter 11, Fourth Edition

Frank Underwood, PhD, MPT, ECS
Associate Professor, Department of
Physical Therapy
University of Evansville
Clinical Electrophysiologist
Rehabilitation Service
Orthopaedic Associates, Inc.
Evansville, Indiana

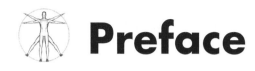

Preface

Physical therapists, athletic trainers, occupational therapists, physical therapy assistants, occupational therapy assistants, physical therapy aides, and chiropractors use a wide variety of therapeutic techniques in the treatment and rehabilitation of their patients. A thorough treatment regimen often involves the use of therapeutic modalities. At one time or another, virtually all clinicians make use of some type of modality. This may involve a relatively simple technique such as using an ice pack for an acute injury or more complex techniques such as the stimulation of nerve and muscle tissue by electrical currents. There is no question that therapeutic modalities are useful tools in injury rehabilitation. When used appropriately, these modalities can greatly enhance the patient's chances for complete recovery. Unfortunately, the clinicians' rationale for using a particular modality is too often based on habit rather than on logic or analysis of effectiveness. For the clinician, it is essential to possess knowledge regarding the scientific basis and the physiologic effects of the various modalities on a specific injury. When this theoretical basis is applied to practical experience, it has the potential to become an extremely effective clinical method.

It must be emphasized that the use of therapeutic modalities in any treatment program is an inexact science. If you were to ask 10 different clinicians what combination of modalities and therapeutic exercise they use in a given treatment program, you would likely get 10 different responses. There is no way to "cookbook" a treatment plan that involves the use of modalities. Thus, what this book will attempt to do is to present the basis for use of each different type of modality and allow the clinician to make his or her own decision as to which will be most effective in a given situation. Some recommended protocols developed through the experiences of the contributing authors will be presented.

The following are a number of reasons why this text should be adopted for use.

COMPREHENSIVE COVERAGE OF THERAPEUTIC MODALITIES USED IN A CLINICAL SETTING

The purpose of this text is to provide a theoretically based but practically oriented guide to the use of therapeutic modalities for the practicing clinician and their students. It is intended for use in courses where various clinically oriented techniques and methods are presented.

The chapters in this text are divided into six parts. Each chapter discusses (1) the physiologic basis for use, (2) clinical applications, (3) specific techniques of application through the use of related laboratory activities, and (4) relevant individual case studies for each therapeutic modality.

Part I—Foundations of Therapeutic Modalities begins with a chapter that discusses the scientific basis for using therapeutic modalities and classifies the modalities according to the type of energy each uses. Guidelines for selecting the most appropriate modalities for use in different phases of the healing process are presented. A chapter that deals specifically with the role of therapeutic modalities in wound healing is followed by a discussion of pain in terms of the neurophysiologic mechanisms of pain and the role of therapeutic modalities in pain management.

Part II—Electrical Energy Modalities includes detailed discussions of the principles of electricity, and electrical stimulating currents, iontophoresis, and biofeedback. A chapter that deals with the principles of electrophysiologic evaluation and testing is included. Although this is not a therapeutic modality per se, electrophysiologic testing is commonly taught in classes that cover electrical modalities and thus the decision was made to include this topic in this text.

Part III—Thermal Energy Modalities discusses those modalities that produce a change in tissue temperatures through conduction, including thermotherapy and cryotherapy.

Part IV—Sound Energy Modalities discusses those modalities that utilize acoustic energy to produce a therapeutic effect. These include therapeutic ultrasound and a lesser known modality, extracorporal shockwave therapy.

Part V—Electromagnetic Energy Modalities includes chapters on both the diathermies and low-level laser therapy.

Part VI—Mechanical Energy Modalities includes chapters on traction, intermittent compression, and therapeutic massage.

BASED ON SCIENTIFIC THEORY

This text discusses various concepts, principles, and theories that are supported by scientific research, factual evidence, and previous experience of the authors in dealing with various conditions. The material presented in this text has been carefully researched by the contributing authors to provide up-to-date information on the theoretical basis for employing a particular modality in a specific injury situation. Additionally, the manuscript for this text has been carefully reviewed by educators, researchers, and practicing clinicians who are considered experts in their field to ensure that the material reflects factual and current concepts for modality use.

TIMELY AND PRACTICAL

Certainly, therapeutic modalities used in a clinical setting are important tools for the clinician. This text provides a comprehensive resource that should be used in student instruction on the theoretical basis and practical application of the various modalities. It should serve as a needed guide for the student who is interested in knowing not only how to use a modality but also why that particular modality is most effective in a given situation.

The authors who have contributed to this text have a great deal of clinical experience. Each of these individuals has also at one time or another been involved with the formal academic preparation of the student clinician. Thus, this text has been directed at the student who will be asked to apply the theoretical basis of modality use to the clinical setting.

Several other texts are available that discuss the use of selected physical modalities in various patient populations. This is the most comprehensive text on therapeutic modalities available in any specific discipline.

PEDAGOGIC AIDS

The aids this text uses to facilitate its use by students and instructors include:

Objectives These goals are listed at the beginning of each chapter to introduce students to the points that will be emphasized.

Figures and Tables Essential points on each chapter are illustrated with clear visual materials.

Summary Each chapter has a summary that outlines the major points covered.

Clinical Decision-Making Exercises The scenarios help the clinician develop decision-making abilities about how a specific modality may best be used clinically.

Review Questions Designed to help the student review the material presented in each chapter by answering a series of thought-provoking questions.

Self-Test Questions A set of true/false and multiple choice questions is provided in each chapter to help the student prepare for a written examination and to assess student comprehension.

Glossary of Key Terms Each chapter contains a glossary of terms for quick reference.

References A list of up-to-date references is provided at the end of each chapter for the student who wishes to read further on the subject being discussed.

Case Studies A series of clinically based case studies are presented to enhance student understanding of how these modalities may be applied to a specific patient.

Lab Activities Lab activities are included to guide the student through the setup and application of the various modalities.

Appendices A chart of trigger points and a comprehensive list of manufacturers of therapeutic modality equipment are provided.

HOW TO USE THE LABORATORY ACTIVITIES

There are a wide variety of laboratory activities found throughout this book.

Theory, biophysical principles, and range of potential clinical medicine applications for the various physical agent modalities will be found in this text. The activities are intended to provide the student or interested reader with a systematic and sequential method of completing a therapeutic modality application. The initial performance of a therapeutic procedure should proceed in a logical stepwise fashion. They are structured to allow both the instructor or supervisor and the student the ability to assess competency in a partial or complete fashion culminating in the independent ability to safely and effectively provide a therapeutic modality treatment.

Each therapeutic modality application has a separate sequential checklist. Similarities will be noted in certain aspects of treatment application and completion. Space is provided for up to three separate instructors/supervisors to "sign off" (initial and date) the successful completion and demonstration of each element of the complete application. A Master Competency Check List is provided to document the successful completion of the individual therapeutic modality checklist and when the student is deemed competent to independently provide that treatment. This system documents the acquisition of skills necessary for effective physical agent modality application and ensures accountability by the student and instructor/supervisor to patients and other concerned parties.

Competency in the skillful application of therapeutic modalities is gained through diligent and frequent practice. Use of these activities in the manner described will guide the user in productive practice and successful acquisition of essential skills. Students are encouraged to practice each of the procedures on themselves first, thereby gaining an appreciation of the sensations associated with that particular modality. Further practice with a variety of lab partners will result in the development of the desired competence and confidence with any manufacturer's equipment.

Acknowledgments

I would like to thank my editor at McGraw-Hill, Joe Morita, for his assistance in this project from the very beginning. His advice and direction have certainly helped in its completion.

I would also like to thank my wife, Tena, and our two boys, Brian and Zachary, for putting up with me when I get going with a project like this. Sometimes it's not easy.

MASTER COMPETENCY CHECKLIST

THERAPEUTIC MODALITY	EXAMINER		
	1	2	3
Positioning			
Electrical Stimulation			
Analgesia			
Muscle reeducation			
Muscle strengthening			
Iontophoresis			
Biofeedback			
Shortwave diathermy			
Thermotherapy			
Hydrocollator pack			
Paraffin bath			
Infrared Lamp			
Cryotherapy			
Ice massage			
Ice pack			
Gel cold pack			
Vapocoolant spray			
Cryo/Cuff			
Hydrotherapy			
Warm whirlpool			
Cold whirlpool			
Contrast bath			
Fluidotherapy			
Low power laser			
Ultrasound			
Direct contact			
Bladder coupling			
Underwater coupling			
Phonophoresis			
Mechanical traction			
Cervical			
Lumbar			
Intermittent compression			
Massage			

PART ONE

Foundations of Therapeutic Modalities

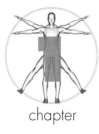

chapter

The Basic Science of Therapeutic Modalities

William E. Prentice and Bob Blake

OBJECTIVES

Following completion of this chapter, the student will be able to:

➤ List and describe the different forms of energy used with therapeutic modalities.

➤ Classify the various modalities according to the type of energy utilized by each.

➤ Analyze the relationship between wavelength and frequency for electromagnetic energy.

➤ Discuss the electromagnetic spectrum and how various modalities that use electromagnetic energy are related.

➤ Explain how the laws governing the effects of electromagnetic energy apply to diathermy, laser, and ultraviolet light.

➤ Discuss how the thermal energy modalities, thermotherapy and cryotherapy, transfer heat through conduction.

➤ Explain the various ways electrical energy can be used to produce a therapeutic effect.

➤ Compare and contrast the properties of electromagnetic and sound energy.

➤ Explain how intermittent compression, traction, and massage use mechanical energy to produce a therapeutic effect.

For the clinician who chooses to incorporate a therapeutic modality into his or her clinical practice, some knowledge and understanding of the basic science behind the use of these agents is useful.[1] The interactions between energy and matter are fascinating, and they are the physical basis for the various therapeutic modalities that are described in this book. This chapter will describe the different forms of energy, the ways energy can be transferred, and how energy transfer affects biologic tissues. A strong theoretical knowledge base can help clinicians understand how each therapeutic modality works.

FORMS OF ENERGY

Energy is defined as the capacity of a system for doing work and exists in various forms. Energy is not ordinarily created or destroyed, but it is often transformed from one form to another or transferred from one location to another.[2]

3

There is considerable confusion among even the most experienced clinicians regarding the different forms of energy involved with the various therapeutic modalities. The forms of energy that are relevant to the use of therapeutic modalities are *electromagnetic energy, thermal energy, electrical energy, sound energy,* and *mechanical energy.*[2] Shortwave and microwave diathermy, infrared lamps, ultraviolet light therapy, and low-power lasers utilize electromagnetic energy. Thermotherapy and cryotherapy transfer thermal energy. The electrical stimulating currents, iontophoresis and biofeedback, utilize electrical energy. Ultrasound and extracorporal shockwave therapy utilize sound energy. Intermittent compression, traction, and massage utilize mechanical energy (Table 1–1).

Each of these therapeutic agents transfers energy in one form or another into or out of biologic tissues. Different forms of energy can produce similar effects in biologic tissues. For example, tissue heating is a common effect of several treatments that utilize different types of energy. Electrical currents that pass through tissues will generate heat as a result of the resistance of the tissue to the passage of electricity. Electromagnetic energy such as

Table 1–1   Classification of Therapeutic Modalities Under the Various Forms of Energy

ELECTROMAGNETIC ENERGY MODALITIES

- Shortwave diathermy
- Microwave diathermy
- Infrared lamps
- Ultraviolet therapy
- Low-power laser

THERMAL ENERGY MODALITIES

- Thermotherapy
- Cryotherapy

ELECTRICAL ENERGY MODALITIES

- Electrical stimulating currents
- Biofeedback
- Iontophoresis

SOUND ENERGY MODALITIES

- Ultrasound
- Extracorporal shockwave therapy

MECHANICAL ENERGY MODALITIES

- Intermittent compression
- Traction
- Massage

light waves will heat any tissues that absorb it. Ultrasound treatments will also warm tissues through which the sound waves travel. Although the electrical, electromagnetic, and sound energy treatments all heat tissues, the physical mechanism of action for each is different.[3]

The mechanism of action of each therapeutic modality depends on which form of energy is utilized during its application. Different forms of energy are generated and transferred by different mechanisms. Electromagnetic energy is typically generated by a high-energy source and is transmitted by the movement of photons. Thermal energy can be transferred by conduction, which involves the flow of thermal energy between objects that are in contact with each other. Electrical energy is stored in electric fields and delivered by the movement of charged particles. Acoustic vibrations produce sound waves that can pass through a medium. Each form of energy and the mechanism of its transfer will be discussed in more detail to provide the scientific basis for understanding the therapeutic modalities.[4]

Clinical Decision-Making *Exercise 1–1*

Several modalities can be used to manage pain. Of the modalities discussed, which may be used to modulate pain and which should a clinician recommend as the best to use immediately following injury?

ELECTROMAGNETIC ENERGY

Radiation is a process by which electromagnetic energy travels from its source outward through space.[5] Sunlight is a visible type of radiant energy, and we know that it not only makes objects visible but also produces heat. The sun emits a spectrum of visible and invisible massless radiant energy and ejects high-energy particles as a result of high-intensity chemical and nuclear reactions. The massless radiant energy emissions from the sun are called **photons.** A photon is the energy carrier that composes all electromagnetic radiation. Photons travel as waves at the speed of light, approximately 300 million meters per second. Since photons all travel at the same speed, they are distinguished by their wave properties of wavelength and frequency, as well as the amount of energy carried by each photon.

The Relationship Between Wavelength and Frequency

Wavelength is defined as the distance between the peak of one wave and the peak of either the preceding or succeeding wave. **Frequency** is defined as the number of wave oscillations or vibrations occurring in a particular time unit and is commonly expressed in Hertz (Hz). One Hertz is one vibration per second (Figure 1–1).

Since all forms of electromagnetic radiation travel at a constant velocity through space, photons with longer wavelengths have lower frequencies and photons with shorter wavelengths

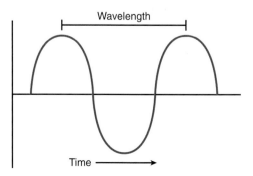

Figure 1–1. Wavelength and frequency.

have higher frequencies.[6] The following equation is useful for doing calculations involving the speed, wavelength, and frequency of waves.

$$\text{Speed} = \text{wavelength} \times \text{frequency}$$

$$c \quad = \quad \lambda \quad \times \quad v$$

An inverse or reciprocal relationship exists between wavelength and frequency. The longer the wavelength of a wave, the lower the frequency of the wave has to be. The velocity of electromagnetic radiation is a constant, 3×10^8 m/s. If we know the wavelength of any wave, the frequency of that wave can also be calculated. Whenever we are dealing with electromagnetic energy of any kind, we can use the speed of light, 3.0×10^8 m/s in that equation. That speed is not appropriate for electrical energy waves or sound energy waves, which do not travel at the speed of light.[7]

The other equation that is important with electromagnetic radiation is the *energy equation*. The energy of a photon is directly proportional to its frequency. This means that the electromagnetic radiation with higher frequency also has higher energy. We will relate this to the effects that each form of electromagnetic radiation can produce in tissues.

$$E = h \times v$$

(The letter *h* is known as *Planck's constant* and has a value of 6.626×10^{-34} Js. When Planck's constant is multiplied by a frequency in vibrations per second, the result has the standard scientific energy unit of Joules.)

The Electromagnetic Energy Spectrum

If a ray of sunlight is passed through a prism, it will be broken down into various colors in a predictable rainbow-like pattern of red, orange, yellow, green, blue, indigo, and violet (Figure 1–2). The range of colors is called a **spectrum**. The colors that we can detect with our eyes are referred to as *visible light* or *luminous radiations*. Each of these colors represents a photon of a different energy. They appear as different colors because the various forms of radiant energy are **refracted** or change direction as a result of differences in wavelength and frequency of each color. When passed through a prism, the type of radiant energy refracted the least appears as the color red, whereas that refracted the most is violet.[7] The longest wavelength light is red in color and low in energy, whereas the shortest wavelength light is violet and relatively higher in energy.

This beam of electromagnetic radiation from the sun that passes through the prism also includes propagating forms of radiant energy that are not visible to our eyes.[2] If a thermometer is placed close to the red end of the visible light spectrum, the thermometer will rise in temperature. This is because there is invisible radiation with longer wavelengths than red light, called **infrared radiation,** which is absorbed by the thermometer. When the infrared

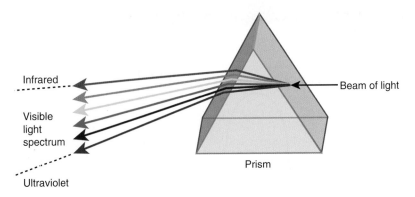

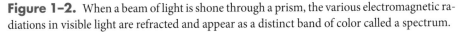

Figure 1–2. When a beam of light is shone through a prism, the various electromagnetic radiations in visible light are refracted and appear as a distinct band of color called a spectrum.

radiation is absorbed by the thermometer, it heats the thermometer, just like the light from the sun can warm your skin as your skin absorbs the light. Likewise, photographic film that is placed close to the violet end of the visible light spectrum can be developed by another form of invisible radiation from the sun, called **ultraviolet radiation**. Infrared radiation is lower in energy than red light (*infra* means lower or below). Ultraviolet radiation is higher in energy than violet light (*ultra* means greater or above). Almost all of the electromagnetic radiation produced by the sun is invisible. The entire electromagnetic spectrum includes radio and television waves, diathermies, infrared rays, visible light rays, ultraviolet rays, x-rays, and gamma rays (Table 1–2).

The electromagnetic spectrum places all of the electromagnetic modalities in order based on wavelengths and corresponding frequencies. It is apparent, for example, that the shortwave diathermies have the longest wavelength and the lowest frequency and, all other factors being equal, they therefore should have the greatest depth of penetration. As we move down the chart, the wavelengths in each region become progressively shorter and the frequencies progressively higher. Diathermy, the various sources of infrared heating, and the ultraviolet regions have progressively less depth of penetration.[8]

Note that the regions labeled as radio and television frequencies, visible light, and high-frequency ionizing and penetrating radiations certainly fall under the classification of electromagnetic radiations. However, they do not have application as therapeutic modalities and, although extremely important to our everyday life, warrant no further consideration in the context of this discussion.

How Is Electromagnetic Energy Produced?

Various forms of electromagnetic radiation can be used by clinicians to treat patients provided that these forms of energy can be produced and directed in safe and economical ways.[9] Traditionally, ultraviolet, infrared, and visible light rays have been produced by heating objects such as a thin filament to very high temperatures. Objects are composed of atoms, which in turn are composed of positively charged nuclei surrounded by negatively charged electrons. As the temperature increases in a particular substance, the charged subatomic particles within the substance vibrate more rapidly due to the increase in available energy. The rapid movement of any charged particles, such as the negatively charged electrons within atoms, produces electromagnetic waves. At higher temperatures, the number of electromagnetic waves produced and the average frequency of those waves increase.[7] This is how incandescent light bulbs in our homes work. The electrical energy heats the filaments to very high temperatures, which causes them to emit radiation. The electromagnetic waves produced by heated filaments include a broad range of radiation and require large amounts of energy to produce. With an improvement in technology, more specific and economical ways to produce electromagnetic radiation have been developed for use in the therapeutic modalities. Electronic tubes or transistors can convert electrical energy into radio waves, and a device called a magnetron can produce focused bursts of microwave radiation.[9,10]

Effects of Electromagnetic Radiations

The effects of electromagnetic radiation on tissues depend on the wavelength, frequency, and energy of the electromagnetic waves that penetrate those tissues. Of the forms of electromagnetic energy used by a clinician, those with longer wavelengths are the most penetrating.[9] At the low-energy end of the electromagnetic spectrum, characterized by low-frequency and long-wavelength radiation, the basic effect is to heat tissues. The electromagnetic radiation with higher amounts of energy per photon can have different, more dramatic effects on tissues. The large regions of radiation with longer wavelengths than infrared radiations are known as the **diathermies**. These include shortwave and microwave radiations. They penetrate tissues more deeply than infrared or visible light. Infrared radiations, such as those produced by luminous and nonluminous infrared lamps, and visible light also heat tissues. These types of radiation are less penetrating than microwave radiation, so the warming effects are more superficial. Ultraviolet radiation is more energetic than visible light and carries enough

Table 1–2 Electromagnetic Energy Spectrum*

REGION	CLINICALLY USED WAVELENGTH	CLINICALLY USED FREQUENCY**	EFFECTIVE DEPTH OF PENETRATION	PHYSIOLOGICAL EFFECTS
Commercial radio and television frequencies‡				
Shortwave diathermy	22 m	13.56 MHz	3 cm	Deep tissue temperature, increased vasodilation, increased blood flow
	11 m	27.12 MHz		
Microwave diathermy	69 cm	433.9 MHz		Deep tissue temperature, increased vasodilation, increased blood flow
	33 cm	915 MHz	5 cm	
	12 cm	2450 MHz		
Infrared				Superficial temperature, increased vasodilation, increased blood flow
Luminous IR (1341°F)	28,860 Å	1.04×10^{13} Hz		
Nonluminous IR (3140°F)	14,430 Å	2.08×10^{13} Hz		
Visible light				
Red laser			5 cm	Pain modulation and wound healing
GaAs	9100 Å	3.3×10^{13} Hz	10–15 mm	
HeNe	6328 Å	4.74×10^{13} Hz		
Violet				
Ultraviolet				
UV-A	3200–4000 Å	9.38×10^{13} to 7.5×10^{13} Hz		Superficial chemical changes, tanning effects, bactericidal
UV-B	2900–3200 Å	1.03×10^{14} to 9.38×10^{13} Hz	1 mm	
UV-C	2000–2900 Å	1.50×10^{14} to 1.03×10^{14} Hz		
Ionizing radiation (x-ray, gamma rays, cosmic rays)‡				

*The only forms of electromagnetic energy included are the ones that obey the equations $C = \lambda \times v$ and $E = h \times v$. Neither electrical currents nor heat traveling by conduction travels at the speed of light.

**Calculated using $C = \lambda \times f$, where C is velocity of light (3×10 m/s), λ is wavelength, and f is frequency.

‡Although these fall under the classification of electromagnetic energy, they have nothing to do with therapeutic modalities and thus warrant no further discussion in this text.

energy to damage tissues. As this radiation is not very penetrating, the result of exposure to ultraviolet radiation is the superficial skin damage that we call sunburn.

Laws Governing the Effects of Electromagnetic Energy

When electromagnetic radiation strikes or comes in contact with various objects, it can be reflected, transmitted, refracted, or absorbed, depending on the type of radiation and the nature of the object it interacts with.[11] The rays that rebound off the material are said to be **reflected**. If a ray passes from one material to another, it changes its path by a process called **refraction**. Rays passing through a material are said to be **transmitted** through the material. A portion of the radiation may be **absorbed** by the material. Any photons that are not absorbed by the tissue will be transmitted to deeper layers. The intensity of a ray depends on how many photons compose the ray (Figure 1–3). Generally, the radiation used in the therapeutic modalities that has the longest wavelength tends to also have the greatest depths of penetration. It must be added, however, that a number of other factors, which are discussed later, can also contribute to the depth of penetration.

Arndt–Schultz Principle

The purpose of using therapeutic modalities is to stimulate body tissue. This stimulation will only occur if the energy produced is absorbed by the tissue.[11,12] The **Arndt–Schultz principle** states that no reactions or changes can occur in the body tissues if the amount of energy absorbed is insufficient to stimulate the absorbing tissues. The goal of the clinician should be to deliver sufficient energy to stimulate the tissues to perform their normal function. An example would be using an electrical stimulating current to create a muscle contraction. To achieve the depolarization of a motor nerve, the intensity of the current must be increased until enough energy is made available and is absorbed by that nerve to facilitate a depolarization. The clinician should also realize that too much energy absorbed in a given period of time may seriously impair normal function and, if severe enough, may cause irreparable damage.[12]

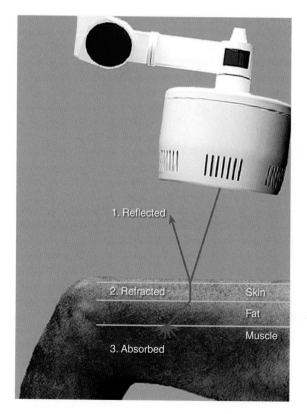

1. Reflected

2. Refracted   Skin

Fat

Muscle

3. Absorbed

Figure 1–3. When electromagnetic radiations contact human tissues, they may be reflected, refracted, or absorbed. Energy that is transmitted through the tissues must be absorbed before any physiological changes can take place.

Law of Grotthus–Draper

The inverse relationship that exists between energy absorption by a tissue and energy penetration to deeper layers is described by the **Law of Grotthus–Draper**. The portion of electromagnetic energy that is not reflected will penetrate into the tissues (skin layers), and some of it will be absorbed superficially. If too much radiation is absorbed by superficial tissues, not enough will be absorbed by the deeper tissues to stimulate the tissues. If the amount of energy absorbed is sufficient to stimulate the target tissue, some physiological response will occur.[11,12] If the target tissue is a motor nerve and your treatment goal is to cause a depolarization of that motor nerve, then enough energy must be absorbed by that nerve to cause the desired depolarization. An example showing application of the Law of Grotthus–Draper is the use of ultrasound treatment to increase tissue temperature in the deeper portions of the gluteus maximus muscle. A clinician could use ultrasound at a frequency of either 1 MHz (long wavelength) or 3 MHz (short wavelength). Using ultrasound treatment at a frequency of 1 MHz would be more effective at penetrating the deeper tissues than ultrasound treatment at 3 MHz, since less energy would be absorbed superficially for the longer wavelength.[13]

Cosine Law

Any reflection of electromagnetic radiation or other waves will reduce the amount of energy that is available for therapeutic purposes. The smaller the angle between the propagating ray and the right angle, the less the radiation reflected and the greater the absorption. Thus, radiant energy is more easily transmitted to deeper tissues if the source of radiation is at a right angle to the area being radiated. This principle, known as the **cosine law**, is extremely important when using the diathermies, ultraviolet light, and infrared heating, since the effectiveness of these modalities is based to a large extent on how they are positioned with regard to the patient (Figure 1–4).[12] An example showing the application of the cosine law could be that, when doing an ultrasound treatment, the surface of the applicator should be kept as flat on the skin surface as possible. This allows the acoustic energy coming from the applicator to strike the surface as close to 90 degrees as possible, thus minimizing the amount of energy reflected.

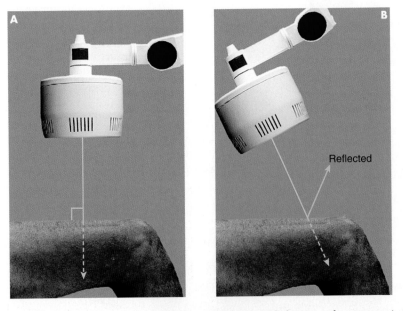

Figure 1–4. The cosine law states that the smaller the angle between the propagating ray and the right angle, the less the radiation reflected and the greater the radiation absorbed. Thus the energy absorbed would be greater in *a* than in *b*.

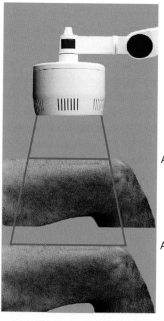

Figure 1–5. The inverse square law states that the intensity of the radiation striking a particular surface varies inversely with the square of the distance from the source.

At 10 cm Intensity is 80 watts

At 20 cm Intensity is 20 watts

Inverse Square Law

The intensity of the radiation striking a particular surface is known to vary inversely with the square of the distance from the source.[14] For example, when using an infrared heating lamp to heat the low back region, the intensity of heat energy at the skin surface with the lamp positioned at a distance of 10 inches will be four times greater than if the lamp is placed at a 20-inch distance. This principle, known as the **inverse square law**, obviously is of great consequence when setting up a specific modality to achieve a desired physiological effect (Figure 1–5). Regardless of the path this transmitted energy takes, the physiological effects are apparent only when the energy is absorbed by a specific tissue. Treatments will only be effective if enough energy is absorbed by the tissues, so modalities are most effective when placed as close to the body as possible.

Electromagnetic Energy Modalities

Diathermy

The diathermies are considered to be high-frequency modalities because they use radiation with more than 1 million cycles per second. When impulses of such a short duration come in contact with human tissue, there is insufficient time for ion movement to take place. Consequently, there is no stimulation of either motor or sensory nerves. The energy of this rapidly vibrating radiation produces heat as it is absorbed by tissue cells, resulting in a temperature increase.[10,15] Shortwave diathermy may be either continuous or pulsed. Both continuous shortwave and microwave diathermy are used primarily for their thermal effects, whereas pulsed shortwave is used for its nonthermal effects.[12,16] Diathermy is discussed in more detail in Chapter 12.

Clinical Decision-Making *Exercise 1–2*

The clinician is treating a patient with a chronic low back strain. At this point it has been decided that heating the area is the treatment of choice. Which of the modalities discussed briefly in this chapter may be used as heating modalities? Which of these modalities would you choose to provide the greatest depth of penetration?

Low-Power Laser

The word *LASER* is an acronym for *light amplification by stimulated emission of radiation* and applies to any instrument that generates light using that technique. There are lasers that produce light in either the infrared or visible light portions of the spectrum.

Lasers can be constructed to operate at certain power levels. High-power lasers are used in surgery for purposes of incision, coagulation of vessels, and thermolysis, owing to their thermal effects. The low-power or cold laser produces little or no thermal effects but seems to have some significant clinical effect on soft-tissue and fracture healing, as well as on pain management, through stimulation of acupuncture and trigger points. The laser as a therapeutic tool is discussed in Chapter 13.

Ultraviolet Light

The ultraviolet portion of the electromagnetic spectrum is higher in energy than violet light. As stated previously, the radiation in the ultraviolet region is undetectable by the human eye. However, if a photographic plate is placed at the ultraviolet end, chemical changes will be apparent. Although an extremely hot source (7000–9000°C) is required to produce ultraviolet wavelengths, the physiological effects of ultraviolet are mainly chemical in nature and occur entirely in the cutaneous layers of skin. The maximum depth of penetration with ultraviolet is about 1 mm.[19]

Clinical Decision-Making   *Exercise 1–3*

With which of the modalities described briefly in this chapter are the cosine law and the inverse square law of greatest consideration?

Due to the availability of oral and topical medications to treat skin lesions, ultraviolet therapy is seldom used as a treatment modality. Its primary application is in wound healing and it will be briefly discussed in Chapter 3.

THERMAL ENERGY

Earlier it was stated that any object heated (or cooled) to a temperature different than the surrounding environment will dissipate (or absorb) heat through conduction to (or from) the other materials with which it comes in contact.

There is confusion over the relationship between electromagnetic energy and thermal energy transfer associated with hot and cold packs. It is correct to think of the *infrared* modalities as those modalities whose primary mechanism of action is the emission of infrared radiation for the purpose of increasing tissue temperatures.[17] All warm objects, including whirlpool baths, emit infrared radiation, but the amount of infrared energy that is radiated from hot and cold baths is very small compared to the amount that transfers to and from them by conduction. Modalities such as hot and cold packs operate by conduction of thermal energy, so they are better described as conductive modalities. The conductive modalities are used to produce a local and occasionally a generalized heating or cooling of the superficial tissues with a maximum depth of penetration of 1 cm or less. Conductive modalities are generally classified into those that produce a tissue temperature increase, which we refer to as **thermotherapy**, and those that produce a tissue temperature decrease, which we call **cryotherapy**.

Earlier we stated that visible light, luminous infrared, and nonluminous infrared lamps are classified as electromagnetic energy modalities. This is because their mechanism of energy transfer is through electromagnetic radiation, not conduction.

The rate of heat transfer from one object to another is proportional to the difference in temperature between them. If two objects are very close in temperature, the transfer of heat will be slow. If there is a great temperature difference between two objects, the heat transfer between them will be very rapid. This has important consequences for the use of hot baths and cold baths. When a cold pack (8°F) is placed in contact with skin (98.6°F), the difference in temperature is approximately 90°F, so the heat flow from the skin to the cold pack is very rapid. This will cool the skin very rapidly and to a greater tissue depth. When tissues are placed in a hot whirlpool (110°F), the difference in temperature is only about 10°F, so the heat transfer from the bath to the skin is much slower. Whirlpools also have other effects, such as the prevention of evaporative cooling of the skin, but the general principle that cold packs work more rapidly and to a greater tissue depth holds true.

It should be added that in addition to producing a tissue temperature increase or decrease, the thermal modalities can elicit either increases or decreases in circulation depending on whether heat or cold is used. They are also known to have analgesic effects as a result of stimulation of sensory cutaneous nerve endings.

Thermal Energy Modalities

Thermotherapy

Thermotherapy techniques are used primarily to produce a tissue temperature increase for a variety of therapeutic purposes. The modalities classified as thermotherapy modalities include warm whirlpool, warm hydrocollator packs, paraffin baths, and fluidotherapy. The specific procedures for applying these techniques are discussed in detail in Chapter 9.

Cryotherapy

Cryotherapy techniques are used primarily to produce a tissue temperature decrease for a variety of therapeutic purposes. The modalities classified as cryotherapy modalities include ice massage, cold hydrocollator packs, cold whirlpool, cold spray, contrast baths, ice immersion, cryo-cuff, and cryokinetics. The specific procedures for applying these techniques are discussed in detail in Chapter 9.

ELECTRICAL ENERGY

In general, electricity is a form of energy that can effect chemical and thermal changes on tissue. Electrical energy is associated with the flow of electrons or other charged particles through an electric field. Electrons are particles of matter that have a negative electrical charge and revolve around the core, or nucleus, of an atom. An electrical current refers to the flow of charged particles that pass along a conductor such as a nerve or wire. Electrotherapeutic devices generate current, which, when introduced into biologic tissue, are capable of producing specific physiological changes.

An electrical current applied to nerve tissue at a sufficient intensity and duration to reach that tissue's excitability threshold will result in a membrane depolarization or firing of that nerve. Electrical stimulating currents affect nerve and muscle tissue in various ways, based on the action of electricity on tissues. Any electrical currents that pass through tissues will warm the tissues based on the resistance of the tissues to the flow of electricity. The clinically used frequencies of electrical currents range from 1 to 4000 Hz. Most stimulators have the flexibility to alter the treatment parameters of the device to elicit a desired physiological response in addition to the warming of tissues.[4]

Electrical Energy Modalities

Electrical Stimulating Currents

The nerve and muscle stimulating currents are capable of (1) modulating pain through stimulation of cutaneous sensory nerves at high frequencies; (2) producing muscle contraction and relaxation or tetany, depending on the type of current and frequency; (3) facilitating soft-tissue and bone healing through the use of subsensory microcurrents low-intensity stimulators; and (4) producing a net movement of ions through the use of continuous direct current and thus eliciting a chemical change in the tissues, which is called iontophoresis (see Chapter 6).[5] The electrical stimulating currents and their various physiological effects are discussed in detail in Chapter 5.

Electromyographic Biofeedback

Electromyographic biofeedback is a therapeutic procedure that uses electronic or electromechanical instruments to accurately measure, process, and feed back reinforcing information via auditory or visual signals. Clinically, it is used to help the patient develop greater voluntary control in terms of either neuromuscular relaxation or muscle reeducation following injury. Biofeedback is discussed in Chapter 7.

SOUND ENERGY

Acoustic energy and electromagnetic energy have very different physical characteristics. Sound energy consists of pressure waves due to the mechanical vibration of particles, whereas electromagnetic radiation is carried by photons. The relationship between velocity, wavelength, and frequency is the same for sound energy and electromagnetic energy, but the speeds of the two types of waves are different. Acoustical waves travel at the speed of sound. Electromagnetic waves travel at the speed of light. Since sound travels more slowly than light, wavelengths are considerably shorter for acoustic vibrations than for electromagnetic radiations at any given frequency.[12] For example, ultrasound traveling in the atmosphere has a wavelength of approximately 0.3 mm, whereas electromagnetic radiations would have a wavelength of 297 m at a similar frequency.

Electromagnetic radiations are capable of traveling through space or vacuum. As the density of the transmitting medium is increased, the velocity of electromagnetic radiation decreases. Acoustic vibrations (sound) will not be transmitted at all through vacuum, since they propagate through molecular collisions. The more rigid the transmitting medium, the greater the velocity of sound will be. Sound has a much greater velocity of transmission in bone tissue (3500 m/s), for example, than in fat tissue (1500 m/s).

Sound Energy Modalities

Ultrasound

A therapeutic modality clinicians frequently use is ultrasound. Ultrasound is the same form of energy as audible sound, except that the human ear cannot detect ultrasound frequencies. Frequencies of ultrasound wave production are between 700,000 and 1 million cycles per second. Frequencies up to around 20,000 Hz are detectable by the human ear. Thus the ultrasound portion of the acoustic spectrum is inaudible. Ultrasound is frequently classified along with the electromagnetic modalities, shortwave and microwave diathermy, as a deep-heating, "conversion"-type modality, and it is certainly true that all of these are capable of producing a temperature increase in human tissue to a considerable depth. However, ultrasound is a mechanical vibration, a sound wave, produced and transformed from high-frequency electrical energy.[12]

Ultrasound generators are generally set at a standard frequency of 1–3 MHz (1000 kHz). The depth of penetration with ultrasound is much greater than with any of the electromagnetic radiations. At a frequency of 1 MHz, 50% of the energy produced will penetrate to a depth of about 5 cm. The reason for this great depth of penetration is that ultrasound travels very well through homogeneous tissue (e.g., fat tissue), whereas electromagnetic radiations are almost entirely absorbed. Thus when therapeutic penetration to deeper tissues is desired, ultrasound is the modality of choice.[13,18]

Therapeutic ultrasound traditionally has been used to produce a tissue temperature increase through thermal physiological effects. However, it is also capable of enhancing healing at the cellular level as a result of its nonthermal physiological effects. The clinical usefulness of therapeutic ultrasound is discussed in greater detail in Chapter 10.

Extracorporeal Shock Wave Therapy

Extracorporeal shock wave therapy (ESWT) is a relatively new noninvasive modality used in the treatment of both soft-tissue and bone injuries. The *shock waves*, in contrast to the connotation of an electrical shock, are actually pulsed high-pressure, short-duration (<1 m/s) sound waves. This sound energy is concentrated in a small focal area (2–8 mm in diameter) and is transmitted through a coupling medium to a target region with little attenuation. Over the past several years, a number of investigators have used this modality successfully in treating plantar fasciitis, medial/lateral epicondylitis, and nonunion fractures. ESWT will be discussed in Chapter 11.

MECHANICAL ENERGY

In all instances in which work is done, there is an object that supplies the force to do the work. When work is done on the object, that object gains energy. The energy acquired by the objects upon which work is done is known as **mechanical energy**.[2] Mechanical energy is the energy possessed by an object due to its motion or position. Mechanical energy can be either **kinetic energy** (energy of motion) or **potential energy** (stored energy of position). Objects have kinetic energy if they are in motion. Potential energy is stored by an object and has the potential to be created when that objected is stretched or bent or squeezed. The kinetic energy created by a clinician's hands moves to apply a force that can stretch, bend, or compress skin, muscles, ligaments, and the like. The stretched, bent, or compressed structure possesses potential energy that can be released when the force is removed.

Mechanical Energy Modalities

Intermittent compression, traction techniques, and massage each use mechanical energy involving a force applied to some soft-tissue structure to create a therapeutic effect. These mechanical energy modalities are discussed in Chapters 14, 15, and 16.

SUMMARY

1. The forms of energy that are relevant to the use of therapeutic modalities are electromagnetic energy, thermal energy, electrical energy, sound energy, and mechanical energy.
2. The various forms of energy may be reflected, refracted, absorbed, or transmitted in the tissues.
3. All forms of electromagnetic energy travel at the same velocity; thus, wavelength and frequency are inversely related.
4. The electromagnetic spectrum places all of the electromagnetic energy modalities including diathermy, laser, ultraviolet light, and luminous infrared lamps in order based on wavelengths and corresponding frequencies.
5. The Arndt–Schultz principle, the Law of Grotthus–Draper, the cosine law, and the inverse square law each can be applied to the electromagnetic energy modalities.
6. Thermotherapy and cryotherapy modalities transfer thermal energy from a heating or cooling source to the body through conduction.
7. Modalities that utilize electrical energy can (1) cause pain modulation through stimulation of cutaneous sensory nerves; (2) produce muscle contraction and relaxation or tetany, depending on the type of current and frequency; (3) facilitate soft-tissue and bone healing through the use of subsensory microcurrents; and (4) produce a net movement of ions, thus eliciting a chemical change in the tissues.
8. Acoustic energy and electromagnetic energy have very different physical characteristics.
9. Mechanical energy can be either kinetic energy (energy of motion) or potential energy (stored energy of position). The kinetic energy created by a clinician's hands moves to apply a force that can stretch, bend, or compress skin, muscles, ligaments, and the like. The stretched, bent, or compressed structure possesses potential energy that can be released when the force is removed.

REVIEW QUESTIONS

1. What are the various forms of energy produced by therapeutic modalities?
2. What is radiant energy and how is it produced?
3. What is the relationship between wavelength and frequency?
4. What are the characteristics of electromagnetic energy?
5. Which of the therapeutic modalities produce electromagnetic energy?
6. What is the purpose of using a therapeutic modality?
7. According to the Law of Grotthus–Draper, what happens to electromagnetic energy when it comes in contact with and/or penetrates human biologic tissue?
8. Explain the cosine and inverse square laws relative to tissue penetration of electromagnetic energy.
9. How do the thermal energy modalities transfer energy?
10. What physiological changes can the use of electrical energy produce in human tissue?
11. Which of the therapeutic modalities produce sound energy?
12. What are the differences between electromagnetic energy and sound energy?
13. What modalities utilize mechanical energy to produce a therapeutic effect?

SELF-TEST QUESTIONS

True or False

1. Wavelength is defined as the number of cycles per second.
2. To achieve deeper tissue penetration, the wavelength must be increased.
3. Continuous shortwave diathermy produces thermal effects.

Multiple Choice

4. Which of the following is NOT an electromagnetic energy modality?
   a. Ultraviolet light
   b. Ultrasound
   c. Low-power laser
   d. Shortwave diathermy
5. Sound or radiation waves that change direction when passing from one type of tissue to another are said to.
   a. Transmit
   b. Absorb
   c. Reflect
   d. Refract
6. The _____ states that if superficial tissue does not absorb energy, it must be transmitted deeper.
   a. Law of Grotthus–Draper
   b. Cosine law
   c. Inverse square law
   d. Arndt–Schultz principle
7. According to the cosine law, to minimize reflection and maximize absorption, the energy source must be at a _____ angle to the surface.
   a. 45 degree
   b. 90 degree
   c. 180 degree
   d. 0 degree
8. Electrical stimulating currents may produce the following effects:
   a. Muscle contraction
   b. Net ion movement

    c. Decrease in pain

    d. All of the above

9. Thermal energy modalities generally affect superficial tissue up to _____ cm deep.

    a. 5 cm

    b. 0.5 cm

    c. 1 cm

    d. 10 cm

10. Based on their different characteristics, which of the following travels at greater velocity through human tissue?

    a. Sound energy

    b. Electromagnetic energy

    c. Both *a* and *b* travel at the same rate.

    d. Neither *a* nor *b* travels through human tissue.

SOLUTIONS TO CLINICAL DECISION-MAKING EXERCISES

1–1

Superficial heat and cold, electrical stimulating currents, and low-power laser may all be effective for modulating pain. However, ice is likely the best choice immediately following injury because it will not only modulate pain but will also cause vasoconstriction and thus help to control swelling.

1–2

The clinician may choose to use infrared heating modalities, shortwave diathermy, or ultrasound—all of which have the ability to produce heat in the tissues. Ultrasound has a greater depth of penetration than any of the electromagnetic or thermal modalities since sound energy is more effectively transmitted through dense tissue than is electromagnetic energy.

1–3

When setting up a patient for treatment using either microwave diathermy or ultraviolet therapy, it is critical that the clinician consider the angle at which the electromagnetic energy is striking the body surface to ensure that most of the energy will be absorbed and not reflected. It is also essential to know the distance that these modalities will be placed from the surface to achieve the right amount of energy in the target tissue.

REFERENCES

1. Nadler SF. Complications from therapeutic modalities: results of a national survey of clinicians. *Arch Phys Med Rehab.* 2003;84(6):849–853.

2. Young H, Freedman R. *Sears and Zemansky's University Physics.* Reading, MA: Addison-Wesley; 2007.

3. De Pinna S. *Transfer of Energy.* Strongsville, OH: Gareth Stevens Publishing; 2007.

4. Sharp T. *Practical Electrotherapy: A Guide to Safe Application.* New York: Elsevier Health Sciences; 2007.

5. Venes D. *Taber's Cyclopedic Medical Dictionary.* Philadelphia: F.A. Davis; 2009.

6. Smith G. *Introduction to Classical Electromagnetic Radiation.* Boston: Cambridge University Press; 1997.

7. Reitz J, Milford F, Christy R. *Foundations of Electromagnetic Theory.* 4th ed. Reading, MA: Addison–Wesley; 2008.

8. Grosswinder L, Jones L, Rogers G. *The Science of Phototherapy: An Introduction.* New York: Springer-Verlag; 2005.

9. Kato M. *Electromagnetics in Biology.* New York: Springer-Verlag; 2007.

10. Habash R. *Bioeffects and Therapeutic Applications of Electromagnetic Energy.* Oxford, UK: Taylor & Francis, Inc.; 2007.

11. Gasos J, Stavroulakis P. *Biological Effects of Electromagnetic Radiation.* New York: Springer-Verlag; 2003.

12. Griffin J, Karselis T. *Physical Agents for Physical Therapists.* Springfield, IL: Charles C Thomas; 1988.

13. Draper D, Sunderland O. Examination of the law of Grotthus-Draper: does ultrasound penetrate subcutaneous fat in humans?. *J Athletic Train.* 1993;28(3):248–250.

14. Goats GC. Appropriate use of the inverse square law. *Physiotherapy.* 1988;74(1):8.

15. Hitchcock RT, Patterson RM. *Radio-frequency and ELF Electromagnetic Energies: A Handbook for Healthcare Professionals.* New York: Van Nostrand Reinhold; 1995.

16. Blank M, ed. *Electromagnetic Fields: Biological Interactions and Mechanisms.* Washington, DC: American Chemical Society; 1995.

17. Lehmann J, ed. *Therapeutic Heat and Cold.* 4th ed. Baltimore: Williams and Wilkins; 1990.

18. Lehmann JF, Guy AW. Ultrasound therapy. *Proceedings of the Workshop on Interaction of Ultrasound and Biological Tissues.* Washington, DC: HEW Pub. (FDA 73:8008); Sept. 1972.

19. Stillwell K. *Therapeutic Electricity and Ultraviolet Radiation.* Baltimore: Williams & Wilkins; 1983.

ADDITIONAL RELATED AND RELEVANT SOURCES

Allen, R: Physical agents used in the management of chronic pain by physical therapists. *Phys Med Rehabil Clin N Am.* 2006;17(2):315–345.

Bracciano A, Mu K. Physical agent modalities: developing a framework for clinical application in occupational therapy practice. *OT Practice.* 2009;14 (11): Suppl.(CE-1-CE-8, 2p)

Cetin N, Aytar A. Comparing hot pack, short-wave diathermy, ultrasound, and TENS on isokinetic strength, pain, and functional status of women with osteoarthritic knees: a single-blind, randomized, controlled trial. *Am J Phys Med Rehabil.* 2008;87(6):443.

Goodgold J, Eberstein A. *Electrodiagnosis of Neuromuscular Diseases.* Baltimore, MD: Williams & Wilkins; 1972.

Habash R. *Bioeffects and Therapeutic Applications of Electromagnetic Energy.* Danvers, MA: CRC Press; 2007.

Jehle H. Charge fluctuation forces in biological systems. *Ann NY Acad Sci.* 1969;158:240–255.

Koracs R. *Light Therapy.* Springfield, IL: Charles C Thomas; 1950.

Licht S, ed. Electrodiagnosis and electromyography. 3rd ed. New Haven, CT: Elizabeth Licht; 1971.

Licht S. *Therapeutic Electricity and Ultraviolet Radiation.* New Haven, CT: Elizabeth Licht; 1959.

Scott P, Cooksey F. *Clayton's Electrotherapy and Actinotherapy.* London: Bailliere, Tindall and Cox; 1962.

GLOSSARY

absorption   Energy that stimulates a particular tissue to perform its normal function.

Arndt–Schultz principle   No reactions or changes can occur in the body if the amount of energy absorbed is not sufficient to stimulate the absorbing tissues.

cosine law   Optimal radiation occurs when the source of radiation is at right angles to the center of the area being radiated.

cryotherapy   A decrease in tissue temperature.

diathermy   The application of high-frequency electrical energy used to generate heat in body tissue as a result of the resistance of the tissue to the passage of energy.

energy   The capacity of a system for doing work.

frequency   The number of cycles or pulses per second.

infrared radiation   The portion of the electromagnetic spectrum associated with thermal changes located adjacent to the red portion of the visible light spectrum.

inverse square law   The intensity of radiation striking a particular surface varies inversely with the square of the distance from the radiating source.

kinetic energy   Energy of motion.

law of Grotthus–Draper   Energy not absorbed by the tissues must be transmitted.

mechanical energy   Energy acquired by the objects upon which work is done.

photon   The energy carrier that composes all electromagnetic radiation.

potential energy   Stored energy of position.

radiation   (1) The process of emitting energy from some source in the form of waves. (2) A method of heat transfer through which heat can be either gained or lost.

reflection   The bending back of light or sound waves from a surface that they strike.

refraction   The change in direction of a wave or radiation wave when it passes from one medium or type of tissue to another.

spectrum   Range of visible light colors.

thermotherapy   An increase in tissue temperature.

transmission   The propagation of energy through a particular biologic tissue into deeper tissues.

ultraviolet radiation   The portion of the electromagnetic spectrum associated with chemical changes located adjacent to the violet portion of the visible light spectrum.

wavelength   The distance from one point in a propagating wave to the same point in the next wave.

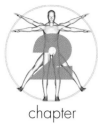

Using Therapeutic Modalities to Affect the Healing Process

William E. Prentice

OBJECTIVES

Following completion of this chapter, the student will be able to:

➤ Define inflammation and its associated signs and symptoms.

➤ Clarify how therapeutic modalities should be used in rehabilitation of various conditions.

➤ Compare the physiological events associated with the different phases of the healing process.

➤ Formulate a plan for how specific modalities can be used effectively during each phase of healing and provide a rationale for their use.

➤ Identify those factors that can interfere with the healing process.

HOW SHOULD THE CLINICIAN USE THERAPEUTIC MODALITIES IN REHABILITATION?

Therapeutic modalities, when used appropriately, can be extremely useful tools in the rehabilitation of the injured patient.[1,2] Like any other tool, their effectiveness is limited by the knowledge, skill, and experience of the clinician using them. For the competent clinician, decisions regarding how and when a modality may best be incorporated should be based on a combination of theoretical knowledge and practical experience. As a clinician, you should not use therapeutic modalities at random, nor should you base their use on what has always been done before. Instead, you must always give consideration to what should work best in a specific injury situation.

There are many different approaches and ideas regarding the use of modalities in injury rehabilitation. Therefore, no "cookbook" exists for modality use. In a given clinical situation, you as a clinician should make your own decision about which modality will be most effective.

In any program of rehabilitation, modalities should be used primarily as adjuncts to therapeutic exercise and certainly not at the exclusion of range-of-motion or strengthening exercises. Rehabilitation protocols and progressions must be based primarily on the physiological responses of the tissues to injury and on an understanding of how various tissues heal (Figure 2–1).[3] Thus, the clinician must understand the healing process to be effective in incorporating therapeutic modalities into the rehabilitative process.

In the physically active population, injuries most often involve the musculoskeletal system and in fewer instances the nervous system.[4,5] Some health care professionals have debated

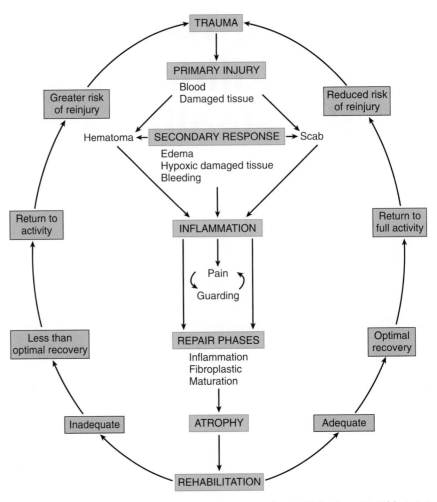

Figure 2–1. A cycle of sport-related injury. (From Booher, J., Thibedeau, G. Athletic Injury Assessment. *St. Louis, McGraw-Hill.* 1994, p 119)

whether the terms *acute* and *chronic* are appropriate in defining injury.[6] At some point all injuries can be considered acute; in other words, there is always some beginning point for every injury. At what point does an acute injury become a chronic injury? Generally injuries occur either from trauma or from overuse. Acute injuries are caused by trauma; chronic injuries can result from overuse as occurs with the repetitive dynamics of running, throwing, or jumping.[7,8] Thus, the terms *traumatic* and *overuse injuries* are more appropriate.

Primary injuries are almost always described as being either traumatic or overuse resulting from *macrotraumatic* or *microtraumatic* forces. Injuries classified as macrotraumatic occur as a result of trauma and produce immediate pain and disability. Macrotraumatic injuries include fractures, dislocations, subluxations, sprains, strains, and contusions.[9] Microtraumatic injuries are most often overuse injuries and result from repetitive overloading or incorrect mechanics associated with continuous training or competition. They include tendinitis, tenosynovitis, bursitis, and so on. A *secondary injury* is essentially the inflammatory or hypoxia response that occurs with the primary injury.[10]

The healing process is a continuum consisting of three phases:
- inflammatory-response phase;
- fibroblastic-repair phase;
- maturation-remodeling phase.

Signs of inflammation are as follows:
- redness;
- swelling;
- tenderness to touch;
- increased temperature;
- loss of function.

Clinical Decision-Making   *Exercise 2–1*

A female soccer player sprains her ankle, and the team physician diagnoses it as a grade 1 sprain. The coach wants to know how long the athlete will be out. On what information should the clinician base his or her response?

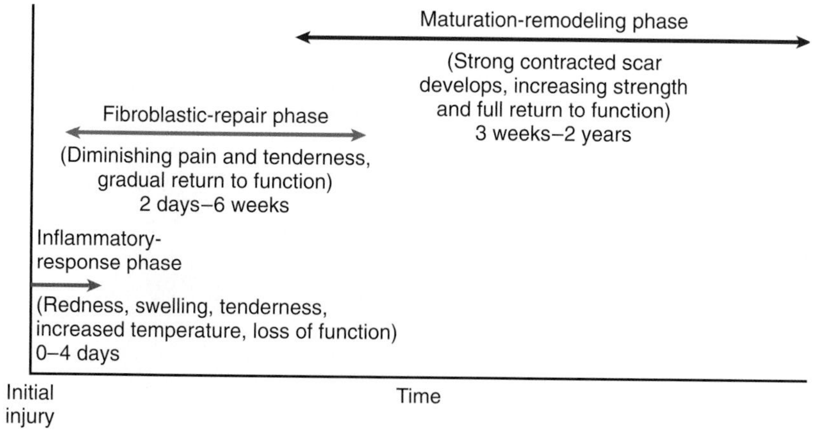

Maturation-remodeling phase

(Strong contracted scar
develops, increasing strength
and full return to function)
3 weeks–2 years

Fibroblastic-repair phase

(Diminishing pain and tenderness,
gradual return to function)
2 days–6 weeks

Inflammatory-
response phase

(Redness, swelling, tenderness,
increased temperature, loss of function)
0–4 days

Initial
injury   Time

Figure 2–2. The three phases of the healing process fall along an overlapping time continuum.

THE IMPORTANCE OF UNDERSTANDING THE HEALING PROCESS

The decisions made by the clinician on how and when therapeutic modalities may best be used should be based on recognition of signs and symptoms as well as some awareness of the time frames associated with the different phases of the healing process.[11,12] The clinician must have a sound understanding of that process in terms of the sequence of the phases of healing that take place.[13]

The healing process consists of the inflammatory-response phase, the fibroblastic-repair phase, and the maturation-remodeling phase. It must be stressed that although the phases of healing are presented as three separate entities, *the healing process is a continuum*. Phases of the healing process overlap one another and have no definitive beginning or end points[14] (Figure 2–2). The clinician should rely primarily on observation of the signs and symptoms to determine how the healing process is progressing.

Inflammatory-Response Phase

When you hear the term *inflammation*, you automatically think of something negative. The fact is that inflammation is a very important part of the healing process.[15] Without the physiological changes that take place during the inflammatory process, the later stages of healing cannot occur. Once a tissue is injured, the process of healing begins immediately.[16] The destruction of tissue produces direct injury to the cells of the various soft tissues. Cellular injury results in altered metabolism and the liberation of materials that initiate the inflammatory response[17] (Figure 2–3).

Signs and Symptoms

The inflammatory-response phase is characterized symptomatically by redness, swelling, tenderness, increased temperature, and loss of function.[11,18]

Cellular Response

Inflammation is a process during which **leukocytes** and other **phagocytic cells** and exudate are delivered to the injured tissue. This cellular reaction is generally protective, tending to localize or dispose of injury by-products (e.g., blood or damaged cells) through phagocytosis, thus setting the stage for repair.[19] Locally, vascular effects, disturbances of fluid exchange, and migration of leukocytes from the blood to the tissues occur.[20]

Chemical Mediators

The events in the inflammatory response are initiated by a series of interactions involving several chemical mediators.[21] Some of these chemical mediators are derived from the invading organism,

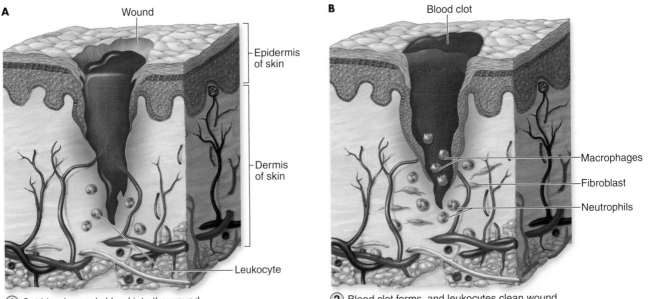

A

Wound

Epidermis
of skin

Dermis
of skin

Leukocyte

(1) Cut blood vessels bleed into the wound.

B

Blood clot

Macrophages

Fibroblast

Neutrophils

(2) Blood clot forms, and leukocytes clean wound.

Figure 2–3. Initial injury and inflammatory-response phase of the healing process. (A) Cut blood vessels bleed into the wound. (B) Blood clot forms, and leukocytes clean wound. Reproduced, with permission, from McKinley M, O'Loughlin VD, Human Anatomy, 2nd ed. New York: McGraw-Hill, 2008.

Chemical mediators are as follows:

- histamine;
- leukotrienes;
- cytokines.

some are released by the damaged tissue, others are generated by several plasma enzyme systems, and still others are products of various white blood cells participating in the inflammatory response. Three chemical mediators, *histamine, leukotrienes*, and *cytokines*, are important in limiting the amount of exudate, and thus swelling, after injury.[22] Histamine, released from the injured mast cells, causes vasodilation and increased cell permeability, owing to a swelling of endothelial cells and then separation between the cells. Leukotrienes and prostaglandins are responsible for *margination*, in which leukocytes (neutrophils and macrophages) adhere along the cell walls.[19] They also increase cell permeability locally, thus affecting the passage of the fluid and white blood cells through cell walls via diapedesis to form exudate. Therefore, vasodilation and active hyperemia are important in exudate (plasma) formation, in supplying leukocytes to the injured area. Cytokines, in particular chemokines and interleukin, are the major regulators of leukocyte traffic and help to attract leukocytes to the actual site of inflammation.[23] Responding to the presence of chemokines, phagocytes enter the site of inflammation within a few hours. The amount of swelling that occurs is directly related to the extent of vessel damage.

Vascular Reaction

The vascular reaction involves vascular spasm, the formation of a platelet plug, blood coagulation, and the growth of fibrous tissue.[24] The immediate response to tissue damage is a vasoconstriction of the vascular walls in the vessels leading away from the site of injury that lasts for approximately 5–10 minutes. This vasoconstriction presses the opposing endothelial wall linings together to produce a local anemia that is rapidly replaced by hyperemia of the area due to vasodilation. This increase in blood flow is transitory and gives way to slowing the flow in the dilated vessels, thus enabling the leukocytes to slow down and adhere to the vascular endothelium. Eventually there is stagnation and stasis. The initial effusion of blood and plasma lasts for 24–36 hours.

The function of platelets. Platelets do not normally adhere to the vascular wall. However, injury to a vessel disrupts the endothelium and exposes the collagen fibers. Platelets adhere to the collagen fibers to create a sticky matrix on the vascular wall, to which additional platelets and leukocytes adhere and eventually form a plug. These plugs obstruct local lymphatic fluid drainage and thus localize the injury response.

The clotting process. The initial event that precipitates clot formation is the conversion of fibrinogen to fibrin.[25] This transformation results from a cascading effect, beginning with

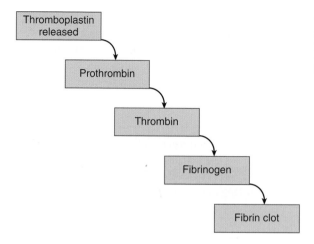

Figure 2–4. The clotting process involves a series of physiological events that require as long as 48 hours to complete.

the release of a protein molecule called thromboplastin, from the damaged cell. Thromboplastin causes prothrombin to be changed into thrombin, which in turn causes the conversion of fibrinogen into a very sticky fibrin clot that shuts off blood supply to the injured area. Clot formation begins around 12 hours following injury and is completed by 48 hours[26] (Figure 2–4).

As a result of a combination of these factors, the injured area becomes walled off during the inflammatory stage of healing. The leukocytes phagocytize most of the foreign debris toward the end of the inflammatory phase, setting the stage for the fibroblastic phase. This initial inflammatory response lasts for approximately 2–4 days following initial injury (Figure 2–5).

Chronic Inflammation

A distinction must be made between the acute inflammatory response as previously described and chronic inflammation. Chronic inflammation occurs when the acute inflammatory response does not respond sufficiently to eliminate the injuring agent and restore tissue to its normal physiological state.[6] Thus, only low concentrations of the chemical mediators are present. The neutrophils that are normally present during acute inflammation are replaced by macrophages, lymphocytes, fibroblasts, and plasma cells. As this low-grade inflammation persists, damage occurs to connective tissue, resulting in tissue necrosis and fibrosis prolonging the healing and repair process. Chronic inflammation involves the production of granulation tissue and fibrous connective tissue. These cells accumulate in a highly vascularized and innervated loose connective

In chronic inflammation, neutrophils are replaced with:
- macrophages;
- lymphocytes;
- fibroblasts;
- plasma cells.

Granulation tissue consists of:
- capillaries;
- collagen;
- fibroblasts.

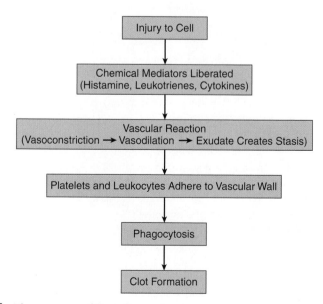

Figure 2–5. The sequence of the inflammatory response.

The extracellular matrix contains:
- collagen;
- elastin;
- ground substance.

tissue matrix in the area of injury.[27] The specific mechanisms that cause an insufficient acute inflammatory response are unknown, but they appear to be related to situations that involve overuse or overload with cumulative microtrauma to a particular structure.[27,28] There is no specific time frame in which the acute inflammation transitions to chronic inflammation. It does appear that chronic inflammation is resistant to both physical and pharmacologic treatments.[29]

Fibroblastic-Repair Phase

During the fibroblastic phase of healing, proliferative and regenerative activity leading to scar formation and repair of the injured tissue follows the vascular and exudative phenomena of inflammation.[30] The period of scar formation referred to as **fibroplasia** begins within the first few hours following injury and may last for as long as 4–6 weeks.

Signs and Symptoms

During this period many of the signs and symptoms associated with the inflammatory response subside. The patient may still indicate some tenderness to touch and will usually complain of pain when particular movements stress the injured structure. As scar formation progresses, complaints of tenderness or pain will gradually disappear.[31]

Revascularization

During this phase, growth of endothelial capillary buds into the wound is stimulated by a lack of oxygen. Thus, the wound is now capable of healing aerobically. Along with increased oxygen delivery comes an increase in blood flow, which delivers nutrients essential for tissue regeneration in the area[32] (Figure 2–6).

Formation of Scar

The formation of a delicate connective tissue called granulation tissue occurs with the breakdown of the fibrin clot. Granulation tissue consists of fibroblasts, collagen, and capillaries. It appears as a reddish granular mass of connective tissue that fills in the gaps during the healing process.

As the capillaries continue to grow into the area, fibroblasts accumulate at the wound site, arranging themselves parallel to the capillaries. Fibroblastic cells begin to synthesize an extracellular matrix, which contains protein fibers of collagen and elastin, a ground substance that consists of

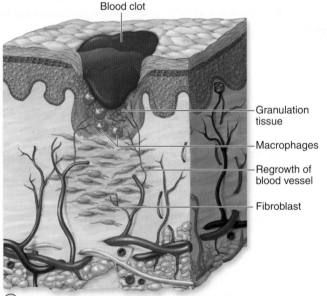

③ Blood vessels regrow, and granulation tissue forms.

Figure 2–6. Blood vessels regrow, and granulation tissue forms in the fibroblastic-repair phase of the healing process. Reproduced, with permission, from McKinley M, O'Loughlin VD, Human Anatomy, 2nd ed. New York: McGraw-Hill, 2008.

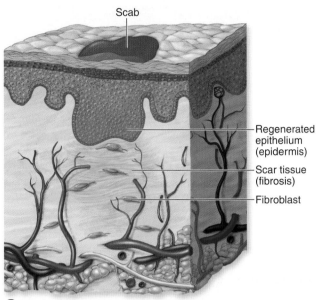

④ Epithelium regenerates, and connective tissue fibrosis occurs.

Figure 2–7. Epithelium regenerates, and connective tissue fibrosis occurs in the maturation-remodeling phase of the healing process. Reproduced, with permission, from McKinley M, O'Loughlin VD, Human Anatomy, 2nd ed. New York: McGraw-Hill, 2008.

nonfibrous proteins called proteoglycans, glycosaminoglycans, and fluid. On about day 6 or 7, fibroblasts also begin producing collagen fibers that are deposited in a random fashion throughout the forming scar. As the collagen continues to proliferate, the tensile strength of the wound rapidly increases in proportion to the rate of collagen synthesis.[39] As the tensile strength increases, the number of fibroblasts diminishes to signal the beginning of the maturation phase.[16]

This normal sequence of events in the repair phase leads to the formation of minimal scar tissue. Occasionally, a persistent inflammatory response and continued release of inflammatory products can promote extended fibroplasia and excessive fibrogenesis that can lead to irreversible tissue damage.[27] Fibrosis can occur in synovial structures, as is the case with adhesive capsulitis in the shoulder; in extra-articular tissues, including tendons and ligaments; in bursa; or in muscle.

A mature scar will be devoid of physiological function, it will have less tensile strength than the original tissue, and it is not as well vascularized.

Maturation-Remodeling Phase

The maturation-remodeling phase of healing is a long-term process. This phase features a realignment or remodeling of the collagen fibers that make up the scar tissue according to the tensile forces to which that scar is subjected (Figure 2–7). Ongoing breakdown and synthesis of collagen occur with a steady increase in the tensile strength of the scar matrix. With increased stress and strain, the collagen fibers will realign in a position of maximum efficiency parallel to the lines of tension.[33] The tissue gradually assumes normal appearance and function, although a scar is rarely as strong as the normal injured tissue. Usually by the end of approximately 3 weeks, a firm, strong, contracted, nonvascular scar exists. The maturation phase of healing may require several years to be totally complete.

FACTORS THAT IMPEDE HEALING

See Table 2–1 for a list of factors that impede healing.

Extent of injury. The nature or amount of the inflammatory response is determined by the extent of the tissue injury. **Microtears** of soft tissue involve only minor damage and are most often associated with overuse. **Macrotears** involve significantly greater destruction of soft tissue and result in clinical symptoms and functional alterations. They are generally caused by acute trauma.

Table 2–1   Factors that Impede Healing
Extent of injury
Edema
Hemorrhage
Poor vascular supply
Separation of tissue
Muscle spasm
Atrophy
Corticosteroids
Keloids and hypertrophic scars
Infection
Humidity, climate, and oxygen tension
Health, age, and nutrition

Edema. The increased pressure caused by swelling retards the healing process, causes separation of tissues, inhibits neuromuscular control, produces reflexive neurological changes, and impedes nutrition in the injured part. Edema is best controlled and managed during the initial first aid management period.[21]

Hemorrhage. Bleeding occurs with even the smallest amount of damage to the capillaries. It produces the same negative effects on healing as does the accumulation of edema, and its presence produces additional tissue damage and thus exacerbation of the injury.[25]

Poor vascular supply. Injuries to tissues with a poor vascular supply heal poorly and at a slow rate. This is likely related to a failure in the delivery of phagocytic cells initially and also of fibroblasts necessary for formation of scar.

Separation of tissue. Mechanical separation of tissue can significantly impact the course of healing. A wound that has smooth edges that are in good apposition will tend to heal by primary intention with minimal scarring. Conversely, a wound that has jagged separated edges must heal by second intention, with granulation tissue filling the defect and causing excessive scarring.[34]

Muscle spasm. Muscle spasm causes traction on the torn tissue, separates the two ends, and prevents approximation. Both local and generalized ischemia may result from spasm.

Atrophy. Wasting away of muscle tissue begins immediately with injury. Strengthening and early mobilization of the injured structure retards atrophy.

Corticosteroids. Use of corticosteroids such as cortisone in the treatment of inflammation is controversial. Steroid use in the early stages of healing has been demonstrated to inhibit fibroplasia, capillary proliferation, collagen synthesis, and increases in tensile strength of the healing scar. Their use in the later stages of healing and with chronic inflammation is debatable.

Keloids and hypertrophic scars. Keloids occur when the rate of collagen production exceeds the rate of collagen breakdown during the maturation phase of healing. This process leads to hypertrophy of scar tissue, particularly around the periphery of the wound, that is out of proportion to normal scarring. The result is a raised, firm, thickened, red scar.

Infection. The presence of bacteria in the wound can delay healing, cause excessive granulation tissue, and frequently cause large deformed scars.

Humidity, climate, and oxygen tension. Humidity significantly influences the process of epithelization. Occlusive dressings stimulate the epithelium to migrate twice as fast without crust or scab formation. The formation of a scab occurs with dehydration of the wound and traps wound drainage, which promotes infection. Keeping the wound moist provides an advantage for the necrotic debris to go to the surface and be shed.

Oxygen tension relates to the neovascularization of the wound, which translates into optimal saturation and maximal tensile strength development. Circulation to the wound can be affected by ischemia, venous stasis, hematomas, and vessel trauma.

Health, age, and nutrition. The elastic qualities of the skin decrease with aging. Degenerative diseases, such as diabetes and arteriosclerosis, also become a concern of the older patient and may affect wound healing. Nutrition is important for wound healing. In particular, vitamins C, K, A, and E, zinc, and amino acids play critical roles in the healing process.

HOW SHOULD THERAPEUTIC MODALITIES BE USED THROUGHOUT THE REHABILITATION PROCESS?

Using Modalities in the Immediate First Aid Management of Injury

Table 2–2 summarizes the various modalities that may be used in the different phases of the healing process. Modality use in the initial treatment of injury should be directed toward limiting the amount of swelling and reducing pain that occurs acutely. The acute phase is marked by swelling, pain to touch or with pressure, and pain on both active and passive motion. In general, the less the initial swelling, the less is the time required for rehabilitation. Traditionally, the modality of choice has been and still is rest, ice, compression, and elevation (*RICE*).

Cryotherapy is known to produce vasoconstriction, at least superficially and perhaps indirectly in the deeper tissues, and thus limits the bleeding that always occurs with injury. Ice bags, cryocuffs, cold packs, and ice massage may all be used effectively. Cold baths should be avoided because the extremities must be placed in a gravity-dependent position. Cold whirlpools also place the extremities in the gravity-dependent position and produce a massaging action that is likely to retard clotting. The importance of applying ice immediately following injury for limiting acute swelling through vasoconstriction has probably been overemphasized. The initial use of ice is more important for decreasing the secondary hypoxic response associated with tissue injury (see Chapter 9). Analgesia, which occurs through stimulation of sensory cutaneous nerves via the gating mechanism, blocks or reduces pain (see Chapter 4).

Immediate compression has been demonstrated to be an effective technique for limiting swelling. An intermittent compression device may be used to provide even pressure around an injured extremity. The pressurized sleeve mechanically reduces the amount of space available for swelling to accumulate. Units that combine both compression and cold have been shown to be more effective in reducing swelling than using compression alone. Regardless of the specific techniques selected (see Chapter 15), cold and compression should always be combined with elevation to avoid any additional pooling of blood in the injured area due to the effects of gravity.

Electrical stimulating currents may also be used in the initial phase for pain reduction. Parameters should be adjusted to maximally stimulate sensory cutaneous nerve fibers, again to take advantage of the gate control mechanism of pain modulation. Intensities that produce muscle contractions should be avoided because they may increase clotting time (see Chapter 5).

Low-intensity ultrasound has been demonstrated to be effective in facilitating the healing process when used immediately following injury and certainly within the first 48 hours. Low intensities produce nonthermal physiological effects that alter the permeability of cell membranes to sodium and calcium ions important in healing (see Chapter 10).

The low-power laser has also been shown to be effective in pain modulation through the stimulation of trigger points and may be used acutely (see Chapter 13).

Table 2–2   Clinical Decision-Making on the Use of Various Therapeutic Modalities in Treatment of Acute Injury

PHASE	APPROXIMATE TIME FRAME	CLINICAL PICTURE	POSSIBLE MODALITIES USED	RATIONALE FOR USE
Initial acute	Injury—day 3	Swelling, pain to touch, pain on motion	CRYO	↓ Swelling, ↓ pain
			ESC	↓ Pain
			IC	↓ Swelling
			LPL	↓ Pain
			ULTRA	Nonthermal effects to ↑ healing
			Rest	
Inflammatory response	Days 2–6	Swelling subsides, warm to touch, discoloration, pain to touch, pain on motion	CRYO	↓ Swelling, ↓ pain
			ESC	↓ Pain
			IC	↓ Swelling
			LPL	↓ Pain
			ULTRA	Nonthermal effects to ↑ healing
			Range of motion	
Fibroblastic-repair	Days 4–10	Pain to touch, pain on motion, swollen	THERMO	Mildly ↑ circulation
			ESC	↓ Pain—muscle pumping
			LPL	↓ Pain
			IC	Facilitate lymphatic flow
			ULTRA	Nonthermal effects to ↑ healing
			Range of motion	
			Strengthening	
Maturation-remodeling	Day 7—recovery	Swollen, no more pain to touch, decreasing pain on motion	ULTRA	Deep heating to circulation
			ESC	↑ Range of motion, ↑ strength
			LPL	↓ Pain
			SWD	↓ Pain
			MWD	Deep heating to ↑ circulation
			Range of motion	Deep heating to ↑ circulation
			Strengthening	
			Functional activities	

CRYO, cryotherapy; ESC, electrical stimulating currents; IC, intermittent compression; LPL, low-power laser; MWD, microwave diathermy; SWD, shortwave diathermy; THERMO, thermotherapy; ULTRA, ultrasound; ↓, decrease; ↑, increase.

The injured part should be rested and protected for at least the first 48–72 hours to allow the inflammatory phase of the healing process to do what it is supposed to do.

Modality Use in the Inflammatory-Response Phase

The inflammatory-response phase begins immediately with injury and may last as long as day 6 following injury. With appropriate care, swelling begins to subside and eventually stops altogether. The injured area may feel warm to the touch, and some discoloration is usually apparent. The injury is still painful to the touch, and pain is elicited on movement of the injured part.

As in the initial injury management stage, modalities should be used to control pain and reduce swelling. Cryotherapy should still be used during the inflammatory stage. Ice bags, cold packs, or ice massages provide analgesic effects. The use of cold also reduces the likelihood of swelling, which may continue during this stage. Swelling does subside completely by the end of this phase.

It must be emphasized that heating an injury too soon is a bigger mistake than using ice on an injury for too long. Many clinicians elect to stay with cryotherapy for weeks following injury; in fact, some never switch to the superficial heating techniques. This procedure is simply a matter of personal preference that should be dictated by experience. Once swelling has stopped, the clinician may elect to begin contrast baths with a longer cold-to-hot ratio.

An intermittent compression device may be used to decrease swelling by facilitating resorption of the by-products of inflammatory process by the lymphatic system. Electrical stimulating currents and low-power laser can be used to help reduce pain.

After the initial stage, the patient should begin to work on active and passive range of motion. Decisions regarding how rapidly to progress exercise should be determined by the response of the injury to that exercise. If exercise produces additional swelling and markedly exacerbates pain, then the level or intensity of the exercise is too great and should be reduced. Clinicians should be aggressive in their approach to rehabilitation, but the healing process will always limit the approach.

Modality Use in the Fibroblastic-Repair Phase

Once the inflammatory response has subsided, the fibroblastic-repair phase begins. This stage may begin as early as 4 days after the injury and may last for several weeks. At this point, swelling has stopped completely. The injury is still tender to the touch but is not as painful as during the last stage. Pain is also less on active and passive motion.

Treatments may change during this stage from cold to heat, once again using increased swelling as a precautionary indicator. Thermotherapy techniques including hydrocollator packs, paraffin, or eventually warm whirlpool may be safely employed. The purpose of thermotherapy is to increase circulation to the injured area to promote healing. These modalities can also produce some degree of analgesia.

Clinical Decision-Making   *Exercise 2–2*

A patient is 8 days poststrain of the quadriceps muscle of the thigh. The clinician feels that it is time to change from cold therapy to some form of heat. What criteria should be used to determine if this patient is ready to change to heat?

Intermittent compression can once again be used to facilitate removal of injury by-products from the area. Electrical stimulating currents can be used to assist this process by eliciting a muscle contraction and thus inducing a muscle pumping action. This aids in facilitating lymphatic flow. Electrical currents can once again be used for modulation of pain, as can stimulation of trigger points with the low-powered laser.

The clinician must continue to stress the importance of range-of-motion and strengthening exercises and progress them appropriately during this phase.

Modality Use in the Maturation-Remodeling Phase

The maturation-remodeling phase is the longest of the four phases and may last for several years, depending on the severity of the injury. The ultimate goal during this maturation stage of the healing process is return to activity. The injury is no longer painful to the touch, although some progressively decreasing pain may still be felt on motion. The collagen fibers must be realigned according to tensile stresses and strains placed on them. Virtually all modalities may be safely used during this stage; thus, decisions should be based on what seems to work most effectively in a given situation.

At this point some type of heating modality is beneficial to the healing process. The deep-heating modalities, ultrasound, or shortwave and microwave diathermy should be used to increase circulation to the deeper tissues. Ultrasound is particularly useful during this period since collagen absorbs a high percentage of the available acoustic energy. Increased blood flow delivers the essential nutrients to the injured area to promote healing, and increased lymphatic flow assists in breakdown and removal of waste products. The superficial heating modalities are certainly less effective at this point.

Electrical stimulating currents can be used for a number of purposes. As before, they may be used in pain modulation. They may also be used to stimulate muscle contractions for the purpose of increasing both range of motion and muscular strength.[35]

Low-power laser can also assist in modulating pain. If pain is reduced, therapeutic exercises may be progressed more quickly.

Clinical Decision-Making   *Exercise 2–3*

In the rehabilitative process for a sprain of the medial collateral ligament in the knee, at what point should the clinician decide to add therapeutic exercises to modality use?

The Role of Progressive Controlled Mobility in the Maturation Phase

Wolff's Law states that bone will respond to the physical demands placed on it, causing it to remodel or realign along lines of tensile force.[36] Although not specified in Wolff's Law, the same response occurs in soft tissue. Therefore, it is critical that injured structures be exposed to progressively increasing loads, particularly during the remodeling phase. Controlled mobilization has been shown to be superior to immobilization for scar formation, revascularization, muscle regeneration, and reorientation of muscle fibers and tensile properties in animal models.[13] However, immobilization of the injured tissue during the inflammatory-response phase will likely facilitate the process of healing by controlling inflammation, thus reducing athletic training symptoms. As healing progresses to the repair phase, controlled activity directed toward return-to-normal flexibility and strength should be combined with protective support or bracing. Generally, clinical signs and symptoms disappear at the end of this phase.

As the remodeling phase begins, aggressive active range-of-motion and strengthening exercises should be incorporated to facilitate tissue remodeling and realignment.[37] To a great extent, pain will dictate rate of progression. With initial injury, pain is intense and tends to decrease and eventually subside altogether as healing progresses. Any exacerbation of pain, swelling, or other symptoms during or following a particular exercise or activity indicates that the load is too great for the level of tissue repair or remodeling. The clinician must be aware of the timelines required for the process of healing and realize that being overly aggressive can interfere with that process.

Clinical Decision-Making   *Exercise 2–4*

The clinician decides to allow a patient with a grade 1 ankle sprain to be full weight bearing immediately following injury. Is this the best decision based on your knowledge of the healing process?

INDICATIONS AND CONTRAINDICATIONS

Table 2–3 presents a summary list of indications for using the various modalities. This list should aid the clinician in making decisions regarding the appropriate use of a therapeutic modality in a given clinical situation.

OTHER CONSIDERATIONS IN TREATING INJURY

During the rehabilitation period following injury, patients must alter their daily routines to allow the injury to heal sufficiently. Consideration must be given to maintaining levels of balance,

Table 2-3 Indications for Therapeutic Modalities

THERAPEUTIC MODALITY	PHYSIOLOGICAL RESOURCES (INDICATIONS FOR USE)
Electrical stimulating currents—high voltage	Pain modulation
	Muscle reeducation
	Muscle pumping contractions
	Retard atrophy
	Muscle strengthening
	Increase range of motion
	Fracture healing
	Acute injury
Electrical stimulating currents—low voltage	Wound healing
	Fracture healing
	Iontophoresis
Electrical stimulating currents—interferential	Pain modulation
	Muscle reeducation
	Muscle pumping contractions
	Fracture healing
	Increase range of motion
Electrical stimulating currents—Russian	Muscle strengthening
Electrical stimulating currents—MENS	Fracture healing
	Wound healing
Shortwave and microwave diathermy	Increase deep circulation
	Increase metabolic activity
	Reduce muscle guarding/spasm
	Reduce inflammation
	Facilitate wound healing
	Analgesia
	Increase tissue temperatures over a large area

(continued)

Table 2–3 (continued)

THERAPEUTIC MODALITY	PHYSIOLOGICAL RESOURCES (INDICATIONS FOR USE)
Cryotherapy—cold packs, ice massage	Acute injury
	Vasoconstriction—decreased blood flow
	Analgesia
	Reduce inflammation
	Reduce muscle guarding/spasm
Thermotherapy—hot whirlpool, paraffin, hydrocollators, infrared lamps	Vasodilation—increased blood flow
	Analgesia
	Reduce muscle guarding/spasm
	Reduce inflammation
	Increase metabolic activity
	Facilitate tissue healing
Low-power laser	Pain modulation (trigger points)
	Facilitate wound healing

neuromuscular control, strength, flexibility, and cardiorespiratory endurance. Modality use should be combined with the use of anti-inflammatory medications prescribed by the physician, particularly during the initial acute and inflammatory-response phases of rehabilitation.[38]

SUMMARY

1. Clinical decisions on how and when therapeutic modalities may best be used should be based on recognition of signs and symptoms, as well as some awareness of the time frames associated with the various phases of the healing process.
2. Once an acute injury has occurred, the healing process consists of the inflammatory-response phase, the fibroblastic-repair phase, and the maturation-remodeling phase.
3. A number of pathologic factors can impede the healing process.
4. Modality use in the initial treatment phase should be directed toward limiting the amount of swelling and reducing pain.
5. It is critical to use logic and common sense based on sound theoretical knowledge when selecting the appropriate modalities to use during the different phases of healing.
6. During the rehabilitation period after injury, patients must alter their normal daily routine to allow the injury to heal sufficiently.

REVIEW QUESTIONS

1. How should the clinician incorporate therapeutic modalities into a rehabilitation program for various injuries?
2. What are the physiological events associated with the inflammatory-response phase of the healing process?

3. How can you differentiate between acute and chronic inflammation?

4. How is collagen laid down in the area of injury during the fibroblastic-repair phase of healing?

5. Explain Wolff's Law and the importance of controlled mobility during the maturation-remodeling phase of healing.

6. What are some of the factors that can have a negative impact on the healing process?

7. Why is the immediate care provided following acute injury so important to the healing process and the course of rehabilitation?

8. What specific modalities may be incorporated into treatment during the inflammatory-response phase?

9. What specific modalities may be incorporated into treatment during the fibroblastic-repair phase?

10. What are the specific indications and contraindications for using the various modalities?

SELF-TEST QUESTIONS

True or False

1. Loss of function is a sign of the inflammatory process.

2. Leukocytes are present in both the acute and chronic inflammatory responses.

3. An injured individual's health, age, and nutrition are factors that influence healing.

Multiple Choice

4. The three phases of the healing process, in order, are as follows:
   a. fibroblastic-repair, inflammatory-response, maturation-remodeling
   b. inflammatory-response, fibroblastic-repair, maturation-remodeling
   c. inflammatory-response, maturation-remodeling, fibroblastic-repair

5. Which of the following type of cell has phagocytic characteristics?
   a. red blood cells
   b. platelets
   c. leukocytes
   d. endothelials

6. The extracellular matrix, formed by fibroblastic cells, consists of
   a. collagen
   b. elastin
   c. ground substance
   d. all of the above

7. During the inflammatory-response phase of the healing process, modalities are used to
   a. control pain
   b. reduce swelling
   c. both *a* and *b*
   d. neither *a* nor *b*

8. _____ states that bone and soft tissue remodel and realign according to the physical demands placed on them.
   a. Wolff's Law
   b. Ohm's Law
   c. Meissner's Law
   d. McGill's Law

9. Approximately how long does the maturation-remodeling phase of the healing process last?
   a. less than 1 week
   b. 1 week
   c. 1–2 weeks
   d. 3 weeks to 2 years

10. Which of the following is *not* a chemical mediator involved in the inflammatory-response phase?
    a. testosterone
    b. histamine
    c. necrosin
    d. leukotaxin

SOLUTIONS TO CLINICAL DECISION-MAKING EXERCISES

2–1

The clinician's response should be based on knowledge of the healing process and an understanding of the time frames necessary in that process.

2–2

At this point, the patient is in transition between the fibroblastic-repair phase and the maturation-remodeling phase. Although there is still some pain on active motion, all of the clinical signs of inflammation (tenderness to touch, increased warmth, redness, and so on) have disappeared, and thus it should be safe to go with heat. If changing to heat causes the patient to have greater difficulty completing strengthening and flexibility exercises, then the change has likely been made too quickly.

2–3

Therapeutic exercises should begin on day 1 following injury. The point is that modalities should be used to facilitate the patient's effort to actively exercise the injured part and not in place of the active exercise.

2–4

Knowing how important it is for the inflammatory-response phase to accomplish what it needs to physiologically without interference, it is likely best to recommend minimal weight bearing for the first 24–48 hours.

REFERENCES

1. Houghton PE. Effects of therapeutic modalities on wound healing: a conservative approach to the management of chronic wounds. *Phys Ther Rev*. 1999;4(3):167–182.
2. Montbriand D. Rehab products: equipment focus. Making progress: modalities can jumpstart the healing process. *Adv Mag Directors Rehabil*. 2002;11(7):69–70, 72, 80.
3. Damjanov I. *Anderson's Pathology*. 10th ed. St. Louis: Mosby; 1996.
4. Allen T. Exercises-induced muscle damage: mechanisms, prevention, and treatment. *Physiother Can*. 2004;56(2):67–79.
5. Clarkson PM, Tremblay I. Exercise-induced muscle damage, repair and adaptation in humans. *J Appl Physiol*. 1988;65:1–6.
6. Grichnick K, Ferrante F. The difference between acute and chronic pain. *Mt Sinai J Med*. 1991;58:217.
7. Weintraub W. *Tendon and Ligament Healing: A New Approach to Sports and Overuse Injury*. St. Paul: Paradigm Publications; 2003.
8. Wilder R. Overuse injuries: tendinopathies, stress fractures, compartment syndrome, and shin splints. *Clin Sports Med*. 2004;23(1):55–81.
9. Soto-Quijano D. Work-related musculoskeletal disorders of the upper extremity. *Crit Rev Phys Rehabil Med*. 2005;17(1):65–82.
10. Peterson L, Renstrom P. Injuries in musculoskeletal tissues. In: Peterson L, ed. *Sports Injuries: Their Prevention and Treatment*. 3rd ed. Champaign, IL: Human Kinetics; 2001.
11. Leadbetter W, Buckwalter J, Gordon S. *Sports-induced Inflammation*. Park Ridge, IL; American Academy of Orthopaedic Surgeons; 1990.
12. Prentice W. *Principles of Athletic Training*. 14th ed. New York: McGraw-Hill; 2010.
13. Arnoczky SP. Physiologic principles of ligament injuries and healing. In: Scott WN, ed. *Ligament and Extensor Mechanism Injuries of the Knee*. St. Louis: Mosby; 1991.
14. Fernandez A, Finlew J. Wound healing: helping a natural process. *Postgrad Med*. 1983;74(4):311–318.

15. Marchesi V. Inflammation and healing. In: Danjanov I, ed. *Anderson's Pathology.* 10th ed. St. Louis: Mosby; 1996.
16. Bryant MW. Wound healing. *CIBA Clin Symp.* 1997;29(3): 2–36.
17. Udermann BE. Inflammation: the body's response to injury. *Int Sports J.* 1999;3(2):19–24.
18. Carrico T, Mehrhof A, Cohen I. Biology and wound healing. *Surg Clin North Am.* 1984;64(4):721–734.
19. Butterfield T, Best T, Merrick M. The dual roles of neutrophils and macrophages in inflammation: a critical balance between tissue damage and repair. *J Athletic Train.* 2006;41 (4):457.
20. Hart J. Inflammation: its role in the healing of acute wounds. *J Wound Care.* 2002;11(6):205–209.
21. Woo SL-Y, Buckwalter J, eds. *Injury and Repair of Musculoskeletal Soft Tissues.* Park Ridge, IL: American Academy of Orthopaedic Surgeons; 1988.
22. Ley K. *Physiology of Inflammation.* Bethesda, MD: American Physiological Society; 2001.
23. Hildebrand K, Behm C, Kydd A. The basics of soft tissue healing and general factors that influence such healing. *Sports Med Arthrosc Rev.* 2005;13(3):136–144.
24. Wahl S, Renstrom P. Fibrosis in soft tissue injuries. In: Leadbetter W, Buckwalter J, Gordon S, eds. *Sports-induced Inflammation.* Park Ridge, IL: American Academy of Orthopaedic Surgeons; 1990.
25. Rywlin A. Hemopoietic system. In: Damjanov I, ed. *Anderson's Pathology.* 10th ed. St. Louis: Mosby; 1996.
26. Houglum P. Soft tissue healing and its impact on rehabilitation. *J Sport Rehabil.* 1992;1(1):19–39.
27. Leadbetter W. Introduction to sports-induced soft-tissue inflammation. In: Leadbetter W, Buckwalter J, Gordon S, eds. *Sports-induced Inflammation.* Park Ridge, IL: American Academy of Orthopaedic Surgeons; 1990.
28. Fantone J. Basic concepts in inflammation. In: Leadbetter W, Buckwalter J, Gordon S, eds. *Sports-induced Inflammation.* Park Ridge, IL: American Academy of Orthopaedic Surgeons; 1990.
29. Hubbel S, Buschbacher R. Tissue injury and healing: using medications, modalities, and exercise to maximize recovery. In: Bushbacher R, Branddom R, eds. *Sports Medicine and Rehabilitation: A Sport Specific Approach.* Philadelphia: Lippincott Williams and Wilkins; 2008.
30. Hettinga D. Inflammatory response of synovial joint structures. In: Gould J, Davies G, eds. *Orthopaedic and Sports Physical Therapy.* St. Louis: Mosby; 1990.
31. Riley W. Wound healing. *Am Fam Phys.* 1981;24:5.
32. Cheng N. The effects of electrocurrents on A.T.P. generation, protein synthesis and membrane transport. *J Orthop Relat Res.* 1982;171:264–272.
33. Young T. The healing process. *Pract Nurs.* 2001;22(10):38, 40, 43.
34. Robbins S, Cotran R, Kumar V. *Pathologic Basis of Disease.* 8th ed. Philadelphia: WB Saunders; 2009.
35. Fleischli JG, Laughlin TJ. Electrical stimulation in wound healing. *J. Foot Ankle Surg.* 1997;36:457.
36. Wolff J. *Gesetz der transformation der knochen.* Berlin: Aug. Hirschwald; 1892.
37. Zachezewski J. Flexibility for sports. In: Sanders B, ed. *Sports Physical Therapy.* Norwalk, CT: Appleton & Lange; 1990.
38. Biederman R. Pharmacology in rehabilitation: nonsteroidal anti-inflammatory agents. *J Orthop Sports Phys Ther.* 2005; 35(6):356–367.
39. Wahl S, Renstrom P. Fibrosis in soft-tissue injuries. In: Leadbetter W, Buckwalter J, Gordon S, eds. *Sports-induced Inflammation.* Park Ridge, IL: American Academy of Orthopaedic Surgeons; 1990.

GLOSSARY

acute injury An injury in which active inflammation is present that includes the classic symptoms of tenderness, swelling, redness, and so on.

chronic injury An injury in which the normal cellular response in the inflammatory process is altered, replacing leukocytes with macrophages and plasma cells, along with degeneration of the injured structure.

fibroplasia The period of scar formation that occurs during the fibroblastic-repair phase.

leukocytes A white blood cell that is the primary effector cell against infection and tissue damage that functions to clean up damaged cells.

macrotears Significant damage to the soft tissues caused by acute trauma that results in clinical symptoms and functional alterations.

microtears Minor damage to soft tissue most often associated with overuse.

phagocytic cell A cell that has the ability to destroy and ingest cellular debris.

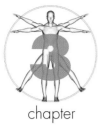

The Role of Therapeutic Modalities in Wound Healing

Pamela E. Houghton

OBJECTIVES

Following completion of this chapter, the student will be able to:

➤ Explain cellular and physiological actions of commonly used modalities on wound healing. Review clinical research evidence of effectiveness of modalities for delayed or nonhealing wounds.

➤ Describe application techniques, stimulus parameters, and treatment schedules commonly used when treating chronic wounds with these modalities.

➤ Review indications, contraindications, and potential risks of each of the modalities.

➤ Use information provided in the chapter to select the best modality for a particular type of chronic wound.

INTRODUCTION

The cellular and physiological processes triggered by tissue injury are often divided into three phases, namely, inflammation, proliferation, and remodeling phases (refer to Chapter 2). Briefly, soon after injury, blood loss is minimized through hemostatic changes that involve a cascade of events involving the platelet that result in fibrin clot formation. Chemical mediators released by the activated platelet and mechanical trauma attract leukocytes, including macrophages and neutrophils, to the site of injury where they exit the blood vessel and enter the injured tissue. Phagocytic activities of these inflammatory cells act to debride necrotic and foreign material present in the damaged tissue. White blood cells also release growth factors that have potent mitogenic and chemoattractant properties that are responsible for mediating migration and proliferation of fibroblasts, endothelial cells, and epithelial cells. Fibroblasts and endothelial cells direct collagen synthesis and angiogenesis, respectively, and migration and proliferation of epithelial cells results in the formation of a new epidermal barrier. During the final remodeling phase, turnover and reorganization of collagen and other components of the extracellular matrix optimizes tissue integrity and strength and helps to prevent future wound breakdown.

Impairments in soft tissue healing are caused by a number of complicating factors that collectively interfere with the normal tissue repair process. Medical, pharmacological, social, and environmental factors that interfere with oxygen perfusion, cause repetitive trauma, promote bacterial growth, or limit the ability of cells involved in tissue response to stimuli will ultimately delay the normal healing process. In addition, there is recent experimental evidence

37

that delayed healing is associated with chronic inflammation that causes elevated levels of inflammatory mediators that promote tissue destruction and interfere with new tissue formation.[1] Therefore, therapies that halt the destructive chronic inflammatory process and help restore the normal balance of tissue promoters and inhibitors may accelerate closure of chronic wounds.

To determine the best modality for the treatment of that particular chronic wound, it is imperative to have an awareness of the experimental research evidence available that provides information about the cellular and systemic effects of these modalities on the biological systems in general and on the processes of wound healing specifically. Understanding how and where these modalities work within the healing processes allows the clinician to make a better choice of modality on this condition.

SUPERFICIAL HOT AND COLD

Both superficial hot and cold therapies are commonly used to treat musculoskeletal conditions following injuries.

Effects of Hot and Cold Agents on Blood Flow

When cold is applied to the skin, vasoconstriction of cutaneous arterioles is stimulated immediately. Reduction in blood vessel lumen diameter causes a significant restriction of local blood flow to the subcutaneous tissue. Local vasoconstriction induced by hypothermia reduces fluid filtration into the interstitium and thus reduces the potential for edema to develop. In addition, the slower metabolism that occurs when tissue temperatures are lowered results in the release of fewer inflammatory mediators and reduced edema formation following tissue injury. Lower rates of metabolism also reduce oxygen demand of tissues and minimize the chances of further injury of tissues with limited blood perfusion due to ischemia. Both human[2] and animal[3] studies have shown that mild tissue cooling is effective in reducing acute inflammation and tissue swelling.

While cold application may be beneficial to control excess inflammation during the early phases of tissue repair, it has been shown to impair bactericidal effects of neutrophils,[4] increase the incidence of wound infection,[5] and interfere with the coagulation cascade.[6] In addition, continued hypothermia throughout the healing process can interfere with the development of optimal tissue strength[7] and limit recovery postoperatively.[8] Persistent inhibition of the inflammatory process deprives the healing process of key chemical mediators responsible for stimulating new tissue formation. In addition, vasoconstriction produced by cryotherapy reduces local blood flow at the site of injury and interferes with the delivery of oxygen to fuel tissue healing.

Elevation of local tissue temperature at the site of tissue in the later stages of the healing process has been purported to accelerate tissue repair. A key mechanism of action by which a thermal agent accelerates the healing process is via heat-induced vasodilation that provides increased blood supply and improved tissue oxygenation.[9] Other beneficial effects of therapeutic heat include alteration of enzymatic activity of chronic wound fluid,[10] stimulation of fibroblast proliferation and metabolism,[11] accelerated proliferation of microvascular endothelial cells,[12] and improved phagocytic activity of inflammatory cell.[13] Preoperative warming of patients undergoing elective surgery was associated with a significant reduction in complications with wound site infection.[14] Application of heat to methicillin-resistant *Staphylococcus aureus* (MRSA) taken from pressure sores eradicated this antibiotic-resistant strain of bacteria.[15]

Modalities capable of producing local increases in tissue temperature include: continuous shortwave diathermy, infrared lamps, continuous ultrasound, hydrocollator packs, and immersion in warm whirlpools. Improved healing of chronic wounds has also been produced by applying heat locally to the wound using a specially designed noncontact dressing that creates a moist wound environment and delivers sufficient thermal energy so as to maintain normal tissue temperature.[9] Petrofsky et al demonstrated increased local blood flow surrounding chronic wounds by global warming using a heat lamp.[16] The 74.5% wound size reduction produced after 4 weeks of treatment of subjects with diabetes was higher in subjects who underwent global warming rather than healing rates produced by local wound heating that produced skin temperatures of 37°C (normothermia = 55.3% in 4 weeks).[16]

Hydrotherapy

One method of delivering superficial heat or cold to healing tissues is by immersing the affected body part or limb in hydrotherapy tanks filled with warm, tepid, or cool water. Wound cleansing using hydrotherapy removes necrotic and devitalized tissue, cleanses the wound surface of loosely adherent yellow fibrinous or gelatinous exudate, and takes away any unwanted dirt, foreign contaminants, or harmful residues of topical agents. Niederhuber et al[17] and Bohannon[18] reported whirlpool with agitation removed surface bacteria especially when whirlpool treatment is followed by spraying of the skin surface. Hydrotherapy treatments have also been shown to increase the rate of granulation tissue formation.[19] Meeker demonstrated in a controlled trial without randomization that patients who received whirlpool therapy in 72-hour postabdominal surgery experienced reduced pain and decreased wound inflammation.[20]

The removal of foreign matter and nonviable tissue using this nonspecific type of mechanical debridement will aid wound healing indirectly and help reduce bacterial burden within the wound.

Additional benefits of hydrotherapy treatments of wounds covered with thick eschar are that the immersion will help soften the eschar and help facilitate subsequent debridement, provided it is carried out soon after hydrotherapy. Based on this mechanism of action of hydrotherapy, this therapeutic modality is indicated for open nonhealing wounds that have substantial amounts of necrotic tissue. According to clinical practice guidelines jointly produced by collaboration between the European Pressure Ulcer Advisory Panel and the NPUAP in the USA, an international panel of experts, a course of whirlpool therapy for wound cleansing facilitates healing and reduces wound bioburden and infection (strength of evidence = C—primarily based on expert opinion).[21] It is also recommended that whirlpool treatments should be discontinued when debriding objectives have been met (i.e., the wound bed is clean).

Elevating water temperature of the whirlpool can have additional therapeutic benefits including increasing changes in local circulation and reducing the patient's perception of pain. Some suggest hydrotherapy treatments may be useful for persons with mild arterial compromise. However, increased cellular activity produced by immersion in warm water could produce relative tissue ischemia if arterial disease is pronounced and local vascular supply cannot meet increased demands for nutrients and oxygen. In addition, heat-induced vasodilation and release of vasoactive substances can also be detrimental if treating persons with concurrent venous disease. McCulloch and Boyd reported that prolonged hydrotherapy treatment (greater than 5 minutes) of chronic venous leg ulcers when the unbandaged lower extremity is immersed in the dependent position can result in increased venous hypertension and vascular congestion leading to limb edema.[22] Ogiwara demonstrated recently that ankle dorsiflexion/plantarflexion exercises performed while the limb was immersed in the whirlpool tank were unable to offset edema formation due to limb dependency during hydrotherapy.[23]

Nonimmersion hydrotherapy techniques have become more popular recently. Pulsed lavage involves the delivery of an irrigating solution under pressure produced by an electronically powered device combined with suction to remove effluent. Haynes et al reported that hydrotherapy delivered using this nonimmersion pulsed lavage technique has greater improvements in granulation tissue formation and removes surface contaminants more completely than traditional hydrotherapy treatments using only limb immersion.[19] Using an animal model, Svoboda et al demonstrated that pulsed lavage produced better removal of bacteria than a similar volume of fluid delivered at a lower pressure using a bulb syringe.[24] However, subsequent experiments showed that bacteria levels rebound back to 95% of original levels within 48 hours of pulsed lavage treatment, suggesting these cleansing effects of this form of hydrotherapy are only transient.[25] Pulsed lavage has been suggested to cleanse deep wounds with undermining. This form of nonimmersion hydrotherapy treatment may be useful with persons who have physical limitations or medical conditions that prevent water immersion.

Most published protocols for the use of whirlpool on chronic wounds suggest that the limb should be immersed in water of a neutral temperature (92–96°F) for 10–20 minutes. Treatment times should be reduced if tissue maceration is produced. Water temperature is often selected based on arterial blood supply and venous return of the patient's limb. Warm water can be used to help improve blood supply and help with patient discomfort, whereas water temperatures should be employed with individuals at risk of developing venous congestion. However, whirlpools using water temperatures above or below body surface temperature should only be used on healthy individuals in whom local circulation is not compromised and cardiovascular status is normal. Hydrotherapy treatments should be discontinued once the wound bed is clean and devoid of necrotic tissue. Rinsing the limb after the limb is removed from the hydrotherapy tank is recommended to further aid the removal of bacteria and contaminants on the skin and wound surface.

Care must be taken to ensure that agitation produced by the turbines within the hydrotherapy tank does not result in excessive pressures that can cause mechanical damage to fragile new tissue deposited in the wound bed. Pressures produced by whirlpool turbines have not been documented and may vary greatly between manufactured models. There are reports in the literature of increased wound infection such as *Pseudomonas aeruginosa* for individuals using whirlpool.[26] In addition, Wheeler et al studied the potential damage and particle penetration produced by pulsed lavage in artificially produced wounds.[27] This was one of the first reports that raised concerns about the use of higher pressures when irrigating wounds. This may occur because prolonged water immersion causes superhydration of the skin and can interfere with the normal skin defenses to bacteria. Appropriate protocols outlined by the Centers for Disease Control are employed for cleaning, disinfecting, sterilizing, and culturing of the hydrotherapy units and should be carried out to reduce the occurrence of these waterborne infections. Other safety considerations when using this modality include the use of appropriate grounding of turbine units, the use of ground fault circuit breakers, and caution when transferring a patient to and from the tank.

ELECTRICAL STIMULATION

Endogenous bioelectrical potentials have been measured across the skin of many animals including humans.[28] This potential formed by the separation of charged ions across the epidermis is believed to be responsible for the formation of a current of injury that occurs whenever the insulative skin layer is disrupted by injury allowing charged particles to move down their concentration gradient. The presence of this small, but measurable, current of injury within a wound is strongly correlated with successful healing outcomes.[29] McCaig et al have written an excellent review of historical and recent research that collectively provides very compelling evidence for the important role of electrical signals in the development, regeneration, and repair of biological tissues.[30] They reviewed the expansive body of literature that demonstrates profound effects of bioelectricity on cell behavior and describe how these small electrical fields influence epithelial and vascular endothelial cell orientation and proliferation that are known to be key cellular processes underlying re-epithelialization and angiogenesis during wound healing.

In vitro studies have demonstrated that electrical stimulation can promote several activities of the inflammatory cells involved in the initial phases of tissue repair. It can induce cell migration to the site of injury through galvanotaxis,[31] stimulate inflammatory cell degranulation,[32] and release important chemical mediators such as growth factors and chemoattractants.[33] Electrical stimulation can also induce inflammatory cell proliferation so that a greater number of these cells are able to respond to the tissue injury.[34] These cellular actions of electrical currents on the inflammatory cells can speed the resolution of the inflammatory phase of tissue repair so that new tissue formation may begin sooner following injury.

Electrically induced activity of inflammatory cells may also underlie reduced edema formation observed following injury in animal models treated with electrical stimulation.[35,36] Reed documented that the application of electrical current reduces microvessel leakage and limits posttraumatic edema formation.[37] Whether electrical stimulation can produce similar effects on posttraumatic edema in clinical situation with human subjects has not been investigated sufficiently. In one clinical study that examined swelling postacute injury in humans, treatment using high-voltage pulsed current (HVPC) was found to be as effective as compression therapy at reducing posttraumatic swelling.[38]

Experimental research performed using various animal models has revealed that local application of electrical current to wounded skin[39-43] or surgically incised ligaments[44-46] and tendons[47,48] results in improved collagen deposition,[39,40,44,47] accelerated collagen maturation and organization,[35] and greater tensile strength.[43,45,48,49] Stimulation of new tissue formation may in part be due to direct action of electrical currents on fibroblasts. Application of electrical current to cultured fibroblasts has been shown to enhance collagen synthesis and secretion,[34,50] stimulate fibroblast proliferation,[34] increase the number of receptor sites for certain growth factors,[51] and direct fibroblast migration.[52,53]

Possible intracellular mechanisms that underlie these fibroblastic responses to electrical currents include activation of transcription and translation of mRNA to make available important protein precursors,[54] increased ATP production to supply necessary energy demands,[50] membrane permeability that would allow increased intracellular stores of calcium,[33] and production of membrane receptors for important cytokines such as epidermal growth factor.[51]

Epithelial cell activity during repair also seems to be affected by electrical current. In particular, in vitro studies have shown that epithelial cell proliferation[55] and differentiation[56] can be activated in epidermal cells by electrical stimulation. In addition, keratinocyte migration can be influenced by the application of an electrical field,[55,57] and the synthesis and secretion of growth factors by epithelial cells can be stimulated to a greater extent by the application of an electrical current.[33] Correspondingly, several authors have reported that exogenous application of electrical currents to various animal models can accelerate wound re-epithelialization.[41,42,107]

In addition to accelerated activities of fibroblasts and epithelial cells during the proliferative stage of healing, electrical current has also been shown to augment angiogenesis. Clinical studies have detected a greater density of capillaries within newly formed granulation tissue analyzed in tissue biopsies taken from individuals with chronic venous leg wounds when they were pretreated with electrical current.[58]

Results from studies in which electrical currents have been applied to cultures of bacteria commonly found in chronic wounds suggest that electrical current may have bactericidal properties. Kincaid and Lavoie[59] and Szuminsky et al[60] showed HVPC applied using a negative electrode can directly affect bacterial growth and replication. However, the high intensity required to produce these bactericidal properties would likely not be tolerated in a clinical situation. Daeschlein et al recently confirmed that ES applied using a clinically relevant dose to bacterial cultures of gram-positive and gram-negative organisms significantly reduced bacterial growth.[61] Wolcott et al were the first to suggest that bacteria counts in chronic wounds were reduced by treatment with cathodal DC current.[62] Subsequently, Rowley et al demonstrated bacterial growth was reduced when cathodal DC current was applied to wounds in rabbits that were infected with *P. aeruginosa*.[63] Both in vitro[64] and in vivo[65] experimental studies have demonstrated greater bacterial inhibition when DC current was combined with silver ions in the active electrode. This potential synergistic action of electrotherapy and silver dressings was demonstrated in a clinical trial where faster closure of full thickness of burns was documented in wounds treated with ES plus silver nylon dressing compared with ES alone.[66]

Increased local vasodilation and improved tissue oxygenation have been reported to occur in individuals with peripheral vascular disease following treatment with electrical current.[67] Gilcreast et al[68] and Faghri et al[69] have demonstrated that electrical stimulation can enhance perfusion of ischemic limbs. In addition, Im et al[70] showed enhanced survival rates of skin flaps pretreated with electrical stimulation that was attributed to improved blood perfusion observed in skin flaps under the negatively charged cathode.

Treatment with high-voltage pulsed current (HVPC) with negative polarity produced greater increases in local blood flow of rats than did positive-polarity stimulation.[35] Some reports suggest elevations in blood flow can be enhanced by stimulating the muscle pump with the use of relatively high-intensity stimulation that is sufficient to produce intermittent neuromuscular contraction.[69] However, there are also reports that suggest only low-intensity stimulation without muscle contraction can produce significant blood flow changes.[71] Both biphasic and monophasic forms of electrical current have been shown to stimulate blood flow and significantly increase transcutaneous oxygen tension in the sacral region of patients with spinal cord injury (SCI) who were at a high risk of developing pressure sores.[72,73] Goldman et al treated a small group of individuals with critically ischemic wounds ($TcPO_2$ <20 mm Hg) with sham and real HVPC and produced a significant increase in $TcPO_2$.[74] Complete wound closure was accomplished in 90% of the wounds treated with HVPC compared with only 29% in the control group.[75] These results provide strong support that electrical stimulation therapy facilitates microcirculation and this was associated with better healing outcomes. Restoration of impaired local circulation by application of electrical currents would promote tissue healing by supplying required nutrients including oxygen and help to wash out accumulated waste products produced by the injured tissue. Improved local circulation would also help remove inflammatory mediators that may contribute to local edema and pain.

In addition to the benefits of electrical stimulation on the tissue healing process, transcutaneous electrical nerve stimulation (TENS) has long been recognized to have analgesic properties. There are several published clinical reports that have shown electrical currents that are similar to those used to treat delayed healing can reduce an individual's perception of pain (refer to Chapter 5). Reducing pain caused by injuries or nonhealing wounds can indirectly aid the healing process by offsetting many of the adverse effects of stress on the healing process and ultimately improving the patient's quality of life.

The most common application technique for electrical stimulation of chronic wounds involves using a monopolar setup in which the active electrode placed directly into the wound bed using specialized electrodes composed of sterile conductive material with a larger dispersive electrode is placed on intact skin proximal to the wound (refer to Figure 3–1). This

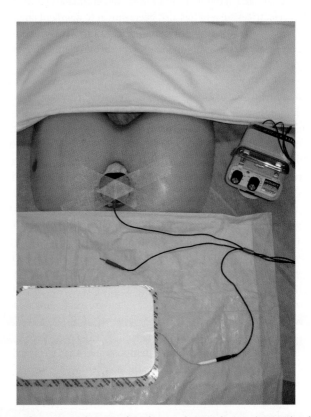

Figure 3–1. Application technique for electrical stimulation (HVPC) where the active electrode is applied directly to the wound bed while a large dispersive electrode is placed on intact skin distant from the wound site.

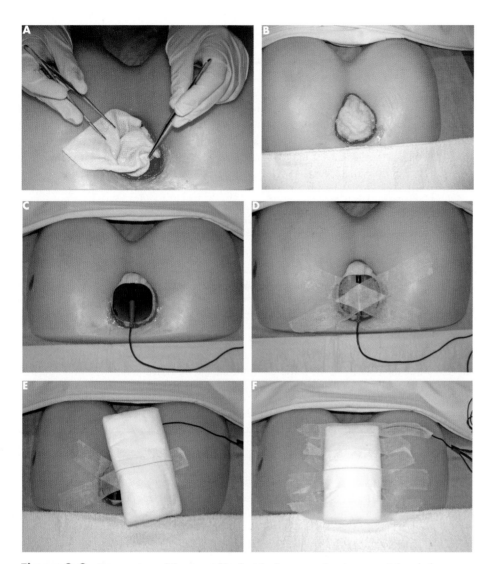

Figure 3–2. Preparation of the wound bed with electroconductive material and placement of the active electrode in the wound bed. (a and b) Gauze soaked in hydrogel is loosely packed into the wound bed; (c and d) a clean electrode is placed over the wound packing and secured in place with tape; (e and f) the active electrode is further held in place by covering with a large cotton dressing.

direct application technique involves preparing the wound bed with electroconductive material. This is usually done by packing the wound loosely with gauze soaked with hydrogel and/or saline (Figure 3–2). Careful removal of wound dressings and judicious use of universal precautions and equipment decontamination procedures are also required so as to avoid wound manipulation, cross-contamination of equipment, and infection of the therapist. Recent reports suggest that a three-electrode setup produced more even current dispersion and deeper electrical current penetration than does the conventional two-electrode setup.[76] Suh et al used this electrode setup in conjunction with local heat therapy in a pilot study with 18 subjects with chronic wounds and produced 57% wound volume reduction after 4 weeks of treatment.[77] This application technique remains to be tested in a larger-scale, properly controlled clinical trial.

Several different stimulus parameters have been shown to be effective in accelerating wound closure. Stimulus intensity and frequency are adjusted so as to produce a strong tingling sensation, or in the case of desensate skin, the stimulus intensity is adjusted to a submotor level. Recommendations regarding the polarity that should be used for the active electrode,

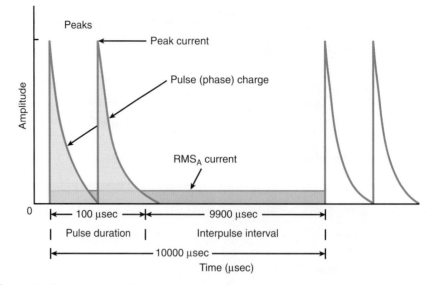

Figure 3–3. Waveform of high-voltage pulsed current (HVPC).

which is placed into the wound bed, vary greatly. A recent review by Kloth and McCulloch suggested that the polarity of the active electrode should be varied at different times during the wound healing process depending on the stage of wound repair and the type of cell you wish to attract into the wound area.[78]

Clinical Decision-Making   *Exercise 3–1*

A patient is reporting a tingling sensation under the larger dispersive electrode rather than the smaller active electrode located over the wound. What could possibly explain this?

Initially, low-intensity direct current (LIDC) was the electrical waveform utilized predominantly in several earlier studies, whereas pulsed currents have since been employed more recently due to greater comfort and less risk of causing tissue pH changes. HVPC is a common type of pulsed current employed in the treatment of chronic wounds. It is a specialized form of pulsed current that has a twin-peaked monophasic waveform composed of two pulses of very short duration and relatively high amplitude (Figure 3–3). The unidirectional flow of ions produced by this form of monophasic pulsed current produces a small net charge under the active electrode that is thought to be important in producing physiological responses such as edema reduction, circulatory changes, and bactericidal effects, and directing cell motility by galvanotaxis. In two studies performed by Baker et al,[79,80] three different ES waveforms were compared with control wounds (biphasic symmetrical, biphasic asymmetrical, and a third ES that was administered at a low level insufficient to produce sensation [MENS]). In both studies involving diabetic foot ulcers[80] and pressure ulcers[79] due to SCI, wounds treated with biphasic asymmetrical current produced significantly better results than controls, whereas the other forms of ES did not. Whether these waveforms produce different amounts of electrical charge in the underlying tissues has been debated; however, these results do suggest that the type of ES used can influence healing outcomes. While the optimal stimulus parameters and treatment schedules for the use of electrical stimulation on chronic wounds have not yet been agreed upon, it appears that beneficial results can be obtained regardless of stimulus parameters used, provided 300–500 µC/s of electrical charge is delivered.[81]

Treatment schedules reported in the literature vary from as little as 1-hour treatments given three times weekly for 4 weeks to as much as 8 hours daily.[82,83] Ahmad evaluated healing

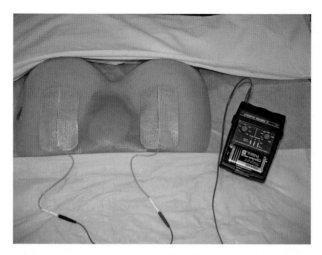

Figure 3–4. Application technique for electrical stimulation where two equally sized electrodes are placed on either side of the wound and connected to a stimulator that delivers asymmetrical biphasic current.

in response to ES applied for three different treatment times (45, 60, and 120 minutes).[84] Faster healing rates were reported when treatment times were increased from 45 to 60 minutes daily, but there was no further increase when treatment time was increased beyond 60 minutes daily.[84] Thus, there seems to be a threshold of exposure time after which continued ES treatment does not produce added benefit. Therefore, extended ES treatment times used by previous studies[82,83] may not be warranted.

It should be noted that to achieve optimal results with this modality, wound desiccation and the use of petrolatum-based products in the wound bed must be avoided. In addition, it may be best to optimize the wound environment by coordinating electrotherapy treatments with the timing of wound dressing changes.

Electrical currents are applied using asymmetrical biphasic waveforms applied through electrodes on the periulcer skin,[79,80] and distance acupuncture points[85] (refer to Figure 3–4). More recently, HVPC applied for extended periods of time using garments made of specialized conductive material has also been shown to accelerate healing of a variety of types of chronic wounds. Both of these indirect application techniques have an obvious practical advantage; however, the treatment protocols often require longer or more frequent application times (1.5–8 hours per day). Studies comparing healing times produced by direct and indirect application techniques of electrical current have not yet been performed.

Adverse effects associated with electrical stimulation of chronic wounds include only minor discomforts associated with tingling sensations that are produced. The risk of electrical shock is minimal, especially considering that most portable electrical stimulation devices are battery powered. Chemical burns induced by pulsed electrical current are very unlikely since tissue pH changes have been shown to be minimal during application of HVPC.[86]

CASE STUDY 3–1
ELECTRICAL STIMULATION: WOUND CARE

Background: A 57-year-old woman sustained a complete SCI at the T3 level in a motor vehicle accident 15 years ago. She has developed a stage III pressure ulcer over the right greater trochanter, and has been referred for wound care. The ulcer is circular, 8 cm in diameter, and 3 cm deep at the deepest point. There is a moderate amount of yellow and green exudate with a mild odor. The wound bed is yellow, the wound margins are intact, and there is no

(continued)

CASE STUDY 3–1   *(continued)*
ELECTRICAL STIMULATION: WOUND CARE

undermining detected. The patient notes that the wound is not painful.

Impression: Stage III pressure ulcer.

Treatment Plan: The source of the ulcer appears to be an improperly fitted wheelchair, resulting from a gradual weight gain over the past 10 years. Therefore, the initial treatment is to obtain a wheelchair of the correct width to relieve pressure on the ulcer. Wound care was initiated on a daily schedule, consisting of pulsed lavage to debride the necrotic tissue. Following each session, the wound was dressed with gauze, which was removed at the next session using the lavage (wet-to-wet dressings).

Response: After seven treatment sessions, there was no exudate and the wound bed was red. Pulsed lavage was then discontinued, and a hydrogel dressing was applied, with changes as needed. After 6 weeks, the wound size and appearance were unchanged. Therefore, treatment with pulsatile monophasic (high voltage) electrical stimulation was initiated on a 5-day per week schedule. Treatment parameters were negative polarity (cathode) for the treatment electrode, 100 pps (continuous mode), 200-V amplitude, and 60-minute duration. The treatment electrode was formed by packing the wound with sterile gauze moistened with sterile saline. The dispersive electrode (anode) was a moistened pad with a surface area of 75 cm² (three times the active electrode size) placed over the anterior thigh. The wound was dressed with sterile gauze following each treatment, with a hydrogel dressing used for weekend periods. After 20 sessions (4 weeks), the wound had decreased to 1.6 cm in diameter (an 80% reduction), and was 0.5 cm deep. Electrical stimulation was discontinued, and a foam sheet dressing

was used. The wound was completely closed 6 weeks later, and the patient was discharged.

Discussion Questions

- What tissues were injured/affected?
- What symptoms were present?
- What phase of the injury-healing continuum did the patient present for care in? What are the physical agent modality's biophysical effects (direct/indirect/depth/tissue affinity)?
- What are the physical agent modality's indications/contraindications?
- What are the parameters of the physical agent modality's application/dosage/duration/frequency in this case study?
- What other physical agent modalities could be utilized to treat this injury or condition? Why? How?
- Why was electrical stimulation not used from the beginning of the episode of care? Why was sharp debridement not used to remove the necrotic tissue?
- What is the role of nutrition in the treatment of this patient?
- What other wound care products (dressings) would have been appropriate?
- Why was the wheelchair issue addressed first in the care of this patient?

The rehabilitation professional employs physical agent modalities to create an optimum environment for tissue healing while minimizing the symptoms associated with the trauma or condition.

ULTRASOUND

A key mechanism of action of ultrasound is through cavitation or compression, and movement of tiny bubbles causes several changes to cellular and subcellular activities. The activity of cells known to be important in the inflammatory phase of healing has been induced by application of ultrasound waves to in vitro cell cultures. Stimulation of phagocytic activity of inflammatory cells such as macrophages and neutrophils has been reported.[87] This debridement action of ultrasound would be important in the initial stages of recovery from injury to clear the area of dead or devitalized material. Ultrasound has been shown to stimulate degranulation of inflammatory cells such as macrophages[88] and mast cells.[89] This results in the release of numerous chemical mediators that in turn have been shown to activate other key cells in the healing process such as fibroblasts.[90] Thus, the effects of ultrasound during inflammation appear to help to reactivate the healing process by stimulating the natural debridement process and by causing the release of the body's endogenous source of growth factors and other cytokines at the local site of injury. A recent hypothesis called the frequency resonance theory suggests that ultrasound can be absorbed by genetic material and cellular protein molecules, resulting in conformational changes that would in turn stimulate a broad range of cellular effects.[91]

Examination of the temporal pattern of changes in the histological composition of tissues obtained from animal models following injury and treated with ultrasound shows that these tissues are in the inflammatory phase of repair for a much shorter period of time following injury.[90] Some researchers have referred to the effects of ultrasound on this phase of repair as "anti-inflammatory."[92] Although it is probably more likely the "proinflammatory" effects of ultrasound that are responsible for stimulating progression through the inflammatory phase of healing, which would allow more rapid deposition of new tissue at the site of injury and faster completion of the repair process. Fyfe and Chahl (1985) reported that application of similar treatment regimen to edema produced experimentally in rat ankle joint caused an initial augmentation of swelling at 30 minutes posttreatment and this was followed by a greater reduction in swelling in ultrasound-treated ankles compared with control animals at 48 hours posttreatment.[93] This temporal pattern of changes to ankle joint swelling following ultrasound treatment is consistent with the theory that ultrasound initially stimulates the inflammatory phase of repair that in turn results in a more rapid resolution of the edema and progression to subsequent phases of tissue repair.

Ultrasound has been found to affect several processes within the fibroblast—a key cell responsible for controlling production and degradation of extracellular matrix postinjury. Cell culture studies have shown that ultrasound can stimulate fibroblasts to synthesize and secrete collagen.[94] Ultrasound can also stimulate fibroblasts to proliferate, resulting in a greater number of fibroblasts available to produce more collagen.[95] Further study of the mechanisms underlying ultrasound-induced fibroblastic activity has revealed that ultrasound can act directly to alter fibroblast function by producing calcium influx[96] and altering plasma membrane permeability.[97] Ultrasound treatment of experimentally placed skin lesions in animals has been shown in many studies to be associated with elevated levels of markers of collagen production such as procollagen mRNA expression, and hydroxyl–proline concentrations.[98] Studies examining the effects of ultrasound on healing tendons have revealed that collagen laid down under the direction of ultrasound is better organized and of greater tensile strength.[99-101] Producing scar tissue of greater breaking strength is an important functional advantage when referring to the healing of soft tissues such as ligaments and tendons. However, care needs to be taken when extrapolating to the clinical situation any results obtained using experimentally produced injuries of ligaments and tendons of animals.

While many sources describe changes in local circulation as one of the physical effects of ultrasound, an examination of research studies performed to assess changes in skeletal blood flow in response to ultrasound treatments has produced inconclusive results.[102] Some reports suggest that ultrasound induces vascular changes such as production of blood stasis,[103] hemolysis,[104] increased vascular permeability, transient vasoconstriction,[102] and production of oxygen free radicals.[105] All of these effects on blood vessels could interfere with local tissue perfusion. However, most of these potentially deleterious effects of ultrasound were associated with the application of quite high intensities of ultrasonic energy (2–3 W/cm^2).[103,104]

A recent review by Ennis et al described the effects of ultrasound on nitric oxide (NO) metabolism.[106] NO is a substrate involved in a multistep cellular reaction that is purported to respond to various forms of applied external energy, including the mechanical energy delivered by ultrasound. In conjunction with other growth factors, such as erythropoietin and vascular endothelial growth factor (VEGF), NO released by US treatment may be a potent stimulator of new blood vessel growth and development at the site of injury. These potent angiogenic effects of ultrasound have been recorded in diabetic mice and would result in greater oxygen perfusion of wounds in the longer term.[102]

In summary, ultrasound has been shown to alter scar tissue formation through its actions on cellular processes in all phases of tissue repair but during the inflammatory phase of repair in particular. Ultrasound promotes the release of chemical mediators from inflammatory cells that in turn attract and activate fibroblasts to the site of injury by directly stimulating collagen production during the proliferative stage of repair. Some research that is available suggests improved healing is more often associated with ultrasound treatments administered

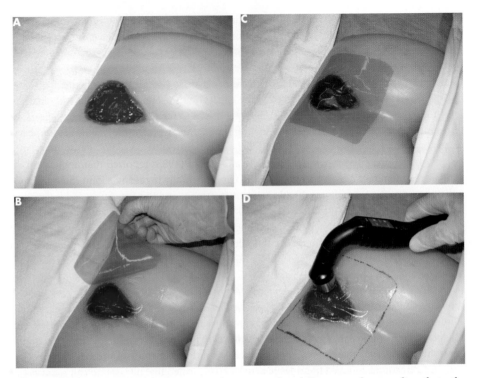

Figure 3–5. Ultrasound application technique used to deliver sound waves directly to the wound bed. (a) Wound bed is filled with sterile hydrogel; (b and c) covered with transparent hydrogel sheet dressing; (d) ultrasound gel is applied over dressing and the sound head is applied to the gel to deliver sound waves directly to the wound bed.

early in the healing process.[108] Jackson et al[99] demonstrated that ultrasound administered soon after tissue injury during the inflammatory phase of repair produced improved tendon breaking strength and that continued ultrasound treatments throughout the healing phase did not produce any further improvements in tensile strength of repaired tendons. Gan et al[100] demonstrated that improvements obtained when ultrasound was administered within 7 days of injury were not observed if the commencement of ultrasound treatments was delayed. Therefore, it is possible that the proinflammatory effect of ultrasound occurring early in the healing process that causes the body to produce its own mediators of tissue repair is the critical action of this modality and is sufficient to kick start scar tissue formation and optimize collagen production, organization, and ultimately functional strength.

Sound waves have been administered to chronic wounds using both direct and indirect application techniques. With either application method, the same ultrasound equipment used for other musculoskeletal disorders can be employed to treat chronic wounds. With the direct application technique, the wound bed is filled with sterile hydrogel and covered with a specialized dressing (Figure 3–5) that is used as a conducting medium to deliver mechanical energy produced by ultrasound directly to the base of the wound bed. Ultrasound can also produce beneficial effects by application of low levels of ultrasound (SATP = 1.0 W/cm^2; duty cycle = 20%; 3 MHz) to the periulcer skin for 5 min/5 cm^2 (Figure 3–6). This indirect application method of pulsed ultrasound to the periulcer skin has tremendous practical advantages since it prevents the risk of wound contamination, and the tissue dehydration and cooling that can occur when wound dressings are removed. Applying ultrasound to the periulcer skin employs similar equipment and application techniques as are used by therapists to treat other musculoskeletal disorders. Therefore, minimal specialized training is required to use therapeutic ultrasound in wound care. Franek et al compared the effects of low-intensity (0.5 W/cm^2) and high-intensity (1.0 W/cm^2) pulsed ultrasound administered through a water bath and found that the low dose of ultrasound produced a significant reduction in wound surface area and improvement in wound appearance compared with control-treated wounds.[109] Accelerated

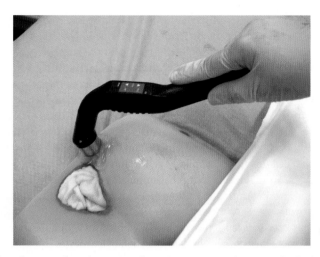

Figure 3–6. Ultrasound application technique using an indirect method where ultrasound is applied through gel to the periulcer skin. Wound packing is left in the wound during treatment to keep unwanted gel from the wound bed.

wound closure has also been achieved by delivering low-frequency sound waves (30 kHz) from a large stationary sound head immersed in a water bath.[110,111] Ultrasound MIST therapy (MIST, Celleration, Eden Prairire, MN) is a relatively new modality available to accelerate healing.[112] It is a low-frequency noncontact ultrasound therapy that uses acoustic pressure transmitted by ultrasound to stimulate cells[113] and remove bacteria.[114] This therapy system received Food and Drug Administration 510K clearance in June 2005 to "promote wound healing through wound cleansing and maintenance debridement by removal of yellow slough, fibrin tissue exudates, and bacteria."[112]

Although high doses of ultrasound have the potential to cause tissue cavitation, use of relatively low doses of ultrasound in wound treatment protocols has not yielded any reports of ultrasound-induced adverse effects. The risks of burns produced by this modality are minimal since it is used in a pulsed or interrupted mode that minimizes the accumulation of heat within the tissue.

LASER
Effects of Laser on Tissue Repair

There are several in vitro studies performed using cultures of various types of cells known to be important in facilitating the healing process including macrophages,[115] neutrophils, mast cells,[116] and lymphocytes,[117] as well as fibroblasts,[118-120] endothelial cells,[115] and epithelial cells.[121]

Biological processes observed to be altered by administration of laser to cell cultures include protein synthesis,[120] cell growth and differentiation,[119] cell proliferation,[117] cell motility,[118] phagocytosis,[122] and cell degranulation.[115,121] Intracellular mechanisms of action to produce these cellular changes have also been investigated and proposed. They include activation of DNA synthesis to facilitate cell proliferation,[117,120] increase in transcription and translation of mRNA to make available important protein precursors,[121] and change in membrane permeability to stimulate physiological changes such as nerve depolarization and stimulation of the influx of extracellular stores of calcium.[125] Calcium influx is, in turn, known to be an important intracellular signal for numerous cell processes including cell movement and phagocytosis, secretion of cytoplasmic granules containing potent chemical mediators, alteration in receptor binding affinity to facilitate intercellular communication, and activation of mitochondrial production of ATP via oxidative metabolism to make available energy to fuel increased needs of the photoactivated cell.

These direct actions of laser observed in these in vitro studies are believed to underlie several cell processes known to be important during the inflammatory phase of tissue repair.[123] Several reports have documented the ability of laser to stimulate cell degranulation causing the release of potent inflammatory mediators such as prostaglandins, growth factors,[124] and histamine[125] from various different types of leukocytes involved in the inflammatory phase of tissue repair. Laser irradiation of rat skin stimulated mast cell accumulation at the site of irradiation, and a greater percentage of those mast cells present was found to be degranulated in previously traumatized skin.[125] Laser applied to macrophages in culture stimulates the release of chemical mediators into the cell culture supernatant that in turn was shown to be capable of activating fibroblast cell function.[115] Similarly, cell cultures of T lymphocytes exposed to laser were found to release an angiogenic factor that stimulated endothelial cell proliferation.[126]

Other effects of laser on white blood cells include the ability of laser to activate the phagocytic abilities, stimulate leukocyte proliferation, and promote migration of white blood cells toward the site of injury.[122] This laser-induced activation of many processes within the inflammatory phase of repair would promote the natural debridement action of leukocytes and help to clean foreign or dead and devitalized tissues within the injury site. Some reports suggest that laser effects are anti-inflammatory. Laser was found to produce a small but significant decrease in experimentally induced inflammation and edema produced by the inflammatory irritant carrageenan.[127]

Laser treatment of animals with injured tissues has resulted in increased collagen deposition,[128] and this augmentation of collagen production was associated with a concomitant improvement in the tensile strength of surgically incised skin[129,130] and tendons.[131] There also exist several other studies that have reported no benefit of laser on wound healing and breaking strength.[132–135] These negative findings tend to occur more commonly in studies where laser treatment regimens result in the administration of relatively low amounts of light energy to the wound bed (less than 1 J/cm^2)[136,137] or where the sham control group to which the effects of laser treatments are compared has been located within the same animal.[120,132,138]

Some reports suggest that laser can alter growth and replication of bacteria commonly found in chronic wounds.[139] However, recent reports have shown that the effects of laser applied to cultures of bacteria are dependent on the amount of laser energy delivered and wavelength of the light source with certain treatment protocols actually causing a stimulation of bacterial growth.[140] This research was continued with studies on excisional wound placed in rat that was inoculated with various types of bacteria.[141] They reported certain wavelengths and energy levels of laser were associated with lower bacterial counts; however, these bactericidal effects were necessarily associated with a significant delay in wound closure. Until factors that control the response of bacteria to laser are more completely understood, the use of laser on wounds contaminated with bacteria should be done cautiously.

Monochromatic infrared energy (MIRE) has been proposed to be preferentially absorbed by hemoglobin present in erythrocyte and release NO that in turn stimulates healing by increased microcirculation.[142] The effects of MIRE were recently examined on tissue oxygenation in people with diabetic neuropathy.[143] These researchers were unable to detect a difference in transcutaneous oxygen values between active and placebo MIRE-treated groups.[143] Furthermore, they did not detect a significant difference in pain perception between groups.[143]

Although there are numerous research studies that suggest laser therapy can have profound physiological effects on tissue healing, there are a number of factors that can impact the tissue response to laser irradiation. Some stimulus parameters believed to influence the effects of laser therapy include laser wavelength, energy density, power density, pulse frequency, and treatment schedule. In addition to the laser parameters provided by the equipment, the biological response to laser is also affected by changes within the host tissue such as tissue type and hydration, skin pigmentation, local blood flow, and basal level of tissue activity. More research is required to fully appreciate the influence that these and other factors have on the ability of laser therapy to produce the desired response.

A similar laser application technique used for the treatment of other musculoskeletal disorders has been described for the treatment of chronic wounds. Laser sources are often applied in contact to points equally distributed around the periulcer skin (Figure 3–7). A transparent film barrier is often employed in conjunction with a contact point application

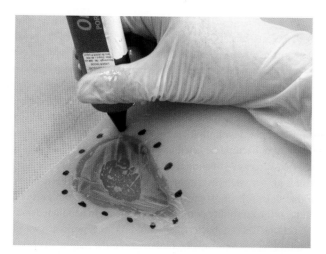

Figure 3–7. Laser application technique where laser tip is applied perpendicularly in contact with periulcer skin covered with transparent film. This procedure is carried for a specified period of time depending on the desired light energy delivered to the wound and is repeated to points evenly distributed around the wound.

technique in order to prevent cross-contamination of the laser equipment. As with all light therapies, it is important to keep the angle and distance from the light source consistent when applying laser treatments. A noncontact, sweeping technique can also be used to deliver laser energy to the wound base; however, this would result in significantly less light energy delivered to the wound tissue and therefore laser treatment doses used with this noncontact application technique need to be increased accordingly. A multitude of different laser sources, wavelengths of light, dosimetry, treatment techniques, and treatment schedules have been reported in the literature. As a result, recommendations for treatment parameters to be used with laser treatments of chronic wounds cannot be provided at this time.

While scarcity of good clinical research evidence to support the use of laser in the treatment of chronic wounds is a disadvantage, an advantage of using this modality is the relatively minor safety precautions and risk. Saltmarche reported that low-level laser therapy was well accepted by untrained staff of an extended care facility.[144] Treatment of both acute and chronic wounds in this case series resulted in complete closing of 42.8% wounds, and no negative responses were recorded in this elderly frail population.[144] There are few medical conditions for which laser therapy is contraindicated for use. Nausea and dizziness have been reported to occur in 2% of patients following laser treatments.[145] Light therapies used in wound care do not produce tissue temperature elevation; therefore, the risk of causing skin burns is minimal. However, exposure to eyes can cause severe retinal damage and therefore both the therapist and patient must wear appropriate eye protection during treatment.

Regardless of the treatment protocol slated to treat with laser therapy, careful documentation of treatment setup and parameters is critical. This documentation will help provide consistent delivery of laser energy and limit the number of variable that may be inadvertently changed during laser treatments. In this way, the clinician can systematically change laser treatment parameters while monitoring improvement in wound status in order to optimize a protocol for the patient who has a particular set of host factors.

ULTRAVIOLET LIGHT

The type of ultraviolet light is important in determining the tissue response. Light of shorter wavelength (180–250 nm) named ultraviolet light C (UVC) is the type of ultraviolet light most commonly used in the treatment of chronic wounds. Effects of ultraviolet light that would be beneficial to the wound healing cascade include stimulation of epithelial migration and proliferation, release of chemical mediators that in turn produce stimulate local cutaneous blood flow or erythema,[146,147] and bactericidal effects.[148] Bactericidal effects are greatest for shorter wavelengths of light (UVC) due to direct effects of UVC on nuclear material of the bacterium.[148] UVC exposure inhibits growth of in vitro cultures of bacteria commonly found to colonize chronic wounds.[149] Furthermore, a dose-dependent inhibition of UVC treatment on bacteria colonization of chronic pressure ulcers has been reported previously.[150] Recently, UVC has been shown to inhibit the in vitro growth of antibiotic-resistant bacteria (MRSA and vancomycin-resistant *Enterococcus faecalis* [VRE]).[150] Thai et al have demonstrated that a single exposure of UVC applied to superficial chronic wounds colonized with multiple bacteria including MRSA resulted in a significant reduction in the amount of bacteria detected using semiquantitative swabs.[151] In addition, it has been demonstrated that successive treatments of UVC lasting 180 seconds each could eliminate MRSA detected using surface swabs in chronic infected wounds.[152] This result is extremely exciting given the fact that one of the most pressing problems today in both acute care hospital and extended care settings is the morbidity or mortality occurring in debilitated patients as a result of MRSA and VRE infections. This antibacterial effect of UVC that peaks at a wavelength of 254 nm is believed to speed healing via removal of a bioburden to the natural debridement system and thereby allowing more rapid progress through the inflammatory phase of wound healing.

Clinical Decision-Making *Exercise 3–2*

Your patient has a wound that is colonized with MRSA and you wish to apply UVC to help reduce bacteria in wound. How do you need to adjust the UVC treatment time to compensate for his or her darkly pigmented skin?

Small, portable, relatively cost-effective lamps that deliver ultraviolet light at specific wavelengths are available commercially (254 nm). By using filter-specific wavelength of UVC, potentially carcinogenic effects of UVA and UVB wavelengths can be reduced and the risks of skin burns can be virtually eliminated. Since even thin transparent dressings have been shown to block the transmission of shorter wavelengths of light such as UVC, wound dressings must be removed and the wound must be properly cleansed prior to the UVC treatment. The amount of light energy delivered is known to be dependent on the duration of the treatment, the distance, and angle of the light source.

Application methods for UVC in wounds are simplified by maintaining the UVC lamp at a consistent angle (perpendicular to the body surface) and distance (approximately 2.5 cm or 1 in) from the wound (refer to Figure 3–8). In this way, the desired response can be obtained

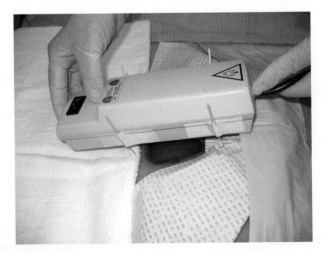

Figure 3–8. Ultraviolet light C (UVC) application technique. A small portable lamp that delivers only light at a wavelength of 254 nm is held in a perpendicular angle 1 in from the wound edge for 180 seconds in duration.

by altering only the treatment time. In vitro studies have shown that bacteria kill rates of 100% can be obtained after 90-second exposure to UVC.[150] Clinical case studies suggest that repeated treatments of longer durations (180 seconds) are required to reduce bacteria counts from chronic wounds.[151,152] This same exposure time can be used daily throughout the treatment period until the clinical signs of wound infection are no longer observed. Cotton drapes and/or a thick petroleum jelly covering are often used on the periulcer skin to ensure that UVC is only delivered to the infected wound bed and the periulcer skin is protected (Figure 3–9). This noncontact application technique is often preferred since chronic infected ulcers are often very painful and cross-contamination of equipment can be minimized. Judicious use of universal precautions and equipment decontamination procedures are critical when using this modality to treat infected wounds.

Some treatment protocols recommend that the ultraviolet light should also be applied to the unprotected periulcer skin. However, there is limited evidence to suggest that treatment of the periulcer skin with a minimal erythemic dose can stimulate local blood flow and enhance epithelial growth from the wound edge. If this method of application is chosen, a standardized skin test must be performed on each individual prior to the onset of ultraviolet light treatment to determine that individual's response to light. Since factors that affect an individual's response to light (skin melanin and epidermal thickness) are located in the outer epidermal layer of the skin, a similar skin test might not be required when treating only the base of an open chronic infected ulcer using the setup shown in Figure 3–8.

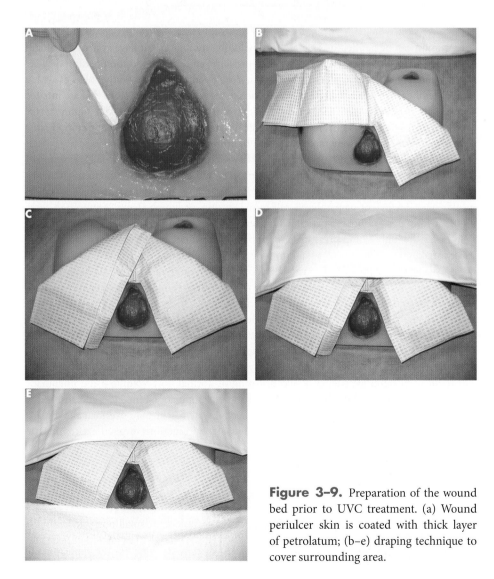

Figure 3–9. Preparation of the wound bed prior to UVC treatment. (a) Wound periulcer skin is coated with thick layer of petrolatum; (b–e) draping technique to cover surrounding area.

Concerns regarding the carcinogenic effects of ultraviolet rays present in sunlight have deterred many from using UVC to treat chronic infected wounds. It should be noted that carcinogenic effects of ultraviolet light are dependent on the wavelength, depth of penetration of the light, and duration of light exposure, and are related to the occurrence of sunburns.[153] UVC is known to have potent effects on the DNA material; however, it is believed to have minimal ability to induce skin cancer since it evokes only minimal erythemic response and penetrates through only the superficial layers of tissue that are often soon to be sloughed off. An extensive literature search has not revealed a single research report that links treatments using this form of ultraviolet light (UVC) with an increased incidence of skin cancer. However, given that the incidence of skin cancer development is related to the duration of light exposure, prolonged treatment times should be avoided and UVC treatments should be discontinued when surface contamination in the wound is removed. Although the risks of tumorigenesis and skin burns are minimal, even short exposure of the eye with UVC can cause severe retinal damage. Therefore, both therapist and patient must wear appropriate eye protection during UVC treatments.

PNEUMATIC COMPRESSION THERAPY

Administration of external pressure using compression therapy to reduce tissue edema is considered essential standard therapy for the treatment of chronic leg wounds due to venous insufficiency.[154,155] Compression therapy is believed to aid wound healing through reducing venous congestion, which may be mediated by promoting systemic fibrinolytic activity. External compression can be applied in several ways including multilayer bandage systems, standard or custom-fitted stockings with gradations of pressure, and pneumatic compression devices. Several different pneumatic devices have been developed that employ either sleeves with a single chamber that is inflated intermittently or sleeves with several divisions that are inflated sequentially from a distal to proximal direction. The application of relatively high external pressures to an edematous extremity using intermittent or sequential pneumatic compression devices can produce relatively rapid reduction in limb girth (within hours).[156]

Pneumatic compression therapy is indicated for chronic wounds that are likely caused by excessive edema such as chronic venous ulcers. It should be used in conjunction with compression stockings or bandages to help remove residual edema in patients with chronic venous insufficiency, inefficient or paralyzed calf muscle pump, or lymphedema. Application techniques involve positioning the patient with edematous limb elevated and applying a neoprene sleeve over the limb. Pump pressures are set based on patient comfort and generally do not exceed maximum pressures of 40–60 mm Hg. Most commercial units have a preset on: off cycle, usually around 90 seconds on and 30 seconds off. Treatment times needed to produce a clinically significant reduction in limb volume will vary depending on the extent and duration of the edema and may last for a period of 1–4 hours.

When applying pneumatic compression devices, the therapist must determine the source of limb edema. There are many medical conditions that can manifest as lower limb edema for which compression therapy can be harmful. For example, patients with congestive heart failure will have a backup of fluid in the venous system and if the venous congestion is sufficient will result in bilateral leg edema. Rapid restoring of normal limb volume using pneumatic compression would not be advisable with this patient population since it could result in a relatively rapid return of fluid to the cardiovascular system that may overload the already compromised heart. Other contraindications and safety precautions of pneumatic compression are listed in a previous chapter.

REVIEW OF CLINICAL RESEARCH EVIDENCE

In addition to the knowledge about biological effects of each modality, awareness about the clinical research evidence that supports the use of the modality is essential. Clinical research evidence should be obtained from clinical trials that directly test whether the application of the particular modality is effective in persons with chronic wounds of known etiology. Proper design of clinical trials is critical if we are to know if adding treatments with a modality is going to speed healing of chronic wounds. The clinical studies must assess objectively whether improvements in valid outcome measures of wound healing are greater than those observed in an appropriate control group that received placebo treatments and/or similar concurrent standard wound therapies.

Many clinical reports exist in the recent literature that consistently demonstrate the ability of electrical current to accelerate wound closure rate of chronic pressure ulcers. At least 20 of these clinical trials that evaluated the effect of electrical current are properly designed randomized controlled studies that involve over 1000 subjects with chronic wounds.[79,80,82–84,157–170] Chronic pressure ulcers were most commonly studied type of chronic wound, and seven of the reports specifically demonstrated that electrical current could accelerate closure of pressure ulcers occurring in people with SCI.[79,82,161,165,166,169] Electrical currents have also been shown to speed healing of foot ulcers in people with diabetic neuropathy[80,83,162] and in people with chronic venous leg ulcers.[164,168,170] In 1999, Gardner et al performed a meta-analysis in which the results from several clinical reports were combined and concluded there was a positive benefit of electrical stimulation on chronic wounds of mixed etiology.[170] More recently, Houghton and Woodbury completed a meta-analysis in 2007 and concluded that chronic wounds treated with electrical current were almost four times more likely to heal compared with control wounds receiving either standard wound care (SWC) or SWC plus placebo electrical current.[171] Currently, a protocol that is examining the effect of electrical current on healing rate and number of wounds closed is being completed for the Cochrane Wounds Group.[173] It was based on the strong clinical and experimental research evidence that several recently published clinical practice guidelines have recommended electrical stimulation for use on delayed or nonhealing wounds.[174,175] Research supporting the effectiveness of all wound therapies was recently reviewed by a large international panel of wound care experts in the production of the combined EPUAP/NPUAP guidelines for the treatment of pressure ulcers.[21] Within this international guideline ES was the only adjunctive wound therapy assigned the highest level of evidence (level = A), and the recommended practice in the guidelines was "to consider the application of direct contact ES in the management of recalcitrant stage II to IV pressure ulcers to stimulate wound healing."[21]

At least 12 controlled clinical studies have assessed the effectiveness of ultrasound in the treatment of chronic pressure ulcers,[176–178] and venous leg ulcers.[110,111,176–184] These clinical studies have produced results that suggest ultrasound treatments can accelerate closure of chronic pressure ulcers and venous leg ulcers. However, some well-designed clinical trials have failed to detect a significant benefit of ultrasound over healing rates observed in similar control subjects.[182,184] These positive and negative findings have been pooled in two separate meta-analyses and both reported subjects treated with ultrasound increased healing compared with appropriate control subjects.[185,186] The *Cochrane* review concluded that these results need interpreting with caution[186] and that clinical trials examining healing effects of therapeutic ultrasound on pressure ulcers provided no added benefits.[187]

A large multicenter, randomized, double-blind clinical trial found a statistically significant difference in the proportion of diabetic foot wounds that closed in the active compared with sham-treated MIST group.[188] Subsequently, a retrospective analysis[189] and a prospective noncontrolled study[190] suggested that other types of chronic wounds (pressure, diabetic, ischemic, venous, inflammatory) may also benefit from this innovative treatment. Use of this modality on burns demonstrated how this therapy may be used effectively to debride very painful burn wounds.[191]

At least five well-controlled clinical trials involving over 200 subjects have tested the effect of either sequential or pneumatic compression on healing of chronic venous ulcers.[38,192–195] These reports have produced inconsistent findings. A recent narrative review by O'Sullivan and Houghton[196] summarized the effects of PCT on lower leg ulcers and suggested that PCT may be a valuable adjunct to aid in the treatment of individuals with cardiosynchronous PCT and may be beneficial for leg ulcers due to arterial insufficiency. It should be considered for those people who are not compliant with compression bandaging or those at risk of limb amputation.[196] Other clinical benefits of PCT include an increase in transcutaneous oxygen tension, improved arterial flow, and reduced edema.[195] Improved healing rates of chronic venous ulcers have been documented following treatments with pneumatic compression pumps with both sequential and intermittent inflating chambers. There can be few or several chambers located in sequential compression pumps. While it is probable that machines with a greater number of chambers are more comfortable, it is not known whether increasing the number of chambers is associated with improved outcomes of chronic venous ulcers.

Controlled clinical trials have been published to document the benefits of treating infected pressure ulcers with UVC.[197-199] A dose-dependent inhibition of UVC treatment on bacteria colonizing chronic pressure ulcers has been reported previously.[199] UVC treatment of chronic superficial wounds of mixed etiology has also been shown to produce significant reduction in several bacteria including MRSA. Accelerated wound closure has also been demonstrated in two small randomized controlled clinical trials of UVC treatment of chronic infected wounds[198] and UVC combined with ultrasound treatment of chronic pressure ulcers.[197] These promising clinical results together with experimental research that suggests an inhibitory action of UVC on antibiotic-resistant strains of bacteria will hopefully promote further research needed to determine if this modality can promote healing of chronic wounds infected with troublesome bacteria such as MRSA and/or VRE.

Hydrotherapy is commonly used by physical therapists to aid healing of chronic wounds. This practice is supported by a recent controlled clinical trial that demonstrated that whirlpool therapy plus conservative wound care produced a faster rate of healing compared with control subjects who were not treated with whirlpool. A recent systematic review and analysis that examined various forms of wound cleansing concluded that whirlpool therapy was effective in reducing inflammation and pain in surgical wounds.[200] Clinical reports exist to suggest that hydrotherapy can reduce bacterial contamination of chronic ulcers.[17,18] However, these cleansing properties of hydrotherapy were not associated with a reduced incidence of wound infection. There is one report that demonstrates pulsed lavage can promote greater granulation tissue formation better than other forms of hydrotherapy.[19] The ability of either nonimmersion hydrotherapy or whirlpool treatments to promote healing of chronic wounds has not been shown in properly designed controlled clinical trials.

Clinical Decision-Making *Exercise 3–3*

A patient is being seen in an outpatient clinic three times weekly to have high compression bandages reapplied. Which modality would you recommend to treat a chronic venous leg ulcer that is relatively shallow and covered in 100% adherent slough?

The application of superficial heat using specialized dressings has been shown to maintain wound temperatures and prevent wound cooling. There are at least four clinical reports,[201-205] and two randomized controlled clinical trials.[206,207] Alvarez and colleagues demonstrated that diabetic foot ulcers treated with noncontact normothermic wound therapy for 12 weeks had a greater mean percent wound closure and a higher proportion of subjects with complete ulcer healing compared with control-treated ulcers.[39] Kloth et al also found a significantly greater healing rate for pressure ulcers receiving this warming therapy.[206] Similar promising findings have been reported in recent noncontrolled clinical trials.[204,205]

Although there are numerous case reports that laser therapy can accelerate healing of several types of skin wounds,[207-210] the benefits of laser on chronic wounds have not been confirmed using properly designed randomized controlled clinical trials. There have been at least nine controlled clinical trials involving over 300 subjects published to date that have examined the healing potential of laser therapy.[211-219] Only two of these controlled trials reported a statistically significant improvement in wound size or wound closure rates with laser treatment.[212,217] Both of these studies involved very low subject numbers and had very poor methodological quality.[212,217] Some suggest that these negative findings are due to uncontrolled factors that affect the biological response to laser[208] and that laser was not administered at a sufficiently high dose to stimulate healing processes.[217] While differences in the laser treatment protocols might explain inconsistent findings, there appears to be mounting evidence that laser therapy provides no added benefit toward healing chronic wounds.

CHOOSING THE BEST MODALITY FOR THE TREATMENT OF DELAYED OR NONHEALING WOUNDS

When deciding whether a modality should be used on a particular individual with delayed healing, the clinician should complete a thorough assessment of the patient to determine the underlying cause of wound. In particular, it is important to review the current wound management program to determine whether the current wound management program has addressed the underlying etiology (malnutrition, excessive pressure, persistent edema). The importance of appropriate "wound bed preparation" where the wound environment has been optimized such as appropriate moisture control with dressings, management of bacterial burden, and unwanted necrotic or foreign material has been debrided. These basic needs of the wound should be taken care of before applying adjunctive wound therapy. Treating wounds without sufficient wound bed preparation or those whose etiology has not been determined and causative factors have not been addressed will limit the effectiveness of these potential modalities.

After assuring that the patient has a chronic wound with a known etiology that is being appropriately addressed in the current wound program and that he or she does not possess any of the medical conditions that would contraindicate the use of any of the therapeutic modalities, the clinician needs to begin the process of deciding on the most appropriate electrotherapeutic modality.

Various therapies accelerate the healing process through different primary mechanisms. Electrical current has been associated with cellular actions that would benefit virtually all phases of repair. In addition, recent evidence is building to suggest that electrical current would also indirectly promote healing by reducing bacteria and promoting circulation to and from the wound area. The experimental and clinical evidence suggests that this modality can be used in all phases of repair and all common types of chronic wounds (pressure, venous, ischemic, and diabetic).

Ultrasound has been shown to stimulate healing by promoting inflammatory processes leading to improved wound debridement and more rapid progression into latter phases of wound repair. Recalcitrant wounds with signs of chronic inflammation and pronounced slough and/or fibrin may be best treated with this therapy. This is a common scenario in venous leg ulcers and the clinical research evidence supports that therapeutic ultrasound is of benefit for healing this type of wound. Lower leg ulcers can often be confused between the common venous ulcer and other rare forms of inflammatory ulcers. Clinicians should take care to ensure that they are aware of the underlying etiology since the proinflammatory effects of ultrasound would surely exacerbate the clinical manifestation of inflammatory ulcers. The practical advantages of using standard techniques and equipment to apply ultrasound to the periulcer skin may also cause some clinicians to choose to use this modality. The relatively comfortable and gentle application procedure associated with noncontact MIST therapy may be the rationale used to choose this form of low-frequency ultrasound to promote wound debridement.

UVC is indicated in the treatment of infected or heavily colonized wounds since it has been shown to have an antibacterial effect on several types of bacteria including MRSA and VRE. It has not been well established that UVC can promote healing processes in wounds where bacterial bioburden is not an issue. Therefore, continued exposure of tissues to UVC light after wound infection has resolved is not advised.

Hydrotherapy will cleanse the wound of surface contaminants and help remove loose necrotic tissue. It will also soften eschar so as to facilitate subsequent debridement techniques. This form of mechanical debridement is nonselective and therefore care must be taken to ensure viable tissue is not damaged with excessive pressures. Continued application of whirlpool after wounds are free of necrotic tissue is not warranted and may result in inadvertent contamination of wounds with water-borne bacteria. Several reports suggest local application of electrical currents will induce vasodilation and improve tissue oxygenation. Studies where electrical current was applied around ischemic wounds showed $TcPO_2$ levels were elevated significantly for up to[30] minutes after treatment. Thus, electrical currents may be beneficial for ischemic wounds that cannot be surgically repaired and are not well managed by any other adjunctive therapy. Angiogenesis promoted by electrical currents and ultrasound therapies may also improve wounds delayed in healing because of poor perfusion.

Pneumatic compression therapy is a modality that can be used in conjunction with compression bandages or stockings for the treatment of chronic venous ulcers. Venous insufficiency associated with these types of chronic wounds invariably results in dependent edema around the feet and ankles. PCT can rapidly reduce lower limb edema, and preliminary findings in small clinical trials suggest this may result in an improved healing rate of venous ulcers.

In all cases when using therapeutic modalities to accelerate the healing of chronic wounds, changes in wound status should be monitored at least weekly using valid and reliable outcome measures. Lack of progression of chronic wounds may also be a missed causative agent and therefore another assessment of patient to review underlying causes and current wound care therapists is warranted. If wound improvements are not detected after a few weeks of treatment with chosen modality, then alteration in stimulus parameters should be initiated. If this continues, then another treatment modality should be offered to the client.

Contraindications

Although there are potential harmful effects associated with the use of each of these therapeutic modalities, these risks are considered minimal provided they are administered by a health care professional who has received sufficient training. However, certain medical conditions do increase the likelihood of producing adverse reactions and therefore prevent or contraindicate the use of some or all of the therapeutic modalities. Commonly cited contraindications for each modality are presented in Table 3–1. It should be pointed out that there is not always

Table 3–1   Conditions that should not be Treated with the Modality (Contraindication) or should be Treated with Caution (Precaution)

CONDITIONS	US	ESTIM	UVC	LLLT	HEAT	HYDROTHERAPY	PEMF	IPC
Pregnancy	C-local	C-local APL	S	C-local	P	P	C	P
Impaired circulation	P	P	S	S	C-local	P	P	C
Impaired sensation	P	P	S	S	C-local	P	S	P
Impaired cognition or communication	P	P	P	P	C	P	P	C
Malignancy History of skin cancer	C-local P	C-local P	C C	C-local P	C-local P	C-local P	C-local P	C P
Wound infection	P	C-local	S	P	C-local	C	P	C
Inflammatory conditions and ulcers (e.g., PG, vasculitis)	C	C	C	P	C	P	C	P
Recently radiated tissue	C-local	C-local	C-local	P	C-local	P	C-local	P
Hemorrhagic conditions	C	C	P	C	C	C	C	C
Active deep vein thrombosis or thrombophlebitis	C-local	C	P	C-local	C	C	C	C

CONDITIONS	US	ESTIM	UVC	LLLT	HEAT	HYDROTHERAPY	PEMF	IPC
Dermatological conditions (e.g., eczema, psoriasis)	P	C-local	C	S	C	P	P	P
Active epiphysis	P	P	S	S	S	S	P	S
Photosensitivity	S	S	C	P	S	S	S	S
Cardiac failure	S	C-local	P	S	P	C	S	C
Hypertension	S	S	P	S	S	C	S	C
Systemic lupus erythematosis/HIV	S	S	C	P	S	P	S	S
Implants/grafts								
Fresh skin grafts	P	P	C	P	P	C	P	C-local
Electronic device	C-local	C-local	S	S	S	S	C	S
Metal implant	S	S	S	S	S	S	S	S
Plastic, cement implant	P	S	S	S	S	S	S	S
Local areas								
Eyes	C	C	C	C	P	Na	P	Na
Reproductive organs	C	C	S	C	C	P	S	Na
Chest, heart	S	P	S	S	S	P	C	Na
Anterior neck, carotid sinus	C	C	S	P	P	P	C	Na
Regenerating nerves	P	P	S	S	S	P	P	Na
Head	S	C	S	S	S	P	S	Na

C = contraindication when modality is applied anywhere on the body
C-local = contraindicated when applied directly over the site
P = precaution—modality can be applied with extra caution (lower intensity or careful monitoring)
S = safe; modality can be used by qualified personnel with normal risks ever present
Na = not applicable—there is no clinical indication to use the modality in this location or condition

US: pulsed mode ultrasound; has duty cycle less than 50% and usually does not produce net accumulation of heat in the tissues.
Estim: electrical stimulation used to stimulate healing of chronic wounds; it is applied in the area of affected tissues at a subsensory or sensory level of stimulation.
LLLT = low-level laser therapy, includes all class II and III lasers and noncoherent light sources.
Heat = includes noncontact normothermic devices, and other superficial, conductive, heating agents that add heat to superficial tissues (within 3 cm of the skin surface).
PEMFs = electromagnetic fields applied using noncontact coil electrodes at an intensity that produces neither muscle contraction nor tissue heating.
Hydrotherapy: application of water via immersion tanks or local irrigation devices at a neutral temperature and using pressures that do not

agreement on which medical conditions should be included in the list of contraindications for a particular modality. A recent review of the research regarding contraindications for various modalities was compiled.[220] These extensive reports included a consensus process among several experts in the field who are involved in instructing electrophysical agents to physical therapy students across Canada.

SUMMARY

1. Before applying therapeutic modality to individuals with chronic wounds, review the wound management program and ensure that the wound environment is optimized and the primary etiology of the wound has been sufficiently addressed.

2. The list of contraindications for various modalities varies greatly across resources. Consult the literature provided with specific equipment in use.

3. Before selecting a modality to accelerate a chronic wound, the clinician should understand the primary action of the modality on the healing process.

4. Hydrotherapy is indicated to help cleanse necrotic tissue and surface contaminants from chronic wounds and should be discontinued when the wound is clean.

5. Administration of pulsed ultrasound during the inflammatory phase of repair can accelerate natural debridement and release chemical mediators that can stimulate subsequent steps involved in tissue repair.

6. Comparatively, electrical stimulation therapy presently has the greatest number of well-designed randomized controlled clinical trials documenting its ability to accelerate healing and promote closure of chronic wounds.

7. Many best practice recommendations and guidelines produced in North America suggest that electrotherapy should be considered to treat individuals with chronic pressure ulcers.

8. Pneumatic compression therapy combined with stockings and bandages can reduce chronic edema associated with chronic venous ulcers.

9. UVC can kill bacteria and may be helpful in the treatment of wounds contaminated with bacteria that are resistant to other antimicrobial therapy.

REVIEW QUESTIONS

Select answers for questions 1–6 from the choice of modalities listed as follows:

    A. pneumatic compression therapy
    B. UVC therapy
    C. laser therapy
    D. electrical stimulation therapy
    E. pulsed ultrasound
    F. hydrotherapy

1. What modalities require direct application of the emitted energy to the wound bed and therefore require prior removal of all wound dressings?

2. What modalities need to be applied perpendicular to the tissue surface in order to optimize energy delivery to the target structure?

3. What modalities could be used on patients with wounds in which the wound and surrounding skin are very painful to touch?

4. What modalities would be best to treat
    a. chronic wounds that are delayed in healing because of an excessive bacterial load?
    b. wounds filled with necrotic tissue?
    c. deep wounds requiring new tissue formation to fill in wound defect?
    d. diabetic foot wounds in individuals with concurrent mild peripheral vascular disease?

5. What modalities act on the wound healing process to
    a. activate the inflammatory process?
    b. improve local blood flow?
    c. stimulate new tissue formation?
    d. improve wound strength?
    e. reduce tissue edema?

6. For what modality is the best clinical research evidence available to support its use on
    a. chronic pressure ulcers?
    b. chronic venous ulcers?

7. Describe a clinical scenario in which a patient would most likely benefit from the use of therapeutic modalities to accelerate wound closure.

8. What factors can alter the biological response to laser therapy and should be monitored, controlled, and documented with each treatment?

SELF-TEST QUESTIONS

True or False

1. Stimulation of endothelial cell function and angiogenesis will promote healing by improving tissue oxygen perfusion.
2. Rinsing the limb after hydrotherapy tank use will help to reduce bacterial colonization on the surface of wounds.

Multiple Choice

3. Which of the following modalities have been shown to be most likely to kill bacteria when applied to in vitro cultures of bacteria that are commonly found in chronic wounds?
   a. pneumatic compression
   b. laser
   c. noncontact, nonthermal ultrasound (MIST)
   d. hydrotherapy
   e. UVC
4. Which of the following modalities help to heal wounds by removing foreign or devitalized tissues (debridement)?
   a. electrical stimulation
   b. laser
   c. noncontact, nonthermal ultrasound (MIST)
   d. hydrotherapy
   e. UVC
5. The highest level of research evidence is available for which of the following modalities to treat pressure ulcers in people with SCI?
   a. negative pressure therapy
   b. hyperbaric oxygen therapy
   c. therapeutic ultrasound
   d. electrical stimulation
   e. laser therapy
6. Which physiological response requires the strongest electrical stimulus or greatest electrical charge?
   a. subsensory
   b. submotor (just below the level required to produce a muscle contraction)
   c. motor (muscle twitch)
   d. noxious or painful stimuli
   e. sensory (pins and needles sensation)
7. Which of the following changes would promote a greater depth of penetration of an electrical signal when using a monopolar electrode setup? Select all the correct answers.
   a. Increase the size of the active electrode.
   b. Improve the conductivity of the wound packing material.
   c. Move the dispersive electrode closer to the active electrode.
   d. Decrease the electrical pulse frequency.
   e. Increase the intensity of the electrical signal.
8. Which of the following modalities require the longest application time (not including time taken for setup and cleanup)?
   a. therapeutic ultrasound
   b. hydrotherapy tank
   c. UVC
   d. laser
   e. electrical stimulation
9. Which of the following mechanisms are believed to underlie the healing response to electrical stimulation?
   a. galvanotaxis
   b. epithelial migration

    c. fibroblast proliferation
    d. bactericidal effects
    e. all of the above

10. Which of the following modalities are not generally thought to stimulate inflammatory cell function (e.g., macrophages)?
    a. therapeutic ultrasound
    b. pneumatic compression therapy
    c. laser
    d. electrical stimulation
    e. hydrotherapy

11. Your patient has an arterial ulcer located on the distal end of her great toe. Which of the following modalities is not contraindicated?
    a. therapeutic ultrasound
    b. pneumatic compression therapy
    c. heat therapy
    d. hydrotherapy
    e. electrical stimulation

SOLUTIONS TO CLINICAL DECISION-MAKING EXERCISES

3-1

When electrical stimulus is applied using a monopolar electrode, it would be expected to produce sensory stimulation under the active electrode first because the current density is greater under this smaller electrode. However, this could be reversed (1) if the volume of the dressing material around the active electrode is larger than the total size of the dispersive electrode or (2) if the dispersive electrode has become smaller than the active one. The effective size of the dispersive electrode can become smaller when skin cells and oils accumulate in self-adhesive electrodes that are used for a prolonged time or if part of the dispersive electrode lifts off the skin.

3-2

Studies show that 180-second treatment applied directly to the wound bed from a UVC lamp that is placed 1 in from the wound surface can significantly reduce the amount of bacteria, including MRSA, in the wound. You do not have to adjust UVC treatment times based on the patient's response to light. This treatment protocol involves protecting the skin surrounding the wound; therefore, changes in a person's response to light due to skin pigmentation and thickness do not affect one's UVC exposure.

3-3

The level of research evidence is highest for the use of therapeutic ultrasound on nonhealing venous ulcers. Ultrasound can be applied to intact periulcer skin using a gel couplant and standard application techniques.

REFERENCES

1. Trengove NJ, Stacey MC, MacAuley S, et al. Analysis of acute and chronic wound environments: the role of proteases and their inhibitors. *Wound Repair Regen.* 1999;7(6):442–452.
2. Weston M, Taber C, Casagranda L, Cornwall M. Changes in local blood volume during gel pack application to traumatized ankles. *J Orthop Sports Phys Ther.* 1994;19:197–199.
3. McMaster WC, Liddle S. Cryotherapy influence on post-traumatic limb edema. *Clin Orthop.* 19080;150:283–287.
4. Akriotis V, Biggar WD. The effect of hypothermia on neutrophil function in vitro. *J Leukoc Biol.* 1985;37:51–61.
5. Kurz A, Sessler KI, Lenhardt R. Perioperative normothermia to reduce the incidence of surgical-wound infection and shorten hospitalization. *N Engl J Med.* 1996;334:1209–1215.
6. Rohrer MJ, Natale AM. Effect of hypothermia on the coagulation cascade. *Crit Care Med.* 1992;10:1402–1405.

7. Esclamado RM, Damiano GA, Cummings CW. Effect of local hypothermia on early wound repair. *Arch Otolaryngol Head Neck Surg.* 1990;116:803–808.

8. Scott EM, Leaper DJ, Clark M, Kelly PJ. Effects of warming therapy on pressure ulcers—a randomised trial. *AORN J.* 2001;73(5):921–938.

9. Rabkin JM, Hunt TK. Local heat increases blood flow and oxygen tension in wounds. *Arch Surg.* 1987;122:221–225.

10. Park H, Phillips T, Kroon C, Murali J, Seah CC. Noncontact thermal wound therapy counteracts the effects of chronic wound fluid on cell cycle regulatory proteins. *Wounds.* 2001;13(6):216–222.

11. Xia Z, Sato A, Hughes MA, Chery GC. Stimulation of fibroblast growth in vitro by intermittent radiant warming. *Wound Repair Regen.* 2000;8:138–144.

12. Hughes MA, Tang C, Cherry GC. Effect of intermittent radiant warming on proliferation of human dermal endothelial cells in vitro. *J Wound Care.* 2003;12:135–137.

13. Price P, Bale S, Crook H, Harding KG. The effect of a radiant heat dressing on pressure ulcers. *J Wound Care.* 2000;9:201–205.

14. Melling AC, Ali B, Scott EM, Leaper DJ. Effects of perioperative warming on the incidence of wound infection after clean surgery: a randomized controlled trial. *Lancet.* 2001;358:878–880.

15. Ellis SL, Finn P, Noone M, Leaper DJ. Eradication of methicillin-resistant *Staphylococcus aureus* from pressure sores using warming therapy. *Surg Infect.* 2003;41(1):53–55.

16. Petrofsky JS, Lawson D, Such HY, et al. The influence of local versus global heat on the healing of chronic wounds in patients with diabetes. *Diab Technol Ther.* 2007;9(6):535–544.

17. Niederhuber S, Stribley RF, Koepke GH. Reduction of skin bacterial load with use of therapeutic whirlpool. *Phys Ther.* 1975;55(5):482–486.

18. Bohannon RW. Whirlpool versus whirlpool rinse for removal of bacteria from a venous stasis ulcer. *Phys Ther.* 1982;62:304–308.

19. Haynes LJ, Brown MH, Handley BC, et al. Comparison of Pulsavac and sterile whirlpool regarding the promotion of tissue granulation [abstract]. *Phys Ther.* 1994;74 (suppl):54.

20. Meeker J. Whirlpool therapy on postoperative pain and surgical wound healing: an exploration. *Patient Educ Counsel.* 1998;33:39–48.

21. European Pressure Ulcer Advisory Panel, National Pressure Ulcer Advisory Panel. *Treatment of Pressure Ulcers: Quick Reference Guide.* Washington, DC: National Pressure Ulcer Advisory Panel; 2009.

22. McCulloch JM, Boyd VB. The effects of whirlpool and the dependent position on lower extremity volume. *J Orthop Sports Phys Ther.* 1992;16(4):169–173.

23. Ogiwara S. Calf muscle pumping and rest positions during and/or after whirlpool therapy. *J Phys Ther Sci.* 201;13(2):99–105.

24. Svoboda SJ, Bice TG, Gooden HA, Brooks DE, Thomas DB, Wenke JC. Comparison of bulb syringe and pulsed lavage irrigation with use of a bioluminescent musculoskeletal wound model. *J Bone Joint Surg.* 2006;88A(10):2167–2174.

25. Owens BD, White DW, Wenke JC. Comparison of irrigation solutions and devices in a contaminated musculoskeletal wound survival model. *J Bone Joint Surg.* 209;91(1):92–98.

26. Solomon SL. Host factors in whirlpool-associated *Pseudomonas aeruginosa* skin disease. *Infect Control.* 1985;16:402–406.

27. Wheeler CB, Rodeheaver GT, Thacker JG. Side effects of high pressure irrigation. *Surg Gynecol Obstet.* 1976;31:842–848.

28. Foulds IS, Barker AT. Human skin battery potentials and their possible role in wound healing. *Br J Dermatol.* 1983;109:515–522.

29. McGinnis ME, Vanable JW. Wound epithelium controls stump currents. *Dev Biol.* 1986;116(1)174–183.

30. McCaig CD, Rajnicek AM, Song B, Zhoa M. Controlling cell behavior electrically: current views and future potential. *Physiol Rev.* 2005;85:943–978.

31. Orida N, Feldman JD. Directional protrusive pseudopodial activity and motility in macrophages induced by extracellular electric fields. *Cell Motil.* 1982;2:243–255.

32. Reich JD, Cazzaniga AL, Mertz PM, Kerdel FA, Eaglstein WH. The effect of electrical stimulation on the number of mast cells in healing wounds. *J Am Acad Dermatol.* 1991;25:40–46.

33. Zhuang H, Wang W, Seldes RM, Tahernia AD, Fan H, Brighton CT. Electrical stimulation induces the level of TGF-β1 mRNA in osteoblastic cells by a mechanism involving calcium/calmodulin pathway. *Biochem Biophys Res Commun.* 1997;237:225–229.

34. Bourguignon GJ, Bourguignon LYW. Electric stimulation of protein and DNA synthesis in human fibroblasts. *FASEB J.* 1987;1:398–402.

35. Taylor K, Fish DR, Mendel FC, Burton HW. Effect of a single 30-minute treatment of high voltage pulsed current on edema formation in frog hind limbs. *Phys Ther.* 1992;72:63–68.

36. Cook HA, Morales M, La Rosa EM, et al. Effects of electrical stimulation on lymphatic flow and limb volume in the rat. *Phys Ther.* 1994;74:1040–1046.

37. Reed BV. Effect of high voltage pulsed electrical stimulation on microvascular permeability to plasma proteins. *Phys Ther.* 1988;4:491–495.

38. Griffin JW, Newsome LS, Stralka SW, Wright PE. Reduction of chronic posttraumatic hand edema: a comparison of high voltage pulsed current intermittent pneumatic compression, and placebo treatments. *Phys Ther.* 1990;170:279–286.

39. Alvarez O, Mertz P, Smerbeck R, Eaglstein W. The healing of superficial skin wounds is stimulated by external electrical current. *J Invest Dermatol.* 1983;81:144–148.

40. Bach S, Bilgrav K, Gottrup F, Jorgensen TE. The effect of electrical current on healing skin incision. *Eur J Surg.* 1991;157:171–174.

41. Mertz PM, Davis SC, Cazzaniga AL, Cheng K, Reich JD, Eaglstein WH. Electrical stimulation: acceleration of soft tissue repair by varying the polarity. *Wounds.* 1993;55(3):153–159.

42. Chu CS, McManus AT, Manson AD, Okerberg CV, Pruitt BA. Multiple graft harvestings from deep partial-thickness scald wounds healed under the influence of weak direct current. *J Trauma.* 1990;30:1044–1050.

43. Burgess E, Hollinger J, Bennett S, et al. Charged beads enhance cutaneous wound healing in Rhesus non-human primates. *Plast Reconstr Surg.* 1998;102:2395–2403.

44. Fujita M, Hukuda S, Doida Y. The effect of constant direct electrical current on intrinsic healing in the flexor tendon in vitro. *J Hand Surg Br.* 1992;17:94–98.

45. Litke DS, Dahners LE. Effects of different levels of direct current on early ligament healing in a rat model. *J Orthop Res.* 1994;12:683–688.

46. Akai M, Oda H, Shirasaki Y, Tateishi T. Electrical stimulation of ligament healing. *Clin Orthop.* 1988; Oct;(235):296–301.

47. Nessler JP, Mass DP. Direct-current electrical stimulation of tendon healing in vitro. *Clin Orthop.* 1987; Apr;(217):303–312.

48. Owoeye I, Spielholz NI, Nelson AJ. Low-intensity pulsed galvanic current and the healing of tenotomized rat Achilles tendons: preliminary report using load-to-break measurements. *Arch Phys Med Rehabil.* 1987;68:415–418.

49. Smith J, Romansky N, Vomero J, Davis R. The effect of electrical stimulation on wound healing in diabetic mice. *J Am Podiatr Assoc.* 1984;74:71–75.

50. Cheng N, Hoof HV, Bockx E, et al. The effects of electric currents on ATP generation, protein synthesis, and membrane transport in rat skin. *Clin Orthop.* 1982;171:264–272.

51. Falanga V, Bourguignon GJ, Bourguignon LYW. Electrical stimulation increases the expression of fibroblast receptors for transforming growth factor-beta. *Wound Repair and Regeneration.* 1987;88:488 [abstract].

52. Dunn MG, Doillon CJ, Berg RA, Olson RM, Silver FH. Wound healing using a collagen matrix: effect of DC electrical stimulation. *J Biomed Mater Res Appl Biomater.* 1988;22:191–206.

53. Erickson CA, Nuccitelli R. Embryonic fibroblast motility and orientation can be influenced by physiological electric fields. *J Cell Biol.* 1984;98:296–307.

54. Zhao M, Dick A, Forrester JV, McCaig CD. Electric field-directed cell motility involves up-regulated expression and asymmetric redistribution of the epidermal growth factor receptors and is enhanced by fibronectin and laminin. *Mol Biol Cell.* 1999;10:1259–1276.

55. Zhao M, McCaig CD, Fernandez AA, Forrester JV, Araki-Sasaki K. Human corneal epithelial cells reorient and migrate cathodally in a small applied electric field. *Curr Eye Res.* 1997;16:973–984.

56. Hinsenkamp M, Jercinovic A, de Graef C, Wilaert F, Heenen M. Effects of low frequency pulsed electrical current on keratinocytes in vitro. *Bioelectromagnetics.* 1997;18:250–254.

57. Cooper MS, Schilwa M. Electrical and ionic controls of tissue cell locomotion in DC electric field. *J Neurosci Res.* 1985;13:223–244.

58. Junger M, Zuder D, Steins A, Hahn M, Klyscz T. Treatment of venous ulcers with low frequency pulsed current (Dermapulse): effects on cutaneous. *Der Hautarzt.* 1997;18:897–903.

59. Kincaid CB, Lavoie KH. Inhibition of bacterial growth in vitro following stimulation with high voltage, monophasic, pulsed current. *Phys Ther.* 1989;69:651–655.

60. Szuminsky NJ, Alberts AC, Unger P, Eddy JG. Effect of narrow, pulsed high voltages on bacterial viability. *Phys Ther.* 1984;74:660–667.

61. Daeschlein G, Assadian O, Kloth LC, Meinl C, Ney F, Kramer A. Antibacterial activity of positive and negative polarity low voltage pulsed current (LVPC) on six typical Gram positive and Gram negative bacterial pathogens of chronic wounds. *Wound Repair Regen.* 2007;15:399–403.

62. Wolcott L, Wheeler P, Hardwicke H, et al. Accelerated healing of skin ulcers by electrotherapy: preliminary clinical results. *S Afr Med J.* 1969;62:795–801.

63. Rowley B, McKenna J, Chase G, et al. The influence of electrical current on an infecting micro-organism in wounds. *Ann N Y Acad Sci.* 1974;238:543–551.

64. Ong P, Laatsch L, Kloth L. Antibacterial effects of a silver electrode carrying microamperage direct current in vitro. *J Clin Electrophysiol.* 1994;6(1):14–18.

65. Thibodeau E, Handelman S, Marquis R. Inhibition and killing of oral bacteria by silver ions generated with low intensity direct current. *J Dent Res.* 1978;57:922–926.

66. Huckfeldt R, Flick AB, Mikkelson D, Lowe C, Finley PJ. Wound closure after split thickness grafting is accelerated by continuous direct anodal microcurrent applied to silver nylon contact dressings. *J Burn Care Res.* 2007;28(5):703–707.

67. Dodgen PW, Johnson BW, Baker LL, Chambers RB. The effects of electrical stimulation on cutaneous oxygen supply in diabetic older adults. *Phys Ther.* 1987;67(9):793.

68. Gilcreast D, Stotts NA, Froelicher E, Baker L, Moss K. Effect of electrical stimulation on foot skin perfusion in persons with or at risk for diabetic foot ulcers. *Wound Repair Regen.* 1998;6:434–441.

69. Faghri P, Votto J, Hovorka C. Venous hemodynamics of the lower extremities in response to electrical stimulation. *Arch Phys Med Rehabil.* 1998;79:842–848.

70. Im MJ, Lee WPA, Hoopes JE. Effect of electrical stimulation on survival of skin flaps in pigs. *Phys Ther.* 1990;70:37–40.

71. Mohr T, Akers TK, Wessman HC. Effect of high voltage stimulation on blood flow in the rat hind limb. *Phys Ther.* 1987;67:526–533.

72. Gagnier K, Manix N, Baker L, et al. The effect of electrical stimulation on cutaneous oxygen supply in paraplegics. *Phys Ther.* 1987;68(5):835–839.

73. Mawson A, Siddiqui F, Connolly B, et al. Effect of high voltage pulsed galvanic stimulation on sacral transcutaneous oxygen tension levels in the spinal cord injured. *Paraplegia.* 1993;31:311–319.

74. Goldman R, Brewley B, Golden M. Electrotherapy reoxygenates inframalleolar ischemic wounds on diabetic patients. *Adv Skin Wound Care.* 2002;15(3):112–120.

75. Goldman R, Rosen M, Brewley B, et al. Electrotherapy promotes healing and microcirculation of infrapopliteal wounds: a prospective pilot study. *Adv Skin Wound Care.* 2004;17:284–290.

76. Suh H, Petrofsky J, Fish A, et al. A new electrode design to improve outcomes in the treatment of chronic healing wounds in diabetes. *Diab Technol Ther.* 2009;11(5):315–322.

77. Suh H, Petrofsky J, Lo T, et al. The combined effect of a 3-electrode delivery system with local heat on healing of chronic wounds. *Diab Technol Ther.* 2009;11(10):681–688.

78. Kloth LC, McCulloch JM. Promotion of wound healing with electrical stimulation. *Adv Wound Care.* 196;9: 42–45.

79. Baker L, Rubayi S, Villar F, DeMuth S. Effect of electrical stimulation waveform on healing of ulcers in human beings with spinal cord injury. *Wound Repair Regen.* 1996;4:21–28.

80. Baker L, Chambers R, DeMuth S, Villar F. Effects of electrical stimulation on wound healing in patients with diabetic ulcers. *Diab Care.* 1997;20:405–412.

81. Kloth LC. *Proceedings of Symposium on Advanced Wound Care. 13th Annual Meeting of the American Association of Wound Care (AAWC) and Medical Research Forum, Dallas, Texas, USA.* April 1–6, 2000.

82. Houghton P, Campbell KE, Fraser C, et al. Electrical stimulation therapy increases healing of pressure ulcers in community dwelling people with spinal cord injury. *Arch Phys Med Rehabil.* 2010. 91(5):669-678

83. Peters EJ, Armstrong DG, Wunderlich RP, Bosma J, Stacpoole-Shea S, Lavery LA. The benefit of electrical stimulation to enhance perfusion in persons with diabetes mellitus. *J Foot Ankle Surg.* 1998;37(5):396–400.

84. Ahmad ET. High voltage pulsed galvanic stimulation: effect of treatment durations on healing of chronic pressure ulcers. *J Physiother Occup Ther.* 2008;2(3):1–5.

85. Kaada B. Promoted healing of chronic ulceration by transcutaneous nerve stimulation (TNS). *Vasa.* 1983;12:262–269.

86. Newton R, Karselis T. Skin pH following high voltage pulsed galvanic stimulation. *Phys Ther.* 1983;63:1593–1596.

87. Crowell JA, Kusserow BK, Nyborg WL. Functional changes in white blood cells after microsonation. *Ultrasound Med Biol.* 1997;3:185.

88. Young SR, Dyson M. Macrophage responsiveness to therapeutic ultrasound. *Ultrasound Med Biol.* 1990;16:809–816.

89. Dyson M, Luke DA. Induction of mast cell degranulation in skin by ultrasound. *IEEE Trans UFFC.* 1986;133:194–201.

90. Young SR, Dyson M. Effect of therapeutic ultrasound on the healing of full-thickness excised skin lesions. *Ultrasonics.* 1990;28:175–179.

91. Johns LD. Nonthermal effects of therapeutic ultrasound: the frequency resonance hypothesis. *J Athletic Train.* 2002;37: 293–299.

92. Hashish I, Harvey W, Harris M. Anti-inflammatory effects of ultrasound therapy: evidence for a major placebo effect. *Br J Rheumatol.* 1986;25:77–81.

93. Fyfe MC, Chahl LA. The effect of single or repeated applications of "therapeutic" ultrasound on plasma extravasation during silver nitrate induced inflammation of the rat hindpaw ankle joint in vivo. *Ultrasound Med Biol.* 1985;11:273–283.

94. Harvey W, Dyson M, Pond J, Grahame R. The 'in vitro' stimulation of protein synthesis in human fibroblasts by therapeutic levels of ultrasound. *In: "Proceedings of the Second European Congress on Ultrasonics in Medicine", Excerpta Medica International Congress Series.* 1975: No.363:10–21

95. De Deyne P, Kirsch-Volders M. In vitro effects of therapeutic ultrasound on the nucleus of human fibroblasts. *Phys Ther.* 1995;75:629–634.

96. Al-Karmi AM, Dinno MA, Stoltz DA, Crum LA, Matthews JC. Calcium and the effects of ultrasound on frog skin. *Ultrasound Med Biol.* 1994;20:73–81.

97. Dinno MA, Dyson M, Young SR, Mortimer AJ, Hart J, Crum LA. The significance of membrane changes in the safe and effective use of therapeutic and diagnostic ultrasound. *Phys Med Biol.* 1989;34:1543–1552.

98. Dyson M, Pond JB, Joseph J, Warwick R. The stimulation of tissue regeneration by means of ultrasound. *Clin Sci.* 1968;35:273–285.

99. Jackson BA, Schwane JA, Starcher BC. Effect of ultrasound therapy on the repair of Achilles tendon injuries in rats. *Med Sci Sports Exerc.* 1991;23:171–176.

100. Gan BS, Huys S, Sherebrin MH, Scilley CG. The effects of ultrasound treatment on flexor tendon healing in the chicken limb. *J Hand Surg.* 1995;20B:809–814.

101. Stevenson JH, Pang CY, Lindsay WK, Zuker RM. Functional, mechanical and biochemical assessment of ultrasound therapy on tendon healing in the chicken toe. *Plast Reconstr Surg.* 1986;77:965–970.

102. Rubin MJ, Etchison MR, Condra KA, Franklin TD, Snoddy AM. Acute effects of ultrasound on skeletal muscle oxygen tension, blood flow and capillary density. *J Med Biol.* 1990;16:271–277.

103. Dyson M, Woodward B, Pond JB. Flow of red blood cells stopped by ultrasound. *Nature.* 1971;232:572–573.

104. Williams AR, Miller DL, Gross DR. Haemolysis in vivo by therapeutic intensities of ultrasound. *Ultrasound Med Biol.* 1986;12:501–509.

105. Maxwell L. Therapeutic ultrasound: its effects on the cellular and molecular mechanisms of inflammation and repair. *Physiotherapy.* 1992;78:421–426.

106. Ennis WJ, Lee C, Meneses P. A biochemical approach to wound healing through the use of modalities. *Clin Dermatol.* 2007;25:63–72.

107. Thawer HA, Houghton PE. Effects of electrical stimulation on histological properties of wounds of diabetic mice. *Wound Repair Regen*. 2001;9(2):107–115.

108. Turner SM, Powell ES, Ng CSS. The effect of ultrasound on the healing of repaired cockerel tendon: is collagen cross-linkage a factor? *J Hand Surg*. 1989;14B:428–433.

109. Franek A, Chmielewska D, Brzezinska-Wcislo L, Slezak A, Blaszczak E. Application of various power densities of ultrasound in the treatment of leg ulcers. *Scand J Rehabil Med*. 1990;22:195–197.

110. Weichenthal M, Mohr P, Stegmann W, Brejtbart EW. Low frequency ultrasound treatment of chronic venous ulcers. *Wound Repair Regen*. 1997;5:18–22.

111. Peschen M, Weichenthal M, Schopf E, Vanscheidt W. Low frequency ultrasound treatment of chronic venous leg ulcers in an outpatient therapy. *Acta Derm Venereol (Stockh)*. 1997;77:311–314.

112. Unger PG. Low-frequency, noncontact, nonthermal ultrasound therapy: a review of the literature. *Ostomy Wound Manage*. 2008;54(1):57–60.

113. Serena T, Lee SK, Attar P, Meneses P, Ennis W. The impact of noncontact nonthermal low frequency ultrasound on bacterial counts in experimental and chronic wounds. *Ostomy Wound Manage*. 2009;55(1):22–30.

114. Thawer HA, Houghton PE. Effects of ultrasound mist therapy on wound size and histological composition in mice with experimental diabetes. *J Wound Care*. 2004;13(5):1–6.

115. Bolton P A, Young S R, Dyson M: Macrophage responsiveness to light therapy. A dose response study. *Low Level Laser Therapy*. 1990;2:101–106.

116. Bouma MG, Buurman WA, van den Wildenberg FAJM. Low energy laser irradiation fails to modulate the inflammatory function of human monocytes and endothelial cells. *Lasers Surg Med*. 1996;19:207–221.

117. Ohta A, Abergel RP, Uitto J. Laser modulation of human immune system: inhibition of lymphocyte proliferation by a gallium–arsenide laser at low energy. *Lasers Surg Med*. 1987;7:199–201.

118. Noble PB, Shields ED, Blecher PDM, Bentley KC. Locomotory characteristics of fibroblasts within a three-dimensional collagen lattice: modulation by a helium/neon soft laser. *Lasers Surg Med*. 1992;12:669–674.

119. Pourreau-Schneider N, Ahmed A, Soudry M, et al. Helium–neon laser treatment transforms fibroblasts into myofibroblasts. *Am J Pathol*. 1990;137:171–178.

120. Skinner S, Gage J, Wilce P, Shaw R. A preliminary study of the effects of laser radiation on collagen metabolism in cell culture. *Aust Dent J*. 1996;41:188–192.

121. Yu H-S, Chang K-L, Yu C-L, Chen J-W, Chen G-S. Low-energy helium–neon laser irradiation stimulates interleukin-1 alpha and interleukin-8 release from cultured human keratinocytes. *J Invest Dermatol*. 1996;107:593–596.

122. Karu Ti, Ryabykh TP, Fedoseyeva GE, Puchkova NI. Helium–neon laser induced respiratory burst of phagocytic cells. *Lasers Surg Med*. 1989;9:585–588.

123. Enwemeka CS. Laser biostimulation of healing wounds: specific effects and mechanisms of action. *Journal of Orthopedic and Sports Physical Therapy*. 1988;9(10):333–338.

124. Young S, Bolton P, Dyson M, Harvey W, Diamantopoulos C. Macrophage responsiveness to light therapy. *Lasers Surg Med*. 1989;9:497–505.

125. El Sayed SO, Dyson M. Effect of laser pulse repetition rate and pulse duration on mast cell number and degranulation. *Lasers Surg Med*. 1996;19:433–437.

126. Agaiby AD, Ghali LR, Wilson R, Dyson M. Laser modulation of angiogenic factor production by T-lymphocytes. *Lasers Surg Med*. 2000;26:357–363.

127. Honmura A, Yanase M, Obata J, Haruki E. Therapeutic effect of Ga–Al–As diode laser irradiation on experimentally induced inflammation in rats. *Lasers Surg Med*. 1992;12:441–449.

128. Bischt D, Gupta SC, Misra V, Mital VP, Sharma P. Effect of low intensity laser radiation on healing of open skin wounds in rats. *Indian J Med Res*. 1994;100:43–46.

129. Kovacs I, Mester E, Gorog P. Laser-induced stimulation of the vascularization of the healing wound. An ear chamber experiment. *Experientia*. 174;15:341–343.

130. Braverman B, McCarthy RJ, Ivankovich AD, Forde DE, Overfield M, Bapna MS. Effect of helium–neon and infrared laser irradiation of wound healing in rabbits. *Lasers Surg Med*. 1989;9:50–58.

131. Reddy GK, Stehno-Bittel L, Enwemeka CS. Laser photostimulation of collagen production in healing rabbit Achilles tendons. *Lasers Surg Med*. 1998;22:281–287.

132. Hall G, Anneroth G, Schennings T, Zetterqvist L, Ryden H. Effect of low level energy laser irradiation on wound healing. An experimental study in rats. *Swed Dent J*. 1994;18:29–34.

133. Surinchak JS, Alago ML, Bellamy RF, Stuck BE, Belkin M. Effects of low-level energy lasers on the healing of full-thickness skin defects. *Lasers Surg Med*. 1983;2:267–274.

134. Broadley C, Broadley KN, Disimone G, Reinisch L, Davidson JM. Low-energy helium–neon laser irradiation and the tensile strength of incisional wounds in the rat. *Wound Repair Regen*. 1995;3:512–517.

135. Allendorf JDF, Bessler M, Huang J, et al. Helium–neon laser irradiation at fluences of 1, 2 and 4 J/cm^2 failed to accelerated wound healing as assessed by both wound contracture rate and tensile strength. *Lasers Surg Med*. 1997;20:340–345.

136. Saperia D, Glassberg E, Lyons RF, et al. Demonstration of elevated type I and type III procollagen mRNA levels in cutaneous wounds treated with helium–neon laser. *Biochem Biophys Res Commun*. 1986;138:1123–1128.

137. Hunter J, Leonard L, Wilson R, Snider G, Dixon J. Effects of low energy laser on wound healing in a porcine model. *Lasers Surg Med*. 1984;3:285–290.

138. McCaughan J, Bethel B, Johnston T, Janssen W. Effect of low-dose argon irradiation on rate of wound closure. *Lasers Surg Med*. 1985;5:607–614.

139. Wilson M, Yianni C. Killing of methicillin-resistant *Staphylococcus aureus* by low power laser light. *J Med Microbiol*. 1997;42:62–66.

140. Nussbaum EL, Lilge L, Mazzulli T. Effects of 630, 660, 810, and 905 nm laser irradiation delivering radiant exposure of 1–50 J/cm² on three species of bacteria in vitro. *J Clin Laser Med Surg*. 2002;20(6):325–333.

141. Nussbaum EL, Mazzulli T, Pritzker KPH, Las Heras F, Jing F, Lilge L. Effects of low intensity laser irradiation during healing of skin lesions in the rat. *Lasers Surg Med*. 2009;41:373–381.

142. Burke TJ. Questions and answers about MIRE treatment. *Adv Skin Wound Care*. 2003;16:369–371.

143. Franzen-Korzendorfer H, Backinton M, Rone-Adams S, McCulloch J. The effect of monochromatic infrared energy on transcutaneous oxygen measurements and protective sensation: results of a controlled, double-blind, randomized clinical study. *Ostomy Wound Manage*. 2008;54(6):16–31.

144. Saltmarche AE. Low level laser therapy for healing acute and chronic wounds—the extendicare experience. *Int Wound J*. 2008;5(2):351–360.

145. Gogia PP. Low-energy laser in wound management. In: Gogia PP, ed. *Clinical Wound Management*. Thorofare, NJ: Slack Inc; 1995:165–172.

146. Rosario R, Mark GJ, Parrish JA, Mihm MC. Histological changes produced in skin by equally erythemogenic doses of UV-A, UV-B, UV-C and UV-A with psoralens. *Br J Dermatol*. 1979;101:299–308.

147. Sachsenmaier C, Radler-Pohl A, Zinck R, et al. Involvement of growth factor receptors in the mammalian UVC response. *Cell*. 1994;78:963–972.

148. Hall JD, Mount DW. Mechanism of DNA replication and mutagenesis in ultraviolet-irradiated bacteria and mammalian cells. *Prog Nucleic Acid Res Mol Biol*. 1981;25:53–126.

149. High AS, High JP. Treatment of infected skin wounds using ultra-violet radiation: an in vitro study. *Physiotherapy*. 1983;89:359–360.

150. Conner Kerr TA, Sullivan PK, Gaillard J, Franklin ME, Jones RM. The effects of ultraviolet radiation on antibiotic resistant bacteria in vitro. *Ostomy Wound Manage*. 1990;44(10):50–56.

151. Thai TP, Houghton PE, Campbell KE, Keast DH, Woodbury MG. Effects of ultraviolet light C (UVC) on bacterial colonization of chronic wounds. *Ostomy Wound Manage*. 2004. In press.

152. Thai TP, Houghton PE, Campbell KE, Keast DH, Woodbury MG. The role of ultraviolet light C (UVC) in the treatment of chronic wounds with MRSA. *Ostomy Wound Manage*. 2002;48(11):52–60.

153. Mackie RM, Elwood JM, Hawk JLM. Links between exposure to ultraviolet radiation and skin cancer. *J R Coll Physicians Lond*. 1987;21:91–96.

154. Cullum N, Nelson EA, Fletcher AW, Sheldon TA. Compression for venous leg ulcers. *Cochrane Database of Systematic Reviews*. 2001, Issue 2.

155. Kunimoto B, Gulliver W, Cooling M, Houghton P, Orsted, H., Sibbald RG. Recommendations for practice: prevention and treatment of venous leg ulcers. *Ostomy Wound Manage*. 2001;47(2):34–50.

156. McCulloch JM, Marler KC, Neal MB, et al. Intermittent pneumatic compression improves venous ulcer healing. *Adv Wound Care*. 1994;7:22–26.

157. Carley PJ, Wainapel SF. Electrotherapy for acceleration of wound healing: low intensity direct current. *Arch Phys Med Rehabil*. 1985;66:443–446.

158. Kloth L, Feedar J. Acceleration of wound healing with high voltage, monophasic, pulsed current. *Phys Ther*. 1988;68:503–508.

159. Feedar J, Kloth L, Gentzkow G. Chronic dermal ulcer healing enhanced with monophasic pulsed electrical stimulation. *Phys Ther*. 1991;71:639–649.

160. Mulder GD. Treatment of open-skin wounds with electric stimulation. *Arch Phys Med Rehabil*. 1991;72:375–377.

161. Griffin J, Tooms R, Mendius R, Clifft J, Vander Zwaag R, El-Zeky F. Efficacy of high voltage pulsed current for healing of pressure ulcers in patients with spinal cord injury. *Phys Ther*. 1991;71:433–444.

161. Lundeberg TCM, Eriksson SV, Malm M. Electrical nerve stimulation improves healing of diabetic ulcers. *Ann Plast Surg*. 1992;29:328–330.

162. Wood JM, Evans PE, Schallreuter KU, et al. A multicenter study on the use of pulsed low-intensity direct current for healing chronic stage II and stage III decubitus ulcers. *Arch Dermatol*. 1993;129:999–1009.

163. Houghton PE, Kincaid CB, Lovell M, et al. Effect of electrical stimulation on chronic leg ulcer size and appearance. *Phys Ther*. 2003;83(1):17–28.

164. Adegoke BOA, Badmos KA. Acceleration of pressure ulcer healing in spinal cord injured patients using interrupted direct current. *Afr J Med Sci*. 2001;30:195–197.

165. Adunsky A, Ohry A. Decubitus direct current treatment (DDCT) of pressure ulcers: results of a randomized double blinded placebo controlled study. *Arch Gerontol Geriatr*. 2005;41:261–269.

166. Absorjornsen G, Hernaes B, Molvaer G. The effect of transcutaneous electrical nerve stimulation on pressure sores in geriatric patients. *J Clin Exp Gerontol*. 1990;12(4):209–214.

167. Jankovic A, Binic I. Frequency rhythmic electrical modulation system in the treatment of chronic painful leg ulcers. *Arch Dermatol Res*. 2008;300:377–383.

168. Jercinovic A, Karba R. Low frequency pulsed current and pressure ulcer healing. *IEEE Trans Rehabil Eng*. 1994;2(4):225–233.

169. Junger M, Arnold A, Zuder D, Hans-Werner S, Heising S. Local therapy and treatment costs of chronic, venous leg ulcers with electrical stimulation (Dermapulse): a prospective, placebo controlled, double blind trial. *Wound Repair Regen*. 2008;16:480–487.

170. Gardner SE, Frantz RA, Schmidt FL. Effect of electrical stimulation on chronic wound healing: a meta analysis. *Wound Repair Regen.* 1999;7;495–503.

171. Houghton PE, Woodbury MG. The effect of electrical stimulation on rate of wound healing of chronic wounds. A meta-analysis. *Wounds.* 2007;19(3):A27 [abstract].

172. Fernandez-Chimeno M, Houghton P, Holey L. Electrical stimulation for chronic wounds (Protocol for Cochrane Review). *Cochrane Database Syst Rev.* 2004;(1):CD004550.

173. Keast DH, Parslow N, Houghton PE, Norton L, Fraser C. Best practice recommendations for the prevention and treatment of pressure ulcers. *Adv Skin Wound Care.* 2007;20(8): 390–405.

174. Paralyzed Veterans of America. Pressure ulcer prevention and treatment following spinal cord injury: *A clinical practice guideline for health care professionals. Washington (DC): Paralyzed Veterans of America;.* 2000:43–45.

175. Ovington LG. Dressings and adjunctive therapies: AHCPR guidelines revisited. *Ostomy Wound Manage.* 1999;45(1A): 94S–106S.

176. Dyson M, Suckling J. Stimulation of tissue repair by ultrasound: a survey of the mechanisms involved. *Physiotherapy.* 1978;64:105–108.

177. Roche C, West J. A controlled trial investigating the effect of ultrasound on venous ulcers referred from general practitioners. *Physiotherapy.* 1984;12:475–477.

178. McDiarmid T, Burns PN, Lewith GT, Machin D. Ultrasound and the treatment of pressure sores. *Physiotherapy.* 1985;71:66–70.

179. Callam MJ, Dale JJ, Harper DR, Ruckley CV. A controlled trial of weekly ultrasound therapy in chronic leg ulceration. *Lancet.* 1987;2(8552):204–206.

180. Lundeberg T, Nordstrom F, Brodda-Jansen G, Eriksson SV, Kjartansson J, Samuelson UE. Pulsed ultrasound does not improve healing of venous ulcers. *Scand J Rehabil Med.* 1990;22:195–197.

181. Eriksson SV, Lundenberg T, Malm M. A placebo controlled trial of ultrasound therapy in chronic leg ulceration. *Scand J Rehabil Med.* 1991;23:211–213.

182. Roche, C, West,J. A controlled trial investigating the effect of ultrasound on venous ulcers referred from general practitioners. *Physiotherapy.* 1984; 70:475–477.

183. ter Riet G, Kessels AGH, Knipschild P. A randomized clinical trial of ultrasound in the treatment of pressure ulcers. *Phys Ther.* 1996;76(12):1301–1311.

184. Taradaj J, Franek A, Brzezinska-Wcislo L, et al. The use of therapeutic ultrasound in venous leg ulcers: a randomized controlled clinical trial. *Phlebology.* 2008;23(4): 178–183.

185. Johannsen F, Nyholm A, Karlsmark T. Ultrasound therapy in chronic leg ulceration: a meta-analysis. *Wound Repair Regen.* 1998;6:121–126.

186. Akbari Sari A, Flemming K, Cullum N, Wollina U. Therapeutic ultrasound for pressure ulcers. *Cochrane Database Syst Rev.* 2006;(3):CD001275.

187. Al-Kurdi D, Bell Syer SEM, Flemming K. Therapeutic ultrasound for venous leg ulcers. *Cochrane Database Syst Rev.* 2008;(1):CD001180.

188. Ennis WJ, Formann P, Mozen N, Massey J, Conner-Kerr T, Meneses P. Ultrasound therapy for recalcitrant diabetic foot ulcers: results of a randomized, double-blind, controlled, multicenter study. *Ostomy Wound Manage.* 2005;51(8):24–39.

189. Ennis WJ, Valdes W, Gainer M, Meneses P. Evaluation of clinical effectiveness of MIST ultrasound therapy for the healing of chronic wounds. *Adv Skin Wound Care.* 2006;19:437–446.

190. Kavros SJ, Leidl DA, Boon AJ, Miller JL, Hobbs JA, Andrews KL. Expedited wound healing with non contract, low frequency ultrasound therapy in chronic wounds: a retrospective analysis. *Adv Skin Wound Care.* 2008;21(9):416–423.

191. Waldorf K, Serfass A. Sound evidence. Clinical effectiveness of non contact, low frequency, nonthermal ultrasound in burn care. *Ostomy Wound Manage.* 2008;54(6):66–69.

192. Kolari PI, Pekanmaki K. Intermittent pneumatic compression in healing of venous ulcers. *Lancet.* 1986;2:1108.

193. Coleridge-Smith P, Sarin S, Hasty J, Scurr JH. Sequential gradient pneumatic compression enhances venous ulcer healing: a randomized trial. *Surgery.* 1990;108:871–875.

194. Mulder G, Robinson J, Seeley J. Study of sequential compression treatment of non healing chronic venous ulcers. *Wounds.* 1990;3:111–115.

195. Pekanmaki K, Kolari PJ, Kiistala U. Intermittent pneumatic compression treatment for post-thrombotic leg ulcers. *Clin Exp Dermatol.* 1987;12:350–335.

196. O'Sullivan D, Houghton PE. Intermittent pneumatic compression in the treatment of chronic ulcers. *Phys Ther Rev.* 2009;14(2):81–91.

197. Nussbaum EL, Biemann I, Mustard B. Comparison of ultrasound/ultraviolet-C and laser for treatment of pressure ulcers in patients with spinal cord injury. *Phys Ther.* 1994;74: 812–825.

198. Wills E, Anderson T, Beattie B, Scott A. A randomized placebo-controlled trial of ultraviolet light in the treatment of superficial pressure sores. *J Am Geriatr Soc.* 1983;31:131–133.

199. Burger A, Jordaan AJ, Schoombee GE. The bactericidal effect of ultraviolet light on infected pressure sores. *S Afr J Physiother.* 1985;41(2):55–57.

200. Hydrotherapy systematic review.

201. Kloth LC, Berman JE, Dumit-Minkel S, et.al. Effects of normothermic dressing on pressure ulcer healing. *Adv Skin Wound Care.* 2000;13:69–74.

202. Cherry GW, Wilson J. The treatment of ambulatory venous ulcer patients with warming therapy. *Ostomy Wound Manage.* 1999;45:65–70.

203. Santilli SM, Valusek PA, Robinson C. Use of a noncontact radiant heat bandage for the treatment of chronic venous stasis ulcers. *Adv Wound Care.* 1999;12:89–93.

204. McCulloch J, Knight CA. Noncontact normothermic wound therapy and offloading in the treatment of neutropathic foot ulcers in patients with diabetes. *Ostomy Wound Manage.* 2002;48(3):38–44.

205. Whitney JD, Salvadalena G, Higa L, Mich M. Treatment of pressure ulcers with noncontact normothermic wound therapy: healing and warming effects. *J Wound Continence Nurs.* 2001;28:244–252.

206. Kloth LC, Berman JE, Nett M, Papanek PE, Dumit-Minkel S. A randomized controlled clinical trial to evaluate the effects of noncontact normothermic wound therapy on chronic full thickness pressure ulcers. *Adv Skin Wound Care.* 2002;15(6):270–276.

207. Horwitz LR, Burke TJ, Carnegie D. Augmentation of wound healing using monochromatic infrared energy. *Adv Wound Care.* 1999;12(1):35–40.

208. Schindl A, Schindl M, Schindl L. Successful treatment of a persistent radiation ulcer by low power laser therapy. *J Am Acad Dermatol.* 1997;37:646–649.

209. Mester AF, Mester A. Wound healing. *Low Level Laser Therapy (LLLT).* 1:7–15.

210. Shuttleworth E, Banfield K. Light relief. *Wound Care.* 1996:70–78.

211. Malm M, Lundeberg T. Effect of low power gallium arsenide laser on healing of venous ulcers. *Scand J Plast Reconstr Hand Surg.* 1991;25:249–251.

212. Gupta AK, Filonenko N, Salansky N, Sauder DN. The use of low energy photon therapy (LEPT) in venous leg ulcers: a double-blind, placebo-controlled study. *Dermatol Surg.* 1998;24:1383–1386.

213. Santoianni P, Monfrecola G, Martellotta D, Ayala F. Inadequate effect of helium–neon laser on venous leg ulcers. *Photodermatology.* 1984;1:245–249.

214. Lucas C, van Gemert MJC, de Haan RJ. Efficacy of low-level laser therapy in the management of stage III decubitus ulcers: a prospective, observer-blinded multicentre randomized clinical trial. *Lasers Med Sci.* 2003;18(2):72–77.

215. Franek A, Krol P, Kucharzewski M. Does low output laser stimulation enhance the healing of crural ulceration? Some critical remarks. *Med Eng Phys.* 2002;24(9):607–615.

216. Lagan KM, McKenna T, Witherow A, Johns J, McDonough SM, Baxter GD. Low-intensity laser therapy/combined phototherapy in the management of chronic ulceration: a placebo-controlled study. *J Clin Laser Med Surg.* 2002;20(3):109–116.

217. Kopera D, Kokol R, Berger C, Haas J. Does the use of low-level laser influence wound healing in chronic venous leg ulcers? *J Wound Care.* 2005;14(8):391–394.

218. Taly AB, Nair KPS, Murali T, John A. Efficacy of multi-wavelength light therapy in the treatment of pressure ulcers in subjects with disorders of the spinal cord: a randomized double-blind controlled trial. *Arch Phys Med Rehabil.* 2004;85(10):1657–1661.

219. Bihari I, Mester A. The biostimulative effect of low level laser therapy. *Laser Ther.* 1989;1(2):97–98.

220. Houghton PE, Nussbaum E, Hoens A. Electrophysical agents: contraindications and precautions—an evidence-based approach to clinical decision making in physical therapy. *Physiother Can Spec Suppl.* 2010:62(5):5–10

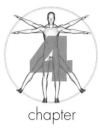

chapter

Managing Pain With Therapeutic Modalities

Craig R. Denegar and William E. Prentice

OBJECTIVES

Following completion of this chapter, the student will be able to:

➤ Compare the various types of pain and appraise their positive and negative effects.

➤ Choose a technique for assessing pain.

➤ Analyze the characteristics of sensory receptors.

➤ Examine how the nervous system relays information about painful stimuli.

➤ Distinguish between the different neurophysiologic mechanisms for pain control for the therapeutic modalities used by clinicians.

➤ Predict how pain perception can be modified by cognitive factors.

UNDERSTANDING PAIN

The International Association for the Study of Pain defines pain as "an unpleasant sensory and emotional experience associated with actual or potential tissue damage, or described in terms of such damage."[1] Pain is a subjective sensation with more than one dimension and an abundance of descriptors of its qualities and characteristics. In spite of its universality, pain is composed of a variety of human discomforts, rather than being a single entity.[2] The perception of pain can be subjectively modified by past experiences and expectations.[37] Much of what we do to treat patients' pain is to change their perceptions of pain.[3]

Pain does have a purpose. It warns us that something is wrong and can provoke a withdrawal response to avoid further injury. It also results in muscle spasm and guards or protects the injured part. Pain, however, can persist after it is no longer useful. It can become a means of enhancing disability and inhibiting efforts to rehabilitate the patient.[4] Prolonged spasm, which leads to circulatory deficiency, muscle atrophy, disuse habits, and conscious or unconscious guarding, may lead to a severe loss of function.[5] Chronic pain may become a disease state in itself. Often lacking an identifiable cause, chronic pain can totally disable a patient.

Research in recent years has led to a better understanding of pain and pain relief. This research also has raised new questions, while leaving many unanswered. We now have better explanations for the analgesic properties of the physical agents we use, as well as a better understanding of the psychology of pain. Newer physical agents, such as laser, and recent improvements to older agents such as diathermy and transcutaneous electrical nerve simulators offer new approaches to the treatment of musculoskeletal injury and pain.[6] The evolution of the treatment of pain is, however, incomplete. Not even the mechanisms for the analgesic response to the simplest therapeutic modalities, heat and cold, have been fully described.[7]

The control of pain is an essential aspect of caring for an injured patient. The clinician can choose from several therapeutic agents with analgesic properties.[8] The selection of a therapeutic agent should be based on a sound understanding of its physical properties and physiologic effects. This chapter will not provide a complete explanation of neurophysiology, pain, and pain relief. Several physiology textbooks provide extensive discussions of human neurophysiology and neurobiology to supplement this chapter. Instead, this chapter presents an overview of some theories of pain control, intended to provide a stimulus for the clinician to develop his or her own rationale for using modalities in the plan of care for patients he or she treats. Ideally, it will also facilitate growth in the body of evidence from which improved responses to the therapeutic agents used in the treatment of pain can be derived.

Many of the modalities discussed in later chapters have analgesic properties. Often, they are employed to reduce pain and permit the patient to perform therapeutic exercises. Some understanding of what pain is, how it affects us, and how it is perceived is essential for the clinician who uses these modalities.[8]

Types of Pain

Acute versus Chronic Pain

Traditionally, pain has been categorized as either *acute* or *chronic*. Acute pain is experienced when tissue damage is impending and after injury has occurred. Pain lasting for more than 6 months is generally classified as chronic.[9] More recently, the term *persistent pain* has been used to differentiate chronic pain that defies intervention from conditions where continuing (persistent) pain is a symptom of a treatable condition.[10,11] More research is devoted to chronic pain and its treatment, but acute and persistent pain confronts the clinician most often.[12]

Referred Pain

Referred pain, which also may be either acute or chronic, is pain that is perceived to be in an area that seems to have little relation to the existing pathology. For example, injury to the spleen often results in pain in the left shoulder. This pattern, known as Kehr's sign, is useful for identifying this serious injury and arranging prompt emergency care. Referred pain can outlast the causative events because of altered reflex patterns, continuing mechanical stress on muscles, learned habits of guarding, or the development of hypersensitive areas, called **trigger points**.

Radiating Pain

Irritation of nerves and nerve roots can cause *radiating pain*. Pressure on the lumbar nerve roots associated with a herniated disc or a contusion of the sciatic nerve can result in pain radiating down the lower extremity to the foot.

Deep Somatic Pain

Deep somatic pain is a type that seems to be **sclerotomic** (associated with a sclerotome, a segment of bone innervated by a spinal segment). There is often a discrepancy between the site of the disorder and the site of the pain.

PAIN ASSESSMENT

Pain is a complex phenomenon that is difficult to evaluate and quantify because it is subjective and is influenced by attitudes and beliefs of the clinician and the patient. Quantification is hindered by the fact that pain is a very difficult concept to put into words.[13]

Obtaining an accurate and standardized assessment of pain is problematic. Several tools have been developed. These pain profiles identify the type of pain, quantify the intensity of pain, evaluate the effect of the pain experience on the patient's level of function, and/or assess the psychosocial impact of pain.

The pain profiles are useful because they compel the patient to verbalize the pain and thereby provide an outlet for the patient and also provide the clinician with a better understanding

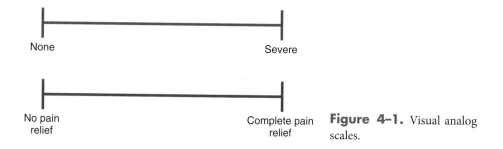

Figure 4–1. Visual analog scales.

of the pain experience. They assess the psychosocial response to pain and injury. The pain profile can assist with the evaluation process by improving communication and directing the clinician toward appropriate diagnostic tests. These assessments also assist the clinician in identifying which therapeutic agents may be effective and when they should be applied. Finally, these profiles provide a standard measure to monitor treatment progress.[10]

Pain Assessment Scales

The following profiles are used in the evaluation of acute and chronic pain associated with illnesses and injuries.

Visual Analog Scales

Visual analog scales are quick and simple tests to be completed by the patient (Figure 4–1). These scales consist of a line, usually 10 cm in length, the extremes of which are taken to represent the limits of the pain experience.[14] One end is defined as "No Pain" and the other as "Severe Pain." The patient is asked to mark the line at a point corresponding to the severity of the pain. The distance between "No Pain" and the mark represents pain severity. A similar scale can be used to assess treatment effectiveness by placing "No Pain Relief" at one end of the scale and "Complete Pain Relief" at the other. These scales can be completed daily or more often as pretreatment and posttreatment assessments.[15]

Pain Charts

Pain charts can be used to establish spatial properties of pain. These two-dimensional graphic portrayals are completed by the patient to assess the location of pain and a number of subjective components. Simple line drawings of the body in several postural positions are presented to the patient (Figure 4–2). On these drawings, the patient draws or colors in areas that

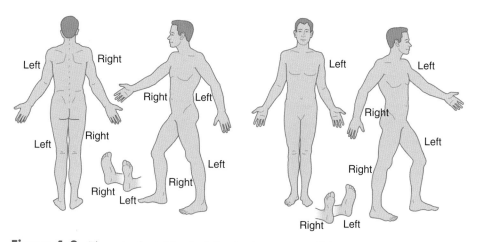

Figure 4–2. The pain chart. Use the following instructions: "Please use all of the figures to show me exactly where all your pains are, and where they radiate to. Shade or draw with *blue marker*. Only the patient is to fill out this sheet. Please be as precise and detailed as possible. Use *yellow marker* for numbness and tingling. Use *red marker* for burning or hot areas, and *green marker* for cramping. Please remember: blue = pain, yellow = numbness and tingling, red = burning or hot areas, green = cramping." Used with permission from Ref.[2].

correspond to his or her pain experience. Different colors are used for different sensations—for example, blue for aching pain, yellow for numbness or tingling, red for burning pain, and green for cramping pain. Descriptions can be added to the form to enhance the communication value. The form could be completed daily.[16]

McGill Pain Questionnaire

The *McGill Pain Questionnaire* (MPQ) is a tool with 78 words that describe pain (Figure 4–3). These words are grouped into 20 sets that are divided into four categories representing dimensions of the pain experience. While completion of the MPQ may take only 20 minutes, it is often frustrating for patients who do not speak English well. The MPQ is commonly administered to patients with low back pain. When administered every 2–4 weeks, it demonstrates changes in status very clearly.[2]

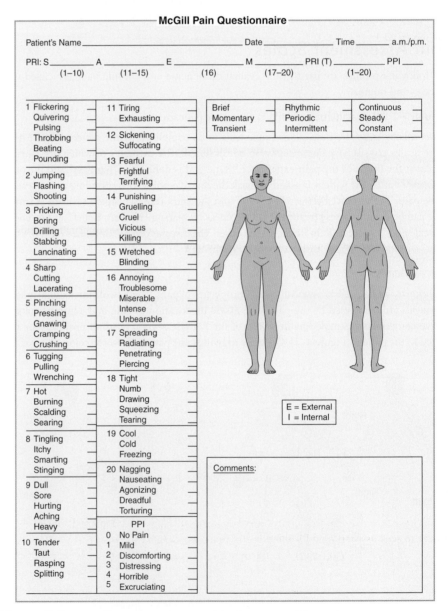

Figure 4–3. McGill Pain Questionnaire. The descriptors fall into four major groups: sensory, 1–10; affective, 11–15; evaluative, 16; and miscellaneous, 17–20. The rank value for each descriptor is based on its position in the word set. The sum of the rank values is the pain rating index (PRI). The present pain intensity (PPI) is based on a scale of 0–5.

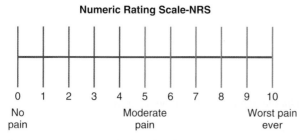

Numeric Rating Scale-NRS

0 1 2 3 4 5 6 7 8 9 10
No   Moderate   Worst pain
pain   pain   ever

Figure 4-4. The *numeric Rating Scale (NRS)* is the most common acute pain profile.

Activity Pattern Indicators Pain Profile

The *Activity Pattern Indicators Pain Profile* measures patient activity. It is a 64-question, self-report tool that may be used to assess functional impairment associated with pain. The instrument measures the frequency of certain behaviors such as housework, recreation, and social activities.[10]

Numeric Pain Scale

The most common acute pain profile is a *numeric pain scale*. The patient is asked to rate his or her pain on a scale from 1 to 10, with 10 representing the worst pain he or she has experienced or could imagine (Figure 4–4). The question is asked before and after treatment. When treatments provide pain relief, patients are asked about the extent and duration of the relief. In addition, patients may be asked to estimate the portion of the day that they experience pain and about specific activities that increase or decrease their pain. When pain affects sleep, patients may be asked to estimate the amount of sleep they got in the previous 24 hours. In addition, the amount of medication required for pain can be noted. This information helps the clinician assess changes in pain, select appropriate treatments, and communicate more clearly with the patient about the course of recovery from injury or surgery.

All of these scales help patients communicate the severity and duration of their pain and appreciate changes that occur. Often in a long recovery, patients lose sight of how much progress has been made in terms of the pain experience and return to functional activities. A review of these pain scales often can serve to reassure the patient; foster a brighter, more positive outlook; and reinforce the commitment to the plan of treatment.

Documentation

The efficacy of many of the treatments used by clinicians has not been fully substantiated. These scales are one source of data that can help clinicians identify the most effective approaches to managing common injuries. These assessment tools can also be useful when reviewing a patient's progress with physicians, and third-party payers. Thus, pain assessments should be routinely included as documentation in the patient's note.

GOALS IN MANAGING PAIN

Regardless of the cause of pain, its reduction is an essential part of treatment. Pain signals the patient to seek assistance and is often useful in establishing a diagnosis. Once the injury or illness is diagnosed, pain serves little purpose. Medical or surgical treatment or immobilization is necessary to treat some conditions, but physical therapy and an early return to activity are appropriate following many injuries. The clinician's objectives are to encourage the body to heal through exercise designed to progressively increase functional capacity and to return the patient to work, recreational, and other activities as swiftly and safely as possible. Pain will inhibit therapeutic exercise. The challenge for the clinician is to control acute pain and protect the patient from further injury while encouraging progressive exercise in a supervised environment.

Pain assessment techniques are as follows:
- visual analog scales;
- pain charts;
- MPQ;
- Activity Pattern Indicators Pain Profile;
- numeric pain scales.

PAIN PERCEPTION

The patient's perception of pain can differ markedly from person to person as can the terminology used to describe the type of pain the patient is experiencing. The clinician commonly asks the patient to describe what his or her pain feels like during an injury evaluation. The patient often uses terms such as *sharp, dull, aching, throbbing, burning, piercing, localized,* and *generalized*. It is sometimes difficult for the clinician to infer what exactly is causing a particular type of pain. For example, "burning" pain is often associated with some injury to a nerve, but certainly other injuries may produce what the patient is perceiving as "burning" pain. Thus, verbal descriptions of the type of pain should be applied with caution.

Sensory Receptors

A nerve ending is the termination of a nerve fiber in a peripheral structure. It may be a sensory ending (receptor) or a motor ending (effector). Sensory endings can be capsulated (e.g., free nerve endings, Merkel's corpuscles) or encapsulated (e.g., end bulbs of Krause or Meissner's corpuscles).

There are several types of sensory receptors in the body, and the clinician should be aware of their existence as well as of the types of stimuli that activate them (Table 4–1). Activation of some of these sense organs with therapeutic agents will decrease the patient's perception of pain.

Six different types of receptor nerve endings are commonly described:

1. Meissner's corpuscles are activated by light touch.
2. Pacinian corpuscles respond to deep pressure.

TABLE 4–1   Some Characteristics of Selected Sensory Receptors

	STIMULUS		RECEPTOR	
TYPE OF SENSORY RECEPTORS	GENERAL TERM	SPECIFIC NATURE	TERM	LOCATION
Mechanoreceptors	Pressure	Movement of hair in a hair follicle	Afferent nerve fiber	Base of hair follicles
		Light pressure	Meissner's corpuscle	Skin
		Deep pressure	Pacinian corpuscle	Skin
		Touch	Merkel's touch corpuscle	Skin
Nociceptors	Pain	Distension (stretch)	Free nerve endings	Wall of gastrointestinal tract, pharynx skin
Proprioceptors	Tension	Distension	Corpuscles of Ruffini	Skin and capsules in joints and ligaments
		Length changes	Muscle spindles	Skeletal muscle
		Tension changes	Golgi tendon organs	Between muscles and tendons
Thermoreceptors	Temperature change	Cold	Krause's end bulbs	Skin
		Heat	Corpuscles of Ruffini	Skin and capsules in joints and ligaments

Reproduced with permission from Previte J. *Human Physiology*. New York: McGraw-Hill Inc;1983.

3. Merkel's corpuscles respond to deep pressure, but more slowly than Pacinian corpuscles, and also are activated by hair follicle deflection.

4. Ruffini corpuscles in the skin are sensitive to touch, tension, and possibly heat; those in the joint capsules and ligaments are sensitive to change in position.

5. Krause's end bulbs are thermoreceptors that react to a decrease in temperature and touch.[17]

6. Pain receptors, called **nociceptors** or *free nerve endings,* are sensitive to extreme mechanical, thermal, or chemical energy.[3] They respond to noxious stimuli—in other words, to impending or actual tissue damage (e.g., cuts, burns, sprains, and so on). The term *nociceptive* is from the Latin *nocere,* to damage, and is used to imply pain information. These organs respond to superficial forms of heat and cold, analgesic balms, and massage.

Proprioceptors found in muscles, joint capsules, ligaments, and tendons provide information regarding joint position and muscle tone. The muscle spindles react to changes in length and tension when the muscle is stretched or contracted. The Golgi tendon organs also react to changes in length and tension within the muscle. See Table 4–1 for a more complete listing.

Some sensory receptors respond to phasic activity and produce an impulse when the stimulus is increasing or decreasing, but not during a sustained stimulus. They adapt to a constant stimulus. Meissner's corpuscles and Pacinian corpuscles are examples of such receptors.

Tonic receptors produce impulses as long as the stimulus is present. Examples of tonic receptors are muscle spindles, free nerve endings, and Krause's end bulbs. The initial impulse is at a higher frequency than later impulses that occur during sustained stimulation.

Accommodation is the decline in generator potential and the reduction of frequency that occur with a prolonged stimulus or with frequently repeated stimuli. If some physical agents are used too often or for too long, the receptors may adapt to or accommodate the stimulus and reduce their impulses. The **accommodation** phenomenon can be observed with the use of superficial hot and cold agents, such as ice packs and hydrocollator packs.

As a stimulus becomes stronger, the number of receptors excited increases, and the frequency of the impulses increases. This provides more electrical activity at the spinal cord level, which may facilitate the effects of some physical agents.

Cognitive Influences

Pain perception and the response to a painful experience may be influenced by a variety of cognitive processes, including anxiety, attention, depression, past pain experiences, and cultural influences.[18] These individual aspects of pain expression are mediated by higher centers in the cortex in ways that are not clearly understood.[3] They may influence both the sensory discriminative and motivational affective dimensions of pain.

Many mental processes modulate the perception of pain through descending systems. Behavior modification, the excitement of the moment, happiness, positive feelings, **focusing** (directed attention toward specific stimuli), hypnosis, and suggestion may modulate pain perception. Past experiences, cultural background, personality, motivation to play, aggression, anger, and fear are all factors that could facilitate or inhibit pain perception. Strong central inhibition may mask severe injury for a period of time.[3] At such times, evaluation of the injury is quite difficult.

Patients with chronic pain may become very depressed and experience a loss of fitness. They tend to be less active and may have altered appetites and sleep habits. They have a decreased will to work and exercise and often develop a reduced sex drive. They may turn to self-abusive patterns of behavior. Tricyclic drugs are often used to inhibit serotonin depletion for the patient with chronic pain.

Just as pain may be inhibited by central modulation, it may also arise from central origins. Phobias, fear, depression, anger, grief, and hostility are all capable of producing pain in the absence of local pathologic processes. In addition, pain memory, which is associated with old injuries, may result in pain perception and pain response that are out of proportion to a new, often minor, injury. Substance abuse can also alter and confound the perception of pain. Substance abuse may cause the chronic pain patient to become more depressed or may lead to depression and psychosomatic pain.

NEURAL TRANSMISSION

Afferent nerve fibers transmit impulses from the sensory receptors toward the brain while **efferent** fibers, such as motor neurons, transmit impulses from the brain toward the periphery.[7] First-order or primary afferents transmit the impulses from the sensory receptor to the dorsal horn of the spinal cord (Figure 4–5). There are four different types of first-order neurons (Table 4–2). Aα and Aβ are large-diameter afferents that have a *high* (fast) conduction velocity, and Aδ and C fibers are small-diameter fibers with *low* (slow) conduction velocity.

Second-order afferent fibers carry sensory messages up the spinal cord to the brain. They are categorized as wide dynamic range or nociceptive specific. The wide dynamic range second-order afferents receive input from Aβ, Aδ, and C fibers. These second-order afferents serve relatively large, overlapping receptor fields. The nociceptive specific second-order afferents respond exclusively to noxious stimulation. They receive input only from Aδ and C fibers. These afferents serve smaller receptor fields that do not overlap. All of these neurons synapse with third-order neurons, which carry information to various brain centers where the input is integrated, interpreted, and acted upon.

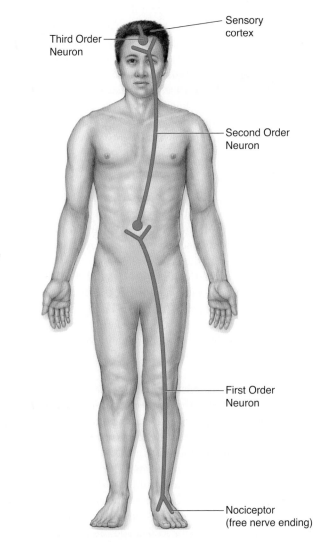

Figure 4–5. Neural afferent transmission. Sensory (pain) information from free nerve endings is transmitted to the sensory cortex in the brain via first-, second-, and third-order neurons.

TABLE 4–2 Classification of Afferent Neurons

SIZE	TYPE	GROUP	SUBGROUP	DIAMETER (MICROMETERS)	CONDUCTION VELOCITY (M/S)	RECEPTOR	STIMULUS
Large	Aα	I	1a	13–22	70–120	Proprioceptive mechanoreceptor	Muscle velocity and length change, muscle shortening of rapid speed
	Aα	I	1b			Proprioceptive mechanoreceptor	Muscle length information from touch and Pacinian corpuscles
	Aβ	II	Muscle	8–13	40–70		
	Aβ	II	Skin			Cutaneous receptors	Touch, vibration, hair receptors
	Aδ	III	Muscle	1–4	5–15	75% mechanoreceptors and thermoreceptors	Temperature change
Small	Aδ	III	Skin			25% nociceptors, mechanoreceptors, and thermoreceptors (hot and cold)	Noxious, mechanical, and temperature (>45°C, <10°C)
	C	IV	Muscle	0.2–1.0	0.2–2.0	50% mechanoreceptors and thermoreceptors	Touch and temperature

Facilitators and Inhibitors of Synaptic Transmission

For information to pass between neurons, a transmitter substance must be released from the end of one neuron terminal (presynaptic membrane), enter the synaptic cleft, and attach to a receptor site on the next neuron (postsynaptic membrane) (Figure 4–6). In the past, all the activity within the synapse was attributed to **neurotransmitters**, such as acetylcholine. The neurotransmitters, when released in sufficient quantities, are known to cause depolarization of the postsynaptic neuron. In the absence of the neurotransmitter, no depolarization occurs.

It is now apparent that several compounds that are not true neurotransmitters can facilitate or inhibit synaptic activity. **Serotonin**, **norepinephrine**, **enkephalin**, **β-endorphin**, **dynorphin**, and **substance P** are each important in the body's pain control mechanism.[19]

Enkephalin is an **endogenous** (made by the body) **opioid** that inhibits the depolarization of second-order nociceptive nerve fibers. It is released from **interneurons**, enkephalin neurons with short axons. The enkephalins are stored in nerve-ending vesicles found in the **substantia gelatinosa (SG)** and in several areas of the brain. When released, enkephalin may bind to presynaptic or postsynaptic membranes.[19]

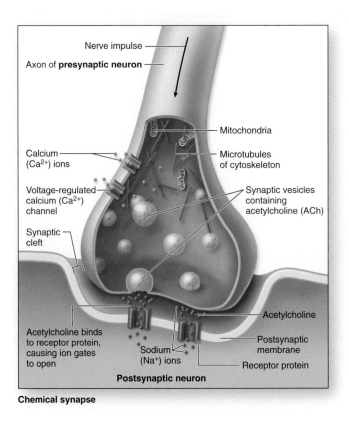

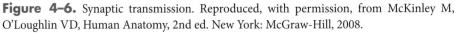

Figure 4–6. Synaptic transmission. Reproduced, with permission, from McKinley M, O'Loughlin VD, Human Anatomy, 2nd ed. New York: McGraw-Hill, 2008.

Norepinephrine is released by the depolarization of some neurons and binds to the postsynaptic membranes. It is found in several areas of the nervous system, including a tract that descends from the pons, which inhibits synaptic transmission between first- and second-order nociceptive fibers, thus decreasing pain sensation.[20]

Other endogenous opioids may be active analgesic agents. These neuroactive peptides are released into the central nervous system and have an action similar to that of morphine, an opiate analgesic. There are specific opiate receptors located at strategic sites, called binding sites, to receive these compounds. β-Endorphin and dynorphin have potent analgesic effects. These are released within the central nervous system by mechanisms that are not fully understood at this time.

Nociception

A nociceptor is a peripheral pain receptor. Its cell body is in the dorsal root ganglion near the spinal cord. Pain is initiated when there is injury to a cell causing a release of three chemicals, *substance P*, *prostaglandin*, and *leukotrienes*, which sensitize the nociceptors in and around the area of injury by lowering their depolarization threshold. This is referred to as *primary hyperalgesia*, in which the nerve's threshold to noxious stimuli is lowered, thus enhancing the pain response.[5] Over a period of several hours, *secondary hyperalgesia* occurs, as chemicals spread throughout the surrounding tissues, increasing the size of the painful area and creating hypersensitivity.

Nociceptors initiate the electrical impulses along two afferent fibers toward the spinal cord. Aδ and C fibers transmit sensations of pain and temperature from peripheral nociceptors. The majority of the fibers are C fibers. Aδ fibers have larger diameters and faster conduction velocities. This difference results in two qualitatively different types of pain, termed acute and chronic.[19] *Acute pain* is rapidly transmitted over the larger, faster-conducting Aδ afferent neurons and originates from receptors located in the skin.[19] It is localized and short, lasting only as long as there is a stimulus, such as the initial pain of an unexpected pinprick. *Chronic pain* is transmitted by the C fiber afferent neurons and originates from both superficial skin tissue and deeper ligament and muscle tissue. This pain is an aching, throbbing, or burning sensation that is poorly localized and less specifically related to the stimulus. There is a delay in the perception of pain following injury, but the pain will continue long after the noxious stimulus is removed.[5]

The various types of afferent fibers follow different courses as they ascend toward the brain. Some Aδ and most C afferent neurons enter the spinal cord through the dorsal horn of the spinal cord and synapse in the SG with a second-order neuron (Figure 4–7).[20] Most nociceptive second-order neurons ascend to higher centers along one of the three tracts—(1) the lateral spinothalamic tract, (2) spinoreticular tract, or (3) spinoencephalic tract—with the remainder ascending along the spinocervical tract.[20] About 80% of nociceptive second-order neurons ascend to higher centers along the lateral spinothalamic tract.[20] Approximately 90%

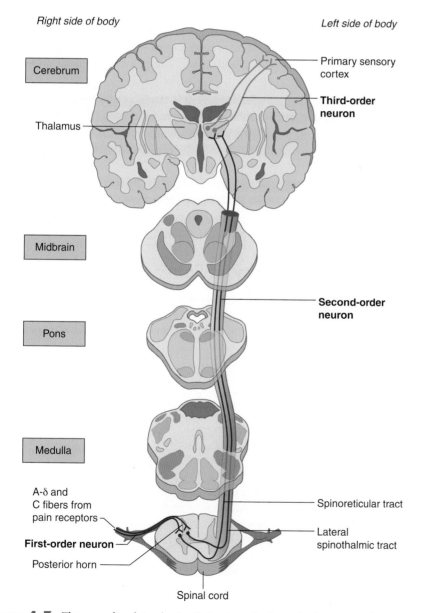

Figure 4–7. The ascending lateral spinothalamic and spinoreticular tract in the spinal cord carries pain information to the cortex.

of the second-order afferents terminate in the thalamus.[20] Third-order neurons project to the sensory cortex and numerous other centers in the central nervous system (see Figure 4–6).

These projections allow us to perceive pain. They also permit the integration of past experiences and emotions that form our response to the pain experience. These connections are also believed to be parts of complex circuits that the clinician may stimulate to manage pain. Most analgesic physical agents are believed to slow or block the impulses ascending along the Aδ and C afferent neuron pathways through direct input into the dorsal horn or through descending mechanisms. These pathways are discussed in more detail in the following section.

NEUROPHYSIOLOGIC EXPLANATIONS OF PAIN CONTROL

The neurophysiologic mechanisms of pain control through stimulation of cutaneous receptors have not been fully explained.[21] Much of what is known—and current theory—is the result of work involving electroacupuncture and transcutaneous electrical nerve stimulation. However, this information often provides an explanation for the analgesic response to other modalities, such as massage, analgesic balms, and moist heat.

The concepts of the analgesic response to cutaneous receptor stimulation presented here were first proposed by Melzack and Wall[22] and Castel.[23] These models essentially present three analgesic mechanisms:

1. Stimulation from ascending Aβ afferents results in blocking impulses at the spinal cord level of pain messages carried along Aδ and C afferent fibers (gate control).
2. Stimulation of descending pathways in the dorsolateral tract of the spinal cord by Aδ and C fiber afferent input results in a blocking of the impulses carried along the Aδ and C afferent fibers.
3. The stimulation of Aδ and C afferent fibers causes the release of endogenous opioids (β-endorphin), resulting in a prolonged activation of descending analgesic pathways.

These theories or models are not necessarily mutually exclusive. Recent evidence suggests that pain relief may result from combinations of dorsal horn and central nervous system activity.[24,25]

The Gate Control Theory of Pain

The gate control theory explains how a stimulus that activates only non-nociceptive nerves can inhibit pain (Figure 4–8).[22] Three peripheral nerve fibers are involved in this mechanism of pain control: Aδ fibers, which transmit noxious impulses associated with intense pain;

Mechanisms of pain control are as follows:
- blocking ascending pathways (gate control);
- blocking descending pathways;
- release of β-endorphin and dynorphin.

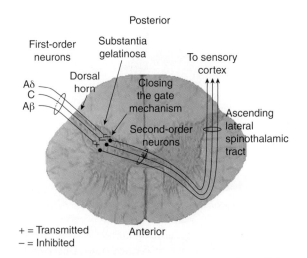

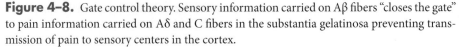

Figure 4–8. Gate control theory. Sensory information carried on Aβ fibers "closes the gate" to pain information carried on Aδ and C fibers in the substantia gelatinosa preventing transmission of pain to sensory centers in the cortex.

C fibers, which carry noxious impulses associated with long-term or chronic pain; and Aβ fibers, which carry sensory information from cutaneous receptors but are non-nociceptive and do not transmit pain. Impulses ascending on these fibers stimulate the SG as they enter the dorsal horn of the spinal cord. Essentially the non-nociceptive Aβ fibers inhibit the effects of the Aδ and C pain fibers, effectively "closing a gate" to the transmission of their stimuli to the second-order interneurons. Thus, the only information that is transmitted on the second-order neurons through the ascending lateral spinothalamic tract to the cortex is the information from the Aβ fibers. The "pain message" carried along the smaller-diameter Aδ and C fibers is not transmitted to the second-order neurons and never reaches sensory centers.

The discovery and isolation of endogenous opioids in the 1970s led to new theories of pain relief. Castel introduced an endogenous opioid analog to the gate control theory.[23] This theory proposes that increased neural activity in Aβ primary afferent pathways triggers a release of enkephalin from **enkephalin interneurons** found in the dorsal horn. These neuroactive amines inhibit synaptic transmission in the Aδ and C fiber afferent pathways. The end result, as in the gate control theory, is that the pain message is blocked before it reaches sensory levels.

The concept of sensory stimulation for pain relief, as proposed by the gate control theory, has empirical support. Rubbing a contusion, applying moist heat, or massaging sore muscles decreases the perception of pain. The analgesic response to these treatments is attributed to the increased stimulation of Aβ afferent fibers. A decrease in input along nociceptive Aδ and C afferents also results in pain relief. Cooling afferent fibers decreases the rate at which they conduct impulses. Thus, a 20-minute application of cold is effective in relieving pain because of the decrease in activity, rather than an increase in activity along afferent pathways.

Descending Pain Control

A second mechanism of pain control essentially expands the original gate control theory of pain control and involves input from higher centers in the brain through a descending system (Figure 4–9).[26] Emotions (such as anger, fear, stress), previous experiences, sensory perceptions, and other factors coming from the thalamus in the cerebrum stimulate the **periaqueductal gray** (PAG) matter of the midbrain. The pathway over which this pain reduction takes place is a dorsal lateral projection from cells in the PAG to an area in the medulla of the brain stem called the **raphe nucleus**. When the PAG fires, the raphe nucleus also fires. Serotonergic efferent pathways from the raphe nucleus project to the dorsal horn along the entire length of the spinal cord where they synapse with enkephalin interneurons located in the substantia gelitanosa.[27] The activation of enkephalin interneuron synapses by serotonin suppresses the release of the neurotransmitter substance P from Aδ and C fibers used by the sensory neurons involved in the perception of chronic and/or intense pain. Additionally, enkephalin is released into the synapse between the enkephalin interneuron and the second-order neuron that inhibits synaptic transmission of impulses from incoming Aδ and C fibers to the second-order afferent neurons that transmit the pain signal up the lateral spinothalamic tract to the thalamus (Figure 4–10).[28]

A second descending, noradrenergic pathway projecting from the pons to the dorsal horn has also been identified.[20] The significance of these parallel pathways is not fully understood. It is also not known if these noradrenergic fibers directly inhibit dorsal horn synapses or stimulate the enkephalin interneurons.

This model provides a physiologic explanation for the analgesic response to brief, intense stimulation. The analgesia following acupressure and the use of some transcutaneous electrical nerve stimulators (TENS), such as point stimulators, is attributed to this descending pain control mechanism.[38,39,40]

Clinical Decision-Making   *Exercise 4–1*

The clinician is interested in an injured patient's subjective perception of pain following a TENS treatment designed to reduce pain. Describe the steps you would take to evaluate pain and suggest which pain scale you might choose to use.

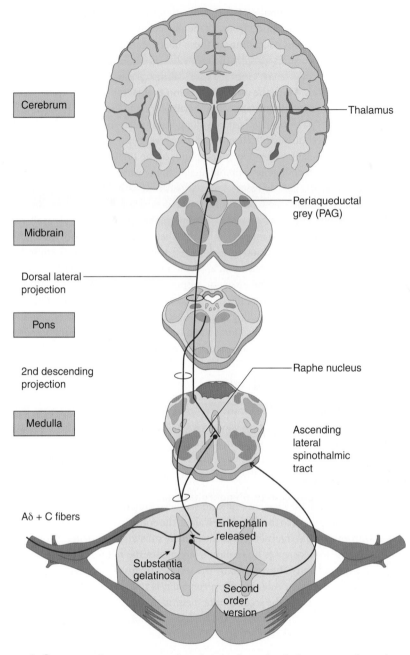

Figure 4–9. Descending pain control. Influence from the thalamus stimulates the periaqueductal gray, the raphe nucleus, and the pons to inhibit the transmission of pain impulses through the ascending tracts.

β-Endorphin and Dynorphin in Pain Control

There is evidence that stimulation of the small-diameter afferents (Aδ and C) can stimulate the release of other endogenous opioids called **endorphins**.[7,17,21,22,25,26,29] β-Endorphin and dynorphin are endogenous opioid peptide neurotransmitters found in the neurons of both the central and peripheral nervous system.[30] The mechanisms regulating the release of β-endorphin and dynorphin have not been fully elucidated. However, it is apparent that these endogenous substances play a role in the analgesic response to some forms of stimuli used in the treatment of patients in pain.

β-Endorphin is released into the blood from the anterior pituitary gland and into the brain and spinal cord from the hypothalamus.[30] In the anterior pituitary gland, it shares a

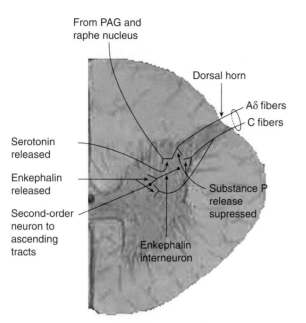

From PAG and
raphe nucleus

Dorsal horn

Aδ fibers

C fibers

Serotonin
released

Enkephalin
released

Substance P
release
supressed

Second-order
neuron to
ascending
tracts

Enkephalin
interneuron

Figure 4–10. The enkephalin interneuron functions to inhibit transmission of pain between the Aδ and C fibers and the second-order neuron to the ascending tracts.

prohormone with adrenocorticotropin (**ACTH**). Thus, when β-endorphin is released, so too is ACTH. β-Endorphin does not readily cross the blood–brain barrier,[19] and thus the anterior pituitary gland is not the sole source of β-endorphin.[31,41]

As stated previously, pain information is transmitted to the brain stem and thalamus primarily on two different pathways, the spinothalamic and spinoreticular tracts. Spinothalamic input is thought to effect the conscious sensation of pain, and the spinoreticular tract is thought to effect the arousal and emotional aspects of pain. Pain stimuli from these two tracts stimulate the release of β-endorphin from the hypothalamus (Figure 4–11). β-Endorphin released into the nervous system binds to specific opiate-binding sites in the nervous system. The neurons in the hypothalamus that send projections to the PAG and noradrenergic nuclei in the brain stem contain β-endorphin. Prolonged (20–40 minutes) small-diameter afferent fiber stimulation via electroacupuncture has been thought to trigger the release of β-endorphin.[21,41] It is likely that β-endorphin released from these neurons by stimulation of the hypothalamus is responsible for initiating the same mechanisms in the spinal cord as previously described with other descending mechanisms of pain control.[36,43] Once again, further research is needed to clarify where and how these substances are released and how the release of β-endorphin affects neural activity and pain perception.

Dynorphin, a more recently isolated endogenous opioid, is found in the PAG, rostroventral medulla, and the dorsal horn.[20] It has been demonstrated that dynorphin is released during electroacupuncture.[32] Dynorphin may be responsible for suppressing the response to noxious mechanical stimulation.[20]

Summary of Pain Control Mechanisms

The body's pain control mechanisms are probably not mutually exclusive. Rather, analgesia is the result of overlapping processes. It is also important to realize that the theories presented are only models. They are useful in conceptualizing the perception of pain and pain relief. These models will help the clinician understand the effects of therapeutic modalities and form a sound rationale for modality application.[8] As more research is conducted and as the mysteries of pain and neurophysiology are solved, new models will emerge. The clinician should adapt these models to fit new developments.

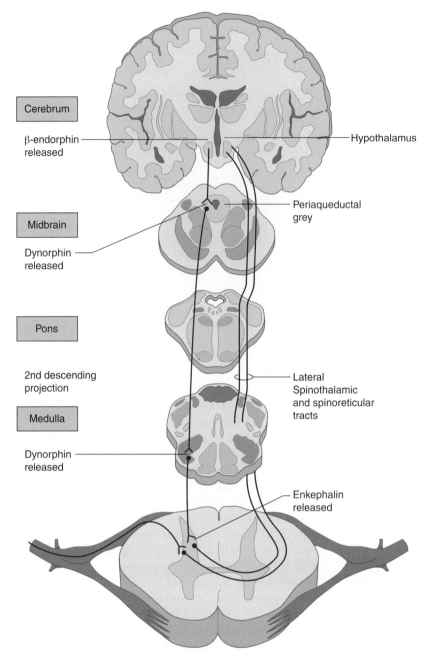

Figure 4–11. β-Endorphin released from the hypothalamus, and dynorphin released from the periaqueductal gray and the medulla modulate.

PAIN MANAGEMENT

How should the clinician approach pain? First, the source of the pain must be identified. Unidentified pain may hide a serious disorder, and treatment of such pain may delay the appropriate treatment of the disorder.[33] Once a diagnosis has been made, many physical agents can provide pain relief. The clinician should match the therapeutic agent to each patient's situation. Casts and braces may prevent the application of ice or moist heat. However, TENS electrodes often can be positioned under a cast or brace for pain relief. Following acute injuries, ice may be the therapeutic agent of choice because of the effect of cold on the inflammatory process. There is not one "best" therapeutic agent for pain control. The clinician must select the therapeutic agent that is most appropriate for each patient, based on the knowledge

CASE STUDY 4–1
MANAGING ACUTE PAIN

Background: Stacey is a 21-year-old college basketball player referred for physical therapy the day after arthroscopic surgery to remove loose bodies and a tear in the medial meniscus of her left knee.

Impression: She is typical of patients presenting the day following acute injury and surgery. She is experiencing considerable discomfort and demonstrates inhibition of the quadriceps muscles and an unwillingness to flex and extend the knee.

Treatment Plan: Stacey was treated with an ice bag around the knee for 20 minutes, being careful to protect the common peroneal nerve on the posterior lateral aspect of the knee. Following cold application, she was encouraged to perform quadriceps setting and heel slides.

Response: Her volitional control of the quadriceps improved and she left the clinic able to perform a straight leg raise without a lag. She was also able to move the knee from extension to 50 degrees of flexion. She was sent home with instructions to use cold three to four times daily followed by the previously described exercises. Stacey demonstrated active range of motion from terminal extension to 115 degrees of flexion and good control of the quadriceps on return to the clinic 5 days later. Her rehabilitation progressed well and she returned to playing basketball within 3 weeks in preparation for the upcoming season.

Surgery results in acute pain and the associated guarding, splinting, and neuromuscular inhibition. When active muscle contractions and range of motion exercises can be performed safely, the use of therapeutic modalities can assist the patient regain function. In this case, cold was selected because of the acute presentation and the ease of use at home. TENS also would have been appropriate, either alone or in combination with cold. It is also important to appreciate the effects of pain-free movement on the recovery process. Movement lessens the sensation of stiffness postoperatively and provides large-diameter afferent input into the dorsal horn, which may relieve pain through a gating mechanism or the stimulation of enkephalin interneurons.

The rehabilitation professional employs physical agent modalities to create an optimum environment for tissue healing while minimizing the symptoms associated with the trauma or condition.

Discussion Questions

- What tissues were injured/affected?
- What symptoms were present?
- What phase of the injury-healing continuum did the patient present for care in?
- What are the physical agent modality's biophysical effects (direct/indirect/depth/tissue affinity)?
- What are the physical agent modality's indications/contraindications?
- What are the parameters of the physical agent modality's application/dosage/duration/frequency in this case study?
- What other physical agent modalities could be utilized to treat this injury or condition? Why? How?

of the modalities and professional judgment.[34] In no situation should the clinician apply a therapeutic agent without first developing a clear rationale for the treatment.[35]

In general, physical agents can be used to:

1. stimulate large-diameter afferent fibers ($A\beta$)—this can be done with TENS, massage, and analgesic balms;
2. decrease pain fiber transmission velocity with cold or ultrasound;
3. stimulate small-diameter afferent fibers ($A\delta$ and C) and descending pain control mechanisms with acupressure, deep massage, or TENS over acupuncture points or trigger points;
4. stimulate a release of β-endorphin and dynorphin or other endogenous opioids through prolonged small-diameter fiber stimulation with TENS.[17]

Other useful pain control strategies include the following:

1. Encourage cognitive processes that influence pain perception, such as motivation, tension diversion, focusing, relaxation techniques, positive thinking, thought stopping, and self-control.
2. Minimize the tissue damage through the application of proper first aid and immobilization.

3. Maintain a line of communication with the patient. Let the patient know what to expect following an injury. Pain, swelling, dysfunction, and atrophy will occur following injury. The patient's anxiety over these events will increase his or her perception of pain. Often, a patient who has been told what to expect by someone he or she trusts will be less anxious and suffer less pain.

4. Recognize that all pain, even psychosomatic pain, is very real to the patient.

5. Encourage supervised exercise to encourage blood flow, promote nutrition, increase metabolic activity, and reduce stiffness and guarding if the activity will not cause further harm to the patient.

Clinical Decision-Making *Exercise 4–2*

In addition to managing pain through the use of therapeutic modalities, the clinician should make every effort to encourage the cognitive processes that can influence pain perception. What techniques can be taught to the patient to take advantage of the cognitive aspects of pain modulation?

The physician may choose to prescribe oral or injectable medications in the treatment of the patient. The most commonly used medications are classified as analgesics, anti-inflammatory agents, or both. The clinician should become familiar with these drugs and note if the patient is taking any medications. It is also important to work with the referring physician to assure that the patient takes the medications appropriately.

CASE STUDY 4–2
MANAGING CHRONIC PAIN

Background: Linda is a 31-year-old resident in oral surgery. She was referred for physical therapy for complaints of upper back and neck pain with frequent headaches. She states that she has been experiencing the symptoms off and on for about 2 years. Her symptoms are worse at the end of the work day, especially on days she is in the operating room. There is no history of trauma to the affected region.

Physical exam reveals a forward head, rounded shoulder posture, spasm of the cervical paraspinal and trapezius muscles, and very sensitive trigger points throughout the region.

Impression: Her symptoms were consistent with pain of myofascial origin secondary to posture, job-related stress, and fatigue of the postural muscles.

Treatment Plan: She was treated with TENS over the trigger points using a Neuroprobe, soft tissue mobilization, and instructed in a routine of postural exercises. She was encouraged to perform postural exercises and relaxation activities during breaks in her schedule. Linda returned to the clinic indicating she had experienced near complete relief following her first visit for about 6 hours. The stimulation of trigger points was repeated, and Linda was instructed in the use of a

TENS unit with conventional parameters over her most sensitive trigger point. She had access to the TENS unit through the surgical clinic where she worked.

Response: Linda was seen for two additional visits. She indicated her compliance with the exercise program, which was subsequently expanded into a general conditioning program with an emphasis on upper body endurance. She also indicated that her symptoms were becoming much less severe and less frequent and that the home TENS unit gave her a means of controlling her pain before it became severe enough to affect her activities. Over the subsequent several months, Linda completed her residency without additional care for her neck and upper back.

Myofascial pain or pain of soft tissue origin has several causes, many of which may contribute to a single individual's symptoms. Poor posture, stress, repetitive microtrauma, and acute injuries can combine to cause a pain pattern that is often difficult to understand. The keys to management are to identify the causative factors and help the patient address them. In this case, Linda had to recondition postural muscles to restore balance between antagonistic groups.

(continued)

CASE STUDY 4–2 *(continued)*
MANAGING CHRONIC PAIN

Her long hours of standing over operating tables had contributed to her postural deficits. She also became more aware of how she responded to stressors and began using relaxation techniques with which she was familiar.

Her four visits to physical therapy enabled us to identify the causes of Linda's pain, break the pain spasm cycle, desensitize her trigger points, and initiate a program of progressive, pain-free exercises. Pain control is essential in the management of myofascial pain. Exercise that is painful further sensitizes trigger points and promotes the use of inefficient, antalgic movement patterns.

The rehabilitation professional employs physical agent modalities to create an optimum environment for tissue healing while minimizing the symptoms associated with the trauma or condition.

Discussion Questions

- What tissues were injured/affected?
- What symptoms were present?
- What phase of the injury-healing continuum did the patient present for care in?
- What are the physical agent modality's biophysical effects (direct/indirect/depth/tissue affinity)?
- What are the physical agent modality's indications/contraindications?
- What are the parameters of the physical agent modality's application/dosage/duration/frequency in this case study?
- What other physical agent modalities could be utilized to treat this injury or condition? Why? How?

The clinician's approach to the patient has a great impact on the success of the treatment. The patient will not be convinced of the efficacy and importance of the treatment unless the clinician appears confident about it. The clinician must make the patient a participant rather than a passive spectator in the treatment and rehabilitation process.

The goal of most treatment programs is to encourage early pain-free exercise. The physical agents used to control pain do little to promote tissue healing. They should be used to relieve acute pain following injury or surgery or to control pain and other symptoms, such as swelling, to promote progressive exercise. The clinician should not lose sight of the effects of the physical agents or the importance of progressive exercise in restoring the patient's functional ability.

Clinical Decision-Making *Exercise 4–3*

A patient asks the clinician to explain why electrical stimulation of a trigger point can help reduce pain in his or her shoulder. What is the explanation?

Reducing the perception of pain is as much an art as a science. Selection of the proper physical agent, proper application, and marketing are all important and will continue to be so even as we increase our understanding of the neurophysiology of pain. There is still the need for a good empirical rationale for the use of a physical agent. The clinician is encouraged to keep abreast of the neurophysiology of pain and the physiology of tissue healing to maintain a current scientific basis for selecting modalities and managing the pain experienced by his or her patients.

Clinical Decision-Making *Exercise 4–4*

A patient is complaining of pain in the low back from a muscle strain. The clinician plans to incorporate a modality that will affect the ascending pathways, in effect "closing the gate" to ascending pain fibers. What modalities can be used to take advantage of the gate control theory of pain modulation?

SUMMARY

1. Pain is a response to a noxious stimulus that is subjectively modified by past experiences and expectations.
2. Pain is classified as either acute or chronic and can exhibit many different patterns.
3. Early reduction of pain in a treatment program will facilitate therapeutic exercise.
4. Stimulation of sensory receptors via the therapeutic modalities can modify the patient's perception of pain.
5. Three mechanisms of pain control may explain the analgesic effects of physical agents:
    (a.) dorsal horn modulation due to the input from large-diameter afferents through a gate control system, the release of enkephalins, or both;
    (b.) descending efferent fiber activation due to the effects of small-fiber afferent input on higher centers including the thalamus, raphe nucleus, and PAG region;
    (c.) the release of endogenous opioids including β-endorphin through prolonged small-diameter afferent stimulation.
6. Pain perception may be influenced by a variety of cognitive processes mediated by the higher brain centers.
7. The selection of a therapeutic modality for controlling pain should be based on current knowledge of neurophysiology and the psychology of pain.
8. The application of physical agents for the control of pain should not occur until the diagnosis of the injury has been established.
9. The selection of a therapeutic modality for managing pain should be based on establishing the primary cause of pain.

REVIEW QUESTIONS

1. What is the basic definition of pain?
2. What are the different types of pain?
3. What are the different assessment scales available to help the clinician determine the extent of pain perception?
4. What are the characteristics of the various sensory receptors?
5. How does the nervous system relay information about painful stimuli?
6. Describe how the gate control mechanism of pain modulation may be used to modulate pain.
7. How do the descending pain control mechanisms function to modulate pain?
8. What are the opiatelike substances, and how do they act to modulate pain?
9. How can pain perception be modified by cognitive factors?
10. How can the clinician help modulate pain during a rehabilitation program?

SELF-TEST QUESTIONS

True or False

1. Both sclerotomic and radiating pain may cause pain away from the site of the disorder.
2. Afferent nerve fibers conduct impulses from the brain to peripheral sites.
3. Serotonin and β-endorphin affect synaptic activity.

Multiple Choice

4. Which of the following is *not* a method of pain assessment?
    a. MPQ
    b. Snellen test
    c. visual analog scales
    d. numeric pain scale

5. Pain receptors in the body are called _____.
   a. Meissner's corpuscles
   b. Krause's end bulbs
   c. Pacinian corpuscles
   d. nociceptors

6. Which of the following plays a role in transmitting sensations of pain?
   a. substance P
   b. enkephalin
   c. dynorphin
   d. serotonin

7. Which of the following is/are characteristic(s) of Aδ fibers?
   a. large-diameter fibers
   b. fast conduction velocities
   c. transmission of brief, localized pain
   d. all of the above

8. Stimulation of the SG occurs in the _____ theory of pain.
   a. space
   b. descending
   c. gate control
   d. enkephalin release

9. β-Endorphin, an endogenous opioid, is released from the _____.
   a. hypothalamus
   b. anterior pituitary gland
   c. raphe nucleus
   d. a and b

10. Which of the following cognitive processes may affect pain perception?
    a. depression
    b. past pain experiences
    c. both a and b
    d. neither a nor b

SOLUTIONS TO CLINICAL DECISION-MAKING EXERCISES

4–1

After conducting a detailed evaluation, a number of options are available, including visual analog scales, pain charts, the MPQ, the Activity Pattern Indicators Pain Profile, and numeric pain scales. Numeric pain scales, in which the patient is asked to rate his or her pain on a scale from 1 to 10, are perhaps the most widely used in the athletic training setting.

4–2

The clinician may choose to use relaxation techniques, tension diversion, focusing, positive thinking, thought stopping, and self-control techniques. Certainly the cognitive perception of pain and the ability to control that perception is an aspect of rehabilitation that the clinician should take very seriously.

4–3

The clinician should explain that stimulating the trigger point with an electrical stimulating current will trigger the release of a chemical (β-endorphin) in the brain that will act to modulate pain in the shoulder.

4–4

The modality selected should provide a significant amount of cutaneous input that would be transmitted to the spinal cord along Aβ fibers. The modalities of choice may include various types of heat or cold, electrical stimulating currents, counterirritants (analgesic balms), or massage.

REFERENCES

1. Merskey H, Albe Fessard D, Bonica J. Pain terms: a list with definitions and notes on usage. *Pain*. 1979;6:249–252.
2. Melzack R. Concepts of pain measurement. In: Melzack R, ed. *Pain Measurement and Assessment*. New York: Raven Press; 1983.
3. Beissner K, Henderson C, Papaleontiou M. Physical therapists' use of cognitive–behavioral therapy for older adults with chronic pain: a nationwide survey. *Phys Ther*. 2009; 89(5):456–469.
4. Deleo J. Basic science of pain. *Am J Bone Joint Surg*. 2006; 88(2):58.
5. Kahanov L, Kato M, Kaminski T. Therapeutic modalities. Therapeutic effect of joint mobilization: joint mechanoreceptors and nociceptors. *Athletic Ther Today*. 2007;12(4):28–31.
6. Fedorczyk J. The role of physical agents in modulating pain. *J Hand Ther*. 1997;10:110–121.
7. Willis W, Grossman R. *Medical Neurobiology*. 3rd ed. St. Louis: Mosby; 1981.
8. Aronson P. Pain theories—a review for application in athletic training and therapy. *Athletic Ther Today*. 2002;7(4):8–13.
9. Bowsher D. Central pain mechanisms. In: Wells P, Frampton V, Bowsher D, eds. *Pain Management in Physical Therapy*. Norwalk, CT: Appleton & Lange; 1994.
10. Fishman S, Ballantyne J. *Bonica's Management of Pain*. Philadelphia: Lippincott Williams and Wilkins; 2009.
11. Previte J. *Human Physiology*. New York: McGraw-Hill Inc; 1983.
12. Merskey H, Bogduk N. *Classification of Chronic Pain. Definitions of Chronic Pain Syndromes and Definition of Pain Terms*. 2nd ed. Seattle: International Association for the Study of Pain; 1994.
13. Addison R. Chronic pain syndrome. *Am J Med*. 1985;77:54.
14. Mattacola C, Perrin D, Gansneder B. A comparison of visual analog and graphic rating scales for assessing pain following delayed onset muscle soreness. *J Sport Rehabil*. 1997;6:38–46.
15. Huskisson E. Visual analogue scales. Pain measurement and assessment. In: Melzack R, ed. *Pain Measurement and Assessment*. New York: Raven Press; 1983.
16. Margoles M. The pain chart: spatial properties of pain. Pain measurement and assessment. In: Melzack R, ed. *Pain Measurement and Assessment*. New York: Raven Press; 1983.
17. Saluka K. *Mechanisms and Management of Pain for the Physical Therapist*. Seattle: International Association for the Study of Pain; 2009.
18. Miyazaki T. Pain mechanisms and pain clinic. *Jpn J Clin Sports Med*. 2005;13(2):183.
19. Berne R. *Physiology*. St. Louis: Elsevier Health Sciences; 2004.
20. Jessell T, Kelly D. Pain and analgesia. In: Kandel E, Schwartz J, Jessell T, eds. *Principles of Neural Science*. Norwalk, CT: Appleton & Lange; 1991.
21. Wolf S. Neurophysiologic mechanisms in pain modulation: relevance to TENS. In: Manheimer J, Lampe G, eds. *Sports Medicine Applications of TENS*. Philadelphia: FA Davis Co; 1984.
22. Melzack R, Wall P. Pain mechanisms: a new theory. *Science*. 1965;150:971–979.
23. Castel J. *Pain Management: Acupuncture and Transcutaneous Electrical Nerve Stimulation Techniques*. Lake Bluff, IL: Pain Control Services; 1979.
24. Allen RJ. Physical agents used in the management of chronic pain by physical therapists. *Phys Med Rehabil Clin North Am*. 2006;17(2):315–345.
25. Clement-Jones V, McLaughlin L, Tomlin S. Increased beta-endorphin but not met-enkephalin levels in human cerebrospinal fluid after electroacupuncture for recurrent pain. *Lancet*. 1980;2:946–948.
26. Chapman C, Benedetti C. Analgesia following electrical stimulation: partial reversal by a narcotic antagonist. *Life Sci*. 1979;26:44–48.
27. Millan MJ. Descending control of pain. *Prog Neurobiol*. 2002;66:355–474.
28. Gebhart G. Descending modulation of pain. *Neurosci Biobehav Rev*. 2004;27:729–737.
29. Sjoland B, Eriksson M. Increased cerebrospinal fluid levels of endorphins after electro-acupuncture. *Acta Physiol Scand*. 1977;100:382–384.
30. Stein C. The control of pain in peripheral tissue by opioids. *N Engl J Med*. 1995;332:1685–1690.
31. Denegar G, Perrin D, Rogol A. Influence of transcutaneous electrical nerve stimulation on pain, range of motion and serum cortisol concentration in females with induced delayed onset muscle soreness. *J Orthop Sports Phys Ther*. 1989;11:101–103.
32. Ho W, Wen H. Opioid-like activity in the cerebrospinal fluid of pain athletes treated by electroacupuncture. *Neuropharmacology*. 1989;28:961–966.
33. Cohen S, Christo P, Moroz L. Pain management in trauma patients. *Am J Phys Med Rehabil*. 2004;83(2):142–161.
34. Curtis N. Understanding and managing pain. *Athletic Ther Today*. 2002;7(4):32.
35. Bishop B. Pain: its physiology and rationale for management. *Phys Ther*. 1980;60:13–37.
36. Cheng R, Pomeranz B. Electroacupuncture analgesia could be mediated by at least two pain relieving mechanisms: endorphin and non-endorphin systems. *Life Sci*. 1979;25:1957–1962.
37. Dickerman J. The use of pain profiles in sports medicine practice. *Fam Pract Recertification*. 1992;14(3):35–44.
38. Mayer D, Price D, Rafii A. Antagonism of acupuncture analgesia in man by the narcotic antagonist naloxone. *Brain Res*. 1977;121:368–372.
39. Pomeranz B, Paley D. Brain opiates at work in acupuncture. *New Scientist*. 1975;73:12–13.
40. Pomeranz B, Chiu D. Naloxone blockade of acupuncture analgesia: enkephalin implicated. *Life Sci*. 1976;19(10): 1757–1762.

41. Pomeranz B, Paley D. Electro-acupuncture hypoalgesia is mediated by afferent impulses: an electrophysiological study in mice. *Exp Neurol.* 1979;66:398–402.

42. Salar G, Job I, Mingringo S. Effects of transcutaneous electrotherapy on CSF beta-endorphin content in athletes without pain problems. *Pain.* 1981;10:169–172.

43. Wen H, Ho W, Ling N. The influence of electroacupuncture on naloxone: induces morphine withdrawal: elevation of immunoassayable beta-endorphin activity in the brain but not in the blood. *Am J Clin Med.* 1979;7:237–240.

GLOSSARY

accommodation   Adaptation by the sensory receptors to various stimuli over an extended period of time.

ACTH   Adrenocorticotropic hormone. This hormone stimulates the release of glucocorticoids (cortisol) from the adrenal glands.

afferent   Conduction of a nerve impulse toward an organ.

dynorphin   An endogenous opioid.

efferent   Conduction of a nerve impulse away from an organ.

endogenous opioids   Opiatelike neuroactive peptide substances made by the body.

β-endorphin   A neurohormone similar in structure and properties to morphine.

endorphins   Endogenous opioids whose actions have analgesic properties (i.e., β-endorphin).

enkephalin   Neurotransmitter that blocks the passage of noxious stimuli from first- to second-order afferents. It inhibits the release of substance P and is produced by enkephalinergic neurons.

enkephalin interneurons   Neurons with short axons that release enkephalin. They are widespread in the central nervous system and are found in the substantia gelatinosa, nucleus raphe magnus, and periaqueductal gray matter.

focusing   Narrowing attention to the appropriate stimuli in the environment.

interneurons   Neurons contained entirely in the central nervous system. They have no projections outside the spinal cord. Their function is to serve as relay stations within the central nervous system.

neurotransmitter   Substance that passes information between neurons.

nociceptor   Pain information or signals of pain stimuli.

norepinephrine   A neurotransmitter.

periaqueductal gray   A midbrain structure that plays an important role in descending tracts that inhibit synaptic transmission of noxious input in the dorsal horn.

raphe nucleus   Part of the medulla in the brain stem that is known to inhibit pain impulses being transmitted through the ascending system.

sclerotome   A segment of bone innervated by a spinal segment.

serotonin   A neurotransmitter found in descending pathways. It is thought to play a significant role in pain control.

substance P   The neurotransmitter of small-diameter primary afferent. It is released from both ends of the neuron.

substantia gelatinosa (SG)   The dorsal horn of the gray matter thought to be the mechanism responsible for closing the gate to painful stimuli.

trigger point   Localized deep tenderness in a palpable firm band of muscle. *When stretched, a palpating finger* can snap the band like a taut string, which produces local pain, a local twitch of that portion of the muscle, and a jump by the patient. Sustained pressure on a trigger point reproduces the pattern of referred pain for that site.

PART **TWO**
Electrical Energy Modalities

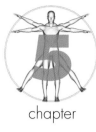

chapter 5

Basic Principles of Electricity and Electrical Stimulating Currents

Daniel N. Hooker and William E. Prentice

OBJECTIVES

Following completion of this chapter, the student will be able to:

➤ Define the most common terminology related to electricity.

➤ Differentiate between monophasic, biphasic, and pulsatile currents.

➤ Categorize various waveforms and pulse characteristics.

➤ Contrast the various types of current modulation.

➤ Discriminate between series and parallel circuit arrangements.

➤ Explain current flow through various types of biologic tissue.

➤ Explain muscle, nerve, and nonexcitatory cell responses to electrical stimulation.

➤ Describe how current flows through biologic tissue.

➤ Discuss the various treatment parameters including frequency, intensity, duration, and polarity that must be considered with electrical stimulating currents.

➤ Differentiate between the various currents that can be selected on many modern generators including high volt, biphasic, microcurrent, Russian, interferential, premodulated interferential, and low volt.

➤ Compare techniques for modulating pain through the use of transcutaneous electrical nerve stimulators.

➤ Be able to create a safe environment when using electrical equipment.

Many of the modalities discussed in this book may be classified as electrical modalities. These pieces of equipment have the capabilities of taking the electrical current flowing from a wall outlet and modifying that current to produce a specific, desired physiologic effect in human biologic tissue.

Understanding the basic principles of electricity usually is difficult even for the clinician who is accustomed to using electrical modalities on a daily basis. To understand how

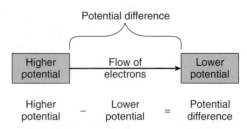

Figure 5–1. The difference between high potential and low potential is potential difference. Electrons tend to flow from areas of higher concentration to areas of lower concentration. A potential difference must exist if there is to be any movement of electrons.

current flow affects biologic tissue, it is first necessary to become familiar with some of the principles and terminology that describe how electricity is produced and how it behaves in an electrical circuit.[172,180,186]

COMPONENTS OF ELECTRICAL CURRENTS

All matter is composed of atoms that contain positively and negatively charged particles called **ions**. These charged particles possess electrical energy and thus have the ability to move about. They tend to move from an area of higher concentration toward an area of lower concentration. An electrical force is capable of propelling these particles from higher to lower energy levels, thus establishing **electrical potentials**. The more ions an object has, the higher its potential electrical energy is. Particles with a positive charge tend to move toward negatively charged particles, and those that are negatively charged tend to move toward positively charged particles (Figure 5–1).[1]

Electrons are particles of matter possessing a negative charge and very small mass. The net movement of electrons is referred to as an **electrical current**. The movement or flow of these electrons will always go from a higher potential to a lower potential.[2] An electrical force is oriented only in the direction of the applied force. This flow of electrons may be likened to a domino reaction.

The unit of measurement that indicates the rate at which electrical current flows is the **ampere**; 1 A is defined as the movement of 1 **C** or 6.25×10^{15} electrons/s. Amperes indicate the rate of electron flow, whereas coulombs indicate the number of electrons. In the case of therapeutic modalities, **current** flow is generally described in milliamperes (1/1000 of an ampere, denoted as mA) or in microamperes (1/1,000,000 of an ampere, denoted as μA).[3]

The electrons will not move unless an electrical potential difference in the concentration of these charged particles exists between two points. The electromotive force, which must be applied to produce a flow of electrons, is called a **volt** and is defined as the difference in electron population (potential difference) between two points.[4]

Voltage is the force resulting from an accumulation of electrons at one point in an electrical circuit, usually corresponding to a deficit of electrons at another point in the circuit. If the two points are connected by a suitable conductor, the potential difference (in electron population) will cause electrons to move from the area of higher population to the area of lower population.

Commercial current flowing from wall outlets produces an electromotive force of either 115 or 220 V. The electrotherapeutic devices used in injury rehabilitation modify voltages. Electrical generators are sometimes referred to as being either low or high volt. These terms are not very useful, although some older texts have referred to generators that produce less than 150 V as *low volt* and those that produce several hundred volts as *high volt*.[4]

Electrons can move in a current only if there is a relatively easy pathway to move along. Materials that permit this free movement of electrons are referred to as **conductors**. **Conductance** is a term that defines the ease with which current flows along a conducting medium and is measured in units called siemens. Metals (copper, gold, silver, aluminum) are

Table 5-1 Electron Flow as Analogous to Water Flow	
ELECTRON FLOW	**WATER FLOW**
Volt	=Pump
Ampere	=Gallon
Ohm (property of conductor)	=Resistance (length and distance of pipe)

good conductors of electricity, as are electrolyte solutions, because both are composed of large numbers of free electrons that are given up readily. Thus, materials that offer little opposition to current flow are good conductors. Materials that resist current flow are called **insulators**. Insulators contain relatively fewer free electrons and thus offer greater resistance to electron flow. Air, wood, and glass are all considered insulators. The number of amperes flowing in a given conductor is dependent both on the voltage applied and on the conduction characteristics of the material.[5]

The opposition to electron flow in a conducting material is referred to as **resistance** or **electrical impedance** and is measured in a unit known as an **ohm**. Thus, an electrical circuit that has high resistance (ohms) will have less flow (amperes) than a circuit with less resistance and the same voltage.[6]

The mathematical relationship between current flow, voltage, and resistance is demonstrated in the following formula:

$$\text{Current flow} = \frac{\text{Voltage}}{\text{Resistance}}$$

The above formula is the mathematical expression of **Ohm's law**, which states that the current in an electrical circuit is directly proportional to the voltage and inversely proportional to the resistance.[7]

An analogy comparing the movement of water with the movement of electricity may help to clarify this relationship between current flow, voltage, and resistance (Table 5–1). For water to flow, some type of pump must create a force to produce movement. Likewise, the volt is the pump that produces the electron flow. The resistance to water flow is dependent on the length, diameter, and smoothness of the water pipe. The resistance to electrical flow depends on the characteristics of the conductor. The amount of water flowing is measured in gallons, whereas the amount of electricity flowing is measured in amperes.

The amount of energy produced by flowing water is determined by two factors: (1) the number of gallons flowing per unit of time and (2) the pressure created in the pipe. Electrical energy or power is a product of the voltage or electromotive force and the amount of current flowing. Electrical power is measured in a unit called a **watt**:

$$\text{Watt} = \text{volts} \times \text{amperes}$$

Simply, the watt indicates the rate at which electrical power is being used. A watt is defined as the electrical power needed to produce a current flow of 1 A at a pressure of 1 V.

ELECTROTHERAPEUTIC CURRENTS

Electrotherapeutic devices generate three different types of current that, when introduced into biologic tissue, are capable of producing specific physiologic changes. These three types of current are referred to as biphasic or alternating (AC), monophasic or direct (DC), or pulsatile (PC).

Monophasic or DC, also referred to in some texts as galvanic current, has an uninterrupted unidirectional flow of electrons toward the positive pole (Figure 5–2a). On most modern DC devices, the polarity and thus the direction of current flow can be reversed.[8] Some

Types of electrical current are as follows:
- biphasic or AC;
- monophasic or DC;
- pulsatile or PC.

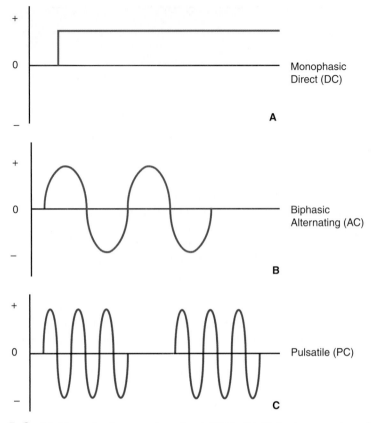

Figure 5–2. (a) Monophasic current or direct (DC). (b) Biphasic current or alternating (AC). (c) Pulsatile current (PC).

generators have the capability of automatically reversing polarity, in which case the physiologic effects will be similar to AC current.[9]

In a **biphasic or AC**, the continuous flow of electrons is bidirectional, constantly changing direction or, stated differently, reversing its polarity. Electrons flowing in an AC always move from the negative to positive pole, reversing direction when polarity is reversed (Figure 5–2b).

PC usually contain three or more pulses grouped together and may be unidirectional or bidirectional (Figure 5–2c). These groups of pulses are interrupted for short periods of time and repeat themselves at regular intervals. PC are used in interferential and so-called Russian currents.[10,11]

GENERATORS OF ELECTROTHERAPEUTIC CURRENTS

A great deal of confusion has developed relative to the terminology used to describe electrotherapeutic currents.[12,175] Basically, all therapeutic electrical generators, regardless of whether they deliver biphasic, monophasic, or PC through electrodes attached to the skin, are **transcutaneous electrical stimulators**. The majority of these are used to stimulate peripheral nerves and are correctly called **transcutaneous electrical nerve stimulators (TENS)**. Occasionally, the terms **neuromuscular electrical stimulator (NMES)** or electrical muscle stimulator (EMS) are used; however, these terms are only appropriate when the electrical current is being used to stimulate muscle directly, as would be the case with denervated muscle where peripheral nerves are not functioning. A **microcurrent electrical nerve stimulator (MENS)** uses current intensities too small to excite peripheral nerves. **Low-intensity stimulator (LIS)** is a term that has also been used to refer to **MENS**.[10,13,14] Currently MENS and LIS are most often referred to simply as **microcurrent**.

Clinical Decision-Making *Exercise 5–1*

A student asks the clinical instructor the difference between a TENS unit and an NMES unit. How should the clinical instructor respond?

Clinical Decision-Making *Exercise 5–2*

An injured lacrosse player has a strain of the right quadriceps muscle group. The clinician has decided to use a high-volt electrical stimulator to induce a muscle contraction and is explaining how the electricity will do this when the athlete becomes fearful that there will be an electrical shock. What should the clinician explain about using electrical current to reassure the patient?

There is no relationship between the type of current the generator delivers to the patient and the type of current the generator uses as a power source (i.e., a wall outlet or battery). Generators that produce electrotherapeutic currents may be driven by either AC or DC. Devices that plug into the standard electrical wall outlet use AC. The commercially produced AC changes its direction of flow 120 times/s. In other words, there are 60 complete cycles/s. The number of cycles occurring in 1 second is called **frequency** and is indicated in hertz, pulses per second (pps), or cycles per second (CPs). The voltage of electromotive force producing this alternating directional flow of electrons is set at a standard 115 or 220 V. Thus, commercial AC is produced at 60 Hz with a corresponding voltage of either 115 or 220 V.

Clinical Decision-Making *Exercise 5–3*

How can the clinician make adjustments in the electrode placement to increase the current density in the deeper tissues?

Other electrotherapeutic devices are driven by batteries that always produce DC, ranging between 1.5 and 9 V, although the devices driven by batteries may, in turn, produce modified types of current.

ELECTRICAL CIRCUITS

The path of current from a generating power source through various components back to the generating source is called an electrical **circuit**.[15] In a closed circuit, electrons are flowing, and in an open circuit, the current flow ceases. Electronic circuits are not ordinarily composed of single elements; they often encompass several branches or components with different resistances. The current in each branch may be easily calculated if the individual resistances are known and if the amount of voltage applied to the circuit is also known.[16]

We all know that with the development of the microelectronics industry, electrical circuits can be extremely complex. However, all electrical circuits have several basic components. There is a power source, which is capable of producing voltage. There is some type of conducting medium or pathway that current travels along and that carries the flowing electrons. Finally, there is some component or group of components that is driven by this flowing current. These driven elements provide resistance to electrical flow.[16]

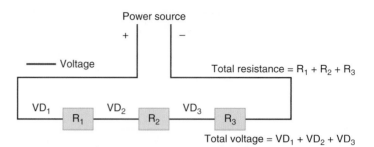

Figure 5–3. In a series circuit, the component resistors are placed end to end. The total resistance to current flow is equal to the resistance of all the components added together. There is a voltage decrease at each component such that the sum of the voltage decreases is equal to the total voltage.

Series and Parallel Circuits

The components that provide resistance to current flow may be connected to one another in one of the two different patterns, a **series circuit** or a **parallel circuit**. The main difference between these two is that in a series circuit there is only one path for current to get from one terminal to another. In a parallel circuit, two or more routes exist for current to pass between the two terminals.

In a series circuit the components are placed end to end (Figure 5–3). The number of amperes of an electrical current flowing through a series circuit is exactly the same at any point in that circuit. The resistance to current flow in this total circuit is equal to the resistance of all the components in the circuit added together:

$$R_T = R_1 + R_2 + R_3$$

Electrical energy is required to force the current through the resistor, and this energy is dissipated in the form of heat. Consequently, there is a decrease in voltage at each component such that the total voltage at the beginning of the circuit is equal to the sum of the voltage decreases at each component:

$$V_T = VD_1 + VD_2 + VD_3$$

In a parallel circuit, the component resistors are placed side by side and the ends are connected (Figure 5–4). Each of the resistors in a parallel circuit receives the same voltage.

The current passing through each component depends on its resistance. Therefore, the total voltage will be exactly the same as the voltage at each component:

$$V_T = V_1 = V_2 = V_3$$

Each additional resistance added to a parallel circuit in effect decreases the total resistance. Adding an alternative pathway, regardless of its resistance to current flow, improves the ability

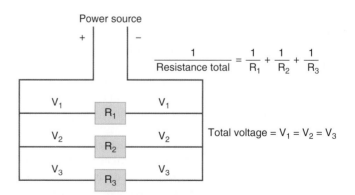

Figure 5–4. In a parallel circuit, the component resistors are placed side by side and the ends are connected. The current flow in each of the pathways is inversely proportional to the resistance of the pathway. The total voltage is the sum of the voltages at each component.

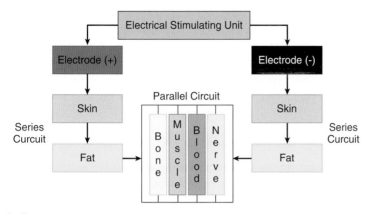

Figure 5–5. The electrical circuit that exists when electrons flow through human tissue is in reality a combination of a series and a parallel circuit.

of the current to get from one point to another. The current will, in general, choose the pathway that offers the least resistance. The formula for determining total resistance in a parallel circuit according to Ohm's law is:

$$\frac{1}{R_T} = \frac{1}{R_1} + \frac{1}{R_2} + \frac{1}{R_3}$$

Thus, component resistors connected in a series circuit have a higher resistance and lower current flow, and resistors in a parallel circuit have a lower resistance and a higher current flow.

The electrical stimulating units, in general, make use of some combination of both series and parallel circuits.[17] For example, to elicit a muscle contraction, the electrodes from an electrical stimulating unit are placed on the skin (Figure 5–5). The current from those electrodes must pass directly through the skin and fat. The total resistance to current flow seen by the electrical stimulating unit is equal to the combined resistances at each electrode. This passage of current through the skin is basically a series circuit.

After the current passes through the skin and fat, it comes in contact with a number of different types of biologic tissues (bone, connective tissue, blood, muscle). The current has several different pathways through which it may reach the muscle to be stimulated. The total current traveling through these tissues is the sum of the currents in each different type of tissue, and because there are additional tissues through which current may travel, the total resistance is effectively reduced. Thus, in this typical application of a therapeutic modality, both parallel and series circuits are used to produce the desired physiologic effect.

Current Flow through Biologic Tissues

As stated previously, electrical current tends to choose the path that offers the least resistance to flow or, stated differently, the material that is the best conductor.[18] The conductivity of the different types of tissue in the body is variable. Typically, tissue that is highest in water content and consequently highest in ion content is the best conductor of electricity.

The skin has different layers that vary in water content, but generally the skin offers the primary resistance to current flow and is considered an insulator. Skin preparation for the purpose of reducing electrical impedance is of primary concern with electrodiagnostic apparatus, but it is also important with electrotherapeutic devices. The greater the impedance of the skin, the higher the voltage of the electrical current must be to stimulate underlying nerve and muscle. Chemical changes in the skin can make it more resistant to certain types of current. Thus, skin impedance is generally higher with DC than with biphasic current.[19]

Blood is a biologic tissue that is composed largely of water and ions and is consequently the best electrical conductor of all tissues. Muscle is composed of about 75% water and depends on the movement of ions for contraction. It tends to propagate an electrical impulse much more effectively in a longitudinal direction than transversely. Muscle tendons are considerably more dense than muscle, contain relatively little water, and are considered poor conductors. Fat contains only about 14% water and is thought to be a poor conductor.

Peripheral nerve conductivity is approximately six times that of muscle. However, the nerve generally is surrounded by fat and a fibrous sheath, both of which are considered to be poor conductors. Bone is extremely dense, contains only about 5% water, and is considered to be the poorest biologic conductor of electrical current. It is essential for the clinician to understand that many biologic tissues will be stimulated by an electrical current. Selecting the appropriate treatment parameters is critical if the desired tissue response is to be attained.[20]

CHOOSING APPROPRIATE TREATMENT PARAMETERS

To make the treatment options very simple for the clinician, the equipment manufacturers have created preset treatment protocols for each type of current. A clinician may choose the preset protocols or can choose to manually alter a number of treatment parameters including waveforms, current modulation, frequency, intensity, duration, and polarity. He or she must also choose the size and placement location of the electrodes.

WAVEFORMS

Waveform shapes are as follows:
- sinusoidal;
- rectangular;
- square;
- spiked.

The term **waveform** indicates a graphic representation of the shape, direction, **amplitude, duration**, and pulse frequency of the electrical current the electrotherapeutic device produces, as displayed by an instrument called an oscilloscope.

Waveform Shape

Electrical currents may take on a *sinusoidal, rectangular, square,* or *spiked* waveform configuration, depending on the capabilities of the generator producing the current (Figure 5–6). Biphasic, monophasic, and PC may take on any of the waveform shapes.

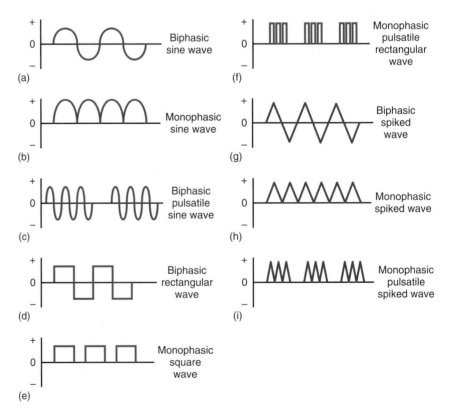

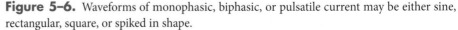

Figure 5–6. Waveforms of monophasic, biphasic, or pulsatile current may be either sine, rectangular, square, or spiked in shape.

Pulses versus Phases and Direction of Current Flow

On an oscilloscope, an individual waveform is referred to as a **pulse**. A pulse may contain one or more **phases**, which is that portion of the pulse that rises in one direction either above or below the baseline for some period of time. Thus, DC is unidirectional and is referred to as *monophasic* current. It produces waveforms that have only a single pulse and phase, which are the same (Figure 5–7a). Because current flow is unidirectional, it always flows in the same direction toward either the positive or negative pole. With DC the terms pulse duration and phase duration only indicate the length of time that current is flowing.

Conversely, AC, referred to as *biphasic current*, produces waveforms that have two separate phases during each individual **cycle**. (*Cycle* applies to biphasic current, whereas *pulse*

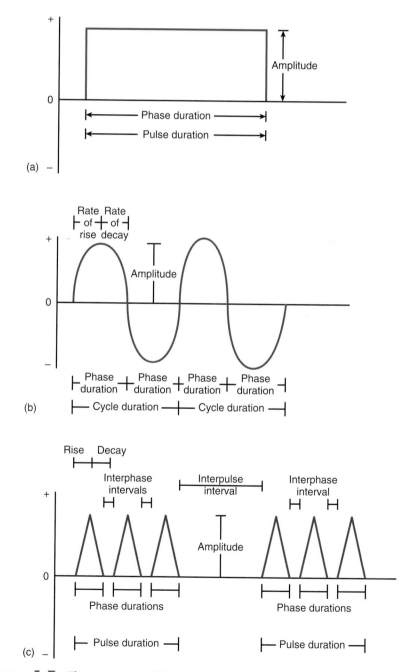

Figure 5–7. Characteristics of (A) monophasic current, (B) biphasic current, and (C) pulsatile current.

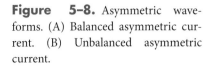

Figure 5–8. Asymmetric waveforms. (A) Balanced asymmetric current. (B) Unbalanced asymmetric current.

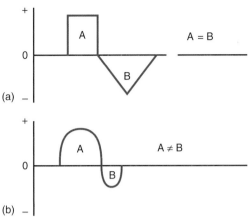

applies to monophasic current.) Current flow is bidirectional, reversing direction or polarity once during each cycle. Biphasic waveforms may be symmetric or asymmetric.[11] A biphasic symmetric waveform has the same shape and size for each phase in both directions (Figure 5–7b). In contrast, a biphasic asymmetric waveform has different shapes for each phase (Figure 5–8a). Asymmetric waveforms can be either balanced or unbalanced. If the phases are balanced, the net charge in each direction is equal. If the phases are unbalanced, one phase has a greater net charge than the other and some movement of ions will occur (Figure 5–8b).

PC waveforms are representative of electrical current that is conducted as a series of pulses of short duration (milliseconds) and may be either monophasic or biphasic. The time that each pulse lasts is called the phase duration. Sometimes single pulses may be interrupted by an **interphase interval**. Pulse duration is the sum of all phases plus the interphase interval. With PC there is always a short period of time when current is not flowing between the two phases called the **interpulse interval** (Figure 5–7c).

Pulse Amplitude

The amplitude of each pulse reflects the intensity of the current, the maximum amplitude being the tip or highest point of each phase (see Figure 5–7). Amplitude is measured in amperes, microamperes, or milliamperes. The term *amplitude* is synonymous with the terms *voltage* and *current intensity*. Voltage is measured in volts, microvolts, or millivolts. The higher the amplitude, the greater the peak voltage or intensity is. However, the peak amplitude should not be confused with the total amount of current being delivered to the tissues.

On electrical generators that produce short-duration pulses, the total current produced (c/s) is low compared with peak current amplitudes owing to long interpulse intervals that have current amplitudes of zero. Thus, the *total current* (average), or the amount of current flowing per unit of time, is relatively low, ranging from as low as 2 mA to as high as 100 mA in some interferential currents (IFC). Total current can be increased by either increasing pulse duration or increasing pulse frequency or by some combination of the two (Figure 5–9).

Pulse Charge

The term **pulse charge** refers to the total amount of electricity being delivered to the patient during each pulse (measured in coulomb or microcoulomb). With monophasic current, the phase charge and the pulse charge are the same and always greater than zero. With biphasic current, the pulse charge is equal to the sum of the phase charges. If the pulse is symmetric, the net pulse charge is zero. In asymmetric pulses the net pulse charge is greater than zero, which is a monophasic current by definition.[10]

Pulse Rate of Rise and Decay Times

The **rate of rise** in amplitude, or the rise time, refers to how quickly the pulse reaches its maximum amplitude in each phase. Conversely, **decay time** refers to the time in which a pulse

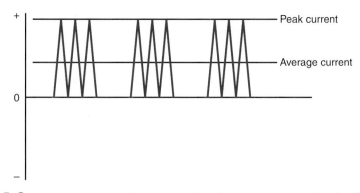

Figure 5–9. Average current is low compared with peak current amplitudes due to long interpulse intervals.

goes from peak amplitude to 0 V. The rate of rise is important physiologically because of the **accommodation** phenomenon, in which a fiber that has been subjected to a constant level of depolarization will become unexcitable at that same intensity or amplitude. Rate of rise and decay times are generally short, ranging from nanoseconds (billionths of a second) to milliseconds (thousandths of a second) (see Figure 5–6):

$$\text{Amplitude} = \text{Voltage} = \text{Current intensity}$$

By observing the different waveforms, it is apparent that the sine wave has a gradual increase and decrease in amplitude for biphasic, monophasic, and PC (see Figure 5–6a–c). The rectangular wave has an almost instantaneous increase in amplitude, which plateaus for a period of time and then abruptly falls off (see Figure 5–6d–f). The spiked wave has a rapid increase and decrease in amplitude (see Figure 5–6g–i). The shape of these waveforms as they reach their maximum amplitude or intensity is directly related to the excitability of nervous tissue. The more rapid the increase in amplitude or the rate of rise, the greater the current's ability to excite nervous tissue is.

Many high-volt monophasic currents make use of a twin peak spiked pulse of very short duration (170 microseconds) and peak amplitudes as high as 500 V (Figure 5–10). Combining a high peak intensity with a short phase duration produces a very comfortable type of current as well as an effective means of stimulating sensory, motor, and pain fibers.[21]

Pulse Duration

The **duration** of each pulse indicates the length of time current is flowing in one cycle. With monophasic current, the phase duration is the same as the pulse duration and is the time from initiation of the phase to its end. With biphasic current, the pulse duration is determined by the combined phase durations. In some electrotherapeutic devices, the duration is preset by

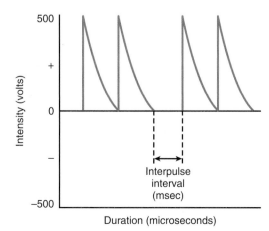

Figure 5–10. Most DC generators produce a twin peak spiked pulse of short duration and high amplitude.

the manufacturer. Other devices have the capability of changing duration. The phase duration may be as short as a few microseconds or may be a long-duration DC that flows for several minutes.

With PC, and in some instances with biphasic and monophasic currents, the current flow is off for a period of time. The combined time of the pulse duration and the interpulse interval is referred to as the **pulse period** (see Figure 5–7).

Pulse Frequency

Pulse frequency indicates the number of pulses or cycles per second. Each individual pulse represents a rise and fall in amplitude. As the frequency of any waveform is increased, the amplitude tends to increase and decrease more rapidly. The muscular and nervous system responses depend on the length of time between pulses and on how the pulses or waveforms are modulated.[22] Muscle responds with individual twitch contractions to pulse rates of less than 50 pps. At 50 pps or greater, a tetanic contraction will result, regardless of whether the current is biphasic, monophasic, or polyphasic.

Currents have been clinically labeled as low, medium, or high frequency, and a great deal of misunderstanding exists over how these frequency ranges are classified.[10] Generally, all stimulating currents are low frequency and deliver between one and several hundred pulses per second. Recently, a number of so-called medium-frequency currents have been developed that have frequencies of 2500 pps to as high as 10,000 pps. However, these so-called medium-frequency pulses are in reality groups of pulses combined as bursts that range in frequency from 1 to 200 pps. These modulated bursts are capable of producing a physiologically effective frequency of stimulation only in this 1–200 pps range owing to the limitations of the absolute refractory period of nerve cell membranes. Therefore, many of the claims of equipment manufacturers relative to medium-frequency currents are inaccurate.[10]

The types of current modulation are as follows:
- continuous;
- burst;
- beat;
- ramping.

Current Modulation

The physiologic responses to the various waveforms depend to a large extent on current modulation. **Modulation** refers to any alteration in the amplitude, duration, or frequency of the current during a series of pulses or cycles.

Continuous Current

With continuous current the amplitude of current flow remains the same for several seconds or perhaps minutes. Continuous current is usually associated with long-pulse-duration monophasic current (Figure 5–11a). With monophasic current, flow is always in a uniform direction. In the discussion of physiologic responses to electrical currents, it was indicated that positive and negative ions are attracted toward poles or, in this case, electrodes of opposite polarity. This accumulation of charged ions over a period of time creates either an acidic or alkaline environment that may be of therapeutic value. This therapeutic technique has been referred to as **medical galvanism**. The technique of **iontophoresis** also uses continuous monophasic current to transport ions into the tissues (see Chapter 6). If the amplitude is great enough to produce a muscle contraction, the contraction will occur only when the current flow is turned on or off. Thus, with direct continuous current, a muscle contraction will occur both when the current is turned on and when it is turned off.

Clinical Decision-Making   *Exercise 5–4*

The clinician is interested in producing a tetanic muscle contraction. What treatment parameter can be adjusted to produce this type of contraction?

Burst Modulation

Burst modulation occurs when PC or biphasic current flows for a short duration (milliseconds) and then is turned off for a short time (milliseconds) in a repetitive cycle (Figure 5–11b and c).

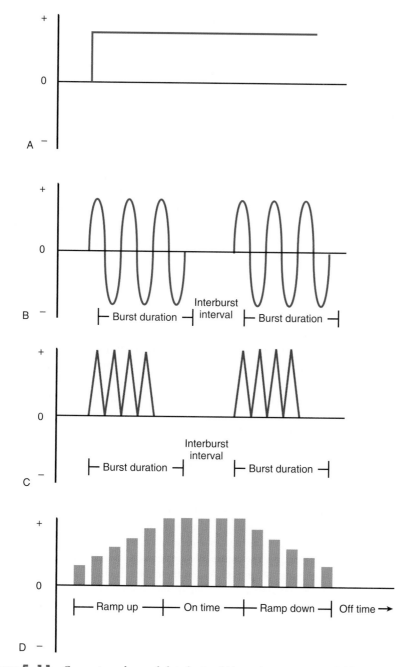

Figure 5–11. Current may be modulated using (A) continuous current, (B) burst-modulated alternating current, (C) burst-modulated pulsatile current, and (D) ramp-up and ramp-down modulation.

With PC, sets of pulses are combined. These combined pulses are most commonly referred to in the literature as **bursts**, but they have also been called *packets, envelopes,* or *pulse trains.*[23] The interruptions between individual bursts are called **interburst intervals**. The interburst interval is much too short to have any effect on a muscle contraction. Thus, the physiologic effects of a burst of pulses will be the same as with a single pulse.[10] Some machines allow the clinician to change the burst duration and/or the interburst interval.

Beat Modulation

A beat modulation will be produced when two interfering biphasic current waveforms with differing frequencies are delivered to two separate pairs of electrodes through separate channels within the same generator (see Figure 5–33). The two pairs of electrodes are set up in a crisscrossed or cloverleaf-like pattern so that the circuits interfere with one another. This interference pattern produces a beat frequency equal to the difference in frequency between the two biphasic current frequencies. As an example, one circuit may have a fixed frequency of 4000 Hz, while the other is set at a frequency of 4100 Hz, thus creating a beat frequency of 100 beats/s. This type of beat-modulated AC is referred to as *IFC* and/or *premodulated interferential* and will be discussed later in this chapter.

Ramping Modulation

In **ramping** modulation, also called surging modulation, current amplitude will increase or ramp up gradually to some preset maximum and may also decrease or ramp down in intensity (Figure 5–11d). Ramp-up time is usually preset at about one third of the on time. The ramp-down option is not available on all machines. Most modern stimulators allow the clinician to set the on and off times between 1 and 10 seconds. Ramping modulation is used clinically to elicit muscle contraction and is generally considered to be a very comfortable type of current since it allows for a gradual increase in the intensity of a muscle contraction.

Frequency

To understand electrically stimulated muscle contractions, we must think in terms of multiple stimuli rather than a simple DC response. The motor nerves are not stimulated by a steady flow of DC. The nerve repolarizes under the influence of the current and will not depolarize again until a sudden change in current intensity occurs. If continuous monophasic current were the only current mode available, we would get a muscle contraction only when the current intensity rose to a stimulus threshold. Once the membrane is repolarized, another change in the current intensity would be needed to force another depolarization and contraction (Figure 5–12).

Frequency indicates the numbers of impulses or cycles produced by an electrical stimulating device in 1 second and is referred to as cycles per second (CPS), pulses per second, or hertz. It can determine the type of muscle contraction elicited. The amount of shortening of the muscle fiber and the amount of recovery allowed to the muscle fiber are a function of the frequency. The mechanical shortening of the single muscle fiber response can be influenced by stimulating again as soon as the tissue membrane repolarizes. Only the membrane has the absolute refractory period; the contractile mechanism operates on a different timing sequence and is just beginning to contract. When the muscle membrane receives a second stimulus, the myofilaments are already overlapping, and the second stimulus causes an increased mechanical shortening of the muscle fiber. This process of superimposing one twitch

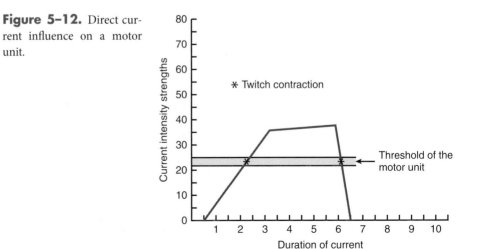

Figure 5–12. Direct current influence on a motor unit.

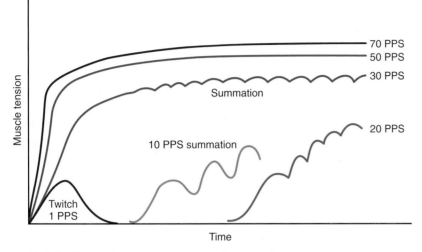

Figure 5–13. Summation of contractions and tetanization.

contraction on another is called *summation of contractions*. As the number of twitch contractions per second increases, single twitch responses cannot be distinguished, and **tetanization** of the muscle fiber is reached (Figure 5–13). The tension developed by a muscle fiber in tetany is much greater than the tension from a twitch contraction.[185] This muscle fiber tetany is strictly a function of the frequency of the stimulating current; it is not dependent on the intensity of the current.[24,25] In general, a higher frequency can be used to produce an increase in muscle tension due to the summative effects, while a lower frequency is more often used for muscle pumping and edema reduction.

Intensity

Increasing the intensity of the electrical stimulus causes the current to reach deeper into the tissue. Depolarization of additional nerve fibers is accomplished by two methods: higher threshold fibers within the range of the stimulus are depolarized by the higher-intensity stimulus and fibers with the same threshold but deeper in the structure are depolarized by the deeper spread of the current. High-volt currents are capable of deeper penetration into the tissue than low-volt currents and may be desirable when stimulating deep muscle tissue. This is one of the most significant differences between high- and low-volt currents.[8,25]

Duration

We also can stimulate more nerve fibers with the same intensity current by increasing the length of time (duration) that an adequate stimulus is available to depolarize the membranes. Greater numbers of nerve fibers then would react to the same intensity stimulus, because the current would be available for a longer period of time.[2,24,26] This method requires the use of a stimulator with an adjustable duration.

Polarity

With any electrical current, the electrode that has a greater number of electrons is called the *negative electrode* or the **cathode**. The other electrode has a relatively lower number of electrons and is called the *positive electrode* or the **anode**. The negative electrode attracts positive ions, and the positive electrode attracts negative ions and electrons. With biphasic waves, these electrodes change polarity with each current cycle.

    With a monophasic current, the clinician can designate one electrode as the negative and one as the positive, and for the duration of the treatment the electrodes will provide that polar

- negative electrode: cathode;
- positive electrode: anode;
- muscle contraction: negative active electrode;
- cathode: distal;
- anode: proximal.

effect. The polar effect can be thought of in terms of three characteristics: (1) chemical effects, (2) ease of excitation, and (3) direction of current flow.[2,24,25,27-29]

Chemical changes occur only with long-duration continuous current.

Clinical Decision-Making   *Exercise 5–5*

A clinician is using an electrical stimulator to induce a muscle contraction of the rectus femoris. The active electrode is placed over the motor point of the muscle and the dispersive electrode is placed under the leg. What changes in the setup of the electrodes and/or changes in current parameters can be made to reach the threshold of depolarization for this muscle?

Chemical Effects

Changes in pH under each electrode, a reflex vasodilation, and the ability to facilitate movement of oppositely charged ions through the skin into the tissue (iontophoresis) are all thought of as chemical effects. A tissue-stimulating effect is ascribed to the negative electrode. To create these effects, longer pulse durations (>1 minute) are required.[27,29-31] The bacteriostatic effect is achieved at either the anode or cathode with intensities in the 5–10 mA range, although at 1 mA or below the greatest bacteriostatic effect was found at the cathode.[32] Another study using treatment times exceeding 30 minutes found some bacteriostatic effect of high-voltage pulsed currents.[33]

Ease of Excitation of Excitable Tissue

The polarity of the active electrode usually should be negative when the desired result is a muscle contraction because of the greater facility for membrane depolarization at the negative pole. However, current density under the positive pole can be increased rapidly enough to create a depolarizing effect. Using the positive electrode as the active electrode is not as efficient, because it will require more current intensity to create an action potential. This may cause the patient to be less comfortable with the treatment. In treatment programs requiring muscle contraction or sensory nerve stimulation, patient comfort should dictate the choice of positive or negative polarity. Negative polarity usually is the most comfortable in this instance.[2,25,34]

Direction of Current Flow

In some treatment schemes, the direction of current flow also is considered important. Generally speaking, the negative electrode is positioned distally and the positive electrode proximally. This arrangement tries to replicate the naturally occurring pattern of electrical flow in the body.[27,35]

The direction of current flow could also influence shifting of the water content of the tissues and movement of colloids (fluid suspension of the intracellular fluid). Neither of these phenomena is well documented or understood, and further study is needed before clinical treatments are designed around these concepts.[2,36,37]

True polar effects can be substantiated when they occur close to the electrodes through which the current is entering the tissue. In laboratory situations in physics, polar effects occur in very close proximity to the electrode. To cause these effects, the current must flow through a medium. If the tissue to be treated is centrally located between the two electrodes, results cannot be assigned to polar effects (Hooker DN, personal communication, January 30, 1994).[27] Clinically, polar effects are an important consideration in iontophoresis, stimulating motor points or peripheral nerves, and the biostimulative effects on nonexcitatory cells.

Current Density

The **current density** (amount of current flow per cubic volume) at the nerve or muscle must be high enough to cause depolarization. The current density is highest where the electrodes meet

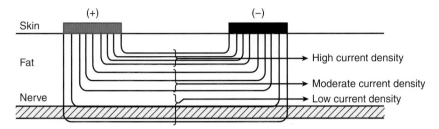

Figure 5–14. Current density using equal size electrodes spaced close together.

the skin and diminishes as the electricity penetrates into the deeper tissues (Figure 5–14).[2,24] If there is a large fat layer between the electrodes and the nerve, the electrical energy may not have a high enough density to cause depolarization (Figure 5–15).

If the electrodes are spaced closely together, the area of highest current density is relatively superficial (Figure 5–16A). If the electrodes are spaced farther apart, the current density will be higher in the deeper tissues, including nerve and muscle (Figure 5–16B).

Electrode size will also change current density. As the size of one electrode relative to another is decreased, the current density beneath the smaller electrode is increased. The larger the electrode, the larger the area over which the current is spread, decreasing the current density (Figure 5–17).[2,8,24,25,38]

Using a large (dispersive) electrode remote from the treatment area while placing a smaller (active) electrode as close as possible to the nerve or muscle motor point will give the greatest effect at the small electrode. The large electrode disperses the current over a large area; the small electrode concentrates the current in the area of the motor point (Figure 5–17).

Electrode size and placement are key elements the clinician controls that will have great influence on results. High current density close to the neural structure to be stimulated makes success more certain with the least amount of current. Electrode placement is probably one of the biggest causes of poor results from electrical therapy (Hooker DN, personal communication, January 30, 1994).

Electrode Placement

Several guidelines will help the clinician select the appropriate sites for electrode placement when using any of the treatment protocols aimed at the electrical stimulation of sensory or motor nerves. Electrodes should be placed where the clinician feels will be the most effective location and then moved in a trial-and-error pattern until a specific treatment goal is achieved. The following patterns may be used:

1. Electrodes may be placed on or around a painful area.
2. Electrodes may be placed over specific dermatomes, myotomes, or sclerotomes that correspond to the painful area.
3. Electrodes may be placed close to the spinal cord segment that innervates a painful area.

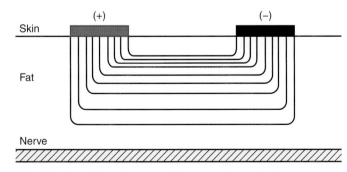

Figure 5–15. Equal size electrodes spaced close together on body part with thick fat layers. Thus, the electrical current does not reach the nerve.

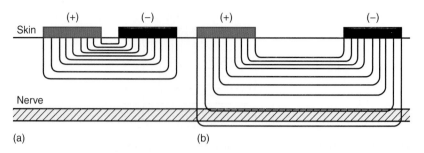
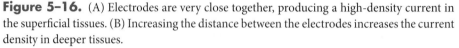

Figure 5–16. (A) Electrodes are very close together, producing a high-density current in the superficial tissues. (B) Increasing the distance between the electrodes increases the current density in deeper tissues.

4. Peripheral nerves that innervate the painful area may be stimulated by placing electrodes over sites where the nerve becomes superficial and can be stimulated easily.

5. Vascular structures contain neural tissue as well as ionic fluids that would transmit electrical stimulating currents and may be most easily stimulated by electrode placement over superficial vascular structures.

6. Electrodes may be placed over trigger point or acupuncture point locations.[39]

7. Electrodes should be placed over motor points of the muscle or at least over the muscle belly of the muscle in which you are trying to elicit a contraction.

8. Both acupuncture and trigger points have been conveniently mapped out and illustrated. A reference on acupuncture and trigger areas is included in Appendix A. The clinician should systematically attempt to stimulate the points listed as successful for certain areas and types of pain. If they are effective, the patient will have decreased pain. These points also can be identified using an ohm meter point locator to determine areas of decreased skin resistance.

9. Combinations of any of the preceding systems and bilateral electrode placement also can be successful.[28,40,41]

10. A **bipolar** application of electrodes uses electrodes of the same size in the same general treatment area (Figure 5–18a). Since the size of the electrodes is the same, the current density under each electrode is essentially the same. Thus, the physiologic effects under each electrode should be the same. However, if one electrode is located over a motor point and the other is not, a muscle contraction may occur at lower current amplitude over the motor point.

11. A **monopolar** application of electrodes uses one or more small active electrodes over a treatment area and a large dispersive electrode placed somewhere else on the body (Figure 5–18b). The higher current density is under the smaller or active electrode, and thus a desired physiologic response will likely occur at the active electrode.

12. A **quadripolar** technique uses two sets of bipolar electrodes, each of which comes from a completely separate channel on the electrical stimulator (Figure 5–18c).

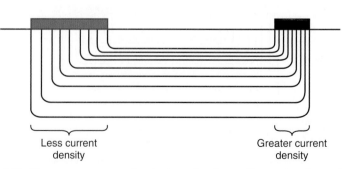

Less current density

Greater current density

Figure 5–17. The greatest current density is under the small or active electrode.

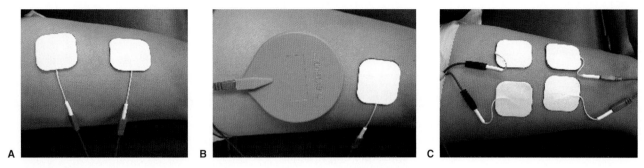

Figure 5–18. Electrode setup: (a) bipolar, (b) monopolar, and (c) quadripolar.

13. Crossing patterns are used with interferential and premodulated IFC. They involve electrode application such that the electrical signals from each set of electrodes add together at some point in the body and the intensity accumulates. The electrodes are usually arranged in a crisscross pattern around the point to be stimulated (Figure 5–19). If you wish to stimulate a specific superficial area, the electrodes should be relatively close together. They should be located so that the area to be treated is central to the location of the electrodes. If pain is poorly localized pain (e.g., general shoulder pain) and seems to be deeper in the joint or muscle area, spread the electrodes farther apart to give more penetration to the current.

The clinician should not be limited to any one system but should evaluate electrode placement for each patient. The effectiveness of sensory or motor stimulation is closely tied in with proper electrode placement. As in all trial-and-error treatment approaches, a systematic, organized search is always better than a "shotgun," hit-or-miss approach. Numerous articles

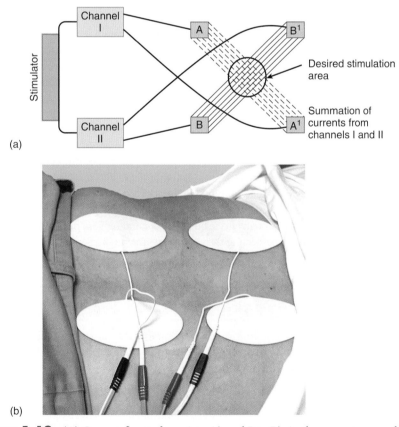

Figure 5–19. (A) Current flow is from A to A^1, and B to B^1. As the currents cross the area of stimulation, they summate in intensity. (B) Typical crossing pattern for electrodes.

have identified some of the best locations for common clinical problems, and these may be used as a starting point for the first approach.[42] If the treatment is not achieving the desired results, the electrode placement should be reconsidered.

Clinical Decision-Making *Exercise 5–6*

A clinician is using electrical stimulation for muscle strengthening following a hamstring muscle strain. What treatment parameters will likely be most effective in improving strength?

Clinical Decision-Making *Exercise 5–7*

How should a clinician go about setting up a conventional TENS treatment for a sore biceps muscle?

On/Off Time

Most electrical generators allow the clinician the capability of setting the ratio of time the electrical current will be on and the time it will be off. The lower the ratio of on time to off time, the less total current the patient will receive. On some generators this on/off time is referred to as the *duty cycle*.

PHYSIOLOGIC RESPONSES TO ELECTRICAL CURRENT

Electricity has an effect on each cell and tissue that it passes through.[43,44] The type and extent of the response are dependent on the type of tissue and its response characteristics (e.g., how it normally functions or changes under normal stress) and the nature of the current applied (current type, intensity, duration, voltage, and density). The tissue should respond to electrical energy in a manner similar to that in which it normally functions.[38]

The effects of electrical current passing through the various tissues of the body may be thermal, chemical, or physiologic.[45] All electrical currents cause a rise in temperature in a conducting tissue.[46] The tissues of the body possess varying degrees of resistance, and those of higher resistance should heat up more when electrical current passes through. As indicated previously, the electrical currents used for stimulation of nerve and muscle have a relatively low average current flow that produces minimal thermal effects.

Clinically, clinicians use electrical currents to produce either muscle contractions or modification of pain impulses through effects on the motor and sensory nerves. This function is dependent to a great extent on selecting the appropriate treatment parameters based on the principles identified in this chapter.[46]

Clinical Decision-Making *Exercise 5–8*

The clinician is treating a myofascial trigger point in the upper trapezius. He decides to use a point stimulator for the purpose of pain modulation. What treatment technique will likely be most effective?

Electrical currents are also used to produce chemical effects. Most biologic tissue contains negatively and positively charged ions. A DC flow will cause migration of these charged particles toward the pole of opposite polarity, producing specific physiologic changes.

Direct and Indirect Physiologic Effects

These physiologic responses to electrical stimulating currents can be broken into direct and indirect effects. There is always a direct effect along the lines of current flow and under the electrodes. Indirect effects occur remote to the area of current flow and are usually the result of stimulating a natural physiologic event to occur.[8,47]

If a certain effect is desired from stimulation, goals must be established to achieve the specific physiologic response as a goal of treatment. These responses can be grouped into two basic physiologic responses: excitatory and nonexcitatory.

The excitatory is the most obvious and the one that has been used the most often in the past in treating patients. In the clinical setting, we spend most of our time trying to get the excitatory response from the nerve cells. Patients perceive excitatory responses as electrical sensation, muscle contraction, and electrical pain. Physiologically, the nerves that affect these perceptions fire in that order as the stimulus intensity is increased gradually. Nerves have very little discriminatory ability. They can tell only if there is electricity in sufficient magnitude to cause a depolarization of the nerve membrane. They have very little regard for the different shapes and polarities of waveforms. To the nerve cell, electricity is electricity. As in all things dealing with higher-level organisms, the range of responses to the same stimulus is wide, depending on the environmental and systemic factors.

Clinical Decision-Making *Exercise 5–9*

When using IFC to treat muscle guarding in the low back, how should the electrodes be placed?

All perception is a product of the brain's activity of receiving the signal that a nerve has been stimulated electrically. This further enlarges the broad range of systemic effects that occur in response to the electrical stimulation.

Stimulation events will change the body's perception. As the strength of the current increases and/or the duration of the current increases, more nerve cells will fire. As the strength of the stimulus increases and these events occur, certain quality judgments about the electrical stimuli are made. Is the current pleasant or unpleasant? Is the intensity of the stimulus weak or strong? The broad range of individual responses to these quality judgments has a significant impact on the beneficial effects of this therapy.

Nerve Responses to Electrical Currents

Nerves and muscles are both excitable tissues. This excitability is dependent on the cell membrane's **voltage-sensitive permeability**. The nerve or muscle cell membrane regulates the exchange of electrically charged ions between the inside of the cell and the environment outside the cell. This voltage-sensitive permeability produces an unequal distribution of charged ions on each side of the membrane, which in turn creates a potential difference between the charge of the interior of the cell and that of the exterior of the cell. The membrane then is considered to be polarized. The potential difference between the inside and outside is known as the **resting potential**, because the cell tries to maintain this electrochemical gradient as its normal homeostatic environment.[43]

Both electrical and chemical gradients are established along the cell membrane, with a greater concentration of diffusable positive ions on the outside of the membrane than on the inside. Using the continuous activity of the sodium pumps in the nerve cell membrane, the nerve cell continually moves Na^+ from inside the cell to outside the cell membrane while voltage-activated potassium channels allow K^+ to move into the cell. This maintains the larger concentration of K^+ on the inside of the cell membrane. The overall charge difference between the inside and the outside of the membrane creates an electrical gradient at its resting level of -70 to -90 mV (Figure 5–20). As Guyton explains, "The potential is proportional to the

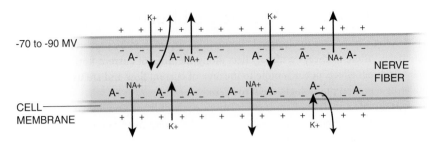

Figure 5–20. Nerve cell membrane with active transport mechanisms maintaining the resting membrane potential.

difference in tendency of the ions to diffuse in one direction versus the other direction."[32] Two conditions are necessary for the membrane potential to develop: (1) the membrane must be semipermeable, allowing ions of one charge to diffuse through the pores more readily than ions of the opposite charge; and (2) the concentration of the diffusable ions must be greater on one side of the membrane than on the other side.[32,43]

The resting membrane potential is generated because the cell is an ionic battery whose concentration of ions inside and outside the cell is maintained by regulatory Na^+K^+ pumps within the cell wall. In addition to the ability of the nerve and muscle cell membranes to develop and maintain the resting potential, the membranes are excitable.[32,48]

To create transmission of an impulse in the nerve tissue, resting membrane potential must be reduced below a threshold level. Changes in the membrane's permeability then may occur. These changes create an **action potential** that will propagate the impulse along the nerve in both directions from the location of the stimulus. An action potential created by a stimulus from chemical, electrical, thermal, or mechanical means always creates the same result, membrane **depolarization**.

Not all stimuli are effective in causing an action potential and depolarization. To be an effective agent, the stimulus must have an adequate intensity and last long enough to equal or exceed the membrane's basic threshold for excitation. The stimulus must alter the membrane so that a number of ions are pushed across the membrane, exceeding the ability of the active transport pumps to maintain the resting potentials. A stimulus of this magnitude forces the membrane to depolarize and results in an action potential.[2,32]

Depolarization

As the charged ions move across the nerve fiber membranes beneath the anode and cathode, membrane depolarization occurs. The cathode usually is the site of depolarization (Figure 5–21A). As the concentration of negatively charged ions increases, the membrane's voltage potential becomes low and is brought toward its threshold for depolarization (Figure 5–21B). The anode makes the nerve cell membrane potential more positive, increasing the threshold necessary for depolarization (Figure 5–21C). The cathode in this example becomes the active electrode; the anode becomes the indifferent electrode (dispersive). The anode and cathode may switch active and indifferent roles under other circumstances.[2,8,24] The number of ions needed to exceed the membrane pump's ability to maintain the normal membrane resting potential is tissue dependent.

Depolarization propagation. Following excitement and propagation of the impulse along the nerve fiber, there is a brief period during which the nerve fiber is incapable of reacting to a second stimulus. This is the **absolute refractory period**, which lasts about 0.5 microsecond. Excitability is restored gradually as the nerve cell membrane repolarizes itself. The nerve then is capable of being stimulated again. The maximum number of possible discharges of a nerve may reach 1000/s, depending on fiber type.[2,24,32,49]

The difference in electrical potential between the depolarized region and the neighboring inactive region causes a small electrical current to flow between the two regions. This forms a complete local circuit and makes the depolarization self-propagating as the process is repeated all along the fiber in each direction from the depolarization site. Energy released by the

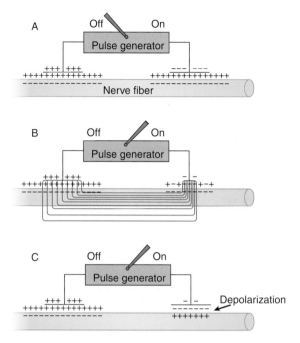

Figure 5-21. (A–C) Depolarization of nerve cell membrane.

cell keeps the intensity of the impulse uniform as it travels down the cell.[2,24,32,49] This process is illustrated in Figure 5–22.

Depolarization effects. As the nerve impulse reaches its effector organ, either another nerve cell or a muscle, the impulse is transferred between the two at a motor endplate or synapse. At this junction, a neurotransmitter substance is released from the nerve. If the effector organ is a muscle, this neurotransmitter substance causes the adjacent excitable muscle to contract, resulting in a single twitch muscle contraction (Figure 5–23).[2,24] This contraction, initiated by an electrical stimulus, is the same as a twitch contraction coming from voluntary activity.

Strength–Duration Curve

The *strength–duration (SD) curve* is a graphic representation of the threshold for depolarization of a particular nerve fiber (Figure 5–24). A sufficient amount of electrical current must be delivered to make a nerve depolarize. As illustrated, there is a nonlinear relationship between current duration and current intensity, in which shorter-duration stimuli require increasing intensities to reach the threshold for depolarization of the nerve. **Rheobase** is a term that identifies the specific *intensity* of current necessary to cause an observable tissue response (i.e., a muscle contraction) given a long current duration. **Chronaxie** identifies the specific length of time or *duration* required for a current of twice the intensity of the rheobase to produce tissue excitation.

Different sizes and types of nerve fibers have different thresholds for depolarization and thus different SD curves (Figure 5–25). Aβ fibers require the least amount of electrical current to reach their threshold for depolarization followed by motor nerve fibers, Aδ fibers, and finally C fibers. The curves are basically symmetric, but the intensity of current necessary to reach the membrane's threshold for excitation differs for each type of nerve fiber.[2,32,41,50]

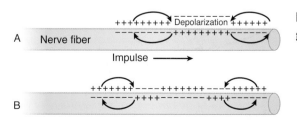

Figure 5-22. (A and B) Propagation of a nerve impulse.

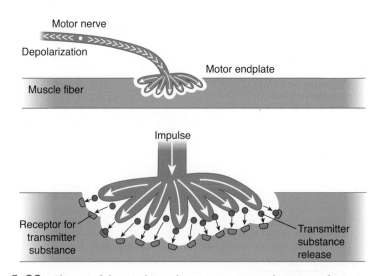

Figure 5–23. Change of electrical impulse to transmitter substance at the motor endplate. When activated, the muscle cell membrane will depolarize and contraction will occur.

By gradually increasing the current intensity and/or current duration, the first physical response would be a tingling sensation caused by depolarization of Aβ fibers, followed by a muscle contraction when motor nerve fibers depolarize, and finally a feeling of pain from depolarization of Aδ fibers and then C fibers.

Equipment manufacturers use the SD curves in choosing their preset pulse durations to be effective in depolarizing nerve fibers.

Muscular Responses to Electrical Current

To reemphasize, normally a muscle contracts in response to depolarization of its motor nerve. Stimulation of the motor nerve is the method used in most clinical applications of electrically stimulated muscle contractions. However, in the absence of muscle innervation, it is possible for a muscle to contract by using an electrical current that causes the muscle membrane, rather than the motor nerve, to depolarize. This will create the same muscle contraction as a natural stimulus.

The **all-or-none response** is another important concept that is relevant when applying electrical current to nerve or muscle tissue. Once a stimulus reaches a depolarizing threshold,

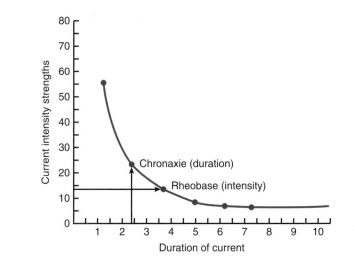

Figure 5–24. Strength–duration curve.

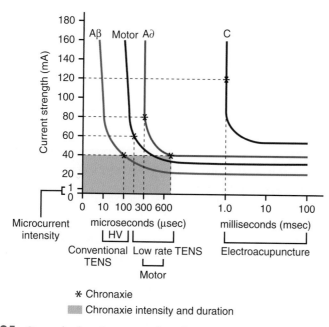

Figure 5–25. Strength–duration curves for Aβ sensory, motor, Aδ sensory, and C (pain) nerve fibers. Durations of several electrical stimulators are indicated along the lower axis. Corresponding intensities would be necessary to create a depolarizing stimulus for any of the nerve fibers. Microcurrent intensity is so low that the nerve fibers will not depolarize. This current travels through other body tissues to create effects.

the nerve or muscle membrane depolarizes, and propagation of the impulse or muscle contraction occurs. This reaction remains the same regardless of increases in the strength of the stimulus used. Either the stimulus causes depolarization (the all) or it does not cause depolarization (the none). There is no gradation of response; the response of the single nerve or muscle fiber is maximal or nonexistent.[2,24,25] This all-or-none phenomenon does not mean that muscle fiber shortening and overall muscle activity cannot be influenced by changing the intensity, pulses per second, or duration of the stimulating current. Adjustments in current parameters can cause changes in the shortening of the muscle fiber and the overall muscle activity.

Stimulation of Denervated Muscle

Electrical currents may be used to produce a muscle contraction in **denervated muscle**. A muscle that is denervated is one that has lost its peripheral nerve supply. The primary purpose for electrically stimulating denervated muscle is to help minimize the extent of atrophy during the period while the nerve is regenerating. Following denervation, the muscle fibers experience a number of progressive anatomic, biochemical, and physiologic changes that lead to a decrease in the size of the individual muscle fibers and in the diameter and weight of the muscle. Consequently, the amount of tension that muscle can generate will decrease and the time required for the muscle to contract will increase.[51,52] These degenerative changes progress until the muscle is reinnervated by axons regenerating across the site of the lesion. If reinnervation does not occur within 2 years, it is generally accepted that fibrous connective tissue will have replaced the contractile elements of the muscle and recovery of muscle function is not possible.[52,174,177]

A review of the literature indicates that the majority of studies support the use of electrical stimulation of denervated muscle. These studies generally indicate that muscle atrophy can be retarded, loss of both muscle mass and contractile strength can be minimized, and muscle fiber size can be maintained by the appropriate use of electrical stimulation.[53–55] Electrically stimulated contractions of denervated muscle may limit edema and venous stasis, thus delaying muscle fiber fibrosis and degeneration.[52] However, there also seems to be general agreement that electrical stimulation has little or no effect on the rate of nerve regeneration or muscle reinnervation.

A few studies have suggested that electrical stimulation of denervated muscle actually may interfere with reinnervation, thus delaying functional return.[56,57] These studies propose that the muscle contraction disrupts the regenerating neuromuscular junction retarding reinnervation, and that electrical stimulation may traumatize denervated muscle since it is more sensitive to trauma than normal muscle.[52,56,58,178]

Treatment Parameters for Denervated Muscle are as Follows:

1. A current with an asymmetric, biphasic waveform with a pulse duration less than 1 millisecond may be used during the first 2 weeks.[59]

2. After 2 weeks, an interrupted square wave DC and a progressive exponential wave DC, each with a long pulse duration of greater than 10 milliseconds, or a sine wave AC with a frequency lower than 10 Hz will produce a twitch contraction.[52] The length of the pulse should be as short as possible but long enough to elicit a contraction.[60]

3. The current waveform should have a pulse duration equal to or greater than the chronaxie of the denervated muscle.

4. The amplitude of the current along with the pulse duration must be sufficient to stimulate a denervated muscle with a prolonged chronaxie while producing a moderately strong contraction of the muscle fibers.

5. The pause between stimuli should be 1:4 or 5 (15–40 mA) longer (about 3–6 seconds) than the stimulus duration to minimize fatigue.[60]

6. Either a monopolar or bipolar electrode setup can be used with the small-diameter active electrode placed over the most electrically active point in the muscle. This may not be the motor point since the muscle is not normally innervated.

7. Stimulation should begin immediately following denervation using three stimulation treatments per day involving three sets of between 5 and 20 repetitions that can be varied according to fatigability of the muscle.[52]

8. The contraction needs to create muscle tension, so joints may need to be fixed or isotonic contraction for end-range positions may be needed.

Biostimulative Effects of Electrical Current on Nonexcitatory Cells

Electrical stimulating currents can have an effect on the function of nonexcitatory cells, which will respond to electrical current in ways consistent with their cell type and tissue function. We have discussed how electrical currents cause depolarization of excitable cells that compose nerve tissue and muscle tissue. Electrical stimulation of the appropriate frequency and amplitude may be able to activate the receptor site on nonexcitable cells and stimulate the same cellular changes as the naturally occurring chemical molecular stimulation. The cell functions by incorporating a multitude of chemical reactions into a living process. It is conceivable that the appropriate electrical signal could create more specific sites for enzymatic activity, thereby changing or stimulating cell function.[15]

Cells seem responsive to steady DC gradients. The cells move or grow toward one pole and away from the other. The electric field created by the monophasic current may help guide the healing process and the regenerative capabilities of injured or developing tissues.[15,59]

Cells also may respond to a particular frequency of current. The cell may be selectively responsive to certain frequencies and unresponsive to other frequencies. Some researchers claim that specific genes for protein manufacture can be activated by a certain shaped electrical impulse. This frequency could change in certain ways according to the cellular state. This phenomenon has been termed the **"frequency window" selectivity** of the cell.[43]

Overall we see that small-amplitude monophasic currents are intrinsic to the ways the body works to grow and repair. Clinically if we can duplicate some of these same signals, we may be successful in using electrotherapy in the most efficient manner.

CLINICAL USES OF ELECTRICAL STIMULATING CURRENTS

Older electrical stimulating units were generally capable of outputting only one type of current and were labeled specifically as a high-volt stimulating unit, a low-volt stimulating unit, or perhaps a microcurrent stimulating unit. Over the years, advances in technology have enabled manufacturers of electrical stimulators to offer sophisticated pieces of equipment that allow the clinician the flexibility of making choices when it comes to selecting the most appropriate type of currents and treatment parameters to accomplish a specific treatment goal.[179] The newest electrical stimulating units are capable of outputting multiple types of current including high volt, biphasic, microcurrent, Russian, interferential, premodulated interferential, and low volt (Figure 5–26). Table 5–2 provides a list of indications and contraindications for using the various types of electrical currents. A detailed discussion of these various types of current follows.

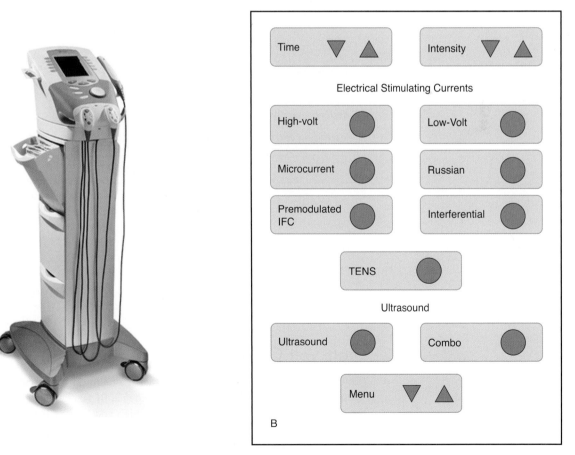

A

B

Figure 5-26. Most electrical stimulating units allow the clinician to choose from a variety of current choices. Some units offer multiple modality options. (A) A combination electrical stimulating unit and ultrasound. (B) Control panel for selecting current options.

Table 5–2 Summary of Indications and Contraindications for Electrical Stimulating Currents

INDICATIONS

Modulating acute, postacute, and chronic pain muscle contraction

Stimulating contraction of denervated muscle reeducation

Retarding atrophy

Muscle strengthening

Increasing range of motion

Decreasing edema

Decreasing muscle spasm

Decreasing muscle guarding

Stimulating the healing process

Wound healing

Fracture healing

Tendon healing

Ligament healing

Stimulating nerve regeneration

Stimulating peripheral nervous system function

Changing membrane permeability

Synthesizing protein

Stimulating fibroblasts and osteoblasts

Regenerating tissue

Increasing circulation through muscle pumping contractions

CONTRAINDICATIONS

Pacemakers

Infection

Malignancies

Pregnancy

Musculoskeletal problems where muscle contraction would exacerbate the condition

High-Volt Currents

High-volt currents are widely used for a variety of clinical purposes: to elicit muscle contractions, for pain control, and for reducing edema. By far the most common application is for producing muscle contraction. Although high-volt current is most commonly used to cause muscle contraction, it should be made clear that other types of electrical currents—Russian, interferential, premodulated interferential, or biphasic—may also be used. While high-volt current can also be used to control pain, it is not the current of modulation. Many of the devices that generate high-volt current are not portable. Thus, TENS would be a better treatment modality choice for long-term pain relief. The efficiency and effectiveness of treatment can be increased by following the protocols as closely as possible with the available equipment. A high-volt current is a twin-peaked pulsed waveform that has a long interpulse interval (see Figure 5–7).

Therapeutic Uses of Electrically Stimulated Muscle Contractions

A variety of therapeutic gains can be made by electrically stimulating a muscle contraction:

1. muscle reeducation;
2. muscle pump contractions;
3. retardation of atrophy;
4. muscle strengthening;
5. increasing range of motion.

Muscle fatigue should be considered when deciding on treatment parameters. The variables that have an influence on muscle fatigue are the following:

1. intensity: combination of the pulse stimulus's amplitude intensity and the pulse duration;

CASE STUDY 5–1
ELECTRICAL STIMULATING CURRENTS: STRENGTHENING OF INNERVATED MUSCLE

Background: A 22-year-old woman sustained a severe grade II MCL sprain of the left knee 3 days ago in an auto accident, and is being treated with plaster immobilization for 3 weeks. She is not able to generate a maximal isometric quadriceps contraction voluntarily. The cast has been modified to accommodate electrodes over the femoral nerve and the motor point of the vastus medialis muscle. There are no restrictions on the amount of force she is allowed to produce during a knee extension effort.

Impression: Grade II MCL sprain of the left knee, with inability to generate maximal isometric force of the knee extensors.

Treatment Plan: A 5-day per week schedule of electrical stimulation was initiated. A polyphasic waveform was selected, with a 2500-Hz carrier wave, with an effective frequency of 50 Hz (10 milliseconds on, 10 milliseconds off). The stimulator was set to ramp the current up for 6 seconds, maintain the current at a specific amplitude for 10 seconds, and then drop to zero with no ramp; rest time was 50 seconds, giving an effective duty cycle of 1:5 (10 seconds on, 50 seconds off). Each treatment session began with 10 repetitions at a comfortable stimulus amplitude, followed by three sets of 10 repetitions each with the maximal amount of current tolerable. A 2-minute rest separated the sets. During the 10 seconds on time, the current amplitude was adjusted to the maximal amount the patient was able to tolerate. The patient was encouraged to contract the quadriceps femoris muscle group as the current was delivered.

Response: The patient's tolerance for the electrical stimulation gradually increased during the first week, and then reached a plateau; this plateau was maintained for the next 2 weeks. On removal of the cast, there was no measurable or visible atrophy of the left thigh. A rehabilitation program of active range of motion, strengthening exercise, and functional activities was initiated, and the patient returned to full, pain-free activity 3 weeks following cast removal.

Discussion Questions

- What tissues were injured or affected?
- What symptoms were present?
- What phase of the injury-healing continuum did the patient present for care in?
- What are the physical agent modality's biophysical effects (direct, indirect, depth, and tissue affinity)?
- What are the physical agent modality's indications and contraindications?
- What are the parameters of the physical agent modality's application, dosage, duration, and frequency in this case study?
- What other physical agent modalities could be used to treat this injury or condition? Why? How?

The rehabilitation professional employs physical agent modalities to create an optimum environment for tissue healing while minimizing the symptoms associated with the trauma or condition.

2. the number of pulses or bursts per second;

3. on time;

4. off time.

Muscle force is varied by changing the intensity to recruit more or less motor units. It can also be varied to a certain degree by increasing the summating quality of the contraction with high burst or pulse rates. The greater the force, the greater the demands on the muscle, the greater the occlusion of muscle blood flow, and the greater the fatigue. If high muscle forces are not required, the intensity and frequency can be adjusted to desired levels but fatigue can still be a factor. To minimize fatigue associated with forceful contractions, a combination of the lowest frequency and the higher intensity will keep the force constant.[61]

If high force levels are desired, then higher frequencies and intensities can be used. To keep the muscle fatigue as low as possible, the rest time between contractions should be at least 60 seconds for each 10 seconds of contraction time. A variable frequency train, in which a high-frequency stimulus and then a low-frequency stimulus is used, will also help minimize fatigue in repetitive functional electrical stimulation (FES).[61]

Neuromuscular-induced contraction at the higher torques is associated with patient perceptions of pain, from either the current used or the intensity of the contraction. This is often a limiting factor in the success of any of the following protocols. Each patient needs supervision and satisfactory clinician confidence for the most effective compliance with the treatment goals (Hooker DN, personal communication, January 30, 1994).[61,62]

When using electrical stimulation for muscle contraction, motor point stimulation can give the best individual muscle contraction. To find the motor point of a muscle, a probe electrode should be used to stimulate the muscle. Stimulation should be started in the approximate location of the desired motor point. (See Appendix A for motor point chart.) The intensity should be increased until contraction is visible, and the current intensity should be maintained at that level. The probe should be moved around until the best visible contraction for that current intensity is found; this is the motor point.[24,63] By choosing this location for stimulation, the current density can be increased in an area where numerous motor nerve fibers can be affected, maximizing the muscular response from the stimulation.

Muscle reeducation. Muscular inhibition after surgery or injury is the primary indication for muscle reeducation.[181] If the neuromuscular mechanisms of a muscle have not been damaged, then central nervous system inhibition of this muscle usually is a factor in loss of control. The atrophy of synaptic contacts that remain unused for long periods is theorized as a source of this sensorimotor alienation. The addition of electrical stimulation of the motor nerve provides an artificial use of the inactive synapses and helps restore a more normal balance to the system as the ascending sensory information will be reintegrated into the patient's movement control patterns. A muscle contraction usually can be forced by electrically stimulating the muscle. Forcing the muscle to contract causes an increase in the sensory input from that muscle. The patient feels the muscle contract, sees the muscle contract, and can attempt to duplicate this muscular response.[24,50,64,65,182] The object here is to reestablish control and not to create a strengthening contraction.

Protocols for muscle reeducation do not list specific parameters to make this treatment more efficient, but the criteria listed in the treatment protocol for muscle reeducation are essential.

Treatment Parameters for Muscle Reeducation are as Follows:

1. Current intensity must be adequate for muscle contraction but comfortable for the patient.

2. Pulse per duration should be set as close as possible to chronaxie for motor neurons (300–600 microseconds).

3. Pulses per second should be high enough to produce a tetanic contraction (35–55 pps) but adjusted so that muscle fatigue is minimized. Higher rates may be more fatigue producing than rates in the midrange of tetanic contraction.

4. On/off cycles should be based on the equipment parameters available and the clinician's preference in teaching the patient to regain control of the muscle. Currents that ramp up or down will require longer on times, so the effective current is on for 2–3 seconds. Off times can either be a 1:1 contraction to recovery ratio or 1:4 or 5, depending on the clinician's preference or the patient's attention span and/or level of fatigue.

5. Interrupted or surged current must be used.

6. The patient should be instructed to allow just the electricity to make the muscle contract, allowing the patient to feel and see the response desired. Next, the patient should alternate voluntary muscle contractions with current-induced contractions.

7. Total treatment time should be about 15 minutes, but this can be repeated several times daily.

8. High-voltage pulsed or medium-frequency biphasic current may be most effective.[24,64,66]

CASE STUDY 5–2
ELECTRICAL STIMULATING CURRENTS: REEDUCATION OF INNERVATED MUSCLE (2)

Background: A 16-year-old male underwent arthroscopic partial medial meniscectomy on the right knee yesterday. He is to begin ambulation with crutches, weight bearing as tolerated, today. Clinic policy states that patients must be able to produce an active quadriceps femoris contraction prior to crutch-walking instruction. However, the patient is unable to produce an active contraction of the quadriceps femoris muscle. There is minimal pain and swelling, but after working with the patient for 15 minutes, he remains unable to contract the quadriceps femoris.

Impression: Status postarthroscopic surgery on the right knee with inhibition of quadriceps femoris control.

Treatment Plan: Using a pulsatile monophasic waveform generator, a course of electrical stimulation was initiated. The cathode (active, negative polarity) was placed over the motor point of the vastus medialis, and the anode (inactive, positive polarity) was placed on the posterior thigh. The frequency was set at 40 pps. Using an uninterrupted (1:0) duty cycle, the amplitude was set to a level that produced a visible contraction, but was below the pain threshold. After establishing the stimulus amplitude, the duty cycle was then adjusted to deliver

15 seconds of stimulus followed by 15 seconds of rest; the current was not ramped, so the effective duty cycle was 1:1. The patient was encouraged to contract the quadriceps femoris during the stimulation for the first five stimulations, and then was asked to contract the quadriceps femoris before the stimulus was delivered.

Response: After 20 repetitions of the stimulus, the patient was able to initiate a contraction of the quadriceps femoris before the current was delivered. The electrical stimulation was discontinued, and the patient was able to continue to contract the quadriceps femoris voluntarily. He was then instructed in crutch walking, and routine postoperative rehabilitation was initiated.

Discussion Questions

- What tissues were injured/affected?
- What symptoms were present?
- What phase of the injury-healing continuum did the patient present for care in?
- What are the physical agent modality's biophysical effects (direct/indirect/depth/tissue affinity)?

(continued)

CASE STUDY 5–2 *(continued)*
ELECTRICAL STIMULATING CURRENTS: REEDUCATION OF INNERVATED MUSCLE (2)

- What are the physical agent modality's indications/contraindications?
- What are the parameters of the physical agent modality's application/dosage/duration/frequency in this case study?
- What other physical agent modalities could be utilized to treat this injury or condition? Why? How?
- Why was the patient unable to contract the quadriceps femoris following surgery?
- Why was the ability to contract the quadriceps femoris a prerequisite to crutch ambulation?
- What is the difference (pathway and physiology) between the voluntary muscle contraction and the induced (stimulated) contraction?

- How did the electrical stimulation assist the patient in regaining the ability to voluntarily contract the muscle?
- What is a viable alternative approach to assisting this patient?
- What would you suspect if there were no responses to the electrical stimulation?
- Why was the amplitude of stimulus set below the pain threshold?

The rehabilitation professional employs physical agent modalities to create an optimum environment for tissue healing while minimizing the symptoms associated with the trauma or condition.

CASE STUDY 5–3
ELECTRICAL STIMULATING CURRENTS: REEDUCATION OF INNERVATED MUSCLE

Background: A 23-year-old man experienced a Sunderland grade V lesion of the left radial nerve as a result of an open fracture of the humerus sustained in a motorcycle accident. The injury occurred 2 years ago. There was an unsuccessful primary repair of the nerve injury; because there was no evidence of reinnervation, a sural nerve graft was completed 1 year ago. Again, there was no evidence of reinnervation, so the distal attachment of the flexor carpi radialis (FCR) was transferred to the posterior aspect of the base of the third metacarpal to provide wrist extension. The tendon transfer was completed 3 weeks ago. The wrist and forearm have been immobilized until yesterday, and the patient has been referred for rehabilitation. The surgeon has cleared the patient for gentle FCR contraction.

Impression: Posttendon transfer with lack of voluntary control.

Treatment Plan: Using a pulsatile biphasic waveform generator, a course of therapeutic electrical stimulation was initiated. A bipolar electrode arrangement was used, with one electrode over the motor point of the FCR and the other electrode approximately 4 cm distal, over the FCR. The pulse rate was set at 40 pps, and the effective duty cycle was set at 5:5 (5 seconds on, 5 seconds off), with a 2-second ramp up and a 2-second ramp down (so the total time the current was delivered was 7 seconds, with 7 seconds between stimulations). The current amplitude was adjusted to achieve a palpable contraction of the FCR, but no wrist motion, and the treatment time was set to 12 minutes, so as to achieve approximately 50 contractions.

Response: Treatment was conducted daily for 3 weeks, with gradual increases in the current amplitude and number of repetitions. At this time, the patient was able to initiate wrist extension independent of the electrical stimulation, and was discharged to a home program.

Discussion Questions
- What tissues were injured or affected?
- What symptoms were present?
- What phase of the injury-healing continuum did the patient present for care in?
- What are the physical agent modality's biophysical effects (direct, indirect, depth, and tissue affinity)?
- What are the physical agent modality's indications and contraindications?

(continued)

CASE STUDY 5–3 (continued)
ELECTRICAL STIMULATING CURRENTS: REEDUCATION OF INNERVATED MUSCLE

- What are the parameters of the physical agent modality's application, dosage, duration, and frequency in this case study?
- What other physical agent modalities could be used to treat this injury or condition? Why? How?
- What structures are involved with a Sunderland grade V peripheral nerve injury?
- What is involved in a sural nerve graft? What was the surgeon trying to achieve?
- What factors led to the failure of the primary radial nerve repair and the sural graft?

- Why did the surgeon wait nearly a year after the primary repair to do the sural graft and nearly a year after the sural graft to perform the tendon transfer?
- Will wrist extension in the absence of extensor digitorum communis function really increase the patient's function? Why or why not?

The rehabilitation professional employs physical agent modalities to create an optimum environment for tissue healing while minimizing the symptoms associated with the trauma or condition.

Muscle pump contractions. Electrically induced muscle contraction can be used to duplicate the regular muscle contractions that help stimulate circulation by pumping fluid and blood through venous and lymphatic channels back into the heart.[67,183] A discussion of edema formation is included in Chapter 15. Using sensory-level stimulation has also been found to decrease edema in sprain and contusion injuries in animals.

Electrical stimulation of muscle contractions in the affected extremity can help in reestablishing the proper circulatory pattern while keeping the injured part protected.[68–71]

Treatment Parameters for Muscle Pumping Contraction to Reduce Edema are as Follows:

1. Current intensity must be high enough to provide a strong, comfortable muscle contraction.
2. Pulse duration is preset on most of the therapeutic generators. If adjustable, it should be set as close as possible to the duration needed for chronaxie (300–600 microseconds) of the motor nerve to be stimulated.
3. Pulses per second should be in the beginnings of tetany range (35–50 pps).
4. Interrupted or surged current must be used.
5. On time should be 5–10 seconds.
6. Off time should be 5–10 seconds.
7. The part to be treated should be elevated.
8. The patient should be instructed to allow the electricity to make the muscles contract. Active range of motion may be encouraged at the same time if it is not contraindicated.
9. Total treatment time should be between 20 and 30 minutes; treatment should be repeated two to five times daily.
10. High-voltage PC or medium-frequency biphasic current may be most effective.[13,36,72–74]
11. Use this protocol in addition to normal ice for best effect.[36,75]

Retardation of atrophy. Prevention or retardation of atrophy has traditionally been a reason for treating patients with electrically stimulated muscle contraction. The maintenance of muscle tissue, after an injury that prevents normal muscular exercise, can be accomplished by substituting an electrically stimulated muscle contraction. The electrical stimulation reproduces the physical and chemical events associated with normal voluntary muscle contraction and helps to maintain normal muscle function. Again, no specific protocols exist. In designing a program, the practitioner should try to duplicate muscle contractions associated with normal exercise routines.

Treatment Parameters for Retardation of Atrophy are as Follows:

1. Current intensity should be as high as can be tolerated by the patient. This can be increased during the treatment as some sensory accommodation takes place. The contraction should be capable of moving the limb through the antigravity range or of achieving 25% or more of the normal **maximum voluntary isometric contraction (MVIC)** torque for the muscle. The higher torque readings seem to have the best results.

2. Pulse duration is preset on most of the therapeutic generators. If it is adjustable, it should be set as close as possible to the duration needed for chronaxie (300–600 microseconds) of the motor nerve to be stimulated.

3. Pulses per second should be in the tetany range (50–85 pps).

4. Interrupted or surge-type current should be used.

5. On time should be between 6 and 15 seconds.

6. Off time should be at least 1 minute.

7. The muscle should be given some resistance, either gravity or external resistance provided by the addition of weights or by fixing the joint, so that the contraction becomes isometric.

8. The patient can be instructed to work with the electrically induced contraction, but voluntary effort is not necessary for the success of this treatment.

9. Total treatment time should be 15–20 minutes, or enough time to allow a minimum of 10 contractions; some protocols have been successful with three sets of 10 contractions. The treatment can be repeated two times daily. Some protocols using battery-powered rather than line-powered units have advocated longer bouts with more repetitions, probably because of low contraction force.

10. High-volt or medium-frequency biphasic current should be used.[50,65,76–78]

Muscle strengthening. Muscle strengthening from electrical muscle stimulation has been used with some good results in patients with weakness or denervation of a muscle group.[79–85] The protocol is better established for this use, but more research is needed to clarify the procedures and allow us to generalize the results to other patient problems.

Treatment Parameters for Muscle Strengthening are as Follows:

1. Current intensity should be high enough to make the muscle develop 60% of the torque developed in an MVIC.

2. Pulse duration is preset on most therapeutic generators. If adjustable, it should be set as close as possible to the duration needed for chronaxie (300–600 microseconds) of the motor nerve to be stimulated. In general, longer pulse durations should include more nerves in response.

3. Pulses per second should be in the tetany range (70–85 pps).

4. Surged or interrupted current with a gradual ramp to peak intensity is most effective.

5. On time should be in the 10- to 15-second range.

6. Off time should be in the 50-second to 2-minute range.

7. Resistance usually is applied by immobilizing the limb. The muscle is then given an isometric contraction torque equal to or greater than 25% of the MVIC torque. The greater the percentage of torque produced, the better the results are.

8. The patient can be instructed to work with the electrically induced contraction, but voluntary effort is not necessary for the success of the treatment.

9. Total treatment time should include a minimum of 10 contractions, but mimicking normal active resistive training protocols of three sets of 10 contractions can also be productive. Fatigue is a major factor in this setup. Electrical stimulation bouts should be scheduled at least three times weekly. Generally, strength gains will continue over the treatment course, but intensities may need to increase to keep pace with the most current maximum voluntary contraction torques.

10. High-volt or a medium-frequency Russian current is the current of choice.[50,61,62,64,65,76–78,86]

CASE STUDY 5–4
ELECTRICAL STIMULATING CURRENTS: STRENGTHENING OF INNERVATED MUSCLE (2)

Background: A 33-year-old woman sustained an isolated rupture of the left anterior cruciate ligament (ACL) 2 weeks ago while skiing. Three days ago, she underwent an arthroscopically assisted intra-articular reconstruction of the ACL using an autologous patellar ligament graft. She is now weight bearing as tolerated with axillary crutches, is using a removable splint, and has been cleared for accelerated rehabilitation.

Impression: Postoperative ACL reconstruction.

Treatment Plan: In addition to the standard active strengthening and range of motion exercise and physical agent modalities to control postoperative pain and swelling, a course of electrical stimulation for strengthening was initiated. The split was removed, and the patient was seated on an isokinetic testing and training device, with the left knee in 65 degrees of flexion and the device set at a speed of 0°/s (isometric). A pulsatile polyphasic electrical stimulator was used, with electrodes placed over the motor points of the vastus medialis and vastus lateralis muscles. The stimulator produced a 2500-Hz carrier wave, with an effective frequency of 50 Hz (10 milliseconds on, 10 milliseconds off). A 2-second ramp-up and then a 2-second ramp-down setting was selected, with a total duty cycle of 10:50 (14 seconds on, 50 seconds off), and the current amplitude was adjusted to maximal tolerance during every third stimulation. Fifteen cycles were administered, and then the patient rested for 5 minutes; this was repeated twice, for a total of 45 contractions per treatment session. The patient was treated three times per week for a total of 5 weeks.

Response: A linear increase in force produced during electrical stimulation, as well as maximal isometric force production, was recorded over the 5 weeks of treatment. The patient's gait and range of motion improved, and she was discharged to a home program at the end of treatment.

(continued)

CASE STUDY 5–4   (continued)
ELECTRICAL STIMULATING CURRENTS: STRENGTHENING OF INNERVATED MUSCLE (2)

Discussion Questions

- What tissues were injured or affected?
- What symptoms were present?
- What phase of the injury-healing continuum did the patient present for care in?
- What are the physical agent modality's biophysical effects (direct, indirect, depth, and tissue affinity)?
- What are the physical agent modality's indications and contraindications?
- What are the parameters of the physical agent modality's application, dosage, duration, and frequency in this case study?
- What other physical agent modalities could be used to treat this injury or condition? Why? How?

- What advantages are there to augmenting the ACL repair with the patellar tendon?
- Why was the training of the quadriceps femoris conducted at 65 degrees of flexion? What biomechanical factors favor training at this joint angle as opposed to full extension of the knee?
- What effect did the electrical stimulation have on the healing rate of the reconstruction? On the patient's return to function?

The rehabilitation professional employs physical agent modalities to create an optimum environment for tissue healing while minimizing the symptoms associated with the trauma or condition.

Increasing range of motion. Increasing the range of motion in contracted joints is also a possible and documented use of electrical muscle stimulation. Electrically stimulating a muscle contraction pulls the joint through the limited range. The continued contraction of this muscle group over an extended time appears to make the contracted joint and muscle tissue modify and lengthen. Reduction of contractures in patients with hemiplegia has been reported, although no studies have reported this type of use in contracted joints from athletic injuries or surgery.

Treatment Parameters for Increasing Range of Motion are as Follows:

1. Current intensity must be of sufficient intensity and duration to make a muscle contract strongly enough to move the body part through its antigravity range. Intensity should be increased gradually during treatment.
2. Pulse duration is preset on most of the therapeutic generators. If it is adjustable, it should be set as close as possible to the duration needed to stimulate chronaxie (300–600 microseconds) of the motor nerve.
3. Pulses per second should be at the beginning of the tetany range (40–60 pps).
4. Interrupted or surged current should be used.
5. On time should be between 15 and 20 seconds.
6. Off time should be equal to or greater than on time because fatigue is a big consideration.
7. The stimulated muscle group should be antagonistic to the joint contracture, and the patient should be positioned so the joint will be moved to the limits of the available range.

8. The patient is passive in this treatment and does not work with the electrical contraction.
9. Total treatment time should be 90 minutes daily. This can be broken into three 30-minute treatments.
10. High-volt PC or Russian currents are the best choices.

CASE STUDY 5–5
ELECTRICAL STIMULATING CURRENTS: PAIN MODULATION

Background: A 47-year-old man sustained a closed crush injury of the right foot in a construction accident 12 weeks ago. Radiographs revealed no bone injury, and the physical examination indicated that the neurovascular structures were intact. A pneumatic immobilization device was applied to the right leg in the emergency department, the patient was supplied with axillary crutches, and he was instructed to avoid weight bearing on the right foot until he was cleared by his family physician. The immobilization device was removed 6 weeks ago, and the patient was instructed to begin progressive weight bearing and to exercise the foot on his own. He has now been referred to you because of a progressive increase in burning pain in the foot and leg, with swelling and extreme sensitivity to touch. The patient refuses to bear weight on the foot and is not wearing a sock or shoe on the right foot.

Impression: Complex regional pain syndrome (CRPS) type I (aka reflex sympathetic dystrophy).

Treatment Plan: A pulsatile biphasic current was delivered to the right leg, with electrodes over the anterior and posterior compartments. The frequency was 2 pps, and the amplitude was above the patient's pain threshold but below pain tolerance; a strong muscular twitch response was elicited. The current was delivered without interruption (duty cycle of 1:0) for 60 seconds. When the current was turned off, the patient's foot was brushed lightly with the therapist's hands. The process was repeated a total of 10 times in the initial treatment session, and the patient was instructed to attempt the brushing process at home.

Response: After the initial 60 seconds of current at the first treatment session, the patient was able to tolerate 5 seconds of light touch. After the 10th period of stimulation, the patient was able to tolerate 45 seconds of moderate touch. Treatment was repeated 3 days per week for 2 weeks, at which time the patient was able to tolerate a sock and shoe, was partial weight bearing, and continued the desensitization process on a home program.

Discussion Questions

- What tissues were injured or affected?
- What symptoms were present?
- What phase of the injury-healing continuum did the patient present for care in?
- What are the physical agent modality's biophysical effects (direct, indirect, depth, and tissue affinity)?
- What are the physical agent modality's indications and contraindications?
- What are the parameters of the physical agent modality's application, dosage, duration, and frequency in this case study?
- What other physical agent modalities could be used to treat this injury or condition? Why? How?
- What is CRPS type I?
- What is the difference between CRPS type I and CRPS type II?
- Why was low-frequency TENS selected for this patient? Would other forms of TENS (e.g., conventional, hyperstimulation) have been effective? Why or why not?
- Is it likely that CRPS could have been prevented in this patient? How?

The rehabilitation professional employs physical agent modalities to create an optimum environment for tissue healing while minimizing the symptoms associated with the trauma or condition.

The Effect of Noncontractile Stimulation on Edema

Ion movement within biologic tissues is a basic theory in the electrotherapy literature. This is clearly seen in the action potential model of nerve cell depolarization. The effects of sensory-level stimulation on edema have been theorized to work on this principle. Research has not documented the effectiveness of this type of treatment, and clinicians should continue to use other more proven mechanisms to decrease edema. See Chapter 15 for a discussion of edema formation.

Since 1987, numerous studies using rat and frog models have helped to more clearly define the effects of electrical stimulation on edema formation and reduction.[7,21,68–70,87] The muscle pumping theory discussed previously has seemed to be the most viable way to affect this problem.[28] Most of the recent studies have focused on a sensory-level stimulation. Early theory supported the use of sensory-level DC as a driving force to make the charged plasma protein ions in the interstitial spaces move in the direction of the oppositely charged electrode. Cook et al demonstrated an increased lymphatic uptake of labeled albumin within rats treated with sensory-level high-voltage stimulation.[67] However, there was no significant reduction in the limb volume. They hypothesized that the electric field introduced into the area of edema facilitated the movement of the charged proteins into the lymphatic channels. When the lymphatic channel volume increased, so too did the contraction rate of the smooth muscle in the lymphatics. They also hypothesized that stimulation of sensory neurons may cause an indirect activation of the autonomic nervous system. This might cause release of adrenergic substances that would also increase the rate of lymph smooth muscle contraction and lymph circulation.

Treatment considerations include:

1. extended treatment times, 1 hour;
2. monophasic current stimulation with polarity arranged in correct fashion;
3. electrodes arranged to pull or push plasma proteins into the lymphatic system and be moved back into the circulatory system via the thoracic duct.

Another proposed mechanism is that a microamp stimulation of the local neurovascular components in an injured area may cause a vasoconstriction and reduce the permeability of the capillary walls to limit the migration of plasma proteins into the interstitial spaces. This would retard the accumulation of plasma proteins and the associated fluid dynamics of the edema exudate. In a study on the histamine-stimulated leakage of plasma proteins, animals treated with small doses of electrical current produced less leakage.[68] The underlying mechanisms were a reduced pore size in the capillary walls and reduced pooling of blood in the capillaries, which could have been initiated by hormonal, neural, mechanical, or electrochemical factors.

Theory on the exact mechanism of edema control from these methods remains cloudy and contradictory, but we do not have enough research findings to support trying an electrical stimulation edema control trial clinically.

Treatment Parameters for Edema Control are as Follows:

1. Current intensity of 30–50 V or 10% less than that needed to produce a visible muscle contraction is most effective.
2. Preset short-duration currents on the high-voltage equipment are effective.
3. High pulse frequencies (120 pps) are most effective.
4. Interrupted monophasic currents are most effective. Biphasic currents showed increases in volume.
5. The animals treated with a negative distal electrode had a significant treatment effect. The animals with a positive distal electrode showed no change.
6. Time of treatment after injury: the best results were reported when treatment began immediately after injury. Treatment started after 24 hours showed an effect on the accumulation of new edema volume but showed no effect on the existing edema volume.

7. A 30-minute treatment showed good control of volume for 4–5 hours.

8. The water immersion electrode technique was effective, but using surface electrodes was not effective.

9. High-volt pulsed generators were effective, and low-volt generators were not effective.[8,18,33,75,88–98]

Clinical Decision-Making *Exercise 5–10*

When installing a whirlpool in the hydrotherapy area, the clinician must always be concerned about the possibility of electrical shock. What measures can be taken to reduce the possibility of electrical shock?

Asymmetric Biphasic Currents (TENS)

Asymmetric biphasic currents are found on the majority of portable TENS units (Figure 5–27). The term *transcutaneous electrical nerve stimulation* has become closely associated with pain control. Clinically, efforts are made to stimulate the sensory nerves to change the patient's perception of a painful stimulus coming from an injured area. A TENS unit consists of an electrical signal generator, a battery, and a set of electrodes. The units are small and programmable, and the generators can deliver trains of stimuli with variable current strengths, pulse rates, and pulse widths. To understand how to maximally affect the perception of pain through electrical stimulation, it is necessary to understand pain perception. The gate control theory, the descending control theory, and the endogenous opiate pain control theory are the theoretical basis for pain reduction phenomena. These theories were covered in depth in Chapter 4.

Therapeutic Uses of Electrical Stimulation of Sensory Nerves (TENS)

Gate control theory. Providing maximum sensory cutaneous stimulation to peripheral sensory Aβ fibers when there is pain in a certain area will generally "close the gate" to painful afferent impulses being transmitted to the spinal cord on Aδ and C fibers at the spinal cord level. As long as the stimuli are applied, the perception of pain is diminished. Electrical

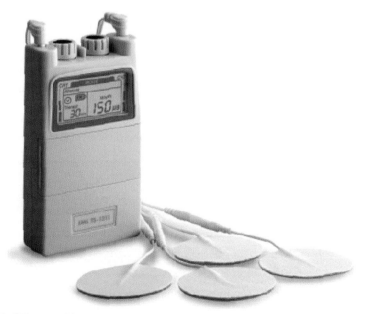

Figure 5–27. Portable TENS unit.

stimulation of sensory nerves will evoke the gate control mechanism and diminish awareness of painful stimuli.[2,35,40,42,46,76,78,99-104] This type of treatment is referred to as a *conventional, high-frequency,* or *sensory-level* TENS treatment and is the most commonly used TENS protocol. The intensity is set only high enough to elicit a tingling sensation but not high enough to cause a muscle contraction. Pain relief lasts while the stimulus is turned on, but it usually abates when the stimulation stops. Normally patients apply the electrodes and leave them in place all day, turning the stimulus on for approximately 30-minute intervals.

Treatment Parameters for Conventional TENS Treatment (Gate Control) are as Follows:

1. Current intensity should be adjusted to tolerance but should not cause a muscular contraction—the higher the better.
2. Pulse duration (pulse width) should be 75–150 microseconds or maximum possible on the machine.
3. Pulses per second should be 80–125, or as high as possible on the machine.
4. A transcutaneous electrical stimulator waveform should be used (most commonly asymmetric biphasic, but it can be symmetric biphasic and less commonly monophasic).
5. On time should be continuous mode.
6. Total treatment time should correspond to fluctuations in pain; the unit should be left on until pain is no longer perceived, turned off, and then restarted when pain begins again.
7. If this treatment is successful, you will have some pain relief within the first 30 minutes of treatment.
8. If it is not successful, but you feel this is the best theoretical or most clinically applicable approach, change the electrode placements and try again. If this is not successful, then using a different theoretical approach may offer more help.
9. Any stimulator that can deliver this current is acceptable. Portable units are better for 24-hour pain control (see Figure 5–21).[40,42,105]

Descending pain control theory. Intense electrical stimulation of the smaller peripheral Aδ and C fibers that transmit pain causes stimulation of the midbrain, pons, and medulla. In turn, this causes the release of enkephalin through descending neurons, which blocks the pain impulses at the spinal cord level (see Figure 3–9).[48] Cognitive input from the cortex relative to past pain perception and experiences also contributes to this descending mechanism control. This type of treatment is referred to as a **low-frequency** or **motor-level** TENS treatment. The intensity is set high enough to elicit both a tingling sensation and a muscle contraction. Pain relief with motor-level TENS should be expected to take longer than with conventional TENS (15–60 minutes), but the relief likely will last longer (>1 hour).

Treatment Parameters for Low-frequency or Motor-level TENS are as Follows:

1. Current intensity should be high enough to elicit a muscle contraction.
2. Pulse duration should be 100–600 microseconds.
3. Pulses per second should be <20 pps.
4. On time should be 30 seconds to 1 minute.

5. Stimulation should be applied over points where it is not difficult to elicit a motor response such as a motor point or even over acupuncture and trigger points.
6. Selection and number of points used vary according to the part treated but they do not necessarily have to be over the area of pain.
7. If this treatment is successful, pain will be relieved in 15–60 minutes but relief may last longer than 1 hour.
8. If this treatment is not successful, try different electrode setups by expanding the treatment points used.

Endogenous opiate pain control theory. Electrical stimulation of sensory nerves may stimulate the release of β-endorphin and dynorphin from the pituitary gland and the hypothalamus into the cerebral spinal fluid. The mechanism that causes the release and then the binding of β-endorphin, dynorphin, and ultimately enkephalin to some nerve cells is still unclear. It is certain that a diminution or elimination of pain perception is caused by applying a noxious electrical current to areas close to the site of pain or to acupuncture or trigger points, both local and distant to the pain area.[48,76,94,106–112]

To use the influence of hyperstimulation analgesia and β-endorphin release, a point stimulation setup must be used.[109] This approach utilizes a large dispersive pad and a small pad or handheld probe point electrode. The point electrode is applied to the chosen site, and the intensity is increased until the patient perceives it. The probe is then moved around the area, and the patient is asked to report relative changes in perception of intensity. When a location of maximum-intensity perception is found, the current intensity is increased to noxious but tolerable levels.[113] This is much the same as finding a motor point, as described earlier.[48,114]

β-Endorphin stimulation may offer better relief for the deep aching or chronic pain similar to the pain of overuse injury. The intensity of the impulse is a function of both pulse duration and amplitude. Comfort is a very important determinant of patient compliance and, thus, the overall success of treatment. Greater pulse widths tend to be more painful. The method of delivering TENS is less tolerable because the impulse intensity is higher.

A combination of noxious point stimulation and transcutaneous electrical nerve stimulation may be used. The transcutaneous electrical nerve stimulation applications should be used as much as needed to make the patient comfortable, and the intense point stimulation should be used on a periodic basis. Periodic use of intense point stimulation gives maximal pain relief for a period of time and allows some gains in overall pain suppression. Daily intense point stimulation may eventually bias the central nervous system and decrease the effectiveness of this type of stimulation.[26]

Treatment Protocols for Noxious-level TENS are as Follows:

1. Current intensity should be high, at a noxious level: muscular contraction is acceptable.
2. Pulse duration should be 100–1000 microseconds.
3. Pulses per second should be between 1 and 5.
4. High-volt pulsed current should be used.
5. On time should be 30–45 seconds.
6. Stimulation should be applied over trigger or acupuncture points.
7. Selection and number of points used vary according to the part and condition being treated.

8. A high-volt PC or a low-frequency, high-intensity machine is best for this effect.[48,102,103]

9. If stimulation is successful, you should know at the completion of the treatment. The analgesic effect should last for several (6–7) hours.

10. If not successful, try expanding the number of stimulation sites. Add the same stimulation points on the opposite side of the body, add auricular (ear) acupuncture points, and add more points on the same limb.

Microcurrent

Generators that produce subsensory-level stimulation were originally called microcurrent electrical neuromuscular stimulators (MENS). However, the stimulation pathway is not the usual neural pathway, and these machines are not designed to stimulate a muscle contraction. Consequently, this type of generator was subsequently referred to as a microcurrent electrical stimulator (MES). *Low-intensity stimulation (LIS)* is another currently used term in an ongoing evolution of terminology relative to this type of stimulation. A review of the current existing literature shows the term *microcurrent* to be the most widely used term to refer to this type of current.

Microcurrent < 1 mA

Perhaps the most important point to emphasize is that microcurrents are not substantially different from the currents discussed previously. These currents still have a direction, and both biphasic and monophasic waveforms are available. The currents also have amplitude (intensity), pulse duration, and frequency. The characteristic that distinguishes this type of current is that the intensity of the stimulus is limited to 1000 μA (1 mA) or less in microcurrent, whereas the intensity of the standard low-voltage equipment can be increased into the milliamp range.[115]

The generators can generate a variety of waveforms from modified monophasic to biphasic square waves with frequencies from 0.3 to 50 Hz. The pulse durations are also variable and may be prolonged at the lower frequencies from 1 to 500 milliseconds. This varies as the frequency changes or is preset when PC are used. Many of these devices are made with an impedance-sensitive voltage that adapts the current to the impedance to keep the current constant as selected.[116]

If the current generator can be adjusted to allow increases of intensity above 1000 μA, the current becomes like those previously described in this text. If the current provokes an action potential in a sensory or motor nerve, the results on that tissue will be the same as previously described for the sensations or muscle contractions caused by other currents.

Most of the literature on microcurrents and subsequently on subsensory stimulators has been generated by researchers interested in stimulating the healing process in fractures and skin wounds. Subsequent research aimed at identifying why and how microcurrents work. The best researched areas of application of microcurrents are in the stimulation of bone formation in delayed union or nonunion of fractures of the long bones. Most of this research was done using implanted rather than surface electrodes, and most has used low-intensity direct current (LIDC) with the negative pole placed at the fracture site.[8,86,117] We are in danger of generalizing treatments for all problems based on success in this one area. These applications were intended to mimic the normal electric field created during the injury and healing process.[38,91] At present, these electrical changes are poorly understood, and the effects of adding additional electrical current to the normal electrical activity created by the injury and healing process are still being investigated.

Microcurrent effects are as follows:
- analgesia;
- fracture healing;
- wound healing;
- ligament and tendon healing.

Microcurrent stimulation has been used for two major effects:

1. analgesia of the painful area[184]

2. biostimulation of the healing process, either for enhancing the process or for acceleration of its stages.[73,173]

CASE STUDY 5–6
ELECTRICAL STIMULATING: ANALGESIA

Background: A 52-year-old woman is 9 months post-hemi-laminectomy and discectomy without fusion at L5-S1 due to a herniated disc with compromise of the S1 nerve root. The surgery resulted in relief of the peripheral pain, weakness, and sensory loss, but persistent pain in the lumbosacral spine and buttock prevents the patient from engaging in rehabilitation exercises effectively.

Impression: Status postspinal surgery with persistent postoperative pain; no neural deficit.

Treatment Plan: The patient was already being treated with a hot pack prior to exercise; conventional TENS was added to the treatment regimen. Electrodes were placed at the L3-4 interspace and over the greater trochanter. A pulsatile biphasic waveform was selected, with a rate of 60 pps, an amplitude between the sensory and motor thresholds, and a duty cycle of 1:0 (uninterrupted). The stimulation was delivered for the 10-minute heat application and remained in place during the therapeutic exercise, as well as for 30 minutes following the exercise.

Response: The patient experienced a 60% reduction in the symptoms during the exercise; this enabled the patient to perform the exercise through a greater range and with a greater effect. The effect of the TENS began to diminish after 8 weeks, but the pain had diminished to manageable levels such that the patient was able to continue the rehabilitation program without the TENS.

Discussion Questions

- What tissues were injured/affected?
- What symptoms were present?
- What phase of the injury-healing continuum did the patient present for care in?
- What are the physical agent modality's biophysical effects (direct/indirect/depth/tissue affinity)?
- What are the physical agent modality's indications/contraindications?
- What are the parameters of the physical agent modality's application/dosage/duration/frequency in this case study?
- What other physical agent modalities could be utilized to treat this injury or condition? Why? How?
- What factors led to the selection of conventional TENS?
- What would be the advantages and disadvantages of low TENS for this patient?
- What is the theoretical mechanism of action of conventional TENS?
- Why did the effect of the TENS diminish over time?
- Would you characterize the patient's pain as chronic or acute? Why? Are there different optimum forms of electrical stimulation for pain relief dependent on the nature of the pain?

The rehabilitation professional employs physical agent modalities to create an optimum environment for tissue healing while minimizing the symptoms associated with the trauma or condition.

Analgesic Effects of Microcurrent

The mechanism of analgesia created by microcurrent does not fit into our present theoretical framework, as sensory nerve excitation is a necessary component of all three models of electroanalgesia stimulation. At best, microcurrent can create or change the constant DC flow of the neural tissues, which may have some way of biasing the transmission of the painful stimulus. LIS may also make the nerve cell membrane more receptive to neurotransmitters that will block transmission. The exact mechanism has not yet been established. The research is not supportive of the effectiveness of microcurrent for pain reduction.[118,119] This lack of consensus and disagreement in the research give the clinician limited security in devising an effective protocol. Most of the research uses delayed onset muscle soreness (DOMS) or cold-induced pain models, and results show no difference between microcurrent and placebo treatments.[54,73,89,103,104,120–130]

Biostimulative Effects on the Healing Process

Promotion of wound healing. Low-intensity monophasic current has been used to treat skin ulcers that have poor blood flow. The treated ulcers show accelerated healing rates when compared with untreated skin ulcers. Other protocols have been successful using the anode in the wound area for the entire time. High-voltage stimulation also has been used in a manner similar to the negative–positive model presented. The intensity was adjusted to give a micro-amp current.

The mechanism by which microcurrent stimulates healing is elusive, but cells are stimulated to increase their normal proliferation, migration, motility, DNA synthesis, and collagen synthesis. Receptor levels for growth factor have also shown a significant increase when wound areas are stimulated.[30,50,100,131–138] The naturally occurring electrical potential gradients are enhanced following electrical stimulation.[54]

Treatment Parameters for Wound Healing are as Follows:

1. Current intensity is 200–400 µA for normal skin and 400–800 µA for denervated skin.
2. Long pulse durations or continuous uninterrupted currents can be used.
3. Maximum pulse frequency.
4. Monophasic DC is best but biphasic DC is acceptable. Microcurrent stimulators can be used but other generators with intensities adjusted to subsensory levels also can be effective. A battery-powered portable unit is most convenient.
5. Treatment time is 2 hours followed by a 4-hour rest time.
6. Utilize two to three treatment bouts per day.
7. The negative electrode is positioned in the wound area for the first 3 days. The positive electrode should be positioned 25 cm proximal to the wound.
8. After 3 days the polarity is reversed and the positive electrode is positioned in the wound area.
9. If infection is present, the negative electrode should be left in the wound area until the signs of infection are not evident. The negative electrode remains in the wound for 3 days after the infection clears.
10. If the wound size decreases to a plateau, then return the negative electrode to the wound area for 3 days.

Promotion of fracture healing. The use of subsensory DC may be an adjunctive modality in the treatment of fractures, especially fractures prone to nonunion. Fracture healing may be accelerated by passing a monophasic current through the fracture site. Getting the current into the bony area without an invasive technique is difficult.[43,46,48,58,86,121,139–141]

Using a standard transcutaneous electrical nerve stimulation unit, Kahn reported favorable results in the electrical stimulation of callus formation in fractures that had nonunions after 6 months.[142] This information is based on a case study. Results of a more extensive population of nonunions have not been documented.

Treatment Protocols for Fracture Healing are as Follows:

1. Current intensity was just perceptible to the patient.
2. Pulse duration was the longest duration allowed on the unit (100–200 milliseconds).
3. Pulses per second were set at the lowest frequency allowed on the unit (5–10 pps).

4. Standard monophasic or biphasic current in the transcutaneous electrical stimulating units was used.

5. Treatment time was from 30 minutes to 1 hour, three to four times daily.

6. A negative electrode was placed close to but distal to the fracture site. A positive electrode was placed proximal to the immobilizing device.

7. If four pads were used, the interferential placement described earlier was used.

8. Results were reassessed at monthly intervals.[142]

Promotion of healing in tendon and ligament. There are only a few research studies on the biostimulative effect of electrical stimulation on tendon or ligament healing. Both tissues have been found to generate strain-generated electrical potentials naturally in response to stress. These potentials help signal the tissue to grow in response to the stress according to Wolff's law.

In an experimental study on partial division of dog patellar tendons treated with 20-μA cathodal stimulation, the stimulated tendons showed 92% recovery of normal breaking strength at 8 weeks.[143]

Tendon stimulated in vitro in a culture medium showed increased fibroblastic cellular activity, tendon cellular proliferation, and collagen synthesis. The rate at which stimulated tendons demonstrated histologic repair at the injury site was also significantly accelerated over the control group.[144] Litke and Dahners studied rat medial collateral ligament (MCL) injuries treated with electrical simulation. The treated group showed statistical significance in the rupture force, stiffness, energy absorbed, and laxity.[56]

As can be seen by the previous sections, microcurrent can be a valuable addition to the clinical armamentarium of the clinician, but it is untested clinically.

Microcurrent is a case where more may not be better. For electricity to produce these effects: (1) cells must be current sensitive; (2) correct polarity orientation may be necessary; and (3) correct amounts of current will cause the cells to be more active in the healing process.

If results are not positive, then reduce the current and/or change polarity. Weak stimuli may increase physiologic activity, whereas very much stronger stimuli abolish or inhibit activity.

Most generators in use today are capable of delivering microcurrent. Simply turn the machine on but do not increase the intensity to threshold levels. This can also be a function of current density using electrode size and placement as well as intensity to keep current in the microampere range. The clinician is certainly entitled to be very skeptical of the manufacturers' claims until more research is reported. Existing protocols for use are not well established, which leaves the clinician with an insecure feeling about this modality.

Russian Currents (Medium-Frequency Current Generators)

This class of current generators was developed in Canada and the United States after the Russian scientist Yadou M. Kots presented a seminar on the use of electrical muscular stimulators to augment strength gain.[145] The stimulators developed after this presentation were termed **Russian current** generators. These stimulators have evolved and presently deliver a medium-frequency (2000–10,000 Hz) pulsatile biphasic waveform. The pulse can be varied from 50 to 250 microseconds; the phase duration will be one half of the pulse duration, or 25–125 microseconds.[146] As the pulse frequency increases, the pulse duration decreases.[45,91,147]

Russian current produces two basic waveforms: a sine wave and a square wave cycle with a fixed intrapulse interval. The sine wave is produced in a burst mode that has a 50% on/off time. According to SD curve data, to obtain the same stimulation effect as the duration of the

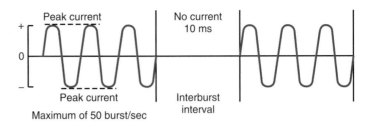

Figure 5–28. Russian current with polyphasic AC waveform and 10-millisecond interburst interval.

stimulus decreases, the intensity must be increased. The intensity associated with this duration of current could be considered painful.

To make this intensity of current tolerable, it is generated in 50-bursts-per-second envelopes with an interburst interval of 10 milliseconds. This slightly reduces the total current but allows enough of a peak current intensity to stimulate muscle very well (Figure 5–28). If the current continued without the burst effect, the total current delivered would equal the lightly shaded area in Figure 5–29. When generated with the burst effect, the total current is decreased. In this case, the total current would equal the darkly shaded area in Figure 5–30. This allows the patient to tolerate greater current intensity. The other factor affecting patient comfort is the effect that frequency will have on the impedance of the tissue. Higher-frequency currents reduce the resistance to the current flow, again making this type of waveform comfortable enough that the patient may tolerate higher intensities. As the intensity increases, more motor nerves are stimulated, increasing the magnitude of the contraction.[80] Because it is a fast-oscillating biphasic current, as soon as the nerve repolarizes it is stimulated again, producing a current that will maximally summate muscle contraction.[23,148] The primary clinical use of Russian current is for muscle strengthening.

The frequency (pulses per second or, in this case, bursts per second) is a variable that can be controlled to make the muscle respond with a twitch rather than a gradually increasing mechanical contraction. Gradually increasing the numbers of bursts interrupts the mechanical relaxation cycle of the muscle and causes more shortening to take place (see Figure 5–13).[25]

Figure 5–29. Russian current without an interburst interval. The lightly shaded area is equal to the total current.

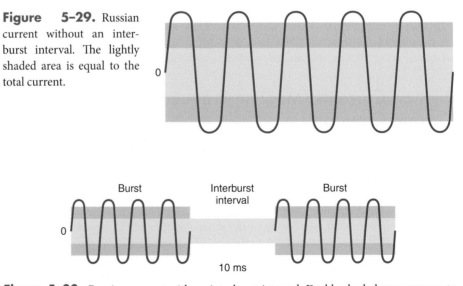

Figure 5–30. Russian current with an interburst interval. Darkly shaded area represents total current, and light shading indicates total current without the interburst interval.

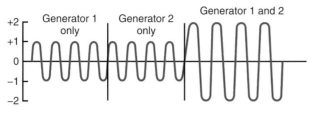

Figure 5–31. Sine wave from generator 1 and sine wave from generator 2 showing a constructive interference pattern.

Interferential Currents

The research on and use of IFC has taken place primarily in Europe. An Austrian scientist, Ho Nemec, introduced the concept and suggested its therapeutic use. The theories and behavior of electrical waves are part of basic physics. This behavior is easiest to understand when continuous sine waves are used as an example.

With only one circuit, the current behaves as described earlier; if put on an oscilloscope, it looks like generator 1 in Figure 5–31. If a second generator is brought into the same location, the currents may interfere with each other. This interference can be summative—that is, the amplitudes of the electrical wave are combined and increase (Figure 5–31). Both waves are exactly the same; if they are produced in phase or originate at the same time, they combine. This is called **constructive interference**.

If these waves are generated out of sync, generator 1 starts in a positive direction at the same time that generator 2 starts in a negative direction; the waves then will cancel each other out. This is called **destructive interference**; in the summation the waves end up with an amplitude of 0 (Figure 5–32).

To make this more complex, assume that one generator has a slightly slower or faster frequency and that the generators begin producing current simultaneously. Initially, the electrical waves will be constructively summated; however, because the frequencies of the two waves differ, they gradually will get out of phase and become destructively summated. When dealing with sound waves, we hear distinct beats as this phenomenon occurs. We borrow the term *beat* when describing this behavior. When any waveforms are out of phase but are combined in the same location, the waves will cause a beat effect. The blending of the waves is caused by the constructive and destructive interference patterns of the waves and is called *heterodyne* (Figure 5–33).[91,149]

The heterodyne effect is seen on an oscilloscope as a cyclic, rising and falling waveform.[150] The peaks or beat frequency in this heterodyne wave behavior occur regularly, according to the difference of each current. With IFC, one generator produces current at a frequency of

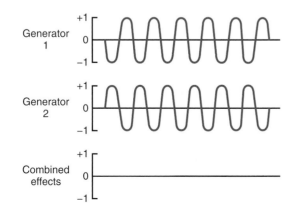

Figure 5–32. Sine wave from generator 1 and sine wave from generator 2 showing a destructive interference pattern.

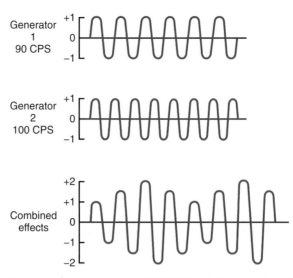

Figure 5–33. Sine wave from generator 1 at 90 CPS and sine wave from generator 2 at 100 CPS showing the heterodyne, or beating pattern, of interference.

4080 pps. The second generator outputs current at a frequency of 4080 pps. Thus, the beat frequency would be 80 pps:

$$4080 \text{ pps} - 4000 \text{ pps} = 80 \text{ pps beat frequency}$$

In electrical currents, this beat frequency is, in effect, the stimulation frequency of the waveform because the destructive interference negates the effects of the other part of the wave. The intensity (amplitude) will be set according to sensations created by this peak.[91] When using an interference current for therapy, the clinician should select the frequencies to create a beat frequency corresponding to his or her choices of frequency when using other stimulators: 20–50 pps for muscle contraction, 50–120 pps for a conventional TENS treatment, and 1 pps for endogenous opiate pain modulation.

When the electrodes are arranged in a square alignment and IFC are passed through a homogeneous medium, a predictable pattern of interference will occur. In this pattern, an electric field is created that resembles a four-petaled flower, with the center of the flower located where the two currents cross and the petals falling between the electrical current force lines. The maximum interference effect takes place near the center, with the field gradually decreasing in strength as it moves toward the points of the petal (Figure 5–34).[91] Because the body is not a homogeneous medium, we cannot predict the exact location of this interference pattern; we must rely on the patient's perception. If the patient has a localized structure that is painful, locating

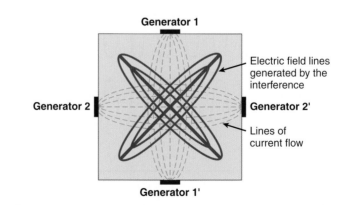

Figure 5–34. Square electrode alignment and interference pattern of current in a homogeneous medium.

CASE STUDY 5–7
ELECTRICAL STIMULATION: CONTROL OF SWELLING

Background: A 43-year-old woman, recreational runner, sustained a grade II ankle sprain (inversion stress) approximately 4 hours prior to presentation for treatment. She is ambulatory in a touch weight-bearing mode with crutches and is not in acute distress. Positive signs are limited to the ankle, which demonstrates 3+/4 swelling, marked restriction in range of motion, and point tenderness over the anterior talofibular and calcaneofibular ligaments. There is no loss of ligamentous stability.

Impression: Grade II ankle sprain, with significant swelling.

Treatment Plan: In addition to therapeutic exercise, electrical stimulation was selected to assist in the reduction of the swelling. A monophasic pulsatile waveform generator was selected, and the cathode (negative polarity) was placed over the anteriolateral aspect of the ankle, with the anode over the posterior leg. The pulse rate was set at 120 pps, with the amplitude between the sensory and motor thresholds. Stimulation was applied for 30 minutes daily.

Response: The swelling was reduced by approximately 30% after the initial treatment, but had returned the next day. Over the next 5 days, the swelling was markedly reduced following treatment, but regressed by about 50% by the next day. Electrical stimulation was discontinued after 7 days. A progressive rehabilitation program was initiated the first day, and the patient returned to full activity after 3 weeks.

Discussion Questions

- What tissues were injured/affected?
- What symptoms were present?
- What phase of the injury-healing continuum did the patient present for care in?
- What are the physical agent modality's biophysical effects (direct/indirect/depth/tissue affinity)?
- What are the physical agent modality's indications/contraindications?
- What are the parameters of the physical agent modality's application/dosage/duration/frequency in this case study?
- What other physical agent modalities could be utilized to treat this injury or condition? Why? How?
- Is electrical stimulation the most effective means to control the swelling in this patient's ankle? What approach might be more or equally effective?
- How will the swelling affect the healing of the injured tissues?
- How will the swelling affect the ability of the patient to perform therapeutic exercise?
- What are the physiologic mechanisms for the swelling? For the resolution of the swelling?
- Why is the term "swelling" used in lieu of "edema" or "effusion?"

The rehabilitation professional employs physical agent modalities to create an optimum environment for tissue healing while minimizing the symptoms associated with the trauma or condition.

---

the stimulation in the correct location is relatively easy. The clinician moves the electrode placement until the patient centers the feeling of the stimulus in the problem area.[91,149] When a patient has poorly localized pain, the task becomes more difficult. See the discussion in the section "Electrode Placement" for a general discussion on the effect of electrode movement. The engineers added features to the generators and created a scanning IFC that moves the flower petals of force around while the treatment is taking place. This enlarges the effective treatment area. Additional technology and another set of electrodes create a three-dimensional flower effect when one looks at the electric field. This is called a **stereodynamic interference current**.[91,149]

All these alterations and modifications are designed to spread the heterodyne effect throughout the tissue. Because it is controlled by a cyclic electrical pattern, however, we actually may be decreasing the current passed through the structures we are trying to treat. The machines seem complex but lack the versatility to do much more than the conventional TENS treatment.[25,151]

Nikolova[152] has used IFC for a variety of clinical problems and found it effective in dealing with pain problems (e.g., joint sprains with swelling, restricted mobility and pain, neuritis, retarded callus formation following fractures, pseudarthrosis).[103] These claims are supported by other researchers. Each of these researchers used slightly different protocols in treating the different clinical problems. To be successful in achieving the desired results with IFC, the clinician must thoroughly review existing protocols and acquire a good working knowledge of the application techniques.

Premodulated Interferential Current

In recent years, a second method of creating the interference effect has been developed, which is referred to as premodulated interferential. Premodulated IFC is available on most of the newer electrical stimulating units. In the premodulated setting, both generators of the unit output a frequency of 4000 Hz. However, each generator has the ability to premodulate or burst the frequency within the unit.[153] The unit has the capability of perfectly synchronizing these bursts in the same polarity, at the same time to create premodulated interferential.[155]

Units that are capable of premodulation are not necessarily premodulated interferential. They may only provide premodulation for the purpose of bipolar (two electrodes) stimulation. While both create the interferential effect, there may be some advantages to the premodulated technique.[155]

The true interferential provides an uninterrupted, constant 4000-Hz frequency to the tissue. This will create a numbness beneath the electrodes that the patient will perceive as a reduction in the intensity of the current. With premodulated interferential, however, since the current is being burst inside the unit itself, numbness does not occur and a larger treatment area is established with the actual therapeutic frequency.[155]

Low-Volt Currents

Medical Galvanism

The application of continuous low-voltage monophasic current causes several physiologic changes that can be used therapeutically. The therapeutic benefits are related to the polar and vasomotor effects and to the acid reaction around the positive pole and the alkaline reaction at the negative pole. The clinician must be concerned with the damaging effects of this variety of current. Acidic or alkaline changes can cause severe skin reactions.[2] These reactions occur only with low-voltage continuous DC and are not likely with the high-voltage pulsed generators. The pulse duration of the high-volt pulsatile generators is too short to cause these chemical changes.[31]

Low-volt currents also have a vasomotor effect on the skin, increasing blood flow between the electrodes. The benefits from this type of DC are usually attributed to the increased blood flow through the treatment area.[2]

Iontophoresis

DC has been used for many years to transport ions from the heavy metals into and through the skin for treatment of skin infections or for a counterirritating effect. Iontophoresis is discussed in detail in Chapter 6.

Treatment Precautions with Continuous Monophasic Currents

Skin burns are the greatest hazard of any continuous monophasic current technique. These burns result from excessive electrical density in any area, usually from direct metal contact with skin or from setting the intensity too high for the size of the active electrode. Both these problems cause a very high density of current in the area of contact.[25,114]

Treatment Protocols for Low-volt Current are as Follows:

1. Current intensity should be to the patient's tolerance; it should be increased as accommodation takes place. These intensities are in the milliampere range.
2. Continuous monophasic current should be used.
3. Pulses per second should be 0.
4. A low-voltage monophasic current stimulator is the machine of choice.

5. Treatment time should be between a 15-minute minimum and a 50-minute maximum.
6. Equal-sized electrodes are used over gauze that has been soaked in saline solution and lightly squeezed.
7. Skin should be unbroken.[25,114,142]

BONE GROWTH STIMULATORS

Generally, bone fractures heal normally with standard care. Occasionally, the healing process stops due to added risks or complications. *Delayed union* refers to a decelerating bone healing process. *Nonunion* is considered to be established when the fracture site shows no visibly progressive signs of healing, without giving any guidance regarding the time frame. A reasonable time period for lack of visible signs of healing is 3 months. It has been shown that electrical current can stimulate bone growth and enhance the healing process.[154]

Several electrical bone growth stimulators are available. These stimulators attempt to produce electromagnetic fields similar to those that normally exist in bone. The *noninvasive type* of stimulator is comprised of coils or electrodes, placed on the skin near the fracture site. Noninvasive bone growth stimulators generate a weak biphasic electrical current within the target site using small electrodes placed on either side of the fracture.[155] These are worn for 24 hours per day until healing occurs or up to 9 months. A second type of noninvasive bone growth stimulator uses pulsed electromagnetic fields delivered via treatment coils placed directly onto the skin and are worn for 6–8 hours per day for 3–6 months. There is also a noninvasive stimulator that uses ultrasound.

The *invasive type* of stimulator includes percutaneous and implanted devices. The percutaneous type involves electrode wires inserted through the skin into the bone while implanted devices include a generator placed under the skin or in the muscles near the fracture site. The implanted devices are surgically placed and later surgically removed. Invasive devices use DC.[155] The implantable device typically remains functional for 6–9 months after implantation. Although the current generator is removed in a second surgical procedure when stimulation is completed, the electrode may or may not be removed. Invasive bone growth stimulation is used only in spinal fusion surgery, and is not used in the appendicular skeleton.

FUNCTIONAL ELECTRICAL STIMULATION

Since the mid-1980s researchers have experimented with using computer-controlled electrical currents that stimulate the peripheral nervous system for the purpose of providing dynamic assistance in functional activities, such as walking or upper extremity function.[156] Used primarily in patients who have sustained spinal cord injury or suffered a stroke, **FES** utilizes multiple-channel electrical stimulators controlled by a microprocessor to recruit muscles in a programmed synergistic sequence that will allow the patient to accomplish a specific functional movement pattern.[113,156] Even though this technique has been used effectively in short-term management of a variety of dysfunctions, there are many practical considerations for use that might impede or limit the long-term independent usefulness of FES by a patient.[157]

Currently, the majority of FES programs are limited to the use of surface electrodes that are difficult to adhere to the skin and to maintain positioning at the appropriate stimulation point.[158] For FES to be useful to the patient on a daily basis, the electrodes, and possibly the stimulator itself, will need to be implanted directly into the muscle or on a nerve.[159] Research is ongoing toward this end, but to date no acceptable system has been developed.

The existing computer control systems for FES also need to be refined if they are to be both useful and safe for the patient. Either the control systems must use a preset activation sequence that will allow the patient to execute a specific task or there must be some type of feedback from the stimulated neuromuscular systems so that the computer can make the appropriate movement corrections to ensure the safety of the patient. The development of a "closed-loop" feedback control system that would allow the computer to compensate for uneven terrain or to adjust the speed and frequency of movement presents a major challenge to researchers working in this area.[160]

Although multichannel microprocessors may be preprogrammed to execute a variety of specific movement patterns, how those programs will be activated presents another obstacle for development of FES systems. Foot switches or crutch switches may potentially be used to trigger a desired response, although there are limitations to the number of switches that a spinal cord or stroke patient would actually be able to use.[113] Some of the upper extremity control devices have used movements of the contralateral shoulder to trigger a response. Verbal commands recognized by the computer also have been used to control stimulation of muscle in various functional tasks.[157]

Presently long-term independent use of FES is practical for only a few problems.[157,176] Certainly as new technologies continue to become available, ongoing clinical research will make FES increasingly practical for various patient populations. The future of FES holds many exciting possibilities for patients and clinicians alike.

Clinical Uses of FES

FES has a number of clinical applications.[161] Initially, FES was used for stroke patients with a foot drop to assist dorsiflexion. Subsequently, it was found to be more useful in treating patients with incomplete spinal cord injury who have good stance stability but are unable to achieve adequate flexion during the swing phase of gait.[157]

FES has been used with some success, enabling patients to stand, transfer, ambulate on level surfaces, and even ascend stairs on a limited basis using a walker or crutches in a closely supervised environment.[107,162–166] Spinal cord patients have used computer-controlled FES to allow them to exercise on bicycle ergometers to improve cardiorespiratory endurance and fitness.[167,168]

Control of muscles in the upper extremity using multiple-channel stimulation has allowed paraplegic patients to use the muscles of the hand and forearm of the paralyzed limb in functional grasp patterns. FES has also been used effectively in managing shoulder subluxation in the hemiplegic patient.[157]

PLACEBO EFFECT OF ELECTRICAL STIMULATION

There is a major placebo effect in all that we do in providing any therapy to our patients. This placebo effect is a basic and extremely important tool to help us achieve the best results. Our attitude toward the patients and our presentation of the therapy to them are crucial. When the clinician demonstrates a sincere interest in the patient's problems, the patient uses that interest to add to his or her own conviction and motivation to get well.

This perceptual change is influenced by many factors at the cognitive and affective levels. When these factors are active, real physiologic changes occur that assist in the healing process. The clinician should not intentionally deceive the patient with a sham treatment but should use the treatment to have the best impact on the patient's perception of the problem and the treatment's effectiveness.

The treatment will work better if the patient has a profound belief in its ability to alleviate the problem. To gain the most from this effect, the patient needs to be intimately involved with the treatment. We must educate, encourage, and empower the patient to get better. Giving the patient the knowledge and ability to feel some control and to be self-determined in healing reduces the stress of injury and enhances the patient's recovery powers. In stressful situations any measure of control lessens the extent of the stress and results in the improvement of disease resistance or injury recovery factors that will improve treatment outcomes.[26]

SAFETY IN THE USE OF ELECTRICAL EQUIPMENT

Electrical safety in the clinical setting should be of maximal concern to the professional clinician. Too often there are reports of patients being electrocuted as a result of faulty electrical circuits in whirlpools. This type of accident can be avoided by taking some basic precautions and acquiring an understanding of the power distribution system and electrical grounds.[169]

The typical electrical circuit consists of a source producing electrical power, a conductor that carries the power to a resistor or series of driven elements, and a conductor that carries the power back to the power source.

Electrical power is carried from generating plants through high-tension power lines carrying 2200 V. The power is decreased by a transformer and is supplied in the wall outlet at 220 or 120 V with a frequency of 60 Hz. The voltage at the outlet is AC, which means that one of the poles, the "hot" or "live" wire, is either positive or negative with respect to other neutral lines. Theoretically, the voltage of the neutral pole should be zero. Actually, the voltage of the neutral line is about 10 V. Thus, both hot and neutral lines carry some voltage with respect to the earth, which has zero voltage. The voltage from either of these two leads may be sufficient to cause physiologic damage.

The two-pronged plug has only two leads, both of which carry some voltage. Consequently, the electrical device has no true **ground**. The term *true ground* literally means the electrical circuit is connected to the earth or the ground, which has the ability to accept large electrical charges without becoming charged itself. The ground will continually accept these charges until the electrical potential has been neutralized. Therefore, any electrical charge that may be potentially hazardous (i.e., any electricity escaping from the circuit) is almost immediately neutralized by the ground. If an individual were to come in contact with a short-circuited instrument that was not grounded, the electrical current would flow through that individual to reach the ground.

Electrical devices that have two-pronged plugs generally rely on the chassis or casing of the power source to act as a ground, but this is not a true ground. Therefore, if an individual were to touch the casing of the instrument while in contact with some object or instrument that has a true ground, an electrical shock may result. With three-pronged plugs, the third prong is grounded directly to the earth and all excess electrical energy theoretically should therefore be neutralized.

By far the most common mechanism of injury from therapeutic devices results when there is some damage, breakdown, or short circuit to the power cord. When this happens, the casing of the machine becomes electrically charged. In other words, there is a voltage leak, and in a device that is not properly grounded electrical shock may occur (Figure 5–35).

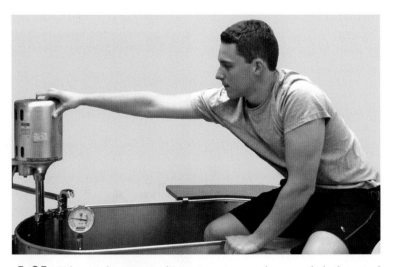

Figure 5–35. When a therapeutic device is not properly grounded, there is danger of electrical shock. This is a major problem in a whirlpool.

Table 5–3 Physiologic Effects of Electrical Shock at Varying Magnitudes

INTENSITY (mA)	PHYSIOLOGIC EFFECTS
0–1	Imperceptible
2–15	Tingling sensation and muscle contraction
16–100	Painful electrical shock
101–200	Cardiac or respiratory arrest
>200	Instant tissue burning and destruction

The magnitude of the electrical shock is a critical factor in terms of potential health danger (Table 5–3). Shock from electrical currents flowing at ≤1 mA will not be felt and is referred to as **microshock**. Shock from a current flow greater than 1 mA is called **macroshock**. Currents that range between 1 and 15 mA produce a tingling sensation or perhaps some muscle contraction. Currents flowing at 15–100 mA cause a painful electrical shock. Currents between 100 and 200 mA may result in fibrillation of cardiac muscle or respiratory arrest. When current flow is above 200 mA, rapid burning and destruction of tissue occur.[170]

Most electrotherapeutic devices (e.g., muscle stimulators, ultrasound, and the diathermies) are generally used in dry environments. All new electrotherapeutic equipment being produced has three-pronged plugs and is thus grounded to the earth. However, in a wet or damp area the three-pronged plug may not provide sufficient protection from electrical shock. We know that the body will readily conduct electricity because of its high water content. If the body is wet or if an individual is standing in water, the resistance to electrical flow is reduced even more. Thus, if a short should occur, the shock could be as much as five times greater in this damp or wet environment. The potential danger that exists with whirlpools or tubs is obvious. The ground on the whirlpool will supposedly conduct all current leakage from a faulty motor or power cord to the earth. However, an individual in a whirlpool is actually a part of that circuit and is subject to the same current levels as any other component of the circuit. Small amounts of current therefore can be potentially harmful, no matter how well the apparatus is grounded. For this reason in 1981 the National Electrical Code required that all health care facilities using whirlpools and tubs install **ground-fault interruptors (GFI)** (Figure 5–36). These devices constantly compare the amount of electricity flowing from the

Figure 5–36. A typical ground-fault interrupter (GFI). Courtesy of *The Family Handyman Magazine.*

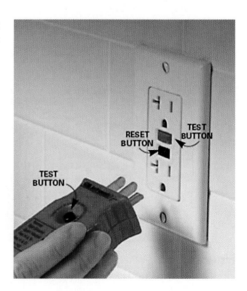

wall outlet with the whirlpool turbine with the amount returning to the outlet. If any leakage in current flow is detected, the ground-fault circuit breaker will automatically interrupt current flow in as little as one fortieth of a second, thus shutting off current flow and reducing the chances of electrical shock.[171] These devices may be installed either in the electrical outlet or in the circuit breaker box.

Regardless of the type of electrotherapeutic device being used and the type of environment, the following safety practices should be considered.

1. The entire electrical system of the building or training room should be designed or evaluated by a qualified electrician. Problems with the electrical system may exist in older buildings or in situations where rooms have been modified to accommodate therapeutic devices (e.g., putting a whirlpool in a locker room where the concrete floor is always wet or damp).

2. It should not be assumed that all three-pronged wall outlets are automatically grounded to the earth. The ground must be checked.

3. The clinician should become very familiar with the equipment being used and any potential problems that may exist or develop. Any defective equipment should be removed from the clinic immediately.

4. The plug should not be jerked out of the wall by pulling on the cable.

5. Extension cords or multiple adaptors should never be used.

6. Equipment should be reevaluated on a yearly basis and should conform to National Electrical Code guidelines. If a clinic or athletic training room is not in compliance with this code, then there is no legal protection in a lawsuit.

7. Common sense should always be exercised when using electrotherapeutic devices. A situation that appears to be potentially dangerous may in fact result in injury or death.

SUMMARY

1. Electrons move along a conducting medium as an electrical current.

2. A volt is the electromotive force that produces a movement of electrons; an ampere is a unit of measurement that indicates the rate at which electrical current is flowing.

3. Ohm's law expresses the relationship between current flow voltage and resistance. The current flow is directly proportional to the voltage and inversely proportional to the resistance.

4. Electrotherapeutic devices generate three different types of current, AC or biphasic, DC or monophasic, or PC or polyphasic, which are capable of producing specific physiologic changes when introduced into biologic tissue.

5. Confusion exists relative to the terminology used to describe electrotherapeutic currents, but all therapeutic electrical generators are transcutaneous electrical stimulators, regardless of whether they deliver biphasic, monophasic, or PC through electrodes attached to the skin.

6. The term *pulse* is synonymous with *waveform*, which indicates a graphic representation of the shape, direction, amplitude, duration, and pulse frequency of the electrical current the electrotherapeutic device produces, as displayed by an instrument called an oscilloscope.

7. Modulation refers to any alteration in the magnitude or any variation in duration of a pulse (or pulses) and may be continuous, interrupted, burst, or ramped.

8. The main difference between a series and a parallel circuit is that in a series circuit there is a single pathway for current to get from one terminal to another, and in a parallel circuit two or more routes exist for current to pass.

9. The electrical circuit that exists when electron flow is through human tissue is in reality a combination of both a series and a parallel circuit.

10. The effects of electrical current moving through biologic tissue may be chemical, thermal, or physiologic.

11. When an electrical system is applied to muscle or nerve tissue, the result will be tissue membrane depolarization, provided that the current has the appropriate intensity, duration, and waveform to reach the tissue's excitability threshold.

12. Muscle and nerve tissue respond in an all-or-none fashion; there is no gradation of response.

13. Muscle contraction will change according to changes in current. As the frequency of the electrical stimulus increases, the muscle will develop more tension as a result of the summation of the contraction of the muscle fiber through progressive mechanical shortening. Increases in intensity spread the current over a larger area and increase the number of motor units activated by the current. Increases in the duration of the current also will cause more motor units to be activated.

14. Nonexcitatory cells and tissues respond to subsensory electrical currents that can alter how the cell functions following injury.

15. The newest electrical stimulating units are capable of producing multiple types of current including high volt, biphasic, microcurrent, Russian, interferential, premodulated interferential, and low volt.

16. Electrically stimulating muscle contractions using primarily high-volt current are used clinically to help with muscle reeducation, muscle contraction for muscle pumping action, reduction of swelling, prevention or retardation of atrophy, muscle strengthening, and increasing range of motion in tight joints.

17. TENS applications are generally used for stimulating sensory nerve fibers and modulating pain. TENS' current parameters can be modified to modulate pain through gate control, descending mechanisms, and endogenous opiate mechanisms of pain control.

18. Microcurrent uses subsensory electrical currents primarily to achieve biostimulative effects in healing of bone and soft tissues.

19. Russian current delivers a medium-frequency biphasic waveform and is used primarily for muscle strengthening.

20. Interferential and premodulated IFC rely on the combined effects of currents produced from two separate generators and are used primarily for pain management.

21. Low-volt currents are continuous monophasic current. Their primary use involves polar effects (acid or alkaline), increased blood flow, bacteriostatic effects (through the negative electrode), and migration and alignment of cellular building blocks in the healing processes.

22. Electrical safety is critical when using electrotherapeutic devices. It is the responsibility of the clinician to make sure that all electrical modalities conform to the National Electrical Code.

REVIEW QUESTIONS

1. How are the following electrical terms defined: *potential difference, ampere, volt, ohm,* and *watt*?

2. What is the mathematical expression of Ohm's law and what does it represent?

3. What are the three different types of electrical current?

4. What is a transcutaneous electrical stimulator and how is it related to a TENS unit?

5. What are the different types of waveforms that electrical stimulating generators may produce?

6. What are the various pulse characteristics of the different waveforms?

7. How can electrical currents be modulated?

8. What are the differences between series and parallel circuits?

9. How does electrical current travel through various types of biologic tissue?

10. What physiologic responses can be elicited by using electrical stimulating currents?

11. Explain the concept of depolarization of muscle and nerve in response to electrical stimulation.

12. What do the SD curves represent?
13. How should electrical stimulating currents be used with denervated muscle?
14. What are the effects of electrically stimulating nonexcitatory cells and tissues?
15. What treatment parameters must be considered when setting up a treatment using electrical stimulating currents?
16. What are the various therapeutic uses of electrically stimulated muscle contractions?
17. How can electrical stimulating currents be used to modulate pain?
18. What are the clinical applications for using low-voltage DC?
19. What are the various physiologic effects of using microcurrent?
20. Are there advantages to using IFC as opposed to other types of electrical stimulating currents?
21. What steps can the clinician take to ensure safety of the patient when using electrical modalities?

SELF-TEST QUESTIONS

True or False

1. Electrons tend to flow from areas of low concentration to areas of high concentration.
2. Insulators resist current flow.
3. The greater the voltage, the greater the amplitude is.
4. The cathode is the negatively charged electrode in a DC system.
5. *Chronaxie* refers to the minimum current intensity needed for tissue excitation if applied for a maximum time.
6. The electrode with the greatest current density is the active electrode.

Multiple Choice

7. A particle of matter with very little mass and a negative charge is a(n)
   a. ion
   b. electron
   c. neutron
   d. proton
8. What is the name of the unit measuring the force necessary to produce electron movement?
   a. ampere
   b. coulomb
   c. volt
   d. watt
9. In _____ current, electron flow constantly changes direction.
   a. alternating
   b. direct
   c. pulsatile
   d. galvanic
10. When the current increases gradually to a maximal amplitude, it is known as
    a. burst
    b. ramping
    c. modulation
    d. galvanic
11. In _____ circuits, electrons have only one path to follow.
    a. galvanic
    b. parallel
    c. resistor
    d. series

12. Physiologic response(s) to electrical current include
    a. thermal
    b. chemical
    c. physiologic
    d. all of the above

13. All whirlpools and tubs in a health care setting must have
    a. GFI
    b. a three-pronged outlet
    c. an insulated cord
    d. a waterproof motor

14. During the absolute refractory period the cell is not capable of
    a. depolarization
    b. an action potential
    c. twitch muscle contraction
    d. all of the above

15. The part of the cell responsible for transmitting messages to other cells via ionic, electrical, or small molecule signals is the
    a. electret
    b. gap junction
    c. dipole
    d. cell membrane pump

16. To _____ current density in deeper tissue, the electrodes must be placed _____.
    a. increase, closer
    b. increase, further apart
    c. decrease, closer
    d. decrease, further apart

17. Electrical stimulation may release enkephalin and endorphin to cause pain relief. What is the name of this pain control method?
    a. gate control theory
    b. central biasing theory
    c. opiate pain control theory
    d. placebo effects

18. Two currents combine and the amplitude decreases. This is called
    a. destructive interference
    b. constructive interference
    c. heterodyne current
    d. beat current

19. Which of the following currents is a pulsatile biphasic wave, generated in bursts, designed to create muscle contraction?
    a. LIS
    b. iontophoresis
    c. IFC
    d. Russian

20. Increased blood flow between electrodes is an effect of which of the following?
    a. IFC
    b. function electrical stimulation
    c. LIS
    d. medical galvanism

SOLUTIONS TO CLINICAL DECISION-MAKING EXERCISES

5–1

The terms *TENS* and *NMES* are for all intents and purposes interchangeable in their physiologic effects. Both units can be used to stimulate peripheral motor or sensory nerves.

5–2

The clinician should make it perfectly clear that even though the generator is producing a high-voltage current, the amperage is very small in the milliamp range and thus the total amount of electrical energy being output to the patient is very small. It is important to explain exactly what the patient will feel, especially if this is the first time that he or she has experienced electrical stimulation.

5–3

The size of the active electrode can be decreased, which will increase current density under that electrode. The active electrodes can be moved further apart. The current intensity can be increased, and the current duration may also be increased.

5–4

The clinician can simply increase current intensity sufficiently to produce a muscle contraction and then adjust the frequency to approximately 50 pulses/s. This will produce a tetanic contraction regardless of whether biphasic, monophasic, or PC is being used.

5–5

The current density under the active electrode could be increased by using a smaller electrode. The current intensity, the current duration, or a combination of the two may be increased to cause a depolarization.

5–6

A medium-frequency AC stimulator should be used. Frequency should be set at 20–30 Hz using an interrupted or surge modulation. On time should be set at about 20 seconds with off time also set at 20 seconds. On most generators of this type, pulse duration is preset. Intensity should be increased to elicit a strong muscle contraction that moves the lower leg through its antigravity range. The patient should be instructed to simultaneously produce a voluntary muscle contraction.

5–7

In a conventional TENS treatment, the goal is to provide as much sensory cutaneous input as possible. Thus, both the frequency and the pulse duration should be set as high as the unit will allow. The intensity should be increased until a muscle contraction is elicited, and then decreased slightly until the patient feels only a tingling sensation. If using a portable unit, the treatment may continue for several hours if necessary or until the pain subsides.

5–8

In treating both trigger points and acupuncture points, the clinician should use a monophasic current with the frequency set between 1 and 5 Hz, and pulse duration between 100 and 1000 microseconds. Intensity should be increased to the point where there is a muscle contraction, and then increased further until it is somewhat painful. The point should be stimulated for 45 seconds.

5–9

The four electrodes should be set up in a square pattern with the target muscle in the center of the square so that the maximum interference will take place where the electric field lines cross at the center of the pattern.

5–10

The four electrodes should be set up in a square pattern with the target muscle in the center of the square so that the maximum interference will take place where the electric field lines cross at the center of the pattern.

5–11

The National Electrical Code requires that all whirlpools have GFI installed to automatically shut off current flow. In addition, the clinician should not allow the patient to turn the whirlpool on and off. This is especially important when the patient is already in contact with the water. Extension cords or multiple adaptors should never be used in the hydrotherapy area.

REFERENCES

1. Licht S. *Therapeutic Electricity and Ultraviolet Radiation.* Vol IV. 2nd ed. Baltimore: Waverly; 1969.
2. Watkins A. *A Manual of Electrotherapy.* 3rd ed. Philadelphia: Lea & Febiger; 1968.
3. Valkenberg V. *Basic Electricity.* Clifton Park, NY: Delmar Learning; 1995.
4. Chamishion R. *Basic Medical Electronics.* Boston: Little, Brown and Company; 1964.
5. Stillwell G. *Therapeutic Electricity and Ultraviolet Radiation.* 3rd ed. Baltimore: Williams & Wilkins; 1983.
6. Bergueld P. *Electromedical Instrumentation: A Guide for Medical Personnel.* Cambridge: Cambridge University Press; 1980.
7. Thornton RM, Mendel FC, Fish DR. Effects of electrical stimulation on edema formation in different strains of rats. *Phys Ther.* 1998;78(4):386–394.
8. Alon G, DeDomeico G. *High Voltage Stimulation: An Integrated Approach to Clinical Electrotherapy.* Chattanooga: Chattanooga Corp; 1987.
9. Shriber W. *A Manual of Electrotherapy.* 4th ed. Philadelphia: Lea & Febiger; 1975.
10. Alon G. Principles of electrical stimulation. In: Nelson R, Currier D, eds. *Clinical Electrotherapy.* Norwalk, CT: Appleton & Lange; 1999.
11. DeDomenico G. *Basic Guidelines for Interferential Therapy.* Sydney, Australia: Theramed; 1981.
12. Holcomb WR. A practical guide to electrical therapy. *J Sport Rehabil.* 1997;6(3):272–282.
13. Myklebust B, Robinson A. Instrumentation. In: Snyder-Mackler L, Robinson A, eds. *Clinical Electrophysiology, Electrotherapy and Electrotherapy and Electrophysiologic Testing.* Baltimore: Lippincott Williams & Wilkins; 2007.
14. Robinson A. Basic concepts and terminology in electricity. In: Snyder-Mackler L, Robinson A, eds. *Clinical Electrophysiology, Electrotherapy and Electro-physiologic Testing.* Baltimore: Lippincott Williams & Wilkins; 2007.
15. Carlos J. Clinical electrotherapy part I: physiology and basic concepts. *Phys Ther.* 1998;6(4):44.
16. Cohen H, Brunilik J. *Manual of Electroneuromyography.* 2nd ed. New York: Harper & Row; 1976.
17. Griffin J, Karselis T. *Physical Agents for Physical Therapists.* Springfield, IL: Charles C Thomas; 1988.
18. Taylor K, Mendel FC, Fish DR. Effect of high-voltage pulsed current and alternating current on macromolecular leakage in cheek pouch microcirculation. *Phys Ther.* 1997;77(12):1729–1740.
19. Kitchen S, Bazin S. *Electrotherapy: Evidence-based Practice.* Wernersville, PA: Harcourt Health Sciences; 2001.
20. Kahn I. *Principles and Practice of Electrotherapy.* Philadelphia: Elsevier Health Sciences; 2001.
21. Wolf S. *Electrotherapy: Clinics in Physical Therapy.* Vol 2. New York: Churchill Livingstone; 1981.
22. Nalty T, Sabbahi M. *Electrotherapy Clinical Procedures Manual.* New York: McGraw-Hill; 2001.
23. McLoda TA, Carmack JA. Optimal burst duration during a facilitated quadriceps femoris contraction. *J Athletic Train.* 2000;35(2):145–150.
24. Benton L, Baker L, Bowman B. *Functional Electrical Stimulation: A Practical Clinical Guide.* Downey, CA: Rancho Los Amigos Hospital; 1981.
25. Nelson R, Currier D. *Clinical Electrotherapy.* Norwalk, CT: Appleton & Lange; 1999.
26. Howson D. *Report on Neuromuscular Reeducation.* Minneapolis: Medical General; 1978.
27. Becker R, Selden G. *The Body Electric.* New York: Harper Collins; 1998.
28. Maurer C. The effectiveness of microelectrical neural stimulation on exercise-induced muscle trauma [abstract R200]. *Phys Ther.* 1992;725:574.
29. Randall B, Imig C, Hines HM. Effect of electrical stimulation upon blood flow and temperature of skeletal muscles. *Arch Phys Med.* 1952;33:73–78.
30. Gault W, Gatens P. Use of low-intensity direct current in management of ischemic skin ulcers. *Phys Ther.* 1976;56:265–269.
31. Newton R, Karselis T. Skin pH following high voltage pulsed galvanic stimulation. *Phys Ther.* 1983;63:1593–1596.
32. Guyton A. *Textbook of Medical Physiology.* Philadelphia: WB Saunders; 2005.
33. Kincaid C, Lavoie K. Inhibition of bacterial growth in vitro following stimulation with high voltage monophasic pulsed current. *Phys Ther.* 1989;69:651–655.
34. Delitto A. A study of discomfort with electrical stimulation. *Phys Ther.* 1992;72:410–424.

35. Melzack R. Prolonged relief of pain by brief, intense transcutaneous electrical stimulation. *Pain.* 1975;1(4):357–373.

36. Mohr T, Akers T, Landry R. Effect of high voltage stimulation on edema reduction in the rat hind limb. *Phys Ther.* 1987;67:1703–1707.

37. Reed B. Effect of high voltage pulsed electrical stimulation on microvascular permeability to plasma proteins: a possible mechanism in minimizing edema. *Phys Ther.* 1988;68:491–495.

38. Alon G. High voltage stimulation: effects of electrode size on basic excitatory responses. *Phys Ther.* 1985;65:890.

39. Travell J, Simon D. *Myofascial Pain and Dysfunction: The Trigger Point Manual.* Baltimore: Williams & Wilkins; 1998.

40. Lampe G. A clinical approach to transcutaneous electrical nerve stimulation in the treatment of chronic and acute pain, Minneapolis, July 1978. *Conference presenation.*

41. Wolf S. *Electrotherapy.* New York: Churchill Livingstone; 1981.

42. Lampe G. Introduction to the use of transcutaneous electrical nerve stimulation devices. *Phys Ther.* 1978;58:1450–1454.

43. Charman R. Bioelectricity and electrotherapy—towards a new paradigm? Part 1, the cell. *Physiotherapy.* 1990;76:452–491; Charman R. Part 2, cellular reception and emission of electromagnetic signals. *Physiotherapy.* 1990;76:502–518; Charman R. Part 3, bioelectric potentials and tissue currents. *Physiotherapy.* 1990;76:643–654; Charman R. Part 4, strain generated potentials in bone and connective tissue. *Physiotherapy.* 1990;76:725–730; Charman R. Part 5, exogenous currents and fields—experimental and clinical applications. *Physiotherapy.* 1990;76:743–750.

44. Selkowitz D. High frequency electrical stimulation in muscle strengthening. *Am J Sport Med.* 198;17:103–111.

45. Charman R. Bioelectricity and electrotherapy—towards a new paradigm. Part 6, environmental current and fields—the natural background. *Physiotherapy.* 1991;77:8–13; Charman R. Part 7, environmental currents and fields—man made. *Physiotherapy.* 1991;77:129–140; Charman R. Part 8, grounds for a new paradigm? *Physiotherapy.* 1991;77:211–221.

46. Brighton C. Bioelectric effects on bone and cartilage. *Clin Orthop.* 1977;124:2–4.

47. Clements F. Effect of motor neuromuscular electrical stimulation on microvascular perfusion of stimulated rat skeletal muscle. *Phys Ther.* 1991;71:397–406.

48. Castel J. *Pain Management with Acupuncture and Transcutaneous Electrical Nerve Stimulation Techniques and Photo Simulation (Laser). Symposium on Pain Management, Walter Reed Army Medical Center;* November 13, 1982.

49. Becker R. The bioelectric factors in amphibian-limb regeneration. *J Bone Joint Surg (Am).* 1961;43-A:643–656.

50. Lomo T, Slater C. Control of acetylcholine sensitivity and synapse formation by muscle activity. *J Physiol.* 1978;275:391.

51. Clemente F, Barron K. Transcutaneous neuromuscular electrical stimulation effect on the degree of microvascular perfusion in autonomically denervated rat skeletal muscle, *Arch Phys Med Rehabil.* 1996;77(2):155–160.

52. Cummings J. Electrical stimulation of denervated muscle. In: Gersch M, ed. *Electrotherapy in Rehabilitation.* Philadelphia: FA Davis; 1992.

53. Chu C. Weak direct current accelerates split-thickness graft healing on tangentially excised second-degree burns. *J Burn Care Rehabil.* 1991;12:285–1293.

54. Gersch MR. *Electrotherapy in Rehabilitation.* Philadelphia: FA Davis; 2000.

55. Gorgey A, Dudley G. The role of pulse duration and stimulation duration in maximizing the normalized torque during neuromuscular electrical stimulation. *J Orthop Sports Phys Ther.* 2008;38(8):508.

56. Litke D, Dahners L. Effect of different levels of direct current on early ligament healing in a rat model. *J Orthop Relat Res.* 1994;12:683–688.

57. Schimrigk K, Mclaughlen J, Gruniger W. The effect of electrical stimulation on the experimentally denervated rat muscle. *Scand J Rehabil Med.* 1977;9:55.

58. *Instruction Manual for Electrostim.* Promatek: Canada; 1989:180–182.

59. Kosman A, Osborne S, Ivey A. Comparative effectiveness of various electrical currents in preventing muscle atrophy in rat. *Arch Phys Med Rehabil.* 1947;28:7.

60. Thom H. Treatment of paralysis with exponentially progressive current. *Br J Phys Med.* 1957;20:49.

61. Binder-MacLeod S, Snyder-Mackler L. Muscle fatigue: clinical implications for fatigue assessment and neuromuscular electrical stimulation. *Phys Ther.* 1993;73:902–910.

62. Dallmann S. Preference for low versus medium frequency electrical stimulation at constant induced muscle forces [abstract R345]. *Phys Ther.* 1992;725:5107.

63. Unger P. A randomized clinical trial of the effects of HVPC on wound healing [abstract R294]. *Phys Ther.* 1991;715:5118.

64. Currier D, Lehman J, Lightfoot P. Electrical stimulation in exercise of the quadriceps femoris muscle. *Phys Ther.* 1979;59:1508–1512.

65. Eriksson E, Haggmark T. Comparison of isometric muscle training and electrical stimulation supplement, isometric muscle training in the recovery after major knee ligament surgery. *Am J Sports Med.* 1979;7:169–171.

66. DeVahl J. Neuromuscular electrical stimulation (NMES) in rehabilitation. In: Gersh M, ed. *Electrotherapy in Rehabilitation.* Philadelphia: FA Davis; 1992.

67. Cook H, Morales M, La Rosa EM, et al. Effect of electrical stimulation on lymphatic flow and limb volume in the rat. *Phys Ther.* 1994;74:1040–1046.

68. Dolan M, Graves P, Nakazawa C. Effects of ibuprofen and high voltage electrical stimulation on acute edema following blunt trauma to hind limb of rats [abstract]. *J Athletic Train.* 2004;39(suppl 2):S–49.

69. Dolan M, Mychaskiw A, Mendel F. Cool-water immersion and high-voltage electric stimulation curb edema formation in rats. *J Athletic Train*. 2003;38(4):225–230.

70. Dolan M, Mychaskiw A, Mattacola C, Mendel F. Effects of cool-water immersion and high-voltage electric stimulation for 3 continuous hours on acute edema in rats. *J Athletic Train*. 2003;38(3):325–329.

71. Hopkins J, Ingersoll C, Edwards J. Cryotherapy and transcutaneous electric neuromuscular stimulation decrease arthrogenic muscle inhibition of the vastus medialis after knee joint effusion. *J Athletic Train*. 2002;37(1):25–31.

72. Cook T, Barr J. Instrumentation. In: Nelson R, Currier D, eds. *Clinical Electrotherapy*. Norwalk, CT: Appleton & Lange; 1999.

73. Denegar C. The effects of low-volt microamperage stimulation on delayed onset muscle soreness. *J Sport Rehabil*. 1993;1:95–102.

74. Reed A, Robertson V, Low J. *Electrotherapy Explained: Principles and Practices*. Burlington, MA: Elsevier Science and Technology; 2006.

75. Flicker MT. *An Analysis of Cold Intermittent Compression with Simultaneous Treatment of Electrical Stimulation in the Reduction of Postacute Ankle Lymphademia* [unpublished master's thesis]. Chapel Hill, NC: University of North Carolina; May 1993.

76. Salar G. Effect of transcutaneous electrotherapy on CSF B-endorphin content in patients without pain problems. *Pain*. 1981;10:169–172.

77. Selkowitz D. Improvement in isometric strength of the quadriceps femoris muscle after training with electrical stimulation. *Phys Ther*. 1985;65:186–196.

78. Siff M. Applications of electrostimulation in physical conditioning: a review. *J Appl Sport Sci Res*. 1990;4:20–26.

79. Holcomb W, Rubley M, Girouard T. Effect of the simultaneous application of NMES and HVPC on knee extension torque [abstract]. *J Athletic Train*. 2004;39(suppl 2):S–47.

80. Holcomb W, Rubley M, Miller M. The effect of rest intervals on knee-extension torque production with neuromuscular electrical stimulation. *J Sport Rehabil*. 2006;15(2):116.

81. Laufer Y, Ries JD, Leininger PM, Alon G. Quadriceps femoris muscle torques and fatigue generated by neuromuscular electrical stimulation with three different waveforms. *Phys Ther*. 2001;81(7):1307–1316.

82. Lewek M, Stevens J, Snyder-Mackler L. The use of electrical stimulation to increase quadriceps femoris muscle force in an elderly patient following a total knee arthroplasty. *Phys Ther*. 2001;81(8):1565–1571.

83. Valma J, Robertson A, Ward R. Vastus medialis electrical stimulation to improve lower extremity function following a lateral patellar retinacular release. *J Orthop Sports Phys Ther*. 2002;32(9):437–446.

84. Van Lunen B, Caroll C, Gratias K. The clinical effects of cold application on the production of electrically induced involuntary muscle contractions. *J Sport Rehabil*. 2003;12(3):240–248.

85. Windley T. The efficacy of neuromuscular electrical stimulation for muscle-strength augmentation. *Athletic Ther Today*. 2007;12(1):9.

86. Currier D, Mann R. Muscular strength development by electrical stimulation in healthy individuals. *Phys Ther*. 1983;63:915–921.

87. Karnes JL, Mendel FC, Fish DR. High-voltage pulsed current: its influence on diameters of histamine-dilated arterioles in hamster cheek pouches. *Arch Phys Med Rehabil*. 1995;76(4):381–386.

88. Bettany J. Influence of high voltage pulsed current on edema formation following impact injury. *Phys Ther*. 1990;70:219–224.

89. Brown S. The effect of microcurrent on edema, range of motion, and pain in treatment of lateral ankle sprains [abstract]. *J Orthop Sports Phys Ther*. 1994;19:55.

90. Cosgrove K, Alon G. The electrical effect of two commonly used clinical stimulators on traumatic edema in rats. *Phys Ther*. 1992;72:227–233.

91. Fish D. Effect of anodal high voltage pulsed current on edema formation in frog hind limbs. *Phys Ther*. 1991;71:724–733.

92. Griffin J. Reduction of chronic posttraumatic hand edema: a comparison of high voltage pulsed current, intermittent pneumatic compression, and placebo treatments. *Phys Ther*. 1990;70:279–286.

93. Lea J. The effect of electrical stimulation on edematous rat hind paws [abstract R379]. *Phys Ther*. 1992;725:5116.

94. Mendel F. Influence of high voltage pulsed current on edema formation following impact injury in rats. *Phys Ther*. 1992;72:668–673.

95. Miller BF, Gruben KG, Morgan BJ. Circulatory responses to voluntary and electrically induced muscle contractions in humans. *Phys Ther*. 2000;80(1):53–60.

96. Miller M, Cheatham C, Holcomb W. Subcutaneous tissue thickness alters the effect of NMES. *J Sport Rehabil*. 2008;17(1):68.

97. Mulder G. Treatment of open-skin wounds with electric stimulation. *Arch Phys Med Rehabil*. 1991;72:375–377.

98. Taylor K. Effect of a single 30-minute treatment of high voltage pulsed current on edema formation in frog hind limbs. *Phys Ther*. 1992;72:63–68.

99. Bishop B. Pain: its physiology and rationale for management. *Phys Ther*. 1980;60:13–37.

100. Cheing G, Hui-Chan C. Analgesic effects of transcutaneous electrical nerve stimulation and interferential currents on heat pain in healthy subjects. *J Rehabil Med*. 2003;35(1):15.

101. Laughman R, Youdes J, Garrett T. Strength changes in the normal quadriceps femoris muscle as a result of electrical stimulation. *Phys Ther*. 1983;63:494–499.

102. Melzack R, Stillwell D, Fox E. Trigger points and acupuncture points for pain: correlations and implications. *Pain*. 1977;3(1):3–23.

103. Melzack R. *The Puzzle of Pain*. New York: Basic Books; 1973.

104. Rolle W, Alon G, Nirschl R. Comparison of subliminal and placebo stimulation in the management of elbow epicondylitis [abstract R280]. *Phys Ther.* 1991;715:5114.

105. Marino A, Becker R. Biologic effects of extremely low-frequency electric and magnetic fields: a review. *Phys Chem.* 1977;9:131–143.

106. Clement-Jones V. Increased β-endorphin but not metenkephalin levels in human cerebrospinal fluid after acupuncture for recurrent pain. *Lancet.* 1980;8:946–948.

107. Evans T, Denegar C. Is transcutaneous electrical nerve stimulation (TENS) effective in relieving trigger point pain? *J Athletic Train.* 2002;37(suppl 2S):S–103.

108. Malezic M, Hesse S. Restoration of gait by functional electrical stimulation in paraplegic patients: a modified programme of treatment. *Paraplegia.* 1995;33(3):126–131.

109. Malizia E. Electroacupuncture and peripheral β-endorphin and ACTH levels. *Lancet.* 1979;8:535–536.

110. Norcross M, Guskiewicz K, Prentice W. The effects of electrical stimulating currents on pain perception, plasma cortisol, and plasma b-endorphin for DOMS [abstract]. *J Athletic Train (Suppl).* 2004;39(2):S–48.

111. Snyder-Mackler L, Garrett M, Roberts M. A comparison of torque generating capabilities of three different electrical stimulating currents. *J Orthop Sports Phys Ther.* 1989;10:297–301.

112. Wolf S. Perspectives on central nervous system responsiveness to transcutaneous electrical nerve stimulation. *Phys Ther.* 1978;58:1443–1449.

113. Denegar C. Influence of transcutaneous electrical nerve stimulation on pain, range of motion, and serum cortisol concentration in females experiencing delayed onset muscle soreness. *J Orthop Sports Phys Ther.* 1989;11:100–103.

114. *Notes on Low Volt Therapy.* White Plains, NY: TECA Corp; 1966.

115. Alon G. "Microcurrent" stimulation: a progress report 1998. *Athletic Ther Today.* 1998;3(6):15.

116. Picker R. Current trends: low volt pulsed microamp stimulation. Parts 1 and 2. *Clin Manage.* 1989;9:11–14, 28–33.

117. Becker R, Bachman C, Friedman H. The direct current control system. *N Y J Med.* 1962;62:1169–1176.

118. Bonacci JA, Higbie EJ. Effects of microcurrent treatment on perceived pain and muscle strength following eccentric exercise. *J Athletic Train.* 1997;32(2):119–123.

119. Tan G, Monga T, Thornby J. Electromedicine: efficacy of microcurrent electrical stimulation on pain severity, psychological distress, and disability. *Am J Pain Manage.* 2000;10(1):35–44.

120. Allen JD, Mattacola CG, Perrin DH. Effect of microcurrent stimulation on delayed-onset muscle soreness: a double-blind comparison. *J Athletic Train.* 1999;34(4):334–337.

121. Ansoleaga E, Wirth V. Microcurrent electrical stimulation may reduce clinically induced DOMS. *J Athletic Train.* 1999;34(2):S–67.

122. Haynie L, Henry L, VanLunen B. Investigation of microcurrent electrical neuromuscular stimulation and high-voltage electrical muscle stimulation on DOMS. *J Athletic Train (Suppl).* 2002;37 (2S):S–102.

123. Hewlett K, Kimura I, Hetzler R. Microcurrent treatment on pain, edema, and decreased muscle force associated with delayed-onset muscle soreness: a double-blind, placebo study [abstract]. *J Athletic Train.* 2004;39(suppl 2):S–48.

124. Jeter J, Valcenta D. The effects of microcurrent electrical nerve stimulation on delayed onset muscle soreness and peak torque deficits in trained weight lifters [abstract PO-R065-M]. *Phys Ther.* 1993;735:5–24.

125. Johnson MI, Penny P, Sajawal MA. Clinical technical note: an examination of the analgesic effects of microcurrent electrical stimulation (MES) on cold-induced pain in healthy subjects. *Physiother Theory Pract.* 1997;13(4):293–301.

126. Kulig K. Comparison of the effects of high velocity exercise and microcurrent neuromuscular stimulation on delayed onset muscle soreness [abstract R284]. *Phys Ther.* 1991;715:5115.

127. Rapaski D. Microcurrent electrical stimulation: comparison of two protocols in reducing delayed onset muscle soreness [abstract R286]. *Phys Ther.* 1991;715:5116.

128. Ross S, Guskiewicz K. Effect of balance training with and without subsensory electrical stimulation on postural stability of subjects with stable ankles and subjects with functional ankle instability [abstract]. *J Athletic Train.* 2005;40(suppl 2):S–70.

129. Wolcot C. A comparison of the effects of high voltage and microcurrent stimulation on delayed onset muscle soreness [abstract R287]. *Phys Ther.* 1991;715:5116.

130. Young S. Efficacy of interferential current stimulation alone for pain reduction in patients with osteoarthritis of the knee: a randomized placebo control clinical trial [abstract R088]. *Phys Ther.* 1991;715:552.

131. Carley P, Wainapel S. Electrotherapy for the acceleration of wound healing: low-intensity direct current. *Arch Phys Med Rehabil.* 1985;66:443–446.

132. Chreng N, Van Houf H, Bockx E. The effects of electric current on ATP generation, protein synthesis, and membrane transport in rat skin. *Clin Orthop Relat Res.* 1982;171:264–272.

133. Gentzkow G. Electrical stimulation to heal dermal wounds. *J Dermatol Surg Oncol.* 1993;19:753–758.

134. Griffin J. Efficacy of high voltage pulsed current for healing of pressure ulcers in patients with spinal cord injury. *Phys Ther.* 1991;71:433–444.

135. Howson DC. Peripheral neural excitability. *Phys Ther.* 1978;58:1467–1473.

136. Leffmann D. The effect of subliminal transcutaneous electrical stimulation on the rate of wound healing in rats [abstract R166]. *Phys Ther.* 1992;725:567.

137. Weiss D, Kirsner R, Eaglstein W. Electrical stimulation and wound healing. *Arch Dermatol.* 1990;126:222–225.

138. Wood J. A multicenter study on the use of pulsed low-intensity direct current for healing chronic stage II and

stage III decubitus ulcers. *Arch Dermatol.* 1993;129: 999–1009.

139. Connolly J, Hahn H, Jardon O. The electrical enhancement of periosteal proliferation in normal and delayed fracture healing. *Clin Orthop.* 1977;124:97–105.

140. Pettine K. External electrical stimulation and bracing for treatment of spondylolysis—a case report. *Spine.* 1993;188:436–439.

141. Szabo G, Illes T. Experimental stimulation of osteogenesis induced by bone matrix. *Orthopaedics.* 1991;14:63–67.

142. Kahn J. *Low-voltage Technique.* 4th ed. Syosset, NY: Joseph Kahn; 1983.

143. Stanish W, Gunnlaugson B. Electrical energy and soft tissue injury healing. *Sport Care Fitness.* 1988;8(5):12–14.

144. Nessler J, Mass P. Direct current electrical stimulation of tendon healing in vitro. *Clin Orthop Relat Res.* 1987;217(3):303–312.

145. Ward A, Shkuratova N. Russian electrical stimulation: the early experiments. *Phys Ther.* 2002;82(10):1019–1030.

146. Delitto A. Introduction to "Russian electrical stimulation": putting this into perspective. *Phys Ther.* 2002;82(10): 1017–1018.

147. Goodgold J, Eberstein A. *Electrodiagnosis of Neuromuscular Diseases.* Baltimore: Williams & Wilkins; 1980.

148. Comeau M, Brown L, Landrum J. The effects of high volt pulsed current vs. Russian current on the achievable percentage of MVIC [abstract]. *J Athletic Train.* 2004;39(suppl 2): S-47–S-48.

149. Franklin ME. Effect of varying the ratio of electrically induced muscle contraction time to rest time on serum creatine kinase and perceived soreness. *J Orthop Sports Phys Ther.* 1991;13:310–315.

150. Svacina L. Modified interferential technique. *Pain Control.* 1978;4(1):1–2.

151. Snyder S. Opiate receptors and internal opiates. *Sci Am.* 1977;236:44–56.

152. Nikolova L. *Treatment with Interferential Current.* New York: Churchill Livingstone; 1987.

153. Draper D, Knight K. Interferential current therapy: often used but misunderstood. *Athletic Ther Today.* 2006;11(4):29.

154. Driban J. Bone stimulators and microcurrent: clinical bioelectrics. *Athletic Ther Today.* 2004;9(5):22.

155. Reiff, M IInterferential Therapy: Tips for effective treatment, http://www.medicalproductsonline.org/inth.html.

156. Larsson L. Functional electrical stimulation. *Scand J Rehabil Ed Suppl.* 1994;30:63–72.

157. Baker L, McNeal D, Benton L. *Neuromuscular Electrical Stimulation.* Downey, CA: Rancho Los Amigos Medical Center; 1993.

158. Heller B, Granat M, Andrews B. Swing-through gait with free-knees produced by surface functional electrical stimulation. *Paraplegia.* 1996;34(1):8–15.

159. Agnew W, McCreery D, Bullara L. Effects of prolonged electrical stimulation of peripheral nerve. In: Agnew W, McCreery D, eds. *Neural Prosthesis: Fundamental Studies.* Englewood Cliffs, NJ: Prentice-Hall; 1990.

160. Yamamoto T, Seireg A. Closing the loop: electrical muscle stimulation and feedback control for smooth limb motion. *Soma.* 1986;4:38.

161. Kumar V, Lau H, Liu J. Clinical applications of functional electrical stimulation. *Ann Acad Med.* 1995;24(3): 428–435.

162. Bogataj U, Gros N, Kljajic M. The rehabilitation of gait in patients with hemiplegia: a comparison between conventional therapy and multichannel functional electrical stimulation therapy. *Phys Ther.* 1995;75(6):490–502.

163. Kagaya H, Shimada Y. Restoration and analysis of standing-up in complete paraplegia utilizing functional electrical stimulation. *Arch Phys Med Rehabil.* 1995;76(9):876–881.

164. Kralj A, Badj T, Turk R. Enhancement of gait restoration in spinal cord injured patients by functional electrical stimulation. *Clin Orthop.* 1988;233:34.

165. Mannheimer J, Lampe G. *Clinical Transcutaneous Electrical Nerve Stimulation.* Philadelphia: FA Davis; 1984.

166. Stallard J, Major R. The influence of orthosis stiffness on paraplegic ambulation and its implications for functional electrical stimulation (FES) walking. *Prosthet Orthot Int.* 1995;19(2):108–114.

167. Bradley M. The effect of participating in a functional electrical stimulation exercise program on affect in people with spinal cord injuries. *Arch Phys Med Rehabil.* 1994;75(6):676–679.

168. Triolo RJ, Bogie K. Lower extremity applications of functional neuromuscular stimulation after spinal cord injury. *Top Spinal Cord Inj Rehabil.* 1999;5(1):44–65.

169. Gersh MR. Microcurrent electrical stimulation: putting it in perspective. *Clin Manage.* 1990;9(4):51–54.

170. Myklebust B, Kloth L. Electrodiagnostic and electrotherapeutic instrumentation: characteristics of recording and stimulation systems and principles of safety. In: Gersh MR, ed. *Electrotherapy in Rehabilitation.* Philadelphia: FA Davis; 2001.

171. Porter M, Porter J. Electrical safety in the training room. *Journal of Athletic Training.* 1981;16(4):263–264.

172. American Physical Therapy Association. *Electrotherapeutic Terminology in Physical Therapy: APTA Section on Clinical Electrophysiology.* Alexandria, VA: American Physical Therapy Association; 2000.

173. Chan H, Fung DT. Effects of low-voltage microamperage stimulation on tendon healing in rats. *J Orthop Sports Ther.* 2007;37(7):399.

174. Cole B, Gardiner P. Does electrical stimulation of denervated muscle continued after reinnervation, influence recovery of contractile function. *Exp Neurol.* 1984;85:52.

175. Cromwell L, Arditti M, Weibell F. *Medical Instrumentation for Health Care.* Englewood Cliffs, NJ: Prentice-Hall; 1991.

176. FDA clears restorative therapies functional electrical stimulation. *J Orthop Sports Phys Ther.* 2008;38(3):163.

177. Gutman E, Guttman L. Effect of electrotherapy on denervated and reinnervated muscles in rabbit. *Lancet.* 1942;1:169.

178. Herbison G, Jaweed M, Ditunno J. Acetylcholine sensitivity and fibrillation potentials in electrically stimulated crush-denervated rat skeletal muscle. *Arch Phys Med Rehabil.* 1983;64:217.

179. Holcomb W, Rubley M. Effect of the simultaneous application of NMES and HVPC on knee extension torque. *J Sport Rehabil.* 2007;16(4):307.

180. Kloth L, Cummings J. *Electrotherapeutic Terminology in Physical Therapy.* Alexandria, VA: Section on Clinical Electrophysiology and the American Physical Therapy Association; 1990.

181. Mintken P, Carpenter K. Early neuromuscular electrical stimulation to optimize quadriceps muscle function following total knee arthroplasty: a case report. *J Orthop Sports Phys Ther.* 2007;37(7):364.

182. Petterson S, Snyder-Mackler L. The use of neuromuscular electrical stimulation to improve activation deficits in a patient with chronic quadriceps strength impairments following total knee arthroplasty. *J Orthop Sports Phys Ther.* 2006;36(9):678–685.

183. Taylor K. Effect of electrically induced muscle contraction on post traumatic edema formation in frog hind limbs. *Phys Ther.* 1992;72:127–132.

184. Weber W. The effect of MENS on pain and torque deficits associated with delayed onset muscle soreness [abstract R034]. *Phys Ther.* 1991;715:535.

185. Wilding S, Miller K, Stone M. Increasing electrical stimulation frequency above cramp threshold frequency increases the strength and duration of electrically induced muscle cramps. *J Athletic Train.* 2009;44(suppl):S89.

186. Zbar P, Rockmaker G, Bates D. *Basic Electricity: a Text-Lab Manual.* New York: McGraw-Hill; 2000.

SUGGESTED READINGS

Abdel-Moty E, Fishbain D, Goldberg M. Functional electrical stimulation treatment of postradiculopathy associated muscle weakness. *Arch Phys Med Rehabil.* 1994;75(6):680–686.

Akyuz G. Transcutaneous electrical nerve stimulation (TENS) in the treatment of postoperative pain and prevention of paralytic ileus. *Clin Rehabil.* 1993;7(3):218–221.

Allen J, Mattacola C, Perrin D. Microcurrent stimulation effect on delayed onset muscle soreness. *J Athletic Train.* 1996;31:S–47.

Alon G. *High Voltage Stimulation: A Monograph.* Chattanooga, TN: Chattanooga Corporation; 1984.

Alon G. *Electrical Stimulators.* Chattanooga, TN: Chattanooga Corporation; 1985 [video presentation].

Alon G, Allin J, Inbar G. Optimization of pulse duration and pulse charge during TENS. *Aust J Physiother.* 1983;29:195.

Alon G, Bainbridge J, Croson G. High-voltage pulsed direct current effects on peripheral blood flow. *Phys Ther.* 1981;61:678.

Alon G, Kantor G, Ho H. Effects of electrode size on basic excitatory responses and on selected stimulus parameters. *J Orthop Sports Phys Ther.* 1994;20(1):29–35.

Alon G, Kantor G, Smith GV. Peripheral nerve excitation and plantar flexion force elicited by electrical stimulation in males and females. *J Orthop Sports Phys Ther.* 1999;29(4):208–217.

American Physical Therapy Association. *Electrotherapeutic Terminology in Physical Therapy.* Alexandria, VA: APTA Publications; 2000.

Andersson S. Pain control by sensory stimulation. In: Bonica JJ, Liebeskind JC, Albe-Fessard DG, eds. *Advances in Pain Research and Therapy.* Vol 3. New York: Raven; 1979:569–584.

Andersson S, Hansson G, Holmgren E. Evaluation of the pain suppression effect of different frequencies of peripheral electrical stimulation in chronic pain conditions. *Acta Orthop Scand.* 1979;47:149.

Arnold P, McVey S. Functional electric stimulation: its efficacy and safety in improving pulmonary function and musculoskeletal fitness. *Arch Phys Med Rehabil.* 1992;73(7):665–668.

Aubin M, Marks R. The efficacy of short-term treatment with transcutaneous electrical nerve stimulation for osteo-arthritic knee pain. *Physiotherapy.* 1995;81(11):669–675.

Baker L. Neuromuscular electrical stimulation in the restoration of purposeful limb movements. In: Wolf SL, ed. *Electrotherapy—Clinics in Physical Therapy.* New York: Churchill Livingstone; 1981.

Baker L, McNeal D, Benton L. *Neuromuscular Electrical Stimulation: A Practical Guide.* Downey, CA: Rancho Los Amigos Medical Center; 2000.

Balogun J, Onilari O. High voltage electrical stimulation in the augmentation of muscle strength: effects of pulse frequency. *Arch Phys Med Rehabil.* 1993;74(9):910–916.

Bending J. TENS relief of discomfort. *Physiotherapy.* 1993;79(11):773–774.

Benton L, Baker L, Bowman B. *Functional Electrical Stimulation: A Practical Clinical Guide.* 2nd ed. Downey, CA: Professional Staff Association of Rancho Los Amigos Medical Center; 1981.

Berlandt S. Method of determining optimal stimulation sites for transcutaneous nerve stimulation. *Phys Ther.* 1984;64:924.

Binder S. Electrical currents. In: Wolf S, ed. *Electrotherapy.* New York: Churchill Livingstone; 1981.

Binder-Macleod S, McDermond L. Changes in the force–frequency relationship of the human quadriceps femoris muscle following electrically and voluntarily induced fatigue. *Phys Ther.* 1992;72(2):95–104.

Bowman B, Baker L. Effects of waveform parameters on comfort during transcutaneous neuromuscular electrical stimulation. *Ann Biomed Eng.* 1985;13:59–74.

Brown I. *Fundamentals of Electrotherapy, Course Guide.* Madison, WI: University of Wisconsin Press; 1971.

Brown M, Cotter M, Hudlicka O. The effects of long-term stimulation of fast muscles on their ability to withstand fatigue. *J Physiol (Lond).* 1974;238:47.

Brown M, Cotter M, Hudlicka O. Metabolic changes in long-term stimulated fast muscles. In: Howland H, Poortmans JR, eds. *Metabolic Adaptation to Prolonged Physical Exercise.* Basel: Birkhauser; 1975.

Burr H, Harvey S. Bio-electric correlates of wound healing. *Yale J Biol Med.* 1938;11(2):103–107.

Burr H, Taffel M, Harvey S. An electrometric study of the healing wound in man. *Yale J Biol Med.* 1940;12:483.

Butterfield DL, Draper DO, Ricard M. The effect of high-volt pulsed current electrical stimulation on delayed-onset muscle soreness. *J Athletic Train.* 1997;32(1):15–20.

Buxton B, Okasaki E, Hetzler R. Self selection of transcutaneous electrical nerve stimulation parameters for pain relief in injured athletes. *J Athletic Train.* 1994;29(2):178.

Byl N, McKenzie A, West J. Pulsed microamperage stimulation: a controlled study of healing of surgically induced wounds in Yucatan pigs. *Phys Ther.* 1994;74(3):201–211.

Caggiano E, Emrey T, Shirley S. Effects of electrical stimulation or voluntary contraction for strengthening the quadriceps femoris muscles in an aged male population. *J Orthop Sports Phys Ther.* 1994;20(1): 22–28.

Campbell J. A critical appraisal of the electrical output characteristics of ten transcutaneous nerve stimulators. *Clin Phys Physiol Meas.* 1982;3:141.

Carmick J. Clinical use of neuromuscular electrical stimulation for children with cerebral palsy, part 1, lower extremity. *Phys Ther.* 1993;73(8):505–513.

Carmick J. Clinical use of neuromuscular electrical stimulation for children with cerebral palsy, part 2, upper extremity. *Phys Ther.* 1993;73(8):514–522.

Chan C, Chow S. Electroacupuncture in the treatment of post-traumatic sympathetic dystrophy (Sudek's atrophy). *Br J Anesth.* 1981;53:899.

Chase J. Elicitation of periods of inhibition in human muscle by stimulation of cutaneous nerves. *J Bone Joint Surg.* 1972;54:173–177.

Cook H, Morales M, La Rosa E. Effects of electrical stimulation on lymphatic flow and limb volume in the rat. *Phys Ther.* 1994;74(11):1040–1046.

Cooperman A. Use of transcutaneous electrical stimulation in the control of post operative pain. Results of a prospective, randomized, controlled study. *Am J Surg.* 1977;133:185.

Curico F, Berweger R. A clinical evaluation of the pain suppressor TENS, Fairleigh Dickinson University School of Dentistry, 1983. *Curr Opin Orthop.* 1993;4(6):105–109.

Currier D, Mann R. Pain complaint: comparison of electrical stimulation with conventional isometric exercise. *J Orthop Sports Phys Ther.* 1984;5:318.

Currier D, Petrilli C, Threlkeld A. Effect of medium frequency electrical stimulation on local blood circulation to healthy muscle. *Phys Ther.* 1986;66:937.

Currier D, Ray J, Nyland J. Effects of electrical and electromagnetic stimulation after anterior cruciate ligament reconstruction. *J Orthop Sports Phys Ther.* 1993;17(4): 177–184.

DeGirardi C, Seaborne D, Goulet F. The analgesic effect of high voltage galvanic stimulation combined with ultrasound in the treatment of low back pain: a one-group pretest/posttest study. *Physiother Can.* 1984;36:327.

Dimitrijevic M. Mesh-glove. 1. A method for whole-hand electrical stimulation in upper motor neuron dysfunction. *Scand J Rehabil Med.* 1994;26(4):183–186.

Dimitrijevic M. Mesh-glove. 2. Modulation of residual upper limb motor control after stroke with whole-hand electric stimulation. *Scand J Rehabil Med.* 1994;26(4):187–190.

Dolan M, Mendel F, Fish D. Effects of high voltage pulsed current on recovery following grade I and II lateral ankle sprains. *J Athletic Train.* 2009;44(suppl):S57.

Draper V, Lyle L, Seymour T. EMG biofeedback versus electrical stimulation in the recovery of quadriceps surface EMG. *Clin Kinesiol.* 1997;51(2):28–32.

Eisenberg B, Gilal A. Structural changes in single muscle fibers after stimulation at a low-frequency. *J Gen Physiol.* 1979;74:1.

Eriksson E, Haggmark T, Kiessling KH. Effect of electrical stimulation on human skeletal muscle. *Int J Sports Med.* 1981;2:18.

Ersek R. Transcutaneous electrical neurostimulation—a new modality for controlling pain. *Clin Orthop Relat Res.* 197;128:314.

Faghri P, Glaser R, Figoni S. Functional electrical stimulation leg cycle ergometer exercise: training effects on cardiorespiratory responses of spinal cord injured. *Arch Phys Med Rehabil.* 1992;73(11):1085–1093.

Faghri P, Rodger M, Glaser R. The effects of functional electrical stimulation on shoulder subluxation, arm function recovery, and shoulder pain in hemiplegic stroke patients. *Arch Phys Med Rehabil.* 1994;75(1):73–79.

Ferguson A, Granat M. Evaluation of functional electrical stimulation for an incomplete spinal cord injured patient. *Physiotherapy.* 1992;78(4):253–256.

Finlay C. TENS: an adjunct to analgesia. *Can Nurse.* 1992;88(8): 24–26.

Fleischli JG, Laughlin TJ. Electrical stimulation in wound healing. *J Foot Ankle Surg.* 1997;36(6):457.

Fourie JA, Bowerbank P. Stimulation of bone healing in new fractures of the tibial shaft using interferential currents. *Physiother Res Int.* 1997;2(4):255–268.

Fox F, Melzack R. Transcutaneous electrical stimulation and acupuncture: comparison of treatment for low back pain. *Pain.* 1976;2:141.

Frank C, Schachar N, Dittrich D. Electromagnetic stimulation of ligament healing in rabbits. *Clin Orthop Relat Res.* 1983;175:263.

Gallien P, Brisso R, Eyssette M. Restoration of gait by functional electrical stimulation for spinal cord injured patients. *Paraplegia.* 1995;33(11):660–664.

Garrison S. *Handbook of Physical Medicine and Rehabilitation.* Philadelphia: Lippincott Williams and Wilkins; 2003.

Geddes L. A short history of the electrical stimulation of excitable tissue. *Physiologist.* 1984;27(suppl):1.

Geddes L, Baler L. *Applied Biomedical Instrumentation.* New York: Wiley; 1975.

Gellman H, Waters R, Lewonski K. Histologic comparison of chronic implantation of nerve cuff and epineural electrodes. *Adv Ext Control Hum Extrem.* 1990;12:160–183.

Godfrey C, Jayawardena H, Quance T. Comparison of electro-stimulation and isometric exercise in strengthening the quadriceps muscle. *Physiother Can.* 1979;31:265.

Gotlin R, Hershkowitz S. Electrical stimulation effect on extensor lag and length of hospital stay after total knee arthroplasty. *Arch Phys Med Rehabil.* 1994;75(9):957–959.

Gould M, Donnermeyer D, Gammon GG. Transcutaneous muscle stimulation to retard disuse atrophy after open meniscectomy. *Clin Orthop Relat Res.* 1983;178:190.

Granat M. Functional electrical stimulation and hybrid orthosis systems. *Paraplegia.* 1996;34(1):24–29.

Greathouse D, Nitz A, Matullonis D. Effects of electrical stimulation on ultrastructure of rat skeletal muscles. *Phys Ther.* 1984;64:755.

Guffey J, Asmussen M. In vitro bactericidal effects of high voltage pulsed current versus direct current against *Staphylococcus aureus. J Clin Electrophysiol.* 1989;1:5–9.

Gum SL, Reddy GK, Stehno-Bittel L, Enwemeka CS. Combined ultrasound, electrical stimulation, and laser promote collagen synthesis with moderate changes in tendon bio-mechanics. *Am J Phys Med Rehabil.* 1997;76(4):288–296.

Halback J, Straus D. Comparison of electromyostimulation to isokinetic training in increasing power of the knee extensor mechanism. *J Orthop Sports Phys Ther.* 1980;2:20.

Hamilton M, Anguish B, Koch D. Effects of high-voltage pulsed electrical current on pain, swelling and function following delayed onset muscle soreness. *J Athletic Train.* 2008;43(suppl):S86.

Higgins M, Eaton C. Nontraditional applications of neuromuscular electrical stimulation. *Athletic Ther Today.* 2005;9(5):6.

Holcomb W, Golestani S, Hill S. AQ comparison of knee extension force production with biphasic versus Russian current. *J Athletic Train.* 1999;34(2):S–17.

Holcomb W, Mangus B, Tandy R. The effect of icing with the Pro-Stim Edema Management System on cutaneous cooling. *J Athletic Train.* 1996;31(2):126–129.

Holcomb W, Rubley M. Periodic increases in neuromuscular electrical stimulation intensity eliminated significant knee extension torque decline. *J Athletic Train.* 2007;42(suppl):S134.

Houghton PE, Kincaid CB, Lovell M, et al. Effect of electrical stimulation on chronic leg ulcer size and appearance. *Phys Ther.* 2003;83(1):17–28.

Ignelzi R, Nyquist J. Excitability changes in peripheral nerve fibers after repetitive electrical stimulation: implications in pain modulation. *J Neurosurg.* 1979;61:824.

Indergand H, Morgan B. Effects of high frequency transcutaneous electrical stimulation on limb blood flow in healthy humans. *Phys Ther.* 1994;74(4):361–367.

Indergand H, Morgan B. Effect of interference current on forearm vascular resistance in asymptomatic humans. *Phys Ther.* 1995;75(5):306–312.

Johnson MI. The mystique of interferential currents when used to manage pain. *Physiotherapy.* 1999;85(6):294–297.

Johnson MI, Tabasam G. A double-blind placebo controlled investigation into the analgesic effects of inferential currents (IFC) and transcutaneous electrical nerve stimulation (TENS) on cold-induced pain in healthy subjects. *Physiother Theory Pract.* 1999;15(4):217–233.

Jones D, Bigland-Ritchie B, Edwards R. Excitation and frequency and muscle fatigue: mechanical responses during voluntary and stimulated contractions. *Exp Neurol.* 1979;64:401.

Kahn J. *Low-volt Technique.* Syosset, NY: Joseph Kahn; 1983.

Karmel-Ross K, Cooperman D. The effect of electrical stimulation on quadriceps femoris muscle torque in children with spina bifida. *Phys Ther.* 1992;72(10):723–730.

Karnes J. Effects of low-voltage pulsed current on edema formation in frog hind limbs following impact injury. *Phys Ther.* 1992;72:273–278.

Karnes J. Influence of high voltage pulsed current on diameters of arterioles during histamine-induced vasodilation [abstract R341]. *Phys Ther.* 1992;725:5105.

Kim K, Saliba S. Effects of neuromuscular electrical stimulation after anterior cruciate ligament reconstruction on quadriceps strength, function, and patient oriented outcomes: a systematic review. *J Athletic Train.* 2009;44(suppl):S87.

Kono T, Ingersoll CD, Edwards JE. A comparison of acupuncture, TENS, and acupuncture with TENS for pain relief during DOMS. *J Athletic Train.* 1999;34(2):S–67.

Kostov A, Andrews B, Popovic D. Machine learning in control of functional electrical stimulation systems for locomotion. *IEEE Trans Biomed Eng.* 1995;42(6):541–551.

Kramer J, Mendryk S. Electrical stimulation as a strength improvement technique: a review. *J Orthop Sports Phys Ther.* 1982;4:91.

Kues J, Mayhew T. Concentric and eccentric force–velocity relationships during electrically induced submaximal contractions. *Phys Ther.* 1996;76(5):S17.

Lainey C, Walmsley R, Andrew G. Effectiveness of exercise alone versus exercise plus electrical stimulation in strengthening the quadriceps muscle. *Physiother Can.* 1983;35:5.

Lane J. Electrical impedances of superficial limb tissue, epidermis, dermis and muscle sheath. *Ann N Y Acad Sci.* 1974;238:812.

Latash M, Yee M, Orpett C. Combining electrical muscle stimulation with voluntary contraction for studying muscle fatigue. *Arch Phys Med Rehabil.* 1994;75(1):29–35.

LeDoux J, Quinones M. An investigation of the use of percutaneous electrical stimulation in muscle reeducation. *Phys Ther.* 1981;61:678.

Leffman D, Arnall D, Holmgren P. Effect of microamperage stimulation on the rate of wound healing in rats: a histological study. *Phys Ther.* 1994;74(3):195–200.

Levin M, Hui-Chan C. Conventional and acupuncture-like transcutaneous electrical nerve stimulation excite similar afferent fibers. *Arch Phys Med Rehabil.* 1993;74(1):54–60.

Licht S. *Electrodiagnosis and Electromyography.* Vol 1. 3rd ed. Baltimore: Waverly; 1971.

Licht S. History of electrotherapy. In: Stillwell GK, ed. *Therapeutic Electricity and Ultraviolet Radiation.* 3rd ed. Baltimore: Williams & Wilkins; 1983.

Litke D, Dahners L. Effects of different levels of direct current on early ligament healing in a rat model. *J Orthop Res.* 1992;12:683–688.

Livesley E. Effects of electrical neuromuscular stimulation on functional performance in patients with multiple sclerosis. *Physiotherapy.* 1992;78(12):914–917.

Loeser J. Nonpharmacologic approaches to pain relief. In: Ng L, Bonica J, eds. *Pain, Discomfort and Humanitarian Care.* New York: Elsevier; 1980.

Loesor J, Black R, Christman A. A relief of pain by transcutaneous stimulation. *J Neurosurg.* 1975;42:308.

Long D. Cutaneous afferent stimulation for relief of chronic pain. *Clin Neurosurg.* 1974;21:257.

Macdonald A, Coates T. The discovery of transcutaneous spinal electroanalgesia and its relief of chronic pain. *Physiotherapy.* 1995;81(11):653–661.

Mannheimer C, Carlsson C. The analgesic effect of transcutaneous electrical nerve stimulation (TENS) in patients with rheumatoid arthritis. A comparative study of different pulse patterns. *Pain.* 1979;6:329.

Mannheimer C, Lund S, Carlsson C. The effect of transcutaneous electrical nerve stimulation (TENS) on joint pain in patients with rheumatoid arthritis. *Scand J Rheumatol.* 1978;7:13.

Mannheimer J. Electrode placements for transcutaneous electrical nerve stimulation. *Phys Ther.* 1978;58:1455.

Mao W, Ghia J, Scott D. High versus low-intensity acupuncture analgesic for treatment of chronic pain: effects on platelet serotonin. *Pain.* 1980;8:331.

Markov M. Electric current and electromagnetic field effects on soft tissue: implications for wound healing. *Wounds Compen Clin Res Pract.* 1995;7(3):94–110.

Marvie K. A major advance in the control of post-operative knee pain. *Orthopedics.* 1979;2:129.

Massey B, Nelson R, Sharkey B. Effects of high frequency electrical stimulation on the size and strength of skeletal muscle. *J Sports Med Phys Fitness.* 1965;5:136.

Mastbergen P, Lawson N, Meyer R. TENS application does not alter vibratory sensory threshold. *J Athletic Train.* 2009;44(suppl):S90.

Matsunaga T, Shimada Y, Sato K. Muscle fatigue from intermittent stimulation with low and high frequency electrical pulses. *Arch Phys Med Rehabil.* 1999;80(1):48–53.

Mattison J. Transcutaneous electrical nerve stimulation in the management of painful muscle spasm in patients with multiple sclerosis. *Clin Rehabil.* 1993;7(1):45–48.

McMiken D, Todd-Smith M, Thompson C. Strengthening of human quadriceps muscles by cutaneous electrical stimulation. *Scand J Rehabil Med.* 1983;15:25.

McQuain M, Sinaki M, Shibley L. Effect of electrical stimulation on lumbar paraspinal muscles. *Spine.* 1993;18(13):1787–1792.

Merrick MA. Research digest. Unconventional modalities: microcurrent. *Athletic Ther Today.* 1999;4(5):53–54.

Meyer G, Fields H. Causalgia treated by selective large fibre stimulation of peripheral nerve. *Brain.* 1972;95:163.

Meyer R, Lawson N, Niemann A. TENS application alters constant pressure sensory threshold. *J Athletic Train.* 2009;44(suppl):S88.

Michlovitz S. Ice and high voltage pulsed stimulation in treatment of acute lateral ankle sprains. *J Orthop Sports Phys Ther.* 1988;9:301–304.

Miller K, Knight K. The relationship between the beginning electrical stimulation frequency and a person's true cramp threshold frequency. *J Athletic Train.* 2009;44(suppl):S89.

Milner-Brown H, Stein R. The relation between the surface electromyogram and muscular force. *J Physiol.* 1975;246:549.

Mohr T, Carlson B, Sulentic C. Comparison of isometric exercise and high volt galvanic stimulation on quadriceps, femoris muscle strength. *Phys Ther.* 1985;65:606.

Mostowy D. An application of transcutaneous electrical nerve stimulation to control pain in the elderly. *J Gerontol Nurs.* 1996;22(2):36–38.

Munsat T, McNeal D, Waters R. Preliminary observations on prolonged stimulation of peripheral nerve in man. *Arch Neurol.* 1976;33:608.

Myklebust J, ed. *Neural Stimulation*. Boca Raton, FL: CRC Press; 1985.

Naess K, Storm-Mathison A. Fatigue of sustained tetanic contractions. *Acta Physiol Scand*. 1955;34:351.

Newing A, Tsang K, Thomas K. Concomitant application of ice and electrical stimulation does not improve pain threshold. *J Athletic Train*. 2008;43(suppl):S85.

Newton R. Electrotherapy: selecting wave form parameters. Paper presented at the American Physical Therapy Association Conference; 1981; Washington, DC.

Newton R. *Electrotherapeutic Treatment: Selecting Appropriate Wave Form Characteristics*. Clinton, NJ: Preston; 1984.

Owens J, Malone T. Treatment parameters of high frequency electrical stimulation as established on the Electrostim 180. *J Orthop Sports Phys Ther*. 1983;4:162.

Packman-Braun R. Misconceptions regarding functional electrical stimulation. *Neurol Rep*. 1995;19(3):17–21.

Perroti A, Bay R, Snyder A. The influence of high volt electrical stimulation on edema formation following acute injury: a systematic review of the literature. *J Athletic Train*. 2008;43(suppl):S87.

Pert V. TENS for pain in multiple sclerosis. *Physiotherapy*. 1991;77(3):227–228.

Petrofsky J. Functional electrical stimulation, a two-year study. *J Rehabil*. 1992;58(3):29–34.

Picaza J, Cannon B, Hunter S. Pain suppression by peripheral stimulation, part I. Observations with transcutaneous stimuli. *Surg Neurol*. 1975;4:105.

Pouran D, Faghri M, Rodgers M. The effects of functional electrical stimulation on shoulder subluxation, arm function recovery, and shoulder pain in hemiplegic stroke patients. *Arch Phys Med Rehabil*. 1994;75(1):73–79.

Procacci P, Zoppi M, Maresca M. Transcutaneous electrical stimulation in low back pain: a critical evaluation. *Acupunct Electrother Res*. 1982;7:1.

Rabischong E, Doutrelot P, Ohanna F. Compound motor action potentials and mechanical failure during sustained contractions by electrical stimulation in paraplegic. *Paraplegia*. 1995;33(12):707–714.

Rack P, Westbury D. The effects of length and stimulus rate on tension in the isometric cat soleus muscle. *J Physiol*. 1969;204:443.

Ray R, Samuelson A. Microcurrent versus a placebo for the control of pain and edema. *J Athletic Train*. 1996;31:S–48.

Reddana P, Moortly C, Govidappa S. Pattern of skeletal muscle chemical composition during in vivo electrical stimulations. *Ind J Physiol Pharmacol*. 1981;25:33.

Reismann M. A comparison of electrical stimulators eliciting muscle contraction. *Phys Ther*. 1984;64:751.

Requena B, Ereline J, Gapeyeva H. Posttetanic potentiation in knee extensors after high-frequency submaximal percutaneous electrical stimulation. *J Sport Rehabil*. 2005;14(3):248–257.

Rieb L, Pomeranz B. Alterations in electrical pain thresholds by use of acupuncture-like transcutaneous electrical nerve stimulation in pain-free subjects. *Phys Ther*. 1992;72(9):658–667.

Rochester L. Influence of electrical stimulation of the tibialis anterior muscle in paraplegic subjects: 1. Contractile properties. *Paraplegia*. 1995;33(8):437–449.

Roeser W, Meeks LW, Venis R, et al. The use of transcutaneous nerve stimulation for pain control in athletic medicine: a preliminary report. *Am J Sports Med*. 1976;4(5):210.

Romero J, Sanford T, Schroeder R. The effects of electrical stimulation of normal quadriceps on strength and girth. *Med Sci Sports Exerc*. 1982;14:194.

Rosch P, Markov M. *Bioelectromagnetic Medicine*. New York: Informa Healthcare; 2004.

Rosenberg M, Vutyid L, Bourbe D. Transcutaneous electrical nerve stimulation for the relief of post-operative pain. *Pain*. 1978;5:129.

Rowley B, McKenna J, Chase G. The influence of electrical current on an infecting microorganism in wounds. *Ann N Y Acad Sci*. 1974;238:543.

Schmitz R, Martin D, Perrin D. The effects of interferential current of perceived pain and serum cortisol in a delayed onset muscle soreness model. *J Athletic Train*. 1994;29(2):171.

Scott P. *Clayton's Electrotherapy and Actinotherapy*. 5th and 7th ed. Baltimore: Williams & Wilkins; 1965 and 1975.

Seib T, Price R, Reyes M. The quantitative measurement of spasticity: effect of cutaneous electrical stimulation. *Arch Phys Med Rehabil*. 1994;75(7):746–750.

Selkowitz D. Improvement in isometric strength of the quadricep femoris muscle after training with electrical stimulation. *Phys Ther*. 1985;65:186.

Shealey C, Maurer D. Transcutaneous nerve stimulation for control of pain. *Surg Neurol*. 1974;2:45.

Simmonds M, Wessel J, Scudds R. The effect of pain quality on the efficacy of conventional TENS. *Physiotherapy (Can)*. 1992;44(3):35–40.

Sjolund B, Eriksson M. The influence of naloxone on analgesia produced by peripheral conditioning stimulation. *Brain Res*. 1979;173:295.

Sjolund B, Terenius L, Eriksson M. Increased cerebrospinal fluid levels of endorphin after electroacupuncture. *Acta Physiol Scand*. 1977;100:382.

Smith B, Betz R, Mulcahey M. Reliability of percutaneous intramuscular electrodes for upper extremity functional neuromuscular stimulation in adolescents with C5 injury. *Arch Phys Med Rehabil*. 1994;75(9):939–945.

Smith B, Mulcahey M, Betz R. Quantitative comparison of grasp and release abilities with and without functional neuro-muscular stimulation in adolescents with tetraplegia. *Paraplegia*. 1996;34(1):16–23.

Snyder K, Meyer R, Neimann A. Transcutaneous electrical nerve stimulation (TENS) does not alter cold sensory detection threshold. *J Athletic Train*. 2009;44(suppl):S89.

Snyder-Mackler L, Delitto A, Stralka S. Use of electrical stimulation to enhance recovery of quadriceps femoris muscle force production in patients following anterior cruciate ligament reconstruction. *Phys Ther.* 1994;74(10):901–907.

Standish W, Valiant G, Bonen A. The effects of immobilization and of electrical stimulation on muscle glycogen and myofibrillar ATPase. *Can J Appl Sports Sci.* 1982;7:267.

Stone JA. Prevention and rehabilitation. "Russian" electrical stimulation. *Athletic Ther Today.* 1997;2(3):27.

Stone JA. Prevention and rehabilitation. Interferential electrical stimulation. *Athletic Ther Today.* 1997;2(2):27.

Stone JA. Prevention and rehabilitation. Microcurrent electrical stimulation. *Athletic Ther Today.* 1997;2(6):15.

Sunderland S. *Nerves and Nerve Injuries.* Baltimore: Williams & Wilkins; 1968.

Szehi E, David E. The stereodynamic interferential current—a new electrotherapeutic technique. *Electromedica.* 1980;48:13.

Szuminsky N, Albers A, Unger P. Effect of narrow pulsed high voltages on bacterial viability. *Phys Ther.* 1994;74(7):660–667.

Taylor M, Newton R, Personius W. The effects of interferential current stimulation for the treatment of subjects with recurrent jaw pain [abstract]. *Phys Ther.* 1986;66:774.

Taylor P, Hallet M, Flaherty L. Treatment of osteoarthritis of the knee with transcutaneous electrical nerve stimulation. *Pain.* 1981;11:233.

Terezhalmy G, Ross G, Holmes-Johnson E. Transcutaneous electrical nerve stimulation treatment of TMJMPDS patients. *Ear Nose Throat J.* 1982;61:664.

Thorsteinsson G, Stonnington H. The placebo effect of transcutaneous electrical stimulation. *Pain.* 1978;5:31.

Tourville T, Connolly D, Reed B. Effects of sensory level high-volt pulsed electrical current on delayed onset muscle soreness. *J Athletic Train.* 2003;38(suppl 2S):S–33.

Vrbov G, Hudlicka O. *Application of Muscle/Nerve Stimulation in Health and Disease.* New York: Springer; 2008.

Wadsworth H, Chanmugan A. *Electrophysical Agents in Physical Therapy.* Marrickville, Australia: Science Press; 1983.

Walsh D, Foster N, Baxter G. Transcutaneous electrical nerve stimulation parameters to neurophysiological and hypoalgesic effects. *Phys Ther.* 1996;76(5):552.

Walsh D, McAdams E. *TENS: Clinical Applications and Related Theory.* Philadelphia: WB Saunders; 1997.

Ward A. *Electricity Waves and Fields in Therapy.* Marrickville, Australia: Science Press; 1980.

Watson T. *Electrotherapy: Evidence Based Practice.* Philadelphia: Churchill Livingstone; 2008.

Weber M, Servedio F, Woddall W. The effects of three modalities on delayed onset muscle soreness. *J Orthop Sports Phys Ther.* 1994;20(5):236–242.

Wheeler P, Wolcott L, Morris J. Neural considerations in the healing of ulcerated tissue by clinical electrotherapeutic application of weak direct current: findings and theory. In: Reynolds D, Sjoberg A, eds. *Neuroelectric Research.* Springfield, IL: Charles C Thomas; 1971:83–96.

Williams G, Krishrian C, Allen E. Torque-based triggering improves stimulus timing precision in activation tests. *J Athletic Train.* 2009;44(suppl):S88.

Windsor R, Lester J. Electrical stimulation in clinical practice. *Phys Sports Med.* 1993;21(2):85–86, 89–92.

Wolf S, Gersh M, Kutner M. Relationship of selected clinical variables to current delivered during transcutaneous electrical nerve stimulation. *Phys Ther.* 1978;58:1478–1483.

Wolf S, Gersh M, Rao V. Examination of electrode placements and stimulating parameters in treating chronic pain with conventional transcutaneous nerve stimulation (TENS). *Pain.* 1981;11:37.

Wong R, Jette D. Changes in sympathetic tone associated with different forms of transcutaneous electrical nerve stimulation in healthy subjects. *Phys Ther.* 1984;64:478.

Yarkony G, Roth E. Neuromuscular stimulation in spinal cord injury: restoration of functional movement of the extremities, part 1. *Arch Phys Med Rehabil.* 1992;73(1):78–86.

Yarkony G, Roth E, Cybulski J. Neuromuscular stimulation in spinal cord injury II: prevention of secondary complications, part 2. *Arch Phys Med Rehabil.* 1992;73(2):195–200.

Zecca L, Ferrario P, Furia G. Effects of pulsed electromagnetic field on acute and chronic inflammation. *Trans Biol Repair Growth Soc.* 1983;3:72.

GLOSSARY

absolute refractory period Brief time period (0.5 microsecond) following membrane depolarization during which the membrane is incapable of depolarizing again.

accommodation Adaptation by the sensory receptors to various stimuli over an extended period of time.

action potential A recorded change in electrical potential between the inside and outside of a nerve cell, resulting in muscular contraction.

all-or-none response The depolarization of nerve or muscle membrane is the same once a depolarizing intensity threshold is reached; further increases in intensity do not increase the response.

alternating current Current that periodically changes its polarity or direction of flow.

ampere Unit of measure that indicates the rate at which electrical current is flowing.

amplitude   The intensity of current flow as indicated by the height of the waveform from baseline.

anode   The positively charged electrode.

biphasic current   Another name for alternating current, in which the direction of current flow reverses direction.

bursts   A combined set of three or more pulses; also referred to as packets or envelopes.

cathode   The negatively charged electrode.

chronaxie   The duration of time necessary to cause observable tissue excitation, given a current intensity of two times rheobasic current.

circuit   The path of current from a generating source through the various components back to the generating source.

conductance   The ease with which a current flows along a conducting medium.

conductors   Materials that permit the free movement of electrons.

constructive interference   The combined amplitude of two distinct circuits increases the amplitude.

coulomb   Indicates the number of electrons flowing in a current.

current density   Amount of current flow per cubic area.

current   The flow of electrons.

cycle   Applies to biphasic current.

decay time   The time required for a waveform to go from peak amplitude to 0 V.

denervated muscle   A muscle that does not have nerve innervation.

depolarization   Process or act of neutralizing the cell membrane's resting potential.

Destructive interference   Combined amplitude of two distinct circuits decreases the amplitude.

direct current   Galvanic current that always flows in the same direction and may flow in either a positive or a negative direction.

duration   Sometimes also referred to as *pulse width*. Indicates the length of time the current is flowing.

electrical current   The net movement of electrons along a conducting medium.

electrical impedance   The opposition to electron flow in a conducting material.

electrical potential   The difference between charged particles at a higher and a lower potential.

electron   Fundamental particles of matter possessing a negative electrical charge and very small mass.

frequency window selectivity   Cellular responses may be triggered by a certain electrical frequency range.

frequency   The number of cycles or pulses per second.

functional electrical stimulation   Utilizes multiple-channel electrical stimulators to recruit muscles in a programmed sequence that produces a functional movement pattern.

ground   A wire that makes an electrical connection with the earth.

ground-fault interruptors (GFI)   A safety device that automatically shuts off current flow and reduces the chances of electrical shock.

insulators   Materials that resist current flow.

interburst intervals   Interruptions between individual bursts.

interphase interval   The interruptions between individual pulses or groups of pulses.

ion   A positively or negatively charged particle.

iontophoresis   Uses continuous direct current to drive ions into the tissues.

low-intensity stimulator (LIS)   Another more current term for MENS.

macroshock   An electrical shock that can be felt and has a leakage of electrical current of greater than 1 mA.

medical galvanism   Creates either an acidic or an alkaline environment that may be of therapeutic value.

microcurrent electrical nerve stimulator (MENS)   Used primarily in tissue healing, the current intensities too small to excite peripheral nerves.

microcurrent   The term most commonly used to refer to MENS or LIS.

microshock   An electrical shock that is imperceptible because of a leakage of current of less than 1 mA.

modulation   Refers to any alteration in the magnitude or any variation in the duration of an electrical current.

monophasic current   Another name for direct current, in which the direction of current flow remains the same.

neuromuscular electrical stimulator (NMES)   Also called an electrical muscle stimulator (EMS), it is used to stimulate muscle directly, as would be the case with denervated muscle where peripheral nerves are not functioning.

ohm   A unit of measure that indicates resistance to current flow.

ohm's law   The current in an electrical circuit is directly proportional to the voltage and inversely proportional to the resistance.

parallel circuit   A circuit in which two or more routes exist for current to pass between the two terminals.

phases   That portion of the pulse that rises above or below the baseline for some period of time.

pulsatile currents   Contain three or more pulses grouped together and can be unidirectional or bidirectional.

pulse charge   The total amount of electricity being delivered to the patient during each pulse.

pulse period   The combined time of the pulse duration and the interpulse interval.

pulse   An individual waveform.

ramping   Another name for surging modulation, in which the current builds gradually to some maximum amplitude.

ramping   Another name for surging modulation, in which the current builds gradually to some maximum amplitude.

rate of rise   How quickly a waveform reaches its maximum amplitude.

resistance   The opposition to electron flow in a conducting material.

resting potential   The potential difference between the inside and outside of a membrane.

rheobase   The specific intensity of current necessary to cause an observable tissue response given a long current duration.

russian current   A medium-frequency (2000–10,000 Hz) pulsatile biphasic wave generated in 50-bursts-per-second envelopes.

series circuit   A circuit in which there is only one path for current to get from one terminal to another.

stereodynamic interference current   Three distinct circuits blending and creating a distinct electrical wave pattern.

tetanization   When individual muscle twitch responses can no longer be distinguished and the responses force maximum shortening of the stimulated muscle fiber.

tetany   Muscle condition that is caused by hyperexcitation and results in cramps and spasms.

transcutaneous electrical stimulator   All therapeutic electrical generators regardless of whether they deliver biphasic, monophasic, or pulsatile currents through electrodes

transcutaneous electrical nerve stimulator (TENS)   A transcutaneous electrical stimulator used to stimulate peripheral nerves.

volt   The electromotive force that must be applied to produce a movement of electrons. A measure of electrical power.

voltage-sensitive permeability   The quality of some cell membranes that makes them permeable to different ions based on the electrical charge of the ions. Nerve and muscle cell membranes allow negatively charged ions into the cell while actively transporting some positively charged ions outside the cell membrane.

voltage   The force resulting from an accumulation of electrons at one point in an electrical circuit, usually corresponding to a deficit of electrons at another point in the circuit.

watt   A measure of electrical power (*watt = volt × ampere*).

waveform   The shape of an electrical current as displayed on an oscilloscope.

LAB ACTIVTY

ELECTRICAL STIMULATION: ANALGESIA

DESCRIPTION

Electroanalgesia is arguably the most common use of therapeutic electricity. The use of therapeutic electricity for analgesia is often referred to as transcutaneous electrical nerve stimulation or TENS; however, all forms of therapeutic electricity that do not use implanted or needle electrodes are "transcutaneous," and many forms stimulate nerves. Therefore, the term TENS should be discouraged. Although there are hundreds of different types of electrical stimulators available for use, there are essentially three levels in the body that may be affected.

The first level is the spinal gate. This level is activated by increasing the input to the spinal cord from large-diameter afferent neurons. The second level is referred to as the central bias mechanism, where intense small fiber afferent input activates a negative feedback loop through connections in the midbrain. Finally, some forms of electrical stimulation appear to stimulate the production of endogenous opiates, the endorphins.

Although stimulators have many different waveforms and modulations, there is no evidence that an "optimal" waveform exists. It is impossible to predict for an individual patient what type of current, electrode configuration, amplitude of stimulation, and so on will provide relief of pain. Therefore, electroanalgesia is somewhat of a trial-and-error phenomenon. This does not mean the approach should be haphazard; a systematic approach, based on clinical experience, is best.

Generally, there are three types of stimulation for electroanalgesia: conventional, low frequency, and hyperstimulation. Conventional generally has a pulse rate of 10–100 pps and is applied at an amplitude between sensory and motor thresholds. Low-frequency stimulation has a pulse rate of 1–5 pps, and an amplitude between motor and pain thresholds. Hyperstimulation generally uses a monophasic PC at a frequency of 1–128 pps and an amplitude to pain tolerance. It is often referred to as point stimulation.

PHYSIOLOGIC EFFECTS

Depolarization of peripheral nerves

THERAPEUTIC EFFECTS

Inhibition of pain perception

INDICATIONS

The obvious indication for electroanalgesia is pain. However, the cause of the pain should be identified prior to the use of electrical stimulation, and it must be remembered that the modulation of pain is not treating the cause of the pain.

CONTRAINDICATIONS

- Pregnancy
- Implanted electrical pacing devices (e.g., cardiac pacemaker, bladder stimulator)
- Cardiac arrhythmia
- Over the carotid sinus area
- Hypersensitivity (i.e., the patient who has a strong aversion to electricity, or the patient with certain types of catheters or shunts)

ELECTRICAL STIMULATION: ANALGESIA			
PROCEDURE	EVALUATION		
	1	2	3
1. Check supplies.			
a. Obtain towels or sheets for draping, and conductant.			
b. Check stimulator, electrodes, and cables for charged battery, broken or frayed insulation, and so on.			
c. Ensure the amplitude controls are at zero.			
2. Question patient.			
a. Verify identity of patient (if not already verified).			
b. Verify the absence of contraindications.			
c. Ask about previous treatments for current condition, and check treatment notes.			
3. Position patient.			
a. Place patient in a well-supported, comfortable position.			
b. Expose body part to be treated.			
c. Drape patient to preserve patient's modesty, and protect clothing, but allow access to body part.			
4. Inspect body part to be treated.			
a. Check light touch perception.			
b. Assess function of body part (e.g., ROM, irritability).			
5a. Apply conventional electrical stimulation.			
a. Place conductant on electrodes as indicated, secure electrodes to patient.			
b. Remind the patient to inform you when he or she feels something. Do not tell the patient what he or she will feel; for example, do not say, "Tell me when you feel a buzz or tingle."			
c. Adjust the pulse rate, pulse width, and mode of stimulation to desired settings if possible.			
d. Turn on the stimulator, and increase the amplitude slowly. Monitor the patient's response, not the stimulator.			

e. After the patient reports the onset of the stimulus, adjust the amplitude to a comfortable level, but make sure it is below motor threshold. If it is impossible to achieve suprasensory threshold stimulation without a motor response, turn the stimulator off and move the electrodes to another location.			
f. Set a timer for the appropriate treatment time and give the patient a signaling device. Make sure the patient understands how to use the signaling device.			
g. Recheck the patient after about 5 minutes. If the sensation has diminished, adjust the amplitude appropriately.			
5b. Apply low-frequency electrical stimulation.			
a. Place conductant on electrodes as indicated, secure electrodes to patient.			
b. Remind the patient to inform you when he or she feels something. Do not tell the patient what he or she will feel; for example, do not say, "Tell me when you feel a buzz or tingle."			
c. Adjust the pulse rate, pulse width, and mode of stimulation to desired settings if possible			
d. Turn on the stimulator, and increase the amplitude slowly. Monitor the patient's response, not the stimulator.			
e. After the patient reports the onset of the stimulus, adjust the amplitude to a comfortable level above motor threshold. The contraction should be just a twitch, not a strong contraction.			
f. Set a timer for the appropriate treatment time and give the patient a signaling device. Make sure the patient understands how to use the signaling device.			
g. Recheck the patient after about 5 minutes. If the sensation has diminished, adjust the amplitude appropriately.			
5c. Apply hyperstimulation electrical stimulation.			
a. Place conductant on "inactive" electrode; have the patient hold the electrode in his or her palm. Apply the conductant to points to be stimulated.			
b. If using electrical resistance to locate stimulation points, set sensitivity of ohm meter; set pulse rate, polarity, and length of stimulation to desired settings.			
c. Move the "active" electrode slowly in the area of the point to be stimulated until the area of minimal resistance is found; the pressure applied to the electrode must be constant.			
d. Tell the patient to report when the amplitude of stimulation is as high as he or she can tolerate. Activate the stimulation current, and increase the amplitude slowly. Monitor the patient's response, not the stimulator.			
e. After the patient reports that the stimulus is as much as he or she can tolerate, maintain constant pressure on the electrode. Stimulate the point two or three times, for 15–30 seconds each time.			
f. Repeat the process for each point to be stimulated.			
6. Complete treatment.			
a. When the treatment time is over, turn the intensity control to zero, and move the generator away from the patient; remove conductant with a towel.			
b. Remove material used for draping; assist the patient in dressing as needed.			

c. Have the patient perform appropriate therapeutic exercise as indicated.			
d. Clean the treatment area and equipment according to normal protocol.			
7. Assess treatment efficacy.			
a. Ask the patient how the treated area feels.			
b. Visually inspect the treated area for any adverse reactions.			
c. Perform functional tests as indicated.			

LAB ACTIVITY

ELECTRICAL STIMULATION: REEDUCATION

DESCRIPTION

Electrical stimulation may be used to assist a patient in regaining the ability to voluntarily control a normally innervated muscle. Sometimes following surgery, a patient temporarily loses the ability to produce a muscle contraction. Probably the most common loss is of the quadriceps femoris following knee surgery. In addition, if a patient has undergone a tendon transfer, he or she may have difficulty recruiting the muscle to perform the new joint action.

The mechanism by which electrical stimulation aids in the recovery of volitional control of skeletal muscle is not clear, nor is the reason why volitional control is lost following surgery. The probable method of action is via stimulation of joint, muscle, and skin proprioceptors when the muscle produces joint motion.

PHYSIOLOGIC EFFECTS

Depolarization of peripheral nerves

THERAPEUTIC EFFECTS

Recovery of volitional control of skeletal muscle

INDICATIONS

The primary indication is loss of volitional control of a skeletal muscle following surgery or a tendon transfer.

CONTRAINDICATIONS

- Pregnancy
- Implanted electrical pacing devices (e.g., cardiac pacemaker, bladder stimulator)
- Cardiac arrhythmia
- Over the carotid sinus area
- Hypersensitivity (i.e., the patient who has a strong aversion to electricity, or the patient with certain types of catheters or shunts)

ELECTRICAL STIMULATION: REEDUCATION

PROCEDURE	EVALUATION		
	1	2	3
1. Check supplies.			
a. Obtain towels or sheets for draping, and conductant.			
b. Check stimulator, electrodes, and cables for charged battery, broken or frayed insulation, etc.			
c. Verify that the intensity control is at zero.			
2. Question patient.			
a. Verify identity of patient (if not already verified).			

b. Verify the absence of contraindications.			
c. Ask about previous exposure to electrotherapy; check treatment notes.			
3. Position patient.			
a. Place patient in a well-supported, comfortable position.			
b. Expose body part to be treated.			
c. Drape patient to preserve patient's modesty, and protect clothing, but allow access to body part.			
4. Inspect body part to be treated.			
a. Check light touch perception.			
b. Assess function of body part (e.g., ROM, irritability).			
5. Apply electrical stimulation for reeducation.			
a. Place conductant on electrodes as needed; secure electrodes to patient. Electrode location will vary depending on desired effect. Usually, the ideal location for the active electrode is over the motor point of the target muscle or the peripheral nerve trunk that supplies the target muscle.			
b. Remind the patient to inform you when he or she feels something. Do not tell the patient what he or she will feel; for example, do not say, "Tell me when you feel a buzz or tingle."			
c. Adjust the pulse rate, pulse width, and mode of stimulation to desired settings if possible.			
d. Turn on the stimulator, and increase the amplitude slowly. Monitor the patient's response, not the stimulator.			
e. After the patient reports the onset of the stimulus, adjust the amplitude to a comfortable level above motor threshold. Encourage the patient to try to volitionally contract the muscle before the stimulator does, and increase the force during the stimulation.			
f. Continue to monitor the patient during the duration of the treatment.			
6. Complete treatment.			
a. When the treatment time is over or the patient is able to control the muscle contraction, turn the intensity to zero, and move the generator away from the patient; remove conductant with a towel.			
b. Remove material used for draping; assist the patient in dressing as needed.			
c. Have the patient perform appropriate therapeutic exercise as indicated.			
d. Clean the treatment area and equipment according to normal protocol.			
7. Assess treatment efficacy.			
a. Ask the patient how the treated area feels.			
b. Visually inspect the treated area for any adverse reactions.			
c. Perform functional tests as indicated.			

LAB ACTIVITY

ELECTRICAL STIMULATION: STRENGTHENING

DESCRIPTION

Electrical stimulation is often used for increasing skeletal muscle strength by itself or in conjunction with active exercise. However, there is no evidence that the electrical stimulation by itself or in conjunction with active exercise is better than active exercise alone for muscle strengthening. Also, the increase in tension-developing capacity does not transfer to functional activities. Because of this, it is sometimes referred to as "electrical stimulation to increase isometric force development capacity."

PHYSIOLOGIC EFFECTS

Depolarization of peripheral nerves

THERAPEUTIC EFFECTS

Increase in isometric force development capacity

INDICATIONS

The primary indication is muscle weakness. However, electrical stimulation is sometimes used in an attempt to prevent disuse atrophy during immobilization of a limb.

CONTRAINDICATIONS

- Pregnancy
- Implanted electrical pacing devices (e.g., cardiac pacemaker, bladder stimulator)
- Cardiac arrhythmia
- Over the carotid sinus area
- Hypersensitivity (i.e., the patient who has a strong aversion to electricity, or the patient with certain types of catheters or shunts)

ELECTRICAL STIMULATION: STRENGTHENING

PROCEDURE	EVALUATION		
	1	2	3
1. Check supplies.			
a. Obtain towels or sheets for draping, and conductant.			
b. Check stimulator, electrodes, and cables for charged battery, broken or frayed insulation, etc.			
c. Verify that the intensity control is at zero.			
2. Question patient.			
a. Verify identity of patient (if not already verified).			
b. Verify the absence of contraindications.			
c. Ask about previous exposure to electrotherapy; check treatment notes.			
3. Position patient.			
a. Place patient in a well-supported, comfortable position.			
b. Expose body part to be treated.			
c. Drape patient to preserve patient's modesty, and protect clothing, but allow access to body part.			
4. Inspect body part to be treated.			

a. Check light touch perception.			
b. Assess function of body part (e.g., ROM, irritability).			
5. Apply electrical stimulation for muscle strengthening.			
a. Place conductant on electrodes as indicated; secure electrodes to patient. Electrode location will vary depending on desired effect. Usually, the ideal location for the active electrode is over the motor point of the target muscle, or the peripheral nerve trunk that supplies the target muscle.			
b. Remind the patient to inform you when he or she feels something. Do not tell the patient what he or she will feel; for example, do not say, "Tell me when you feel a buzz or tingle."			
c. Adjust the pulse rate, pulse width, and mode of stimulation to desired settings if possible.			
d. Turn on the stimulator, and increase the amplitude slowly. Monitor the patient's response, not the stimulator.			
e. After the patient reports the onset of the stimulus, adjust the amplitude to as high a level as the patient can tolerate.			
f. Set a timer for the appropriate treatment time and give the patient a signaling device. Make sure the patient understands how to use the signaling device.			
g. Recheck the patient after about 5 minutes. If the sensation has diminished, adjust the amplitude appropriately.			
6. Complete treatment.			
a. When the treatment time is over, turn the intensity control to zero, and move the generator away from the patient; remove conductant with a towel.			
b. Remove material used for draping; assist the patient in dressing as needed.			
c. Have the patient perform appropriate therapeutic exercise as indicated.			
d. Clean the treatment area and equipment according to normal protocol.			
7. Assess treatment efficacy.			
a. Ask the patient how the treated area feels.			
b. Visually inspect the treated area for any adverse reactions.			
c. Perform functional tests as indicated.Figure 5–30. Russian current with an interburst interval. Darkly shaded area represents total current, and light shading indicates total current without the interburst interval.			

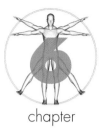

Iontophoresis

William E. Prentice

OBJECTIVES

Following completion of this chapter, the student will be able to:

➤ Differentiate between iontophoresis and phonophoresis.

➤ Explain the basic mechanisms of ion transfer.

➤ Establish specific iontophoresis application procedures and techniques.

➤ Identify the different ions most commonly used in iontophoresis.

➤ Choose the appropriate clinical applications for using an iontophoresis technique.

➤ Establish precautions and concerns for using iontophoresis treatment.

Iontophoresis is a therapeutic technique that involves the introduction of ions into the body tissues by means of a direct electrical current.[1] Originally referred to as **ion transfer**, it was first described by LeDuc in 1903 as a technique of transporting chemicals across a membrane using an electrical current as a driving force.[2] Since that time, the use and popularity of iontophoresis has varied. Recently new emphasis has been placed on iontophoresis, and it has become a commonly used technique in clinical settings. Iontophoresis has several advantages as a treatment technique in that it is a painless, sterile, noninvasive technique for introducing specific ions into a tissue that has been demonstrated to have a positive effect on the healing process.[3]

Although specific statutes relative to the use of iontophoresis vary from state to state, the clinician must be aware that most of the medications used in iontophoresis require a physician's prescription for use.

IONTOPHORESIS VERSUS PHONOPHORESIS

It is critical to point out the difference between iontophoresis and phonophoresis since the two techniques are often confused and occasionally the two terms are erroneously interchanged. It is true that both techniques are used to deliver chemicals to various biologic tissues. Phonophoresis, which is discussed in detail in Chapter 10, involves the use of acoustic energy in the form of ultrasound to drive whole molecules across the skin into the tissues, whereas iontophoresis uses an electrical current to transport ions into the tissues.[97]

Clinical Decision-Making *Exercise 6–1*

A physician sends the clinician a prescription for using topical hydrocortisone to treat plantar fasciitis but does not specify whether phonophoresis or iontophoresis should be used. What should determine the clinician's decision to use one or the other?

BASIC MECHANISMS OF ION TRANSFER

Pharmacokinetics of Iontophoresis

In an ideal drug delivery system, the goal is to maximize the therapeutic effects of a drug while minimizing adverse effects and simultaneously providing a high degree of patient compliance and acceptability.[4] Transdermal iontophoresis delivers medication at a constant rate so that the effective plasma concentration remains within a therapeutic window for an extended period of time. The **therapeutic window** refers to the plasma concentrations of a drug, which should fall between a minimum concentration necessary for a therapeutic effect and the maximum effective concentration above which adverse effects may possibly occur.[4] Iontophoresis is able to facilitate the delivery of charged and high-molecular-weight compounds that cannot be effectively delivered by simply applying them to the skin. It is useful since it appears to overcome the resistive properties of the stratum corneum to charged ions.[4]

Iontophoresis decreases the absorption lag time, while it increases the delivery rate when compared with passive skin application. A primary advantage of iontophoresis is the ability to provide both a spiked and sustained release of a drug, thus reducing the possibility of developing a tolerance to the drug. The rate at which an ion may be delivered is determined by a number of factors including the concentration of the ion, the pH of the solution, molecular size of the solute, current density, and the duration of the treatment.

It appears that mechanisms of absorption of drugs administered by iontophoresis are similar to those of drugs administered via other methods.[4] However, taking medication via transdermal iontophoresis has advantages relative to taking oral medications because the medication is concentrated in a specific area and it does not have to be absorbed within the gastrointestinal tract. Additionally, transdermal administration is safer than administering a drug through injection.

Movement of Ions in Solution

As defined in Chapter 5, **ions** are positively or negatively charged particles. Through the process of **ionization**, soluble compounds such as acids, alkaloids, or salts dissociate or dissolve into ions, which are suspended in some type of solution.[5] Ionic movement occurs in the resulting solutions, called **electrolytes**. Ions move or migrate within this solution according to the electrically charged currents acting on them. The term **electrophoresis** refers to the movement of ions in solution.

At any given instant, the electrode that has the greatest concentration of electrons is negatively charged and is referred to as the negative electrode or cathode. Conversely, the electrode with a lower concentration of electrons is called the positive electrode or anode. Negatively charged ions will be repelled from the negative electrode, and thus they move toward the positive electrode, creating an **acidic reaction**. Positively charged ions will tend to move toward the negative electrode and away from the positive electrode, resulting in an **alkaline reaction**.

The manner in which ions move in solution forms the basis for iontophoresis. Positively charged ions are carried into the tissues from the positive pole, and negatively charged ions are introduced by the negative pole. Once they enter the tissues, the ions are picked up by the body's own charged ions, and electrolytes pick up the electrons and transport them, allowing flow of current between active and dispersive electrodes. Thus, knowing the correct ion polarity and matching it with the appropriate electrode polarity is of critical importance in using iontophoresis.

Movement of Ions Through Tissue

The force that acts to move ions through the tissues is determined by both the strength of the electrical field and the electrical impedance of tissues to current flow. The strength of the electrical field is determined by the current density. The difference in current density between the active and inactive or dispersive electrodes establishes a gradient of potential difference that produces ion migration within the electrical field. (In Chapter 5, the active electrode was defined as the smaller of the two electrodes that has the greater current density. When using iontophoresis, the **active electrode** is defined as the one that is being used to carry the ion into the tissues.) Current density may be altered either by increasing or decreasing current intensity or by changing the size of the electrode. Increasing the size of the electrode will decrease current density under that electrode. It has been recommended that the current density be reduced at the cathode or negative electrode. The accumulation of positively charged ions in a small area creates an alkaline reaction that is more likely to produce tissue damage than an accumulation of negatively charged ions that produces an acidic reaction.[92] Thus, it has been recommended that the negative electrode should be larger, perhaps twice the size of the positive electrode to reduce current density.[5,6] This size relationship should remain the same even when the negative electrode is the active electrode. However, it should be added that this is not usually the case with current electrodes for iontophoresis, which are more likely to be the same size (Figure 6–1).

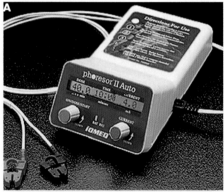

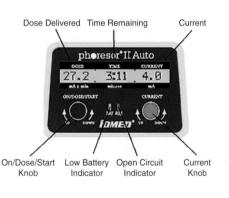

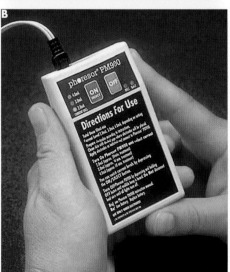

Figure 6–1. Portable iontophoresis units. (a) The Phoresor PM 850 and its control panel. (b) The Phoresor PM 900 is a simpler, more portable unit.

Skin and fat are poor conductors of electrical current, offering greater resistance to current flow. Higher current intensities are necessary to create ion movement in areas where the skin and fat layers are thick, further increasing the likelihood of burns particularly around the negative electrode. However, the presence of sweat glands decreases impedance, thus facilitating the flow of direct current as well as ions. The sweat ducts are the primary paths by which ions move through the skin.[7] As the skin becomes more saturated with an electrolyte and blood flow increases to the area during treatment, overall skin impedance will decrease under the electrodes.[1] Iontophoresis should be considered a relatively superficial treatment, with the medication penetrating no more than 1.5 cm over a 12- to 24-hour period but only 1–3 mm during the duration of the average treatment.

The quantity of ions transferred into the tissues through iontophoresis is determined by the intensity of the current or current density at the active electrode, the duration of the current flow, and the concentration of ions in solution.[5] The number of ions absorbed is directly proportional to the current density. In addition, the longer the current flows, the greater the number of ions transferred to the tissues is. Therefore, ion transfer may be increased by increasing the intensity and duration of the treatment.[95] Unfortunately as treatment duration increases, the skin impedance decreases, thus increasing the likelihood of burns. Even though ion concentration affects ion transfer, concentrations greater than 1–2% are not more effective than medications at lower concentrations.[8,9]

Once the ions have passed through the skin, they recombine with existing ions and free radicals floating in the bloodstream, thus forming the necessary new compounds for favorable therapeutic interactions.[6]

Iontophoresis generators:
- produce continuous DC current.

IONTOPHORESIS EQUIPMENT AND TREATMENT TECHNIQUES
Type of Current Required

Continuous direct current has traditionally been used for iontophoresis. Direct current ensures the unidirectional flow of ions that cannot be accomplished using a bidirectional or alternating current. However, a recent study has shown that drugs can be delivered by AC iontophoresis. Iontophoresis using alternating current avoids electrochemical burns, and delivery of the drug increases with duration of application.[10] Neither high-voltage direct currents nor interferential currents may be used for iontophoresis since the current is interrupted and the current duration is too short to produce significant ion movement. It should be added, however, that modulated pulsed currents have been used with some success in in vivo and in vitro studies on laboratory animals for transdermal delivery of drugs.[11-13]

Iontophoresis Generators

A variety of current generators are available on the market that produce continuous direct current and are specifically used for iontophoresis (Figures 6–1 and 6–2). It should be emphasized that any generator that has the capability of producing continuous direct current may be used for iontophoresis. Some generators are driven by batteries, others by alternating current. Many generators produce current at a constant voltage that gradually reduces skin impedance, consequently increasing current density and thus increasing the risk of burns. The generator should deliver a constant voltage output to the patient by adjusting the output amperage to normal variations that occur in tissue impedance, thereby reducing the likelihood of burns. For safety purposes, the generator should automatically shut down if the skin impedance decreases to some preset limit.

The generator should have some type of current intensity control that can be adjusted between 1 and 5 mA. It should also have an adjustable timer that can be set up to 25 minutes. Polarity of the terminals should be clearly marked, and a polarity reversal switch is desirable.

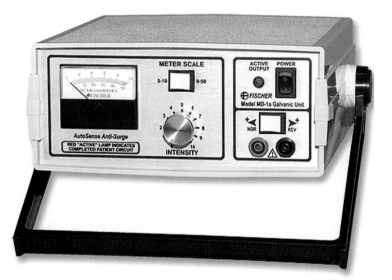

Figure 6–2. The Fischer MD 1a is an example of a less portable unit that can be used for iontophoresis.

The lead wires connecting the electrodes to the terminals should be well insulated and should be checked regularly for damage or breakdown.

Current Intensity

Low-amperage currents appear to be more effective as a driving force than currents with higher intensities.[6,14,15] Higher-intensity currents tend to reduce effective penetration into the tissues. Recommended current amplitudes used for iontophoresis range between 3 and 5 mA.[6,16–18] When initiating the treatment, the current intensity should always be increased very slowly until the patient reports feeling a tingling or prickly sensation. If pain or a burning sensation is elicited, the intensity is too great and should be decreased. Likewise when terminating the treatment, current intensity should be slowly decreased to zero before the electrodes are disconnected.

It has been recommended that the maximum current intensity be determined by the size of the active electrode (Figure 6–3a).[19] Current amplitude is usually set so that the current density falls between 0.1 and 0.5 mA/cm² of the active electrode surface[5] (Figure 6–3b).

The **negative electrode** should be larger than the positive electrode.

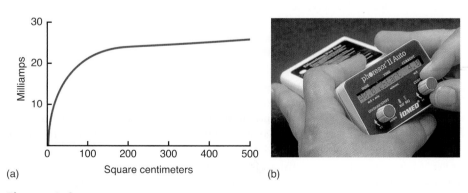

(a)

(b)

Figure 6–3. (a) The maximum current intensity should be determined by the size of the active electrode. (b) Current amplitude is usually set so that the current density falls between 0.1 and 0.5 mA/cm² of the active electrode surface.

Treatment Duration

Recommended treatment durations range between 10 and 20 minutes, with 15 minutes being an average.[20] During this 15-minute treatment, the patient should be comfortable with no reported or visible signs of pain or burning. The clinician should check the patient's skin every 3–5 minutes during treatment, looking for signs of skin irritation. Since skin impedance usually decreases during the treatment, it may be necessary to decrease current intensity to avoid pain or burning.

It should be added that the medicated electrode can be left in place for 12–24 hours to enhance the initial treatment.[20]

Dosage of Medication

An iontophoresis dose of medication delivered during treatment is expressed in milliampere-minutes (mA-min). An mA-min is a function of current and time. The total drug dose delivered (mA-min) = current × treatment time. For example:

40 mA-min dose = 4.0 mA current × 10-minute treatment time
OR
30 mA-min dose = 2.0 mA current × 15-minute treatment time

A typical iontophoretic drug delivery dose is 40 mA-min but can vary from 0 to 80 mA-min depending on the medication.

Electrodes

The continuous direct electrical current must be delivered to the patient through some type of electrode. Many different electrodes are available to the clinician, ranging from those "borrowed" from other electrical stimulators to commercially manufactured, ready-to-use, disposable electrodes made specifically for iontophoresis.[16,21]

The more traditional electrodes are made of tin, copper, lead, aluminum, or platinum backed by rubber and completely covered by a sponge, towel, or gauze that is in contact with the skin. The absorbent material is soaked with the ionized solution to be driven into the tissues. If the ions are contained in an ointment, it should be rubbed into the skin over the target zone and covered by some absorbent material soaked in water or saline before the electrode is applied.

The commercially produced electrodes are sold with most iontophoresis systems. These electrodes have a small chamber, in which the ionized solution is housed, that is covered by some type of semipermeable membrane. The electrode self-adheres to the skin (Figure 6–4). This type of electrode has eliminated the "mess and hassles" that have been associated with electrode preparation for iontophoresis in the past. Some electrodes are available with the ionized solutions already inside. Other electrodes still need to have the medication injected into an electrode cavity (Figure 6–5).

Regardless of the type of electrode used, to ensure maximum contact of the electrodes the skin should be shaved and cleaned prior to attachment of the electrodes. Care should be taken not to excessively abrade the skin during cleaning because damaged skin has a lower resistance to the current so that a burn may more easily occur. Also, caution should be used when treating areas that for one reason or another have reduced sensation.

Once this electrode has been prepared, it then becomes the active electrode, and the lead wire to the generator is attached such that the polarity of the wire is the same as the polarity of the ion in solution. A second electrode, the dispersive electrode, is prepared with water, gel, or some other conductive material as recommended by the manufacturer. Both electrodes must be securely attached to the skin such that uniform skin contact and pressure is maintained under both electrodes to minimize the risk of burns. Electrodes via the lead wires should not be connected to the generator unless both the generator and the amplitude or intensity control are turned off. At the end of the treatment, the intensity control

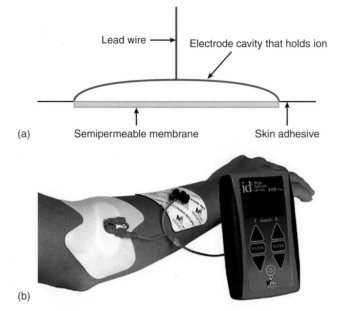

(a)

(b)

Figure 6–4. The commercially produced, self-adhering electrodes used with most iontophoresis systems have a small chamber that is covered by some type of semipermeable membrane that contains the ionized solution.

should be returned to zero and the generator turned off before the electrodes are detached from the patient.

The size and shape of the electrodes can cause a variation in current density and affect the size of the area treated.[22] Smaller electrodes have a higher current density and should be used to treat a specific lesion. Larger electrodes should be used when the target treatment area is not well defined.

Recommendations for spacing between the active and dispersive electrodes seem to be variable. They should be separated by at least the diameter of the active electrode. One source

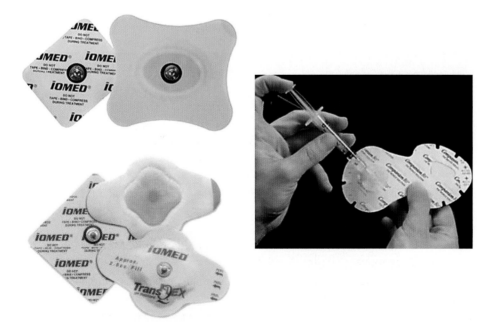

Figure 6–5. Electrodes used for iontophoresis.

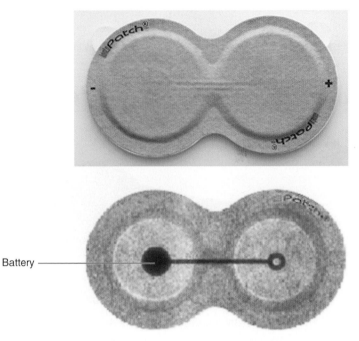

Battery

Figure 6–6. The Iontopatch has a self-contained battery that uses a low-level current to drive ions into the skin.

has recommended spacing them at least 18 in apart.[1] As spacing between the electrodes increases, the current density in the superficial tissues will decrease, perhaps minimizing the potential for burns.

The newest type of electrode utilizes an extended time-released electronic transdermal drug delivery system (Figure 6–6). A self-adhesive patch has a self-contained, built-in battery that produces a low-level electrical current to transport ions to underlying tissue. Drug delivery is shut off automatically when the prescribed dosage has been administered. The patch is single use and disposable.

Treatment Protocols for Iontophoresis are as Follows:

1. Prepare electrodes according to manufacturer's instructions; secure electrodes to patient. Electrode location will vary depending on the drug being phoresed; anionic drugs are repelled from the cathode; cations are repelled from the anode.
2. Remind the patient to inform you when he or she feels something. Do not tell the patient what he or she will feel; for example, do not say, "Tell me when you feel a burning or stinging."
3. Turn on the stimulator, and increase the amplitude slowly. Monitor the patient's response, not the stimulator.
4. After the patient reports the onset of the stimulus, adjust the amplitude to the appropriate intensity.
5. Continue to monitor the patient during the duration of the treatment.

CASE STUDY 6–1
IONTOPHORESIS (1)

Background: A 56-year-old man developed pain in the region inferior to the right patella subsequent to a fall onto the knee while playing tennis. There was immediate mild, localized swelling, which resolved with ice and rest. The acute pain subsided after about 7 days, but the patient then noted significant stiffness following rest, localized tenderness, and pain with climbing stairs, squatting, and kneeling. The physical examination was benign except for mild swelling and point tenderness of the infrapatellar tendon, as well as crepitus to palpation of the tendon during active knee extension.

Impression: Infrapatellar tendinitis.

Treatment Plan: In addition to rest and local ice application, a course of iontophoresis of dexamethasone was initiated. The area was prepared appropriately, and the cathode (negative polarity) was used as the delivery electrode. A total of 60 mA-min of current was delivered on an every-other-day schedule for a total of six treatments.

Response: There was a slight increase in the symptoms following the initial treatment, which persisted for approximately 12 hours following the second treatment. The signs and symptoms then began to diminish, and the patient was symptom-free following the fifth treatment. A progressive increase in physical activity was initiated, and the patient returned to pre-injury function 4 weeks later.

Discussion Questions

- What tissues were injured/affected?
- What symptoms were present?
- What phase of the injury-healing continuum did the patient present for care in?
- What are the physical agent modality's biophysical effects (direct/indirect/depth/tissue affinity)?
- What are the physical agent modality's indications/contraindications?
- What are the parameters of the physical agent modality's application/dosage/duration/frequency in this case study?
- What other physical agent modalities could be utilized to treat this injury or condition? Why? How? What is the pathophysiology of tendinitis?
- What is the mechanism of action of the dexamethasone?
- What is the polarity of the dexamethasone molecule?
- What are the required and ideal characteristics for a molecule to be introduced via iontophoresis?
- What are the advantages and disadvantages of iontophoresis as compared with a needle injection?
- Why did the symptoms increase initially?

The rehabilitation professional employs physical agent modalities to create an optimum environment for tissue healing while minimizing the symptoms associated with the trauma or condition.

CASE STUDY 6–2
IONTOPHORESIS (2)

Background: A 28-year-old woman has a 3-week history of bilateral wrist pain and nocturnal paresthesia in the palmar aspect of the thumb, index, and long fingers. The symptoms started 2 weeks after starting a new job working on the trim line of an automobile manufacturing plant. The job involves repetitive motions with both hands, and a great deal of squeezing to seat weatherstripping in the doors. The paresthesia is provoked with driving, and holding objects, such as a telephone, blow dryer, or newspaper. She attempts to relieve the paresthesia by shaking the hand (flick sign). She has pain with passive wrist and finger extension and resisted finger flexion, and paresthesia is produced with compression over the carpal tunnel for 15 seconds.

She has a positive Tinel sign over the median nerve at the distal wrist crease, and a positive Phalen test at 30 seconds. Crepitus is noted on the anterior wrist with finger flexion.

Impression: Tenosynovitis of the flexor digitorum tendons, with acute carpal tunnel syndrome.

Treatment Plan: The patient was instructed to use resting hand splints at night, and a course of iontophoresis was initiated for the right wrist only. In addition, work restrictions were placed on the patient, to avoid repetitive motion and gripping activities. Dexamethasone was delivered from the cathode (negative polarity), which was placed over the carpal tunnel, with the anode placed over the dorsum of the wrist. A

(continued)

CASE STUDY 6–2 *(continued)*
IONTOPHORESIS (2)

---

total of 45 mA-min of current was delivered 3 days per week for 2 weeks.

Response: The patient's symptoms diminished in both hands over the 2-week period; however, she continued to have a positive carpal compression test, a positive Phalen test, and a positive Tinel sign only on the left. She returned to the trim line with instructions for a 2-week ramp-up period; however, the pain and paresthesia returned in the left wrist. She subsequently underwent a surgical decompression of the left carpal tunnel, and was able to return to work without restrictions following 6 weeks off work and a second 2-week ramp-up period.

Discussion Questions

- What tissues were injured or affected?
- What symptoms were present?
- What phase of the injury-healing continuum did the patient present for care in?
- What are the physical agent modality's biophysical effects (direct, indirect, depth, and tissue affinity)?
- What are the physical agent modality's indications and contraindications?

- What are the parameters of the physical agent modality's application, dosage, duration, and frequency in this case study?
- What other physical agent modalities could be used to treat this injury or condition? Why? How?
- What is the significance of the Tinel sign?
- What is the significance of the Phalen test?
- Why does compression over the carpal tunnel reproduce the symptoms?
- Why does the patient experience nocturnal paresthesia rather than during work?
- What is another potential source of the patient's symptoms?
- If the patient also had cervical pain, would you anticipate a different treatment approach?
- Would electrophysiologic testing be appropriate for this patient? What findings would you anticipate?

The rehabilitation professional employs physical agent modalities to create an optimum environment for tissue healing while minimizing the symptoms associated with the trauma or condition.

Selecting the Appropriate Ion

It is critical that the clinician be knowledgeable in the selection of the most appropriate ions for treating specific conditions (Table 6–1). For a compound to penetrate a membrane such as the skin, it must be soluble in both fat and water. It must be water soluble if it is to remain in an ionized state in solution. However, human skin is relatively impervious to water ions, which are soluble only in water and do not diffuse in the tissues.[24] They must be fat soluble to permeate the tissues of the body.[21] Penetration is relatively superficial and is generally less than 1 mm.[18] The majority of the ions deposited in the tissues are found primarily at the site of the active electrode, where they are stored as either a soluble or insoluble compound. They may be used locally as a concentrated source or transported by the circulating blood, producing more systemic effects.[6]

The tendency of some ions to form insoluble precipitates as they pass into the tissues inhibits their ability to penetrate. This is particularly true with heavy metal ions, including iron, copper, silver, and zinc.[25]

When discussing medical galvanism that uses a continuous low-volt monophasic current (Chapter 5), it was stated that an accumulation of negative ions under the positive pole produces an acidic reaction through the formation of hydrochloric acid. This is sclerotic and produces hardening of the tissues by increasing protein density. In addition, some negative ions can also produce an analgesic effect (salicylates). An accumulation of positive ions under the negative pole produces an alkaline reaction with the formation of sodium hydroxide. Positive ions are sclerolytic; thus, they produce softening of the tissues by decreasing protein density. This is useful in treating scars or adhesions.

In iontophoresis, when using a drug or ion solution, the flow of a monophasic current through the sodium chloride or sodium salicylate solution causes a dissociation in which the positively charged sodium ions migrate toward the negative electrode and the negatively charged chlorine or salicylate ions migrate toward the positive electrode. The presence of these ions causes

Table 6–1   Recommended Ions for Use by Clinicians[23]

POSITIVE

Antibiotics, gentamycin sulfate (+), 8 mg/mL, for suppurative ear chondritis

Calcium (+), from calcium chloride, 2% aqueous solution, believed to stabilize the irritability threshold in either direction, as dictated by the physiologic needs of the tissues. Effective with spasmodic conditions, tics, and "snapping fingers" (joints)

Copper (+), from a 2% aqueous solution of copper sulfate crystals; fungicide, astringent, useful with intranasal conditions, for example, allergic rhinitis or "hay fever," sinusitis, and also dermatophytosis or "athlete's foot"

Hyaluronidase (+), from Wydase crystals in aqueous solution as directed; for localized edema

Lidocaine (+), from Xylocaine 5% ointment; anesthetic/analgesic, especially with acute inflammatory conditions (e.g., bursitis, tendinitis, tic doloreux, and TMJ pain)

Lithium (+), from lithium chloride or carbonate, 2% aqueous solution; effective as an exchange ion with gouty tophi and hyperuricemia

Magnesium (+), from magnesium sulfate ("Epsom Salts"), 2% aqueous solution; an excellent muscle relaxant, good vasodilator, and mild analgesic

Mecholyl (+), familiar derivative of acetylcholine, 0.25% ointment; a powerful vasodilator, good muscle relaxant, and analgesic. Used with discogenic low back radiculopathies and sympathetic reflex dystrophy

Priscoline (+), from benzazoline hydrochloride, 2% aqueous solution; reported effective with indolent ulcers

Zinc (+), from zinc oxide ointment, 20%; a trace element necessary for healing, especially effective with open lesions and ulcerations

NEGATIVE

Acetate (−), from acetic acid, 2% aqueous solution; dramatically effective as a sclerolytic exchange ion with calcific deposits

Chlorine (−), from sodium chloride, 2% aqueous solution; good sclerolytic agent. Useful with scar tissue, keloids, and burns

Citrate (−), from potassium citrate, 2% aqueous solution; reported effective in rheumatoid arthritis

Dexamethasone (−), from Decadron; used for treating musculoskeletal inflammatory conditions

Iodine (−), from Iodex ointment, 4.7%; an excellent sclerolytic agent, as well as bacteriocidal, and a fair vasodilator. Used successfully with adhesive capsulitis ("frozen shoulder"), scars, etc.

Salicylate (−), from Iodex with methyl salicylate, 4.8% ointment; a general decongestant, sclerolytic, and anti-inflammatory agent. If desired without the iodine, may be obtained from Myoflex ointment (trolamine salicylate 10%) or a 2% aqueous solution of sodium salicylate powder. Used successfully with frozen shoulder, scar tissue, warts, and other adhesive or edematous conditions

EITHER

Ringer's solution (+/−), with alternating polarity for open decubitus lesions

Tap water (+/−), usually administered with alternating polarity and sometimes with glycopyrronium bromide in hyperhidrosis

a secondary chemical reaction at these electrodes. They form sodium hydroxide at the negative electrode and hydrochloric acid at the positive electrode, which may be described as a polar effect because it occurs only under the electrodes. The physiologic effects include hardening of tissues under the positive electrode and softening of tissues under the negative electrode.

Table 6–1, modified from a list compiled by Kahn, lists the ions most commonly used with iontophoresis.[26]

Clinical Applications for Iontophoresis

A relatively long list of conditions for which iontophoresis is an appropriate treatment technique has been cited in the literature.[27,99] Clinically, iontophoresis is most often used in the treatment of inflammatory musculoskeletal conditions.[3] It may also be used for analgesic effects, scar modification, wound healing, and in treating edema, calcium deposits, and hyperhidrosis.[96] Many of these published studies are case reports that attempt to establish the clinical efficacy of iontophoresis in treating various conditions.[28,29,98] Table 6–2 provides a list of studies that have treated various conditions using iontophoresis.

Clinical Decision-Making *Exercise 6–2*

A field hockey player is getting her first iontophoresis treatment for patellar tendonitis. Dexamethasone has been prescribed in a dose of 40 mA-min. What can the clinician do to minimize the chances of an adverse sensitivity to this medication during this first-time treatment?

Clinical Decision-Making *Exercise 6–3*

The clinician gets a prescription from the team physician for using dexamethasone, an anti-inflammatory, to treat Achilles tendinitis. What considerations and treatment parameters are important for preparing the patient for this iontophoresis treatment?

Table 6–2 Conditions Treated with Iontophoresis

CONDITION	IONS USED IN TREATMENT
Inflammation	
Bertolucci (1982)[16]	Hydrocortisone, salicylate
Kahn (1981)[26]	Dexamethasone
Chantraine et al (1986)[30]	
Harris (1982)[18]	
Hasson (1991)[31]	
Hasson et al (1992)[32]	
Delacerda (1982)[17]	
Glass et al (1980)[33]	
Zawislak et al. (1966)[34]	
McEntaffer et al (1996)[35]	
Gurney et al (2005)[36]	
Hamann (2006)[37]	
Banta (1995)[38]	
Petelenz et al (1992)[39]	
Panus et al (1999)[40]	Ketoprofen

CONDITION	IONS USED IN TREATMENT
Analgesia	
Evans et al (2001)[41]	
Schaeffer et al (1971)[42]	Lidocaine, magnesium
Russo et al (1980)[43]	
Gangarosa (1993)[44]	
Gangarosa (1974)[91]	
Abell and Morgan (1974)[45]	
Shrivastava and Sing (1977)[46]	
Grice et al (1972)[47]	
Hill (1976)[48]	
Stolman (1987)[49]	
Fungi	
Kahn (1991)[50]	Copper
Haggard et al (1939)[7]	
Open skin lesions	
Cornwall (1981)[51]	Zinc
Jenkinson et al (1974)[23]	
Balogun et al (1990)[52]	
Herpes	
Gangarosa et al. (1989)[90]	
Allergic rhinitis	
Kahn (1991)[50]	Copper
Garzione (1978)[22]	
Pellecchia et al (1994)[53]	
Reid et al (1993)[54]	
Schultz (2002)[55]	
Yarrobino et al (2006)[56]	
Pasero et al (2006)[57]	
Spasm	
Kahn (1975)[58]	Calcium, magnesium
Kahn (1985)[59]	
Ischemia	
Kahn (1991)[50]	Magnesium, mecholyl, iodine
Edema	
Kahn (1991)[50]	Magnesium, mecholyl
Boone (1969)[60]	Hyaluronidase, salicylate
Magistro (1964)[61]	
Schwartz (1955)[62]	

(continued)

Table 6–2 *(continued)*

CONDITION	IONS USED IN TREATMENT
Calcium deposits	
Ciccone (2003)[63]	
Weider (1992)[64]	Acetic acid
Kahn (1982)[65]	
Kahn (1996)[94]	
Psaki and Carol (1955)[66]	
Kahn (1996) (1977)[67]	
Perron and Malouin (1997)[68]	
Tygiel (2003)[69]	
Gard (2004)[70]	
Bringman et al (2003)[71]	
Leduc et al (2003)[72]	
Scar tissue	
Tannenbaum (1980)[73]	Chlorine, iodine, salicylate
Kahn (1985)[59]	
Hyperhidrosis	
Kahn (1973)[6]	Tap water
Levit (1968)[74]	
Gillick et al (2004)[75]	
Gout	
Kahn (1982)[65]	Lithium
Burns	
Rapperport (1965)[76]	Antibiotics
Rigano et al (1992)[77]	
Driscoll et al (1999)[78]	
Reflex sympathetic dystrophy	
Bonezzi et al (1994)[79]	Guanethidine
Lateral epicondylitis	
Demirtas and Oner (1998)[80]	Sodium Salicylate
	Sodium diclofenac
Baskurt (2003)[81]	Naproxen
Plantar fasciitis	
Gudeman et al (1997)[82]	Dexamethasone
Gulick (2000)[83]	Acetic acid
Osborne and Allison (2006)[84]	

CONDITION	IONS USED IN TREATMENT
Patellar tendinitis	
Huggard et al (1999)[85]	Dexamethasone
Rotator cuff	
Preckshot (1999)[86]	Dexamethasone
	Lidocaine
Plantar warts	
Soroko et al (2002)[87]	Sodium salicylate
Epicondylitis	
Nirschl (2003)[88]	Dexamethasone

TREATMENT PRECAUTIONS AND CONTRAINDICATIONS

Problems that might potentially arise from treating a patient using iontophoresis techniques may be avoided for the most part if the clinician (1) has a good understanding of the existing condition to be treated; (2) uses the most appropriate ions to accomplish the treatment goal; and (3) uses appropriate treatment parameters and equipment setup. Poor treatment technique on the part of the clinician is most often responsible for adverse reactions to iontophoresis.[89] A list of indications and contraindications appears in Table 6–3.

Treatment of Burns

Perhaps the single most common problem associated with iontophoresis is a chemical burn, which usually occurs as a result of the direct current itself and not as a result of the ion being used in treatment.[19] Passing a continuous direct electrical current through the tissues creates migration of ions, which alters the normal pH of the skin. The normal pH of the skin is between 3 and 4. In an ***acidic reaction*** the pH falls below 3, whereas in an ***alkaline reaction*** the pH is greater than 5. Although chemical burns may occur under either electrode, they most typically result from the accumulation of sodium hydroxide at the cathode. The alkaline reaction causes sclerolysis of local tissues. Initially, the burn lesion is pink and raised but within hours becomes a grayish, oozing wound.[6] Decreasing current density by increasing the size of the cathode relative to the anode can minimize the potential for chemical burn.

Heat burns may occur as a result of high resistance to current flow created by poor contact of the electrodes with the skin. Poor contact results when the electrodes are not moist enough, there are wrinkles in the gauze or paper towels impregnated with the ionic solution, or there is space between the skin and electrode around the perimeter of the electrode. The patient should not be treated with body weight resting on top of the electrode since this is likely to create some ischemia (reduced circulation) under the electrode. Instead, the electrode should be held firmly in place with adhesive tape, elastic bands, or lightweight sand bags. It is recommended that both chemical burns and heat burns should be treated with sterile dressings and antibiotics.[6]

Clinical Decision-Making *Exercise 6-4*

After having an iontophoresis treatment, a patient comes into the clinic the next day with an area of skin that is red and tender. It is apparent that the treatment has produced a mild burn. What can the clinician do to minimize the likelihood of a reoccurrence?

Table 6–3 Indications and Contraindications for Iontophoresis

INDICATIONS

Inflammation

Analgesia

Muscle spasm

Ischemia

Edema

Calcium deposits

Scar tissue

Hyperhidrosis

Fungi

Open skin lesions

Herpes

Allergic rhinitis

Gout

Burns

Reflex sympathetic dystrophy

CONTRAINDICATIONS

Skin sensitivity reactions

Sensitivity to aspirin (salicylates)

Gastritis or active stomach ulcer (hydrocortisone)

Asthma (mecholyl)

Sensitivity to metals (zinc, copper, magnesium)

Sensitivity to seafood (iodine)

Sensitivity Reactions to Ions

Sensitivity reactions to ions rarely occur; however, they may potentially be very serious. The clinician should routinely question the patient about known drug allergies prior to initiating iontophoresis treatment. During the treatment the clinician should closely monitor the patient, looking for either abnormal localized reactions of the skin or systemic reactions.

Patients who have sensitivity to aspirin may have a reaction when using salicylates. Hydrocortisone may adversely affect individuals with gastritis or an active stomach ulcer. In cases of asthma, mecholyl should be avoided. Patients who are sensitive to metals should not be treated with copper, zinc, or magnesium. Iodine iontophoresis should not be used with individuals who have allergies to seafood or those who have had a bad reaction to intravenous pyelograms.[6]

SUMMARY

1. Iontophoresis is a therapeutic technique that involves the introduction of ions into the body tissues by means of a direct electrical current.

2. The manner in which ions move in solution forms the basis for iontophoresis. Positively charged ions are driven into the tissues from the positive pole, and negatively charged ions are introduced by the negative pole.

3. The force that acts to move ions through the tissues is determined by both the strength of the electrical field and the electrical impedance of tissues to current flow.

4. The quantity of ions transferred into the tissues through iontophoresis is determined by the intensity of the current or current density at the active electrode, the duration of the current flow, and the concentration of ions in solution.

5. Continuous direct current must be used for iontophoresis, thus ensuring the unidirectional flow of ions that cannot be accomplished using a bidirectional or alternating current.

6. Electrodes may be either reusable or commercially produced, self-adhering prepared electrodes that must be securely attached to the skin.

7. It is critical that the clinician be knowledgeable in the selection of the most appropriate ions for treating specific conditions.

8. Clinically, iontophoresis is used in the treatment of inflammatory musculoskeletal conditions, for analgesic effects, scar modification, and wound healing, and in treating edema, calcium deposits, and hyperhidrosis.

9. Perhaps the single most common problem associated with iontophoresis is a chemical burn, which usually occurs as a result of the direct current itself and not because of the ion being used in treatment.

REVIEW QUESTIONS

1. What is iontophoresis and how may it be used?
2. What is the difference between iontophoresis and phonophoresis?
3. How do ions move in solution?
4. What determines the quantity of ions transferred through the tissues during iontophoresis?
5. Why must continuous direct current be used for iontophoresis?
6. What types of electrodes can be used with iontophoresis and how should they be applied?
7. What characteristics should be considered when selecting the appropriate ion for an iontophoresis treatment?
8. What are the various clinical uses for iontophoresis in athletic training?
9. What treatment precautions must be taken when using iontophoresis?

SELF-TEST QUESTIONS

True or False
1. Ionization is the movement of ions in solution.
2. The dispersive electrode contains the ions.
3. pH reactions of greater than 5 are alkaline.

Multiple Choice
4. Which type of current does iontophoresis produce?
   a. biphasic
   b. continuous monophasic
   c. polyphasic
   d. pulsatile
5. What is the recommended range for iontophoresis current amplitude?
   a. 3–5 mA
   b. 5–10 mA
   c. 50–100 mA
   d. 100–150 mA

6. Chemical burn is often associated with iontophoresis and may be attributed to
   a. allergic reaction
   b. poor electrode contact
   c. the medication
   d. continuous direct current
7. Which of the following is *not* an ion used to treat inflammation?
   a. hydrocortisone
   b. salicylate
   c. lidocaine
   d. dexamethasone
8. Skin impedance usually decreases during treatment. _____ should be decreased to avoid pain and burning.
   a. current intensity
   b. electrode size
   c. treatment time
   d. ion dosage
9. What problem do areas of thick fat and skin present?
   a. decreased ion absorption
   b. increased ion absorption
   c. decreased resistance
   d. increased resistance
10. Which of the following is a contraindication for iontophoresis?
   a. inflammation
   b. analgesia
   c. asthma
   d. muscle spasm

SOLUTIONS TO CLINICAL DECISION-MAKING EXERCISES

6-1

If the hydrocortisone comes in an eucerin-based cream preparation or in solution, the clinician should use phonophoresis with the cream preparation to deliver whole molecules. Iontophoresis is more appropriate when ions are suspended in solution and can be carried into the tissues by an electrical current.

6-2

The safest choice is to reduce the intensity of the treatment while increasing the duration. For example, a normal dosage may be delivered at 4 mA for 10 minutes. A setting of 2 mA with a treatment time of 20 minutes would deliver the same dosage at a safer intensity.

6-3

The dexamethasone should be placed under the negative electrode since it is a negatively charged ion. Current intensity should be set between 3 and 5 IDA. Treatment time should be 15 minutes. The clinician should check the skin every 3–5 minutes for a reaction.

6-4

By increasing the size of the cathode relative to the anode, the current density can be decreased. Also, increasing the spacing between the electrodes will decrease current intensity, thus minimizing the chances of a chemical burn.

REFERENCES

1. Costello C, Jeske A. Iontophoresis: applications in transdermal medication delivery. *Phys Ther*. 1995;75(6):554–563.
2. LeDuc S. *Electric Ions and Their Use in Medicine*. Liverpool: Rebman; 1903.
3. Federici P. Injury management update. Treating iliotibial band friction syndrome using iontophoresis. *Athletic Ther Today*. 1997;2(5):22–23.
4. Singh P, Mailbach H. Transdermal iontophoresis: pharmacokinetic considerations. *Clin Pharmacokinet*. 1994;26:327–334.
5. Cummings J. Iontophoresis. In: Nelson RM, Currier DP, eds. *Clinical Electrotherapy*. Norwalk, CT: Appleton & Lange; 1991.
6. Kahn J. Tap-water iontophoresis for hyperhidrosis. Reprinted in *Medical Group News*; August 1973.
7. Haggard H, Strauss M, Greenberg L. Fungus infections of hand and feet treated by copper iontophoresis. *JAMA*. 1939;112:1229.
8. Murray W, Levine L, Seifter E. The iontophoresis of C2 esterified glucocorticoids: preliminary report. *Phys Ther*. 1963;43:579.
9. O'Malley E, Oester Y. Influence of some physical chemical factors on iontophoresis using radioisotopes. *Arch Phys Med Rehabil*. 1955;36:310.
10. Howard J, Drake T, Kellogg D. Effects of alternating current iontophoresis on drug delivery. *Arch Phys Med Rehabil*. 1995;76(5):463–466.
11. Bagniefski T, Burnette R. A comparison of pulsed and continuous current iontophoresis. *J Control Release*. 1990;11:113–122.
12. Sabbahi M, Costello C, Emran A. A method for reducing skin irritation from iontophoresis. *Phys Ther*. 1994;74:S156.
13. Su M, Srinivasan V, Ghanem A. Quantitative in vivo iontophoretic studies. *J Pharm Sci*. 1994;83:12–17.
14. Jacobson S, Stephen R, Sears W. *Development of a New Drug Delivery System (Iontophoresis)*. Salt Lake City, UT: University of Utah; 1980.
15. Mandleco C. *Research: Iontophoresis*. Salt Lake City, UT: Institute for Biomedical Engineering, University of Utah; 1978.
16. Bertolucci L. Introduction of anti-inflammatory drugs by iontophoreses: a double-blind study. *J Orthop Sports Phys Ther*. 1982;4(2):103.
17. Delacerda F. A comparative study of three methods of treatment for shoulder girdle myofascial syndrome. *J Orthop Sports Phys Ther*. 1982;4(1):51–54.
18. Harris P. Iontophoresis: clinical research in musculoskeletal inflammatory conditions. *J Orthop Sports Phys Ther*. 1982;4(2):109–112.
19. Molitor H. Pharmacologic aspects of drug administration by ion transfer. *The Merck Report*: 22–29; January 1943.
20. Anderson CR, Morris RI, Boeh SD, et al. Effects of iontophoresis current magnitude and duration on dexamethasone deposition and localized drug retention. *Phys Ther*. 2003;83(2):161–170.
21. Harris R. Iontophoresis. In: Stillwell K, ed. *Therapeutic Electricity and Ultraviolet Radiation*. Baltimore, MD: Williams & Wilkins; 1983.
22. Garzione J. Salicylate iontophoresis as an alternative treatment for persistent thigh pain following hip surgery. *Phys Ther*. 1978;58(5):570–571.
23. Jenkinson D, McEwan J, Walton G. The potential use of iontophoresis in the treatment of skin disorders. *Arch Phys Med Rehabil*. 1974;94(1):8–12.
24. Boone D. Applications of iontophoresis. In: Wolf S, ed. *Electrotherapy*. New York: Churchill Livingstone; 1981.
25. Gadsby P. Visualization of the barrier layer through iontophoresis of ferric ions. *Med Instrum*. 1979;13:281.
26. Kahn J. Iontophoresis with hydrocortisone for Peyronie's disease. *JAPTA*. 1981;62(7):995.
27. Banga AK, Panus. PC. Clinical applications of iontophoretic devices in rehabilitation medicine. *Crit Rev Phys Rehabil Med*. 1998;10(2):147–179.
28. Glick E, Snyder-Mackler L. Iontophoresis. In: Snyder-Mackler L, Robinson A, eds. *Clinical Electrophysiology and Electrophysiologic Testing*. Baltimore, MD: Lippincott Williams & Wilkins; 2007.
29. Smutok MA, Mayo MF, Gabaree CL, Ferslew KE, Panus PC. Failure to detect dexamethasone phosphate in the local venous blood postcathodic iontophoresis in humans. *J Orthop Sports Phys Ther*. 2002;32(9):461–468.
30. Chantraine A, Lundy J, Berger D. Is cortisone iontophoresis possible? *Arch Phys Med Rehabil*. 1986;67:380.
31. Hasson S. Exercise training and dexamethasone iontophoresis in rheumatoid arthritis: a case study. *Physiotherapy Canada*. 1991;43:11.
32. Hasson S, Wible C, Reich M. Dexamethasone iontophoresis: effect on delayed muscle soreness and muscle function. *Can J Sport Sci*. 1992;17:8–13.
33. Glass J, Stephen R, Jacobsen S. The quantity and distribution of radiolabeled dexamethasone delivered to tissues by iontophoresis. *Int J Dermatol*. 1980;19:519.
34. Zawislak D, Rau C, Lee M. The effects of dexamethasone iontophoresis on acute inflammation using a sports model of treatment. *Phys Ther*. 1966;76(5):5–17.
35. McEntaffer D, Sailor M. The effects of stretching and iontophoretically delivered dexamethasone on plantar fasciitis. *Phys Ther*. 1996;76(5):S68.
36. Gurney B, Wischer D, Chineleison S. The absorption of dexamethasone sodium phosphate into connective tissue of humans using iontophoresis [abstract]. *J Orthop Sports Phys Ther*. 2005;35(1):24.
37. Hamann H. Effectiveness of iontophoresis of anti-inflammatory medications in the treatment of common musculoskeletal inflammatory conditions: a systematic review. *Phys Ther Rev*. 2006;11(3):190–194.

38. Banta C. A prospective nonrandomized study of iontophoresis, wrist splinting, and antiinflammatory medication in the treatment of early mild carpal tunnel syndrome. *J Orthop Sports Phys Ther*. 1995;21(2):120.

39. Petelenz T, Buttke J, Bonds C. Iontophoresis of dexamethasone: laboratory studies. *J Control Release*. 1992;20:55–66.

40. Panus PC, Ferslew KE, Tober-Meyer B, Kao RL. Ketoprofen tissue permeation in swine following cathodic iontophoresis. *Phys Ther*. 1999;79(1):40–49.

41. Evans T, Kunkle J, Zinz K. The immediate effects of lidocaine iontophoresis on trigger-point-pain. *J Sport Rehabil*. 2001;10(4):287.

42. Schaeffer M, Bixler D, Yu P. The effectiveness of iontophoresis in reducing cervical hypersensitivity. *J Peridontol*. 1971;42:695.

43. Russo J, Lipman A, Comstock T. Lidocane anesthesia: comparison of iontophoresis, injection and swabbing. *Am J Hosp Pharm*. 1980;37:843–847.

44. Gangarosa L. Iontophoresis in pain control. *Pain Digest*. 1993;3:162–174.

45. Abell E, Morgan K. Treatment of idiopathic hyperhidrosis by glycopyrronium bromide and tap water iontophoresis. *Br J Dermatol*. 1974;91:87.

46. Shrivastava S, Sing G. Tap water iontophoresis in palm and plantar hyperhidrosis. *Br J Dermatol*. 1977;96:189.

47. Grice K, Sattar H, Baker H. Treatment of idiopathic hyperhidrosis with iontophoresis of tap water and poldine methosulphate. *Br J Dermatol*. 1972;86:72.

48. Hill B. Poldine iontophoresis in the treatment of palmar and plantar hyperhidrosis. *Aust J Dermatol*. 1976;17:92.

49. Stolman L. Treatment of excess sweating of the palms by iontophoresis. *Arch Dermatol*. 1987;123:893.

50. Kahn J. *Practices and Principles of Electrotherapy*. New York: Churchill Livingstone; 1991.

51. Cornwall M. Zinc oxide iontophoresis for ischemic skin ulcers. *Phys Ther*. 1981;61(3):359.

52. Balogun J, Abidoye A, Akala E. Zinc iontophoresis in the management of bacterial colonized wounds: a case report. *Physiother Can*. 1990;42(3):147–151.

53. Pellecchia G, Hamel H, Behnke P. Treatment of infrapatellar tendinitis: a combination of modalities and transverse friction massage versus iontophoresis. *J Sport Rehabil*. 1994;3(2):135–145.

54. Reid K, Sicard-Rosenbaum L, Lord D. Iontophoresis with normal saline versus dexamethasone and lidocaine in the treatment of patients with internal disc derangement of the temporomandibular joint. *Phys Ther*. 1993;73(6):S20.

55. Schultz AA. Safety, tolerability, and efficacy of iontophoresis with lidocaine for dermal anesthesia in ED pediatric patients. *J Emerg Nurs*. 2002;28(4):289–296.

56. Yarrobino T, Kalbfleisch J, Ferslew K. Lidocaine iontophoresis mediates analgesia in lateral epicondylalgia treatment. *Physiother Res Int*. 2006;11(3):152.

57. Pasero C. Pain care. Lidocaine iontophoresis for dermal procedure analgesia. *J Perianesth Nurs*. 2006;21(1):48–52.

58. Kahn J. Calcium iontophoresis in suspected myopathy. *JAPTA*. 1975;55(4):276.

59. Kahn J. *Clinical Electrotherapy*. 4th ed. Syosset, NY: J. Kahn; 1985.

60. Boone D. Hyaluronidase iontophoresis. *J Am Phys Ther Assoc*. 1969;49:139–145.

61. Magistro C. Hyaluronidase by iontophoresis in the treatment of edema: a preliminary clinical report. *Phys Ther*. 1964; 44:169.

62. Schwartz M. The use of hyaluronidase by iontophoresis in the treatment of lymphedema. *Arch Intern Med*. 1955; 95:662.

63. Ciccone CD. Evidence in practice ... Does acetic acid iontophoresis accelerate the resorption of calcium deposits in calcific tendinitis of the shoulder? *Phys Ther*. 2003;83(1):68–74.

64. Weider D. Treatment of traumatic myositis ossificans with acetic acid iontophoresis. *Phys Ther*. 1992;72(2):133–137.

65. Kahn J. A case report: lithium iontophoresis for gouty arthritis. *J Orthop Sports Phys Ther*. 1982;4:113.

66. Psaki C, Carol J. Acetic acid ionization: a study to determine the absorptive effects upon calcified tendinitis of the shoulder. *Phys Ther Rev*. 1955;35:84.

67. Kahn J. Acetic acid iontophoresis for calcium deposits. *JAPTA*. 1977;57(6):658.

68. Perron M, Malouin F. Acetic acid iontophoresis and ultrasound for the treatment of calcifying tendinitis of the shoulder: a randomized control trial. *Arch Phys Med Rehabil*. 1997;78(4):379–384.

69. Tygiel PP. On "Does acetic acid iontophoresis accelerate the resorption of calcium deposits in calcific tendinitis of the shoulder?" *Phys Ther*. 2003;83(7):667–670.

70. Gard K. Treatment of traumatic myositis ossificans in a hockey player using acetic acid iontophoresis [abstract]. *J Orthop Sports Phys Ther*. 2004;34(1):A18.

71. Bringman D, Carver J, Thompson A. The effects of acetic acid iontophoresis on a heel spur: a single-subject design study [poster session]. *J Orthop Sports Phys Ther*. 2003;33(2):A-27.

72. Leduc B, Caya J, Tremblay S. Treatment of calcifying tendinitis of the shoulder by acetic acid iontophoresis: a double-blind randomized controlled trial. *Arch Phys Med Rehabil*. 2003;84(10):1523–1527.

73. Tannenbaum M. Iodine iontophoresis in reduction of scar tissue. *Phys Ther*. 1980;60(6):792.

74. Levit R. Simple device for treatment of hyperhidrosis by iontophoresis. *Arch Dermatol*. 1968;98:505–507.

75. Gillick B, Kloth L, Starsky A. Management of postsurgical hyperhidrosis with direct current and tap water. *Phys Ther*. 2004;84(3):262.

76. Rapperport A. Iontophoresis—a method of antibiotic administration in the burn patient. *Plast Reconstr Surg*. 1965;36(5):547–552.

77. Rigano W, Yanik M, Barone F. Antibiotic iontophoresis in the management of burned ears. *J Burn Care Rehabil*. 1992; 13(4):407–409.

78. Driscoll JB, Plunkett K, Tamari A. The effect of potassium iodide iontophoresis on range of motion and scar maturation following burn injury. *Phys Ther Case Rep.* 1999;2(1):13–18.

79. Bonezzi C, Miotti D, Bettagilo R. Electromotive administration of guanethidine for treatment of reflex sympathetic dystrophy. *J Pain Symptom Manage.* 1994;9(1):39–43.

80. Demirtas RN, Oner C. The treatment of lateral epicondylitis by iontophoresis of sodium salicylate and sodium diclofenac. *Clin Rehabil.* 1998;12(1):23–29.

81. Baskurt F. Comparison of effects of phonophoresis and iontophoresis of naproxen in the treatment of lateral epicondylitis. *Clin Rehabil.* 2003;17(1):96–100.

82. Gudeman SD, Eisele SA, Heidt RS Jr, et al. Treatment of plantar fasciitis by iontophoresis of 0.4% dexamethasone: a randomized, double-blind, placebo-controlled study. *Am J Sports Med.* 1997;25(3):312–316.

83. Gulick DT. Effects of acetic acid iontophoresis on heel spur reabsorption. *Phys Ther Case Rep.* 2000;3(2):64–70.

84. Osborne H, Allison G. Treatment of plantar fasciitis by LowDye taping and iontophoresis: short term results of a double blinded, randomised, placebo controlled clinical trial of dexamethasone and acetic acid. *Br J Sports Med.* 2006;40(6):545–549.

85. Huggard C, Kimura I, Mattacola C. Clinical efficacy of dexamethasone iontophoresis in the treatment of patellar tendinitis in college athletes: a double blind study. *J Athletic Train.* 1999;34(2):S-70.

86. Preckshot J. Iontophoresis with lidocaine and dexamethasone for treating rotator cuff injury in a hockey player. *Int J Pharm Compounding.* 1999;3(6):441.

87. Soroko YT, Repking MC, Clemment JA, et al. Treatment of plantar verrucae using 2% sodium salicylate iontophoresis. *Phys Ther.* 2002;82(12):1184–1191.

88. Nirschl RP. Iontophoretic administration of dexamethasone sodium phosphate for acute epicondylitis: a randomized, double-blind, placebo-controlled study. *Am J Sports Med.* 2003;31(2):189–195.

89. Warden G. Electrical safety in iontophoresis. *Rehab Manage Interdisciplinary J Rehabil.* 2007;20(2):20, 22–23.

90. Gangarosa L, Payne L, Hayakawa K. Iontophoretic treatment of herpetic whitlow. *Arch Phys Med Rehabil.* 1989;70(4):336–340.

91. Gangarosa L. Iontophoresis for surface local anesthesia. *J Am Dent Assoc.* 1974;88:125.

92. Guffey JS, Rutherford MJ, Payne W, Phillips C. Skin pH changes associated with iontophoresis. *J Orthop Sports Phys Ther.* 1999;29(11):656–660.

93. Johnson C, Shuster S. The patency of sweat ducts in normal looking skin. *Br J Dermatol.* 1970;83:367.

94. Kahn J. Acetic acid iontophoresis. *Phys Ther.* 1996;76(5):S68.

95. Kahn J. Iontophoresis: practice tips. *Clin Manage.* 1981;2(4):37.

96. Kahn J. Non-steroid iontophoresis. *Clin Manage Phys Ther.* 1987;7(1):14–15.

97. Roberts D. Transdermal drug delivery using iontophoresis and phonophoresis. *Orthop Nurs.* 1999;18(3):50–54.

98. Sakurai T. Iontophoretic administration of prostaglandin E1 in peripheral arterial occlusive disease. *Ann Pharmacother.* 2003;37(5):747.

99. Van Herp G. Iontophoresis: a review of the literature. *N Z J Physiother.* 1997;25(2):16–17.

SUGGESTED READINGS

Abramowitsch D, Neoussikine B. *Treatment by Ion Transfer.* New York: Grune & Stratton; 1946.

Abramson D. Physiologic and clinical basis for histamine by ion transfer. *Arch Phys Med Rehabil.* 1967;48:583–592.

Agostinucci J, Powers W. Motoneuron excitability modulation after desensitization of the skin by iontophoresis of lidocaine hydrochloride. *Arch Phys Med Rehabil.* 1992;73(2):190–194.

Akins D, Meisenheimer I, Dobson R. Efficacy of the Drionic unit in the treatment of hyperhidrosis *J Am Acad Dermatol.* 1987;16:828.

Barton C, Webster K. Evaluation of the scope and quality of systematic reviews on nonpharmacological conservative treatment for patellofemoral pain syndrome. *J Orthop Sports Phys Ther.* 2008;38(9):529.

Beam J. Topical silver for infected wounds. *J Athletic Train.* 2009;44(5):531.

Brumett A, Comeau M. Local anesthesia of the tympanic membrane by iontophoresis. *Trans Am Acad Otolaryngol.* 1974;78:453.

Chein Y, Banga A. Iontophoretic (transdermal) delivery of drugs: overview of historical development. *J Pharm Sci.* 1989;78:353–354.

Comeau M. Local anesthesia of the ear by iontophoresis. *Arch Otolaryngol.* 1973;98:114–120.

Comeau M. Anesthesia of the human tympanic membrane by iontophoresis of a local anesthetic. *Laryngoscope.* 1978;88:277–285.

Dellagatta E, Thompson E. Changes in skin resistance produced by continuous direct current stimulation utilizing methyl nicotinate. *Phys Ther.* 1994;74(5):S12.

Doyle A, Cheatham C. The effects of dexamethasone iontophoresis on an acute muscle injury of the biceps brachii. *J Athletic Train.* 2007;42(suppl):S133.

Falcone A, Spadaro J. Inhibitory effects of electrically activated silver material on cutaneous wound bacteria. *Plast Reconstr Surg.* 1986;77:455.

Fay M. Indications and applications for iontophoresis. *Today's OR Nurse.* 1989;11(4):10–16, 29–31.

Gangarosa L, Park N, Fong B. Conductivity of drugs used for iontophoresis. *J Pharm Sci*. 1978;67:1439–1443.

Glaviano N, Selkow N, Saliba E. No difference in skin anaesthesia with lidocaine delivered with high or standard doses of iontophoresis. *J Athletic Train*. 2009;44(suppl):S87.

Gordon A. Sodium salicylate iontophoresis in the treatment of plantar warts. *Phys Ther Rev*. 1969;49:869–870.

Haggard H, Strauss M, Greenberg L. Copper, electrically injected, cures fungus diseases. Reprinted in *Science Newsletter*; May 6, 1939.

Henley J. Transcutaneous drug delivery: iontophoresis, phonophoresis. *Phys Med Rehabil*. 1991;2:139.

Jarvis C, Voita D. Low voltage skin burns. *Pediatrics*. 1971; 48:831.

Kahn J. Iontophoresis and ultrasound for post-surgical TMJ trismus and paresthesia. *JAPTA*. 1982;60(3):307.

Kahn J. Iontophoresis in clinical practice. *Stimulus (APTA-SCE)*. 1983;8(3):58.

Kahn J. Phoresor adaptation. *Clin Manage Phys Ther*. 1985;5(4): 50–51.

Kahn J. *Iontophoresis* [video tape]. Pittsburgh: AREN; 1988.

LaForest N, Confrancisco C. Antibiotic iontophoresis in the treatment of ear chondritis. *JAPTA*. 1978;58:32.

Langley P. Iontophoresis to aid in releasing tendon adhesions. *Phys Ther*. 1984;64(9):1395.

Lemming M, Cole R, Howland W. Low voltage direct current burns. *JAMA*. 1970;214:1681.

Lininger M, Miller M, Michael T. An exploratory study of ketoprofen drug concentrations in swine tissue using ultrasound with pluronic lecithin isopropyl palmatate coupling medium. *J Athletic Train*. 2008;43 (suppl):S83.

McFadden E. Iontophoresis for pain management. *J Pediatr Nurs*. 1995;10(5):331.

Nightingale A. *Physics and Electronics in Physical Medicine*. London: F. Bell; 1959.

Nimmo W. Novel delivery systems: electrotransport. *J Pain Symptom Manage*. 1992;7(3):160–162.

Panus P, Campbell J, Kulkami S. Transdermal iontophoretic delivery of ketoprofen through human cadaver skin and in humans. *Phys Ther*. 1996;76(5):S67.

Phipps J, Padmanabhan R, Lattin G. Iontophoretic delivery of model inorganic and drug ions. *J Pharm Sci*. 1989;78:365–369.

Puttemans F, Massart D, Gilles F. Iontophoreses: mechanism of action studied by potentiometry and x-ray fluorescence. *Arch Phys Med Rehabil*. 1982;63:176–180.

Saliba S, Mistry D, Perrin D. Phonophoresis and the absorption of dexamethasone in the presence of an occlusive dressing. *J Athletic Train*. 2007;42(3):349.

Sawyer C. Cystic fibrosis of the pancreas: a study of sweat electrolyte levels in thirty-six families using pilocarpine iontophoresis. *Southern Medical Journal*. 1966;59:197–202.

Shapiro B. Insulin iontophoresis in cystic fibrosis. *Soc Exp Biol Med*. 1975;149:592–593.

Shriber W. *A Manual of Electrotherapy*. 4th ed. Philadelphia: Lea & Febiger; 1975.

Sisler H. Iontophoresis local anesthesia for conjunctival surgery. *Ann Ophthalmol*. 1978;10:597.

Stillwell G. Electrotherapy. In: Kottke F, Stillwell G, Lehman J, eds. *Handbook of Physical Medical and Rehabilitation*. Philadelphia: WB Saunders; 1982.

Teeter C, McKeon P, Saliba E. Effect of duration and amplitude of direct current while lidocaine is delivered by iontophoresis. *J Athletic Train*. 2008;43(suppl):S86.

Tregear R. The permeability of mammalian skin to ions. *J Invest Dermatol*. 1966;46:16–23.

Trubatch J, Van Harrevel A. Spread of iontophoretically injected ions in a tissue. *J Theor Biol*. 1972;36:355.

Waud D. Iontophoretic applications of drugs. *J Appl Physiol*. 1967;28:128.

Zankel H, Cress R, Kamin H. Iontophoreses studies with radioactive tracer. *Arch Phys Med Rehabil*. 1959;40:193–196.

GLOSSARY

acidic reaction The accumulation of negative ions under the positive pole that produces hydrochloric acid.

active electrode The electrode that is used to drive ions into the tissues.

alkaline reaction The accumulation of positive ions under the negative electrode that produces sodium hydroxide.

electrolytes Solutions in which ionic movement occurs.

electrophoresis The movement of ions in solution.

ionization A process by which soluble compounds such as acids, alkaloids, or salts dissociate or dissolve into ions that are suspended in some type of solution.

ions Positively or negatively charged particles.

iontophoresis A therapeutic technique that involves the introduction of ions into the body tissues by means of a direct electrical current.

therapeutic window Refers to the plasma concentrations of a drug, which should fall between a minimum concentration necessary for a therapeutic effect and the maximum effective concentration above which adverse effects may possibly occur.

LAB ACTIVITY

IONTOPHORESIS

DESCRIPTION

Iontophoresis is the use of direct current electricity to introduce various drugs to subcutaneous tissues without using invasive means. Although there are many drugs that may be used, various corticosteroids and local anesthetics are the most commonly used drugs.

It is not possible to use any form of electrical current other than direct current to achieve movement of the drug; the misnamed "high-voltage galvanic stimulators" are not capable of phoresing a drug owing to the very low pulse charge. Because of the possibility of producing an electrolytic burn with direct current, it is recommended that the current amplitude remain below 0.7 mA × number of cm² of electrode.

There are many different electrodes available for iontophoresis. The most rudimentary is to use alligator clips to attach the cables to a tin or aluminum conductor, and use a paper towel soaked with the drug between the electrode and the patient. More commonly, electrodes developed by the manufacturer of the stimulator are used.

It is mandatory that the drug be in an ionic form; otherwise, the electrical current will not be able to move the drug. Many drugs come both in ionized forms and as a suspension. If in doubt, a PDR should be consulted.

PHYSIOLOGIC EFFECTS

Depend on the drug

THERAPEUTIC EFFECTS

Depend on the drug; generally, decreased inflammation and local anesthesia

INDICATIONS

The primary indication is for the control of inflammation and/or pain.

CONTRAINDICATIONS

- Pregnancy
- Implanted electrical pacing devices (e.g., cardiac pacemaker, bladder stimulator)
- Cardiac arrhythmia
- Over the carotid sinus area
- Hypersensitivity (i.e., the patient who has a strong aversion to electricity, or the patient with certain types of catheters or shunts)
- Known problems with medication used in treatment

ELECTRICAL STIMULATION: IONTOPHORESIS

PROCEDURE	EVALUATION		
	1	2	3
1. Check supplies.			
a. Obtain towels or sheets for draping, and conductant.			
b. Check stimulator, electrodes, and cables for charged battery, broken or frayed insulation, and so on.			
c. Verify that the intensity control is at zero.			
2. Question patient.			
a. Verify identity of patient (if not already verified).			
b. Verify the absence of contraindications.			
c. Ask about previous exposure to electrotherapy.			
3. Position patient.			
a. Place patient in a well-supported, comfortable position.			
b. Expose body part to be treated.			

c. Drape patient to preserve patient's modesty, and protect clothing, but allow access to body part.			
4. Inspect body part to be treated.			
a. Check light touch perception.			
b. Assess function of body part (e.g., ROM, irritability).			
5. Apply electrical stimulation for iontophoresis.			
a. Prepare electrodes according to manufacturer's instructions; secure electrodes to patient. Electrode location will vary depending on the drug being phoresed; anionic drugs are repelled from the cathode, and cations are repelled from the anode.			
b. Remind the patient to inform you when he or she feels something. Do not tell the patient what he or she will feel; for example, do not say, "Tell me when you feel a burning or stinging."			
c. Turn on the stimulator, and increase the amplitude slowly. Monitor the patient's response, not the stimulator.			
d. After the patient reports the onset of the stimulus, adjust the amplitude to the appropriate intensity.			
e. Continue to monitor the patient during the duration of the treatment.			
6. Complete treatment.			
a. When the treatment time is over, turn the generator off, and turn the intensity control to zero; remove conductant with a towel.			
b. Remove material used for draping; assist the patient in dressing as needed.			
c. Have the patient perform appropriate therapeutic exercise as indicated.			
d. Clean the treatment area and equipment according to normal protocol.			
7. Assess treatment efficacy.			
a. Ask the patient how the treated area feels.			
b. Visually inspect the treated area for any adverse reactions.			
c. Perform functional tests as indicated.			

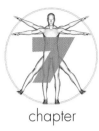

Biofeedback

chapter

William E. Prentice

OBJECTIVES

Following completion of this chapter, the student will be able to:

➤ Define biofeedback and identify its uses in a clinical setting.

➤ Contrast the various types of biofeedback instruments.

➤ Explain physiologically how the electrical activity generated by a muscle contraction can be measured using an electromyograph (EMG).

➤ Break down how the electrical activity picked up by the electrodes is amplified, processed, and converted to meaningful information by the biofeedback unit.

➤ Differentiate between visual and auditory feedback.

➤ Outline the equipment setup and clinical applications for biofeedback.

Electromyographic biofeedback is a modality that seems to be gaining increased popularity in clinical settings. It is a therapeutic procedure that uses electronic or electromechanical instruments to accurately measure, process, and feedback reinforcing information via auditory or visual signals.[1] In clinical practice, it is used to help the patient develop greater voluntary control in terms of either neuromuscular relaxation or muscle reeducation following injury.[32]

ELECTROMYOGRAPHY AND BIOFEEDBACK

Electromyography (EMG) is a clinical technique that involves recording of the electrical activity generated in a muscle for diagnostic purposes. It involves a sophisticated electrodiagnostic study performed in an EMG laboratory, which uses either surface or needle electrodes for measuring not only electrical activity in muscle but also various aspects of nerve conduction. An *electromyogram* is a graphic representation of those electrical currents associated with muscle action. EMG is widely used in the diagnosis of a variety of neuromuscular disorders. Certainly EMG would not be considered a therapeutic modality.[31]

The small portable biofeedback units that will be discussed in this chapter also measure electrical activity in the muscle and are in fact small electromyographs. The discussion in this chapter will be limited to the information on EMG necessary for the clinician to understand to be able to effectively incorporate biofeedback techniques into clinical practice.

Biofeedback instruments measure:
- peripheral skin temperature;
- finger phototransmission;
- skin conductance activity;
- electromyographic activity.

THE ROLE OF BIOFEEDBACK

The term *biofeedback* should be familiar because all clinicians routinely serve as instruments of biofeedback when teaching a therapeutic exercise or in coaching a movement pattern. Using feedback can help the patient to regain function of a muscle that may have been lost or forgotten following injury.[2] Feedback includes information related to the sensations associated with movement itself as well as information related to the result of the action relative to some goal or objective. Feedback refers to the intrinsic information inherent to movement, including kinesthetic, visual, cutaneous, vestibular, and auditory signals collectively termed as response-produced feedback. However, it also refers to extrinsic information or some knowledge of results that is presented verbally, mechanically, or electronically to indicate the outcome of some movement performance. Therefore, feedback is ongoing, in a temporal sense, occurring before, during, and after any motor or movement task. Feedback from some measuring instrument that provides moment-to-moment information about a biologic function is referred to as **biofeedback**.[3]

Perhaps the biggest advantage of biofeedback is that it provides the patient with a chance to make appropriate small changes in performance that are immediately noted and rewarded so that eventually larger changes or improvements in performance can be accomplished. The goal is to train the patient to perceive these changes without the use of the measuring instrument so that he or she can practice independently. Therefore, the patient learns early in the rehabilitation process to do something for himself or herself and not to totally rely on the clinician. This will help him or her to build confidence and increase feelings of self-efficacy. Treatments using biofeedback are useful, particularly in a patient who has difficulty in perceiving the initial small correct responses or who may have a faulty perception of what he or she is doing. Hopefully, the rehabilitating patient will be motivated and encouraged by seeing early signs of slight progress, thus relieving feelings of helplessness and reducing injury-related stress to some extent.[3]

To process feedback information, the patient makes use of a complicated series of interrelated feedback loops involving very complex anatomic and neurophysiologic components.[4] An in-depth discussion of these components is well beyond the scope of this text. Thus, our focus will be oriented toward how biofeedback may best be incorporated in a treatment program.

BIOFEEDBACK INSTRUMENTATION

Biofeedback instruments are designed to monitor some physiologic event, objectively quantify these monitorings, and then interpret the measurements as meaningful information.[5] Several different types of biofeedback modalities are available for use in rehabilitation. These biofeedback units cannot directly measure a physiologic event. Instead they record some aspect that is highly correlated with the physiologic event. Thus, the biofeedback reading should be taken as a convenient indication of a physiologic process but should not be confused with the physiologic process itself.[5]

The most commonly used instruments include those that record *peripheral skin temperatures*, indicating the extent of vasoconstriction or vasodilation; *finger phototransmission units (photoplethysmograph)*, which also measure vasoconstriction and vasodilation; units that record *skin conductance activity*, indicating sweat gland activity; and units that measure *electromyographic activity*, indicating amount of electrical activity during muscle contraction.

Other types of biofeedback units are also available, including electroencephalographs (EEGs), pressure transducers, and electrogoniometers.

Clinical Decision-Making   *Exercise 7–1*

The clinician is beginning rehabilitation day 1 postoperatively following ACL reconstruction. The patient is having a difficult time firing the VMO. Unfortunately, the one biofeedback unit in the clinic is broken. What can the clinician do to help the patient regain voluntary control of the VMO?

Peripheral Skin Temperature

Peripheral skin temperature is an indirect measure of the diameter of peripheral blood vessels. As vessels dilate, more warm blood is delivered to a particular area, thus increasing the temperature in that area. This effect is easily seen in the fingers and toes where the surrounding tissue warms and cools rapidly. Variations in skin temperature seem to be correlated with affective states, with a decrease occurring in response to stress or fear. Temperature changes are usually measured in degrees Fahrenheit.[5]

Finger Phototransmission

The degree of peripheral vasoconstriction can also be measured indirectly using a photoplethysmograph. This instrument monitors the amount of light that can pass through a finger or toe, reflect off a bone, and pass back through the soft tissue to a light sensor. As the volume of blood in a given area increases, the amount of light detected by the sensor decreases, thus giving some indication of blood volume. Only changes in blood volume can be detected because there are no standardized units of measure. These instruments are used most often to monitor pulse.[6]

Skin Conductance Activity

Sweat gland activity can be indirectly measured by determining electrodermal activity, most commonly referred to as the "galvanic skin response." Sweat contains salt that increases electrical conductivity. Thus, sweaty skin is more conductive than dry skin. This instrument applies a very small electrical voltage to the skin, usually on the palmar surface of the hand or the volar surface of the fingers where more sweat glands are located, and measures the impedance of the electrical current in micro-ohm units. Measuring skin conductance is a technique useful in objectively assessing psychophysiologic arousal and is most often used in "lie detector" testing.[5]

ELECTROMYOGRAPHIC BIOFEEDBACK

Electromyographic biofeedback is certainly the most typically used of all the biofeedback modalities in a clinical setting. Muscle contraction results from the more or less synchronous contraction of individual muscle fibers that compose a muscle. Individual muscle fibers are innervated by nerves that collectively comprise a motor unit. The axon of that motor unit conducts an action potential to the neuromuscular junction where a neurotransmitter substance (acetylcholine) is released (Figure 7–1). As this neurotransmitter binds to receptor sites on the sarcolemma, depolarization of that muscle fiber occurs, moving in both directions along the muscle fiber, creating movement of ions and thus an electrochemical gradient around the muscle fiber. Changes in potential difference or voltage associated with depolarization can be detected by an electrode placed in close proximity.

Biofeedback
- measures electrical activity of muscle, not muscle contraction.

CASE STUDY 7–1
BIOFEEDBACK

Background: A 10-year-old female subluxed her left patella while jumping rope at school. There was immediate pain and a localized effusion that resolved with the use of an immobilizer, intermittent ice packs, and rest over a 7-day period. Her pediatrician requested the initiation of quadriceps rehabilitation 2 weeks later after the patient reported no pain and minimal swelling but with a residual stiffness and sensation of weakness in the knee joint. The physical examination was unremarkable except for limited ROM of 10–110 degrees and the inability of the patient to successfully initiate and sustain an isometric contraction of her quadriceps musculature.

(continued)

CASE STUDY 7–1   (*continued*)
BIOFEEDBACK

Impression: Quadriceps inhibition secondary to injury and immobilization.

Treatment Plan: In addition to the initiation of therapeutic exercise—static stretching and active-assistive ROM exercise for the knee joint—biofeedback was initiated for the quadriceps mechanism. Using the vastus medialis muscle as the target muscle, the skin was cleansed and electrodes placed in alignment with the fibers of the muscle. A microvolt threshold of detection slightly above the patient's ability to maximize auditory and visual feedback was chosen. The patient was encouraged to perform isometric quadriceps setting exercises of 6- to 10-second duration attempting to "max out" feedback for the chosen threshold level. The threshold was advanced and the process repeated.

Response: Over the course of the initial rehabilitation session, the patient advanced several threshold levels and "reacquired" the ability to initiate and sustain an isometric quadriceps muscle contraction comparable to her uninvolved extremity. She was rapidly transitioned to limited-range dynamic exercise and a functional closed-chain exercise sequence with emphasis on terminal range knee stability. She returned to unrestricted playground activities several weeks later.

Discussion Questions

- What tissues were injured/affected?
- What symptoms were present?
- What phase of the injury-healing continuum did the patient presented for care in?
- What are the physical agent modality's biophysical effects (direct/indirect/depth/tissue affinity)?
- What are the physical agent modality's indications/contraindications?
- What are the parameters of the physical agent modality's application/dosage/duration/frequency in this case study?

The rehabilitation professional employs physical agent modalities to create an optimum environment for tissue healing while minimizing the symptoms associated with the trauma or condition. What other physical agent modalities could be utilized to treat this injury or condition? Why? How?

Motor Unit Recruitment

The amount of tension developed in a muscle is determined by the number of active motor units. As more motor units are recruited and the frequency of discharge increases, muscle tension increases.

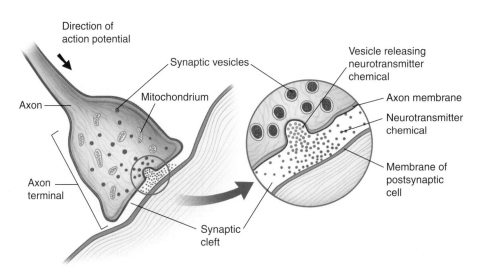

Figure 7–1. The nerve fiber conducts an impulse to the neuromuscular junction where acetylcholine binds to receptor sites on the sarcolemma inducing a depolarization of the muscle fiber, which creates movement of ions and thus an electrochemical gradient around the muscle fiber. Reproduced, with permission, from Van de Graaff KE, Human Anatomy, 6th ed. New York: McGraw-Hill, 2002.

The pattern of motor unit recruitment varies depending on the inherent properties of specific motor neurons, the force required during the activity, and the speed of contraction. Smaller motor units are recruited first and are somewhat limited in their ability to generate tension. Larger motor units generate greater tension because more muscle fibers are recruited.

Motor units are recruited based on the force required in an activity and not on the type of contraction performed. Thus, the firing rate and recruitment of the motor units are dependent on the external force required. The speed of contraction also influences motor unit recruitment. Fast contractions tend to excite larger and depress smaller motor units.

Measuring Electrical Activity

Despite the fact that **biofeedback** is used to determine muscle activity, it does not measure muscle contraction directly. Instead it measures electrical activity associated with muscle contraction. Movement of ions across the membrane creates a depolarization of the muscle membranes, resulting in a reversal in polarity, followed by repolarization. The various stages of membrane activity generate a triphasic electrical signal.[7] Electrical activity of the muscle is measured in volts, or more precisely, microvolts (V = 1,000,000 μV).

Measurement of electrical activity is made in standard quantitative units. Monitoring is useful in detecting changes in electrical activity, although changes cannot be quantified. The advantage of measurement over monitoring is that an objective scale is used; therefore, comparisons can be made between different individuals, occasions, and instruments. Measurement allows *procedures* to be replicated.

Unfortunately, biofeedback units have no universally accepted standardized measurement scale. Each brand of biofeedback unit serves as its own reference standard. Different brands of biofeedback equipment may give different readings for the same degree of muscle contraction. Consequently, biofeedback readings can be compared only when the same equipment is used for all readings.[5]

The biofeedback unit receives small amounts of electrical energy generated during muscle contraction through an electrode. It then separates or filters this electrical energy from other extraneous electrical activity on the skin and amplifies the electrical energy. The amplified activity is then converted to information that has meaning to the user. Most biofeedback units use surface electrodes. Figure 7–2 is a diagram of the various components of a biofeedback unit.

Separation and Amplification of Electromyographic Activity

Once the electrical activity is detected by the electrodes, the extraneous electrical activity, or "**noise**," must be eliminated before the electrical activity is amplified and subsequently

Raw electrical activity may be:
- rectified;
- smoothed;
- integrated.

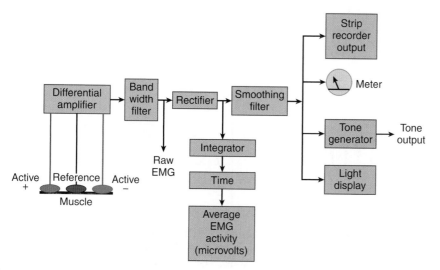

Figure 7–2. The anatomy of a typical biofeedback unit.

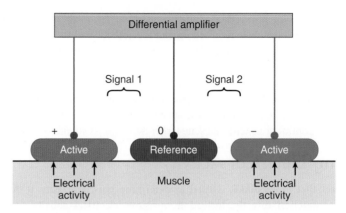

Figure 7–3. The differential amplifier monitors the two separate signals from the active electrodes and amplifies the difference, thus eliminating extraneous noise.

objectified. This is accomplished by using two **active electrodes** and a single ground or **reference electrode** in a **bipolar arrangement** to create three separate pathways from the skin to the biofeedback unit (Figure 7–3). The active electrodes should be placed in close proximity to one another, whereas the reference electrode may be placed anywhere on the body. Typically in biofeedback, the reference electrode is placed between the two active electrodes.

The active electrodes pick up electrical activity from motor units firing in the muscles beneath the electrodes. The magnitude of the small voltages detected by each active electrode will differ with respect to the reference electrode, creating two separate signals. These two signals are then fed to a **differential amplifier** that basically subtracts the signal of one active electrode from the other. This, in effect, cancels out or rejects any components that the two signals have in common coming from the active electrodes, thus amplifying the difference between the signals. The differential amplifier uses the reference electrode to compare the signals of the two active or recording electrodes (see Figure 7–3).

There will always be some degree of extraneous electrical activity created by power lines, motors, lights, appliances, and so on that is picked up by the body and eventually detected by the surface electrodes on the skin. Assuming that this extraneous "noise" is detected equally by both active electrodes, the differential amplifier will subtract the noise detected by one active electrode from the noise detected by the other, leaving only the true difference between the active electrodes. The ability of the differential amplifier to eliminate the common noise between the active electrodes is called the **common mode rejection ratio (CMRR)**.

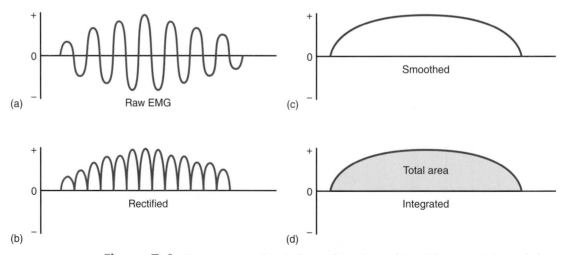

Figure 7–4. Processing an electrical signal involves taking (A) raw activity and then (B) rectifying, (C) smoothing, and (D) integrating it so that the information can be presented in some meaningful format.

External noise can be reduced further by using **filters** that essentially make the amplifier more sensitive to some incoming frequencies and less sensitive to others. Therefore, the amplifier will pick up signals only at those frequencies produced by electrical activity in the muscle within a specific frequency range or **bandwidth**. In general, the wider the bandwidth, the higher the noise readings are.

It must be noted that the clinician is interested in measuring the electrical activity within the muscle. An excessive external noise that is not eliminated by the biofeedback instrument will mask true electrical activity and will significantly decrease the reliability of the information being generated by that device.

Converting Electromyographic Activity to Meaningful Information

After amplification and filtering, the signal is indicative of the true electrical activity within the muscles being monitored. This is referred to as "raw" activity. **Raw EMG** is an alternating voltage that means that the direction or polarity is constantly reversing (Figure 7–4A). The amplitude of the oscillations increases to a maximum, and then diminishes. Biofeedback measures the overall increase and decrease in electrical activity. To obtain this measurement, the deflection toward the negative pole must be flipped upward toward the positive pole; otherwise, the sum total of their deflections would cancel out one another (Figure 7–4B). This process, referred to as **rectification**, essentially creates a pulsed direct current.

Processing the Electromyographic Signal

The rectified signal can be smoothed and integrated. **Smoothing** the signal means eliminating the peaks and valleys or eliminating the high-frequency fluctuations that are produced with a

Raw electrical activity may be:
- rectified;
- smoothed;
- integrated.

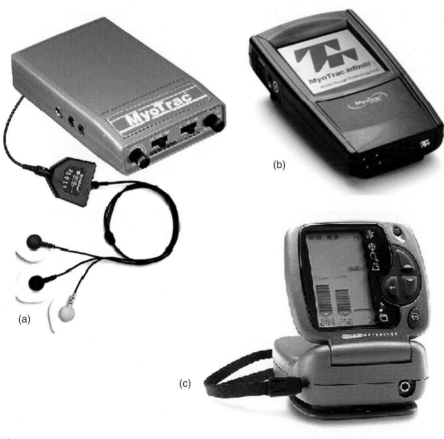

Figure 7–5. Biofeedback units. (a) Myotrac, (b) Myotrac Infiniti, and (c) EMG Retrainer.

changing electrical signal (Figure 7–4C). Once the signal has been smoothed, the signal may be integrated by measuring the area under the curve for a specified period of time. **Integration** forms the basis for quantification of EMG activity (Figure 7–4D).

BIOFEEDBACK EQUIPMENT AND TREATMENT TECHNIQUES

Biofeedback:
- Information may be visual, auditory, or both.

It is imperative that the clinician have some understanding of how biofeedback units monitor and record the electrical activity being produced in a muscle before attempting to set up and use the biofeedback unit in the treatment of a patient (Figure 7–5). Specific treatment protocols involve skin preparation, application of electrodes, selection of feedback or output modes, and selection of sensitivity settings, all of which have been previously discussed. Once these are complete, the clinician should choose to have the patient sitting, lying, or occasionally standing in a comfortable position, depending on the treatment objectives.[30] Generally the clinician should begin with easy tasks and progressively make the activities more difficult. Teaching the patient how to appropriately use the biofeedback unit and briefly explaining what is being measured are essential. In most cases, it is recommended that the clinician attach the biofeedback unit to himself or herself and then demonstrate to the patient exactly what will be done during the treatment.[8]

Treatment Protocols for Biofeedback (Muscle Reeducation) are as Follows:

1. Adjust unit to lowest threshold (µV) that picks up any activity (MUAPs).
2. Adjust audio and visual feedback.
3. Have patient contract target muscle to produce maximum audio and visual feedback.
4. Facilitate target muscle contraction as necessary by tapping, stroking, or contracting opposite like muscle.
5. When maximum feedback is obtained for selected threshold, advance threshold and attempt again.
6. Advance muscle or limb to other positions.
7. Continue muscle contractions for 10–15 minutes per training session or until maximal muscle activation is obtained.

Treatment Protocols for Biofeedback (Muscle Relaxation) are as Follows:

1. Adjust unit to sensitivity threshold (µV) that picks up maximal activity (MUAPs).
2. Adjust audio or visual feedback.
3. Have patient relax target muscle to produce minimum audio or visual feedback.
4. Facilitate target muscle relaxation as necessary by tapping, stroking, or contracting opposite like muscle.
5. When minimum feedback is obtained for selected threshold, reduce threshold and attempt relaxation again.

6. Advance muscle or limb to other functional positions.
7. Continue muscle relaxation for 10–15 minutes per training session or until muscle relaxation is obtained.

Electrodes

Skin-surface electrodes are most often used in biofeedback. Fine-wire in-dwelling electrodes may also be used that permit localized highly accurate measurement of electrical activity. However, these electrodes must be inserted percutaneously and thus are relatively impractical in a clinical setting.

Various types of surface electrodes are available for use with biofeedback units (Figure 7–6). Electrodes are most often made of stainless steel or nickel-plated brass recessed in a plastic holder. These less expensive electrodes are effective in EMG biofeedback applications. More expensive electrodes made of gold or silver/silver chloride also have been used.[9]

The size of the electrodes may range from 4 mm in diameter for recording small muscle activity to 12.5 mm for use with larger muscle groups. Increasing the size of the electrode will not cause an increase in the amplitude of the signal.[8]

Regardless of whether or not electrodes are disposable, some type of conducting gel, paste, or cream with high salt content is necessary to establish a highly conductive connection with the skin. Disposable electrodes come with the appropriate amount of gel and an adhesive ring already applied so that the electrode can be easily connected to the skin. Nondisposable electrodes need to have a double-sided adhesive ring applied. Then enough conducting gel must be added so that it is level with the surface of the adhesive ring before the electrode is applied to the skin.

CASE STUDY 7–2
BIOFEEDBACK

Background: A 19-year-old male suffered a twisting injury to the right knee during football practice. There was immediate pain, effusion, joint line tenderness, and hamstring muscle spasm that prevented full extension of the knee. Initial treatment involved the use of an immobilizer, intermittent application of ice packs, elevation, and rest over the first 24 hours postinjury. Referral for rehabilitation was immediate, and the patient reported to the clinic with residual pain and minimal swelling but with residual hamstring muscle guarding that prevented full active or passive knee extension.

Impression: Hamstring muscle spasm secondary to injury.

Treatment Plan: Therapeutic exercise, PNF contract–relax, was initiated for the knee joint musculature—primarily the hamstrings; biofeedback was also initiated for the hamstring muscles. Using the semimembranosus/semitendinosus muscles as the targets, the skin was cleansed and electrodes placed in alignment with the fibers of the muscles. A microvolt threshold of detection at the level of the patient's current muscle spasm activity was chosen with continuous auditory feedback. The patient was encouraged to isometrically contract

his hamstring muscles, and then consciously think of relaxing the muscles and reducing the level of auditory feedback. When auditory silence was achieved for the chosen microvolt level, the threshold was reduced and the process repeated. The patient was then encouraged to actively and passively extend the knee.

Response: Over the course of the initial rehabilitation session, the patient was able to reduce the threshold level and "relax" the hamstring muscles to achieve full active and passive knee extension comparable to his uninvolved extremity. He was rapidly transitioned to dynamic exercise and a functional closed-chain exercise sequence with emphasis on terminal range knee stability. He returned to football activities several weeks later.

Discussion Questions

- What tissues were injured/affected?
- What symptoms were present?
- What phase of the injury-healing continuum did the patient present for care in?

(continued)

CASE STUDY 7–2 *(continued)*
BIOFEEDBACK

- What are the physical agent modality's biophysical effects (direct/indirect/depth/tissue affinity)?
- What are the physical agent modality's indications/contraindications?
- What are the parameters of the physical agent modality's application/dosage/duration/frequency in this case study?
- What other physical agent modalities could be utilized to treat this injury or condition? Why? How?

Further Discussion Questions

- How would biofeedback assist in this patient's course of rehabilitation?

- What would the goal of the treatment session be?
- How long would you continue the use of biofeedback with this patient?
- Describe how you would integrate PNF techniques with biofeedback.

The rehabilitation professional employs physical agent modalities to create an optimum environment for tissue healing while minimizing the symptoms associated with the trauma or condition.

Skin Preparation

Prior to attachment of the surface electrodes, the skin must be appropriately prepared by removing oil and dead skin along with excessive hair from the surface to reduce skin impedance. Scrubbing with an alcohol-soaked prep pad is recommended.[9] However, if the skin is cleaned until it becomes irritated, it may interfere with biofeedback recording.

Some surface electrodes are permanently attached to cable wires, whereas others may snap onto the wire. Some biofeedback units include a set of three electrodes preplaced on a Velcro band that may be easily attached to the skin.

Electrode Placement

The electrodes should be placed as near to the muscle being monitored as possible to minimize recording extraneous electrical activity. They should be secured with the body part in the position in which it will be monitored so that movement of the skin will not alter the positioning of the electrodes over a particular muscle (Figure 7–7).[9]

The electrodes should be parallel to the direction of the muscle fibers to ensure that a better sample of muscle activity is monitored while reducing extraneous electrical activity.

Spacing the electrodes is also a critical consideration. Electrodes generally detect measurable signals from a distance equal to that of the interelectrode spacing. Therefore, as the distance between the electrodes increases, the signal will include electrical activity not only from muscles directly under the electrodes but also from other nearby muscles.[7]

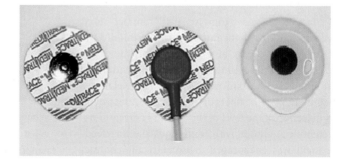

Figure 7–6. Various types of surface electrodes are available for use with biofeedback units.

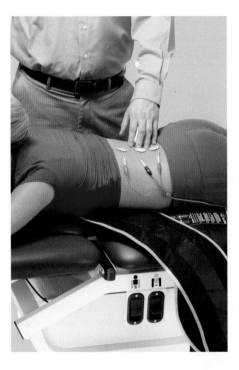

Figure 7-7. The biofeedback unit is connected via a series of electrodes to the skin over the contracting muscle.

Clinical Decision-Making Exercise 7-2

What are the three most important considerations for the clinician who is trying to make a decision regarding the correct placement of electrodes?

Displaying the Information

At this point it is necessary to take this rectified, smoothed, and integrated signal and display the information in a form that has some meaning. Biofeedback units generally provide either visual or auditory feedback relative to the quantity of electrical activity. Some biofeedback units can provide both visual and auditory feedback, depending on the output mode selected.

Visual Feedback

Raw activity is usually displayed visually on an oscilloscope. On most biofeedback units, integrated electrical activity is visually presented, as a line traveling across a monitor, as a light or series of lights that go on and off, or as a bar graph that changes dimension in response to the incoming integrated signal. Some of the newer biofeedback units have incorporated video games as part of their visual feedback system. An electrode attached directly to the skin over a muscle picks up the electrical activity produced by a muscle contraction. If the biofeedback unit uses some type of meter, it may either be calibrated in objective units such as microvolts or simply give some relative scale of measure.[9]

Meters also may be either analog or digital. Analog meters have a continuous scale and a needle that indicates the level of electrical activity within a particular range. Digital meters display only a number. They are very simple and easy to read. However, the disadvantage of a digital meter is that it is more difficult to tell where the signal falls in a given range.

Audio Feedback

On some biofeedback units, raw activity can be listened to and is one type of audio feedback. The majority of biofeedback units have audio feedback that produces some tone—buzzing, beeping, or clicking. An increase in the pitch of a tone, buzz, or beep, or an increase in the frequency of clicking indicates an increase in the level of electrical activity. This would be most useful for individuals who need to strengthen muscle contractions. Conversely, decreases in pitch or frequency indicating a decrease in electrical activity would be most useful in teaching patients to relax.

Setting Sensitivity

Signal sensitivity or **signal gain** may be set by the clinician on many biofeedback units. If a high gain is chosen, the biofeedback unit will have a high sensitivity for the muscle activity signal. Sensitivity may be set at 1, 10, or 100 μV. A 1-μV setting is sensitive enough to detect the smallest amounts of electrical activity and thus has the highest signal gain. High sensitivity levels should be used during relaxation training. Comparatively lower sensitivity levels are more useful in muscle reeducation, during which the patient may produce several hundred microvolts of EMG activity. Generally, the sensitivity range should be set at the lowest level that does not elicit feedback at rest.

CLINICAL APPLICATIONS FOR BIOFEEDBACK

Biofeedback would be useful as a therapeutic modality for a number of clinical conditions. The primary applications for using biofeedback include muscle reeducation, which involves regaining neuromuscular control and increasing muscle strength, relaxation of muscle spasm or muscle guarding, and pain reduction. Table 7–1 lists indications and contraindications for using biofeedback.

Muscle Reeducation

The goal in muscle reeducation is to provide feedback that will reestablish neuromuscular control or promote the ability of a muscle or group of muscles to contract. It may also be used to regain normal agonist/antagonist muscle action and for postural control retraining. Biofeedback is used to indicate the electrical activity associated with that muscle contraction.[10]

When biofeedback is being used to elicit a muscle contraction, the sensitivity setting should be chosen by having the patient perform a maximum isometric contraction of the target muscle. Then the gain should be adjusted so that the patient will be able to achieve the maximum on about two thirds of the muscle contractions. If the patient cannot produce a muscle contraction, the clinician should attempt to facilitate a contraction by stroking or tapping the target muscle. It is also helpful to have the patient look at the muscle when trying to

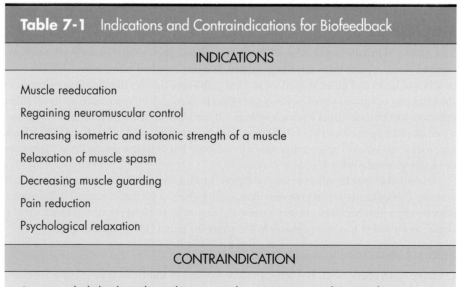

Table 7-1   Indications and Contraindications for Biofeedback
INDICATIONS
Muscle reeducation
Regaining neuromuscular control
Increasing isometric and isotonic strength of a muscle
Relaxation of muscle spasm
Decreasing muscle guarding
Pain reduction
Psychological relaxation
CONTRAINDICATION
Any musculoskeletal condition that a muscular contraction might exacerbate

contract. It may be necessary to move the active electrodes to the contralateral limb and have the patient "practice" the muscle contraction you hope to achieve on the opposite side.

Clinical Decision-Making   *Exercise 7-3*

Two biofeedback units made by different manufacturers are available for use in the clinic. The clinician has been using the same unit to work on muscle strengthening with an injured patient throughout his rehabilitation process. Unfortunately, that generator has broken, and he is forced to use the other one. Can comparisons be made from one unit to another?

The patient should maximally contract the target muscle isometrically for 6–10 seconds. During this contraction, the visual or auditory feedback should be at a maximum and should be closely monitored by both the clinician and patient. Between each contraction the patient should be instructed to completely relax the muscle such that the feedback mode returns to baseline or zero prior to initiating another contraction. A period of 5–10 minutes working with a single muscle or muscle group is most desirable because longer periods tend to produce fatigue and boredom, neither of which is conducive to optimal learning.[11]

As increases in electrical activity occur, the patient should develop the ability to rapidly activate motor units. This can be accomplished by setting the sensitivity level to 60–80% of maximum isometric activity and instructing the patient to reach that level as many times as possible during a given time period (i.e., 10 or 30 seconds). Again, total relaxation must occur between contractions.

It is essential that the treatment be functionally relevant to the patient. Attention to mobility and muscle power cannot be neglected in favor of biofeedback therapy.[11] The clinician should have the patient perform functional movements while observing body mechanics and the related electrical activity. Then recommendations can be made as to how movements can be altered to elicit normal responses.[12] Biofeedback is useful in patients who perform poorly on manual muscle tests. If the patient can only elicit a fair, trace, or zero grade, then biofeedback should be incorporated. Stronger muscles generally should be given resistive exercises rather than biofeedback, although biofeedback has been recommended for increasing the strength of healthy muscle.[11,13]

Relaxation of Muscle Guarding

Often in a clinical setting, patients demonstrate a protective response in muscle that occurs because of pain or fear of movement. This response is most accurately described as **muscle guarding**.

Muscle guarding must be differentiated from those neuromuscular problems arising from central nervous system deficits that result in a clinical condition known as muscle spasticity. For the clinician treating patients exhibiting muscle guarding, the goal is to induce relaxation of the muscle by reducing electrical activity through the use of biofeedback.[11]

Because muscle guarding most often involves fear of pain that may result when the muscle moves, perhaps the most important goal in treatment is to modulate pain. This is best accomplished through the use of other modalities such as ice or electrical stimulation.

Biofeedback treatments should be designed so that the patient experiences success from the first treatment. The patient is now attempting to reduce the visual or auditory feedback to zero. Initially, positioning the patient in a comfortable relaxed position is critical to reducing muscle guarding. A high-sensitivity setting should be selected so that any electrical activity in the muscle will be easily detected.

During relaxation training, the patient should be given verbal cues that will enhance relaxation of individual muscles, muscle groups, or body segments. For example, with individual muscles or small muscle groups, the patient may be instructed to contract, and then relax a specific muscle or to imagine a feeling of warmth within the muscle. For larger muscle groups, using mental imagery or deep breathing exercises may be useful.

As relaxation progresses, the spacing between the electrodes should be increased. Also, the sensitivity setting should move from low to high. Both of these changes will require the patient to relax more muscles, thus achieving greater relaxation. The patient must then apply this newly learned relaxation technique in different positions that are potentially more uncomfortable. Again, the goal is to eliminate muscle guarding during functional activities.[11]

Clinical Decision-Making *Exercise 7–4*

The clinician is using a biofeedback unit for muscle reeducation of the hamstrings following knee surgery. The patient wants to know how the biofeedback unit is going to measure his muscle contraction. How should the clinician respond?

Clinical Decision-Making *Exercise 7–5*

The clinician wishes to use a biofeedback unit to help an injured patient learn to relax muscle guarding in the low back following a contusion. Should the clinician use a high- or low-sensitivity setting and why?

Clinical Decision-Making *Exercise 7–6*

A patient has a sprain of a vertebral ligament in the lumbar region of the low back with accompanying muscle guarding. What modalities might potentially be used to reduce and/or eliminate this muscle guarding?

Pain Reduction

A number of therapeutic modalities discussed in this text are used for the purpose of reducing or modulating pain. As mentioned in the section "Relaxation of Muscle Guarding", biofeedback can be used to relax muscles that are tense secondary to fear of pain on movement. If the muscle can be relaxed, then chances are that pain will also be reduced by breaking the "pain–guarding–pain" cycle. It has been experimentally demonstrated to reduce pain in headaches and low back pain.[12,14–18] Pain modulation is often associated with techniques of imagery and progressive relaxation.

Treating Neurologic Conditions

Biofeedback has been identified as an effective technique for treating a variety of neurologic conditions, including hemiplegia following stroke, spinal cord injury, spasticity, cerebral palsy, fascial paralysis, and urinary and fecal incontinence.[19–29,33–35]

SUMMARY

1. Biofeedback is a therapeutic procedure that uses electronic or electromechanical instruments to accurately measure, process, and feed back reinforcing information by using auditory or visual signals.

2. Perhaps the biggest advantage of biofeedback is that it provides the patient with a chance to make correct small changes in performance that are immediately noted and rewarded so that eventually larger changes or improvements in performance can be accomplished.

3. Several different types of biofeedback modalities are available for use in rehabilitation, with biofeedback being the most widely used in a clinical setting.

4. A biofeedback unit measures the electrical activity produced by depolarization of a muscle fiber as an indicator of the quality of a muscle contraction.

5. The biofeedback unit receives small amounts of electrical energy generated during muscle contraction through active electrodes, and then separates or filters extraneous electrical energy via a differential amplifier before it is processed and subsequently converted to some type of information that has meaning to the user.

6. Biofeedback information is displayed either visually using lights or meters or auditorily using tones, beeps, buzzes, or clicks.

7. High sensitivity levels should be used during relaxation training, whereas comparatively lower sensitivity levels are more useful in muscle reeducation.

8. In a clinical setting, biofeedback is most typically used for muscle reeducation, to decrease muscle guarding, or for pain reduction.

REVIEW QUESTIONS

1. What is biofeedback and how can it be used in injury rehabilitation?
2. What are the various types of biofeedback instruments that are available to the clinician?
3. How can the electrical activity generated by a muscle contraction be measured using biofeedback?
4. What are the important considerations for attaching biofeedback electrodes?
5. How is the electrical activity picked up by the electrodes amplified, processed, and converted to meaningful information by the biofeedback unit?
6. What are the advantages and disadvantages of using visual and auditory feedback?
7. How should sensitivity settings be changed during relaxation training versus during muscle reeducation?
8. What are the most common uses for biofeedback in a rehabilitation setting?

SELF-TEST QUESTIONS

True or False

1. Biofeedback units measure physiologic processes.
2. The reference electrode has no charge associated with it.
3. A high signal gain means the biofeedback unit has a low sensitivity for muscle activity.

Multiple Choice

4. Some biofeedback instruments measure peripheral skin temperature. Which of the following do they also measure?
   a. finger phototransmission
   b. skin conductance activity
   c. electromyographic activity
   d. all of the above

5. Biofeedback electrodes should be placed as near to the muscle of interest as possible. They should also be placed _____ to the muscle.
   a. perpendicular
   b. parallel
   c. obliquely
   d. none of the above

6. What is the principle that allows the biofeedback unit to eliminate common noise between active electrodes?
   a. CMRR
   b. filtering
   c. rectification
   d. integration

7. Raw EMG must be converted to a visual or audio format. What is the order of that conversion?
   a. integrated, rectified, smoothed
   b. smoothed, rectified, integrated
   c. rectified, smoothed, integrated
   d. rectified, integrated, smoothed

8. The goal of using biofeedback in muscle reeducation is to elicit a
   a. twitch response
   b. muscle contraction
   c. decrease in pain
   d. relaxation

9. How long should the average biofeedback period for a single muscle be to avoid fatigue and boredom?
   a. 1–2 minutes
   b. 2–5 minutes
   c. 5–10 minutes
   d. 10–15 minutes

10. What factor(s) must be addressed when using biofeedback to relax muscle guarding?
    a. pain
    b. mental imagery
    c. apprehension
    d. all of the above

SOLUTIONS TO CLINICAL DECISION-MAKING EXERCISES

7–1

The clinician can act as a substitute biofeedback unit. The patient should be instructed to watch the VMO as he or she tries to contract the muscle. This will serve as visual feedback. The clinician can help to facilitate a contraction by tapping or stroking the muscle. Also by maintaining physical contact with the muscle, the clinician, using verbal feedback, can let the patient know when the muscle is actually contracted.

7–2

They should be placed as close to the muscle as possible to minimize "noise." They should be placed parallel to the direction of the muscle fibers. The spacing should be close enough to monitor activity from a specific muscle. If spaced too far apart, electrical activity from other anatomically close muscles may also be detected.

7–3

With biofeedback units, there is no universally accepted or standardized measurement scale. Different machines are likely to give different readings for the same degree of muscle contraction. Each manufacturer has its own reference standards for its particular unit. Thus, information provided from these different units cannot be compared.

7–4

Biofeedback units do not directly measure muscle contraction. Instead, they measure only the electrical activity associated with a muscle contraction. Thus, the patient should understand that the electrical activity infers some information about the quality of a muscle contraction but does not measure the strength of that muscle contraction specifically.

7–5

The clinician should set the signal gain on the biofeedback unit at a high-sensitivity setting whenever the goal is relaxation, while a low-sensitivity setting should be used with muscle reeducation.

7–6

Several modalities could potentially help reduce muscle guarding including thermotherapy, cryotherapy, and electrical stimulation. A recommendation would be to first use electrical stimulation to break the pain–guarding cycle. Once pain has been modulated, a biofeedback unit may be used to help the patient learn to relax the low back muscles and to keep them relaxed as movement occurs.

REFERENCES

1. Olson R. Definitions of biofeedback. In: Schwartz M, ed. *Biofeedback: A Practitioner's Guide*. New York: Guilford Press; 2005.
2. Draper V. Electromyographic feedback and recovery in quadriceps femoris muscle function following anterior cruciate ligament reconstruction. *Phys Ther*. 1990;70:25.
3. Miller N. Biomedical foundations for biofeedback as a part of behavioral medicine. In: Basmajian J, ed. *Biofeedback: Principles and Practice for Clinicians*. Baltimore: Williams & Wilkins; 1989.
4. Wolf S, Binder-Macleod S. Electromyographic feedback in the physical therapy clinic. In: Basmajian JV, ed. *Biofeedback: Principles and Practice for Clinicians*. Baltimore: Williams & Wilkins; 1989.
5. Peek C. A primer of biofeedback instrumentation. In: Schwartz M, ed. *Biofeedback: A Practitioner's Guide*. New York: Guilford Press; 2005.
6. Jennings J, Tahmoush A, Redmond D. Non-invasive measurement of peripheral vascular activity. In: Martin I, Venables PH, eds. *Techniques in Psychophysiology*. New York: Wiley; 1980.
7. Basmajian J. Description and analysis of EMG signal. In: Basmajian J, Deluca C, eds. *Muscles Alive. Their Functions Revealed by Electromyography*. Baltimore: Williams & Wilkins; 1985.
8. LeCraw D, Wolf S. Electromyographic biofeedback (EMG-BF) for neuromuscular relaxation and re-education. In: Gersh M, ed. *Electrotherapy in Rehabilitation*. Philadelphia: FA Davis Company; 1992.
9. Wolf S. Treatment of neuromuscular problems, treatment of musculoskeletal problems. In: Sandweiss J, ed. *Biofeedback: Review Seminars*. Los Angeles, CA: University of California; 1982.
10. Fogel E. Biofeedback-assisted musculoskeletal therapy and neuromuscular reeducation. In: Schwartz MS, ed. *Biofeedback: A Practitioner's Guide*. New York: Guilford Press; 2005.
11. Krebs D. Neuromuscular re-education and gait training. In: Schwartz M, ed. *Biofeedback: A Practitioner's Guide*. New York: Guilford Press; 2005.
12. Bush C, Ditto B, Feuerstein M. Controlled evaluation of paraspinal EMG biofeedback in the treatment of chronic low back pain. *Health Psychol*. 1985;4:307–321.
13. Croce R. The effects of EMG biofeedback on strength acquisition. *Biofeedback Self Regul*. 1986;9:395.
14. Arena J, Bruno G, Hannah S. A comparison of frontal electromyographic biofeedback training, trapezius electromyographic biofeedback training, and progressive muscle relaxation therapy in the treatment of tension headache. *Headache*. 1995;35(7):411–419.
15. Budzynski D. Biofeedback strategies in headache treatment. In: Basmajian J, ed. *Biofeedback: Principles and Practice for Clinicians*. Baltimore: Williams & Wilkins; 1989.
16. Chapman S. A review and clinical perspective on the use of EMG and thermal biofeedback for chronic headaches. *Pain*. 1986;27:1.
17. Nouwen A, Bush C. The relationship between paraspinal EMG and chronic low back pain. *Pain*. 1984;20:109–123.
18. Studkey S, Jacobs A, Goldfarb J. EMG biofeedback training, relaxation training, and placebo for the relief of chronic back pain. *Percept Mot Skills*. 1986;63:1023.
19. Amato A, Hermomeyer C, Kleinman K. Use of electromyographic feedback to increase control of spastic muscles. *Phys Ther*. 1973;53:1063.
20. Asato H, Twiggs D, Ellison S. EMG biofeedback training for a mentally retarded individual with cerebral palsy. *Phys Ther*. 1981;61:1447–1451.
21. Boucher A, Wang S. Effectiveness of a surface electromyographic biofeedback-triggered neuromuscular stimulation on knee rehabilitation: a single case design. *J Orthop Sports Phys Ther*. 2006;36(1):A31.
22. Brucker B, Bulaeva N. Biofeedback effect on electromyography responses in patients with spinal cord injury. *Arch Phys Med Rehabil*. 1996;77(2):133–137.

23. Engardt M. Term effects of auditory feedback training on re-learned symmetrical body weight distribution in stroke patients. A follow-up study. *Scand J Rehabil Med.* 1994;26(2):65–69.

24. Klose K, Needham B, Schmidt D. An assessment of the contribution of electromyographic biofeedback as a therapy in the physical training of spinal cord injured persons. *Arch Phys Med Rehabil.* 1993;74(5):453–456.

25. Moreland J, Thompson M. Efficacy of EMG biofeedback compared with conventional physical therapy for upper extremity function in patients following stroke: a research overview and meta-analysis. *Phys Ther.* 1994;74(6):534–543.

26. Regenos E, Wolf S. Involuntary single motor unit discharges in spastic muscles during EMG biofeedback training. *Arch Phys Med Rehabil.* 1979;60:72–73.

27. Schleenbaker R, Mainous A. Electromyographic biofeedback for neuromuscular reeducation in the hemiplegic stroke patient: a meta-analysis. *Arch Phys Med Rehabil.* 1993;74(12):1301–1304.

28. Sugar E, Firlit C. Urodynamic feedback: a new therapeutic approach for childhood incontinence/infection. *J Urol.* 1982;128:1253.

29. Whitehead W. Treatment of fecal incontinence in children with spina bifida: comparison of biofeedback and behavior modification. *Arch Phys Med Rehabil.* 1986;67:218.

30. Davlin CD, Holcomb WR, Guadagnoli MA. The effect of hip position and electromyographic biofeedback training on the vastus medialis oblique: vastus lateralis ratio. *J Athletic Train.* 1999;34(4):342–349.

31. Draper V, Lyle L, Seymour T. EMG biofeedback versus electrical stimulation in the recovery of quadriceps surface EMG. *Clin Kinesiol.* 1997;51(2):28–32.

32. Linsay KA. Electromyographic biofeedback. *Athletic Ther Today.* 1997;2(4):49.

33. Moreland JD, Thomson MA, Fuoco AR. Electromyographic biofeedback to improve lower extremity function after stroke: a meta-analysis. *Arch Phys Med Rehabil.* 1998;79(2):134–140.

34. Shinopulos NM, Jacobson J. Relationship between health promotion lifestyle profiles and patient outcomes of biofeedback therapy for urinary incontinence. *Urol Nurs.* 1999;19(4):249–253.

35. Wolf S, Binder-Macleod S. Neurophysiological factors in electromyographic feedback for neuromotor disturbances. In: Basmajian JV, ed. *Biofeedback: Principles and Practice for Clinicians.* Baltimore: Williams & Wilkins; 1989.

SUGGESTED READINGS

Angoules A, Balakatounis K. Effectiveness of electromyographic biofeedback in the treatment of musculoskeletal pain. *Orthopedics.* 2008;31(10):980–984.

Baker M, Hudson J, Wolf S. "Feedback" cane to improve the hemiplegic patient's gait: suggestion from the field. *Phys Ther.* 1979;59:170.

Baker M, Regenos E, Wolf S. Developing strategies for biofeedback: applications in neurologically handicapped patients. *Phys Ther.* 1977;57:402–408.

Balliet R, Levy B, Blood K. Upper extremity sensory feedback therapy in chronic cerebrovascular accident patients with impaired expressive aphasia and auditory comprehension. *Arch Phys Med Rehabil.* 1986;67:304.

Basmajian J. Learned control of single motor units. In: Schwartz GE, Beatty J, eds. *Biofeedback: Theory and Research.* New York: Academic Press; 1977.

Basmajian J. Biofeedback in rehabilitation: a review of principles and practice. *Arch Phys Med Rehabil.* 1981;62:469.

Basmajian J. *Biofeedback: Principles and Practice for Clinicians.* Baltimore: Williams & Wilkins; 1989.

Basmajian J, Blumenthal R. Electroplacement in electromyographic biofeedback. In: Basmajian JV, ed. *Biofeedback: Principles and Practice for Clinicians.* 3rd ed. Baltimore: Williams & Wilkins; 1989.

Basmajian J, Kukulka CG, Narayan MC, et al. Biofeedback treatment of foot drop after stroke compared with standard rehabilitation technique: effects on voluntary control and strength. *Arch Phys Med Rehabil.* 1975;56:231–236.

Basmajian J, Regenos E, Baker M. Rehabilitating stroke patients with biofeedback, *Geriatrics.* 1977;32:85.

Basmajian J, Samson J. Special review: standardization of methods in single motor unit training. *Am J Phys Med.* 1973;52:250–256.

Beal M, Diefenbach G, Allen A. Electromyographic biofeedback in the treatment of voluntary posterior instability of the shoulder. *Am J Sports Med.* 1987;15:175.

Bernat S, Wooldridge P, Marecki M. Biofeedback-assisted relaxation to reduce stress in labor. *J Obstet Gynecol Neonatal Nurs.* 1992;(4):295–303.

Biedermann H. Comments on the reliability of muscle activity comparisons in EMG biofeedback research with back pain patients. *Biofeedback Self Regul.* 1984;9:451–458.

Biedermann H, McGhie A, Monga T. Perceived and actual control in EMG treatment of back pain. *Behav Res Ther.* 1987;25:137–147.

Boucher AM, Wang S. Effectiveness of surface EMG biofeedback triggered neuromuscular stimulation on knee joint rehabilitation: a single case design [poster session]. *J Orthop Sports Phys Ther.* 2006;36(1):A31.

Bowman B, Baker L, Waters R. Positional feedback and electrical stimulation. An automated treatment for the hemiplegic wrist. *Arch Phys Med Rehabil.* 1979;60:497.

Brudny J, Grynbaum B, Korein J. Spasmodic torticollis: treatment by feedback display of EMG. *Arch Phys Med Rehabil.* 1974;55:403–408.

Burke R. Motor unit recruitment: what are the critical factors? In: Desmedt J, ed. *Progress in Clinical Neurophysiology.* Vol 9. Basel: Karger; 1981.

Burnside I, Tobias H, Bursill D. Electromyographic feedback in the rehabilitation of stroke patients: a controlled trial. *Arch Phys Med Rehabil.* 1982;63:217.

Burnside I, Tobias H, Bursill D. Electromyographic feedback in the remobilization of stroke patients: a controlled trial. *Arch Phys Med Rehabil.* 1983;63:1393.

Carlsson S. Treatment of temporo-mandibular joint syndrome with biofeedback training. *J Am Dent Assoc.* 1975;91:602–605.

Christie D, Dewitt R, Kaltenbach P. Using EMG biofeedback to signal hyperactive children when to relax. *Except Child.* 1984;50:547–548.

Cox R, Matyas T. Myoelectric and force feedback in the facilitation of isometric strength training: a controlled comparison. *Psychophysiology.* 1983;20:35–44.

Crow J, Lincoln N, De Weerdt N. The effectiveness of EMG biofeedback in the treatment of arm function after stroke. *Intern Disabil Stud.* 1989;11(4):155–160.

Cummings M, Wilson V, Bird E. Flexibility development in sprinters using EMG biofeedback and relaxation training. *Biofeedback Self Regul.* 1984;9:395–405.

Debacher G. Feedback goniometers for rehabilitation. In: Basmajian J, ed. *Biofeedback: Principles and Practice for Clinicians.* Baltimore: Williams & Wilkins; 1983.

Deluca C. Apparatus, detection, and recording techniques. In: Basmajian J, Deluca C, eds. *Muscles Alive: Their Functions Revealed by Electromyography.* Baltimore: Williams & Wilkins; 1985.

Draper V. Electromyographic biofeedback and recovery of quadriceps femoris muscle function following anterior cruciate ligament reconstruction. *Phys Ther.* 1990;70(1):11–17.

Draper V, Ballard L. Electrical stimulation versus electromyographic biofeedback in the recovery of quadriceps femoris muscle function following anterior cruciate ligament surgery. *Phys Ther.* 1991;71(6):455–464.

Dursun N. Electromyographic biofeedback-controlled exercise versus conservative care for patellofemoral pain syndrome. *Arch Phys Med and Rehabil.* 2001;82(12):1692–1695.

English A, Wolf S. The motor unit: anatomy and physiology. *Phys Ther.* 1982;62:1763.

Fagerson TL, Krebs DE. Biofeedback. In: O'Sullivan SB, Schmit TJ, eds. *Physical Rehabilitation: Assessment and Treatment.* Philadelphia: FA Davis Company; 2001.

Fauquier T. Biofeedback. *Phys Ther Prod.* 2008;19(7):18.

Fields R. Electromyographically triggered electric muscle stimulation for chronic hemiplegia. *Arch Phys Med Rehabil.* 1987;68:407–414.

Flom R, Quast J, Boller J. Biofeedback training to overcome poststroke footdrop. *Geriatrics.* 1976;31:47–51.

Flor H, Haag G, Turk D. Long-term efficacy of EMG biofeedback for chronic rheumatic back pain. *Pain.* 1986;27:195–202.

Flor H, Haag G, Turk DC, et al. Efficacy of EMG biofeedback, pseudotherapy, and conventional medical treatment for chronic rheumatic back pain. *Pain.* 1983;17:21–31.

Gaarder K, Montgomery P. *Clinical Biofeedback: A Procedural Manual.* Baltimore: Williams & Wilkins; 1977.

Gallego J, Perez de la Sota A, Vardon G. Electromyographic feedback for learning to activate thoracic inspiratory muscles. *Am J Phys Med Rehabil.* 1991;70(4):186–190.

Glazer H. Biofeedback vs electrophysiology. *Rehab Manage Interdisciplinary J Rehabil.* 2005;18(9):32–34.

Goodgold J, Eberstein A. *Electrodiagnosis of Neuromuscular Diseases.* Baltimore: Williams & Wilkins; 1972.

Green E, Walters E, Green A. Feedback technology for deep relaxation. *Psychophysiology.* 1969;6:371–377.

Hijzen T, Slangen J, van Houweligen H. Subjective, clinical and EMG effects of biofeedback and splint treatment. *J Oral Rehabil.* 1986;13:529–539.

Hirasawa Y, Uchiza Y, Kusswetter W. EMG biofeedback therapy for rupture of the extensor pollicis longus tendon. *Arch Orthop Trauma Surg.* 1986;104:342.

Holtermann A, Mork P. The use of EMG biofeedback for learning of selective activation of intra-muscular parts within the serratus anterior muscle: a novel approach for rehabilitation of scapular muscle imbalance. *J Electromyogr Kinesiol.* 2010;20(2):359.

Honer L, Mohr T, Roth R. Electromyographic biofeedback to dissociate an upper extremity synergy pattern: a case report. *Phys Ther.* 1982;62:299–303.

Horowitz S. Biofeedback applications: a survey of clinical research. *Altern Complement Ther.* 2006;12(6):275–281.

Howard P. Use of EMG biofeedback to reeducate the rotator cuff in a case of shoulder impingement. *J Orthop Sports Phys Ther.* 1996;23(1):79.

Ince L, Leon M. Biofeedback treatment of upper extremity dysfunction in Guillain–Barre syndrome. *Arch Phys Med Rehabil.* 1986;67:30–33.

Ince L, Leon M, Christidis D. Experimental foundations of EMG biofeedback with the upper extremity: a review of the literature. *Biofeedback Self Regul.* 1984;9:371–383.

Ince L, Leon M, Christidis D. EMG biofeedback with upper extremity musculature for relaxation training: a critical review of the literature. *J Behav Ther Exp Psychiatry.* 1985;16:133–137.

Inglis J, Donald M, Monga T. Electromyographic biofeedback and physical therapy of the hemiplegic upper limb. *Arch Phys Med Rehabil.* 1984;65:755–759.

Johnson H, Garton W. Muscle reeducation in hemiplegia by use of electromyographic device. *Arch Phys Med Rehabil.* 1973;54:322–323.

Johnson H, Hockersmith V. Therapeutic electromyography in chronic back pain. In: Basmajian JV, ed. *Biofeedback: Principles and Practice for Clinicians*. 2nd ed. Baltimore, MD: Williams & Wilkins; 1983.

Johnson R, Lee K. Myofeedback: a new method of teaching breathing exercise to emphysematous patients. *J Am Phys Ther Assoc*. 1976;56:826–829.

Kasman G. Long-term rehab. Using surface electromyography: a multidisciplinary tool, sEMG can be a valuable asset to the rehab professional's muscle assessment arsenal. *Rehab Manage*. 2002;14(9):56–59, 76.

Kelly J, Baker M, Wolf S. Procedures for EMG biofeedback training in involved upper extremities of hemiplegic patients. *Phys Ther*. 1979;59:1500.

King A, Ahles T, Martin J. EMG biofeedback-controlled exercise in chronic arthritic knee pain. *Arch Phys Med Rehabil*. 1984;65:341–343.

King T. Biofeedback: a survey regarding current clinical use and content in occupational therapy educational curricula. *Occup Ther J Res*. 1992;12(1):50–58.

Kleppe D, Groendijk H, Huijing P. Single motor unit control in the human mm. abductor pollicis brevis and mylohyoideus in relation to the number of muscle spindles. *Electromyogr Clin Neurophysiol*. 1982;22:21–25.

Krebs D. Biofeedback in neuromuscular reeducation and gait training. In: Schwartz M, ed. *Biofeedback: A Practitioner's Guide*. New York: Guilford Press; 1987.

Large R. Prediction of treatment response in pain patients: the illness self-concept repertory grid and EMG feedback. *Pain*. 1985;21:279–287.

Large R, Lamb A. Electromyographic (EMG) feedback in chronic musculoskeletal pain: a controlled trial. *Pain*. 1983;17:167–177.

Lourençao M, Battistella L. Effect of biofeedback accompanying occupational therapy and functional electrical stimulation in hemiplegic patients. *Int J Rehabil Res*. 2008;31(1):33–41.

Lucca J, Recchiuti S. Effect of electromyographic biofeedback on an isometric strengthening program. *Phys Ther*. 1983;63:200–203.

Madeleine P, Vedsted P. Effects of electromyographic and mechanomyographic biofeedback on upper trapezius muscle activity during standardized computer work. *Ergonomics*. 2006;49(10):921–933.

Mandel A, Nymark J, Balmer S. Electromyographic versus rhythmic positional biofeedback in computerized gait retraining with stroke patients. *Arch Phys Med Rehabil*. 1990;71(9):649–654.

Marinacci A, Horande M. Electromyogram in neuromuscular reeducation. *Bull Los Angeles Neurol Soc*. 1960;25:57–67.

Mims H. Electromyography in clinical practice. *South Med J*. 1956;49:804.

Morasky R, Reynolds C, Clarke G. Using biofeedback to reduce left arm extensor EMG of string players during musical performance. *Biofeedback Self Regul*. 1981;6:565–572.

Morris M, Matyas T, Bach T. Electrogoniometric feedback: its effect on genu recurvatum in stroke. *Arch Phys Med Rehabil*. 1992;73(12):1147–1154.

Mulder T, Hulstijn W. Delayed sensory feedback in the learning of a novel motor task. *Psychol Res*. 1985;47:203–209.

Mulder T, Hulstijn W, van der Meer J. EMG feedback and the restoration of motor control. A controlled group study of 12 hemiparetic patients. *Am J Phys Med*. 1986;65:173–188.

Nafpliotis H. EMG feedback to improve ankle dorsiflexion, wrist extension and hand grasp. *Phys Ther*. 1976;56:821–825.

Ng G, Zhang, A. Biofeedback exercise improved the EMG activity ratio of the medial and lateral vasti muscles in subjects with patellofemoral pain syndrome. *J Electromyogr Kinesiol*. 2008;18(1):128.

Nord S. Muscle learning therapy—efficacy of a biofeedback based protocol in treating work-related upper extremity disorders. *J Occup Rehabil*. 2001;11(1):23–31.

Nouwen A. EMG biofeedback used to reduce standing levels of paraspinal muscle tension in chronic low back pain. *Pain*. 1983;17:353–360.

Pages I. Comparative analysis of biofeedback and physical therapy for treatment of urinary stress incontinence in women. *Am J Phys Med Rehabil*. 2001;80(7):494–502.

Pataky Z, De León Rodriguez D. Biofeedback training for partial weight bearing in patients after total hip arthroplasty. *Arch Phys Med Rehabil*. 2009;90(8):1435–1438.

Peper E, TylovaH. *Biofeedback Mastery: An Experiential Teaching and Self-Training Manual*. Wheat Ridge, CO: Association for Applied Psychology & Biofeedback; 2009.

Petrofsky JS. The use of electromyogram biofeedback to reduce Trendelenburg gait. *Eur J Appl Physiol*. 2001;85(5):135–140.

Poppen R, Maurer J. Electromyographic analysis of relaxed postures. *Biofeedback Self Regul*. 1982;7:491–498.

Pulliam CB. Biofeedback 2003: its role in pain management. *Crit Rev Rehabil Med*. 2003;15(1):65–82.

Russell G, Woolbridge C. Correction of a habitual head tilt using biofeedback techniques—a case study. *Physiother Can*. 1975;27:181–184.

Saunders J, Cox D, Teates C. Thermal biofeedback in the treatment of intermittent claudication in diabetes: a case study. *Biofeedback Self Regul*. 1994;19(4):337–345.

Schulte F. Exercise evaluation via EMG-biofeedback training. *Isokinet Exerc Sci*. 2008;16(3):174.

Smith D, Newman D. Basic elements of biofeedback therapy for pelvic muscle rehabilitation. *Urol Nurs*. 1994;14(3):130–135.

Soderback I, Bengtsson I, Ginsburg E. Video feedback in occupational therapy: its effect in patients with neglect syndrome. *Arch Phys Med Rehabil*. 1992;73(12):1140–1146.

Sousa K, Orfale A. Assessment of a biofeedback program to treat chronic low back pain. *J Musculoskelet Pain.* 2009;17(4):369–377.

Swaan D, van Wiergen P, Fokkema S. Auditory electromyographic feedback therapy to inhibit undesired motor activity. *Arch Phys Med Rehabil.* 1974;55:251.

Winchester P. Effects of feedback stimulation training and cyclical electrical stimulation on knee extension in hemiparetic patients. *Phys Ther.* 1983;63:1097.

Wolf S. Essential considerations in the use of EMG biofeedback. *Phys Ther.* 1978;58:25.

Wolf S. EMG biofeedback application in physical rehabilitation: an overview. *Physiother Can.* 1979;31:65.

Wolf S. Electromyographic biofeedback in exercise programs. *Phys Sports Med.* 1980;8:61–69.

Wolf S. Fallacies of clinical EMG measures from patients with musculoskeletal and neuromuscular disorders. Paper presented at: 14th Annual Meeting of the Biofeedback Society of America; 1983; Denver, CO.

Wolf S. Biofeedback. In: Currier DP, Nelson RM, eds. *Clinical Electrotherapy.* 2nd ed. Norwalk, CT: Appleton & Lange; 1991.

Wolf S, Baker M, Kelly J. EMG biofeedback in stroke: effect of patient characteristics. *Arch Phys Med Rehabil.* 1979;60: 96–102.

Wolf S, Baker M, Kelly J. EMG biofeedback in stroke: a 1-year follow-up on the effect of patient characteristics. *Arch Phys Med Rehabil.* 1980;61:351–355.

Wolf S, Binder-Macleod S. Electromyographic biofeedback applications to the hemiplegic patient. Changes in lower extremity neuromuscular and functional status. *Phys Ther.* 1983;63:1404–1413.

Wolf S, Binder-Macleod S. Electromyographic biofeedback applications to the hemiplegic patient: changes in upper extremity neuromuscular and functional status. *Phys Ther.* 1983;63:1393.

Wolf S, Edwards D, Shutter L. Concurrent assessment of muscle activity (CAMA): a procedural approach to assess treatment goals. *Phys Ther.* 1986;66:218.

Wolf S, Hudson J. Feedback signal based upon force and time delay: modification of the Krusen limb load monitor: suggestion from the field. *Phys Ther.* 1980;60:1289.

Wolf S, LeCraw D, Barton L. A comparison of motor copy and targeted feedback training techniques for restitution of upper extremity function among neurologic patients. *Phys Ther.* 1989;69:719.

Wolf S, Nacht M, Kelly J. EMG feedback training during dynamic movement for low back pain patients. *Behav Ther.* 1982;13:395.

Wolf S, Regenos E, Basmajian J. Developing strategies for biofeedback applications in neurologically handicapped patients. *Phys Ther.* 1977;57:402–408.

Yip S, Ng G. Biofeedback supplementation to physiotherapy exercise programme for rehabilitation of patellofemoral pain syndrome: a randomized controlled pilot study. *Clin Rehabil.* 2006;20(12):1050.

Wong AMK, Lee M, Chang WH, Tang F. Clinical trial of a cervical traction modality with electromyographic biofeedback. *Am J Phys Med Rehabil.* 1997;76(1):19–25.

Young M. Electromyographic biofeedback use in the treatment of voluntary posterior dislocation of the shoulder: a case study. *J Orthop Sports Phys Ther.* 1994;20(3): 173–175.

Zhang Q, Ng G. EMG analysis of vastus medialis obliquus/vastus lateralis activities in subjects with patellofemoral pain syndrome before and after a home exercise program. *J Phys Ther Sci.* 2007;19(2):131.

GLOSSARY

active electrode   An electrode attached directly to the skin over a muscle that picks up the electrical activity produced by a muscle contraction.

bandwidth   A specific frequency range in which the amplifier will pick up signals produced by electrical activity in the muscle.

biofeedback   Information provided from some measuring instrument about a specific biologic function.

bipolar arrangement   Two active recording electrodes placed in close proximity to one another.

common mode rejection ratio (CMRR)   The ability of the differential amplifier to eliminate the common noise between the active electrodes.

differential amplifier   A device that monitors the two separate signals from the active electrodes and amplifies the difference, thus eliminating extraneous noise.

electromyographic biofeedback   A therapeutic procedure that uses electronic or electromechanical instruments to accurately measure, process, and feedback reinforcing information via auditory or visual signals.

filters   Devices that help to reduce external noise that essentially make the amplifier more sensitive to some incoming frequencies and less sensitive to others.

integration   An EMG signal processing technique that measures the area under the curve for a specified period of time, thus forming the basis for quantification of EMG activity.

muscle guarding   A protective response in muscle that occurs owing to pain or fear of movement.

noise   Extraneous electrical activity that may be produced by any source other than the contracting muscle.

raw EMG   A form in which the electrical activity produced by muscle contraction may be displayed and/or recorded before the signal is processed.

rectification   A signal processing technique that changes the deflection of the waveform from the negative to the positive pole, essentially creating a pulsed direct current.

reference electrode   Also referred to as the ground electrode, serves as a point of reference to compare the electrical activity recorded by the active electrodes.

signal gain   Determines the signal sensitivity. If a high gain is chosen, the biofeedback unit will have a high sensitivity for the muscle activity signal.

smoothing   An EMG signal processing technique that eliminates the high-frequency fluctuations that are produced with a changing electrical signal.

LAB ACTIVITY

BIOFEEDBACK

DESCRIPTION

Biofeedback utilizes the body's self-generated motor unit action potentials (MUAP). These signals are recorded by surface electrodes, amplified, and then processed and converted into audio or visual signals to allow an individual to monitor various psychophysiologic processes and recognize appropriate responses.

PHYSIOLOGIC EFFECTS

Increase level of motor unit activation Decrease level of motor unit activation

THERAPEUTIC EFFECTS

Increase level of muscle activation (muscle reeducation) Decrease level of muscle activation (reduce spasticity) General body muscular relaxation

INDICATIONS

Biofeedback is primarily employed by the therapist as an adjunct in the reeducation of muscle function following injury, immobilization, or surgery or as an aid to identifying unwanted levels of muscle activity (spasticity) that may be interfering with the athlete's recovery. Sometimes biofeedback is used as a tool to assess the body's general neuromuscular status as an aid in relaxation to reduce pain and anxiety.

CONTRAINDICATIONS

• Possible skin irritation at electrode site from coupling gel or adhesives

BIOFEEDBACK			
PROCEDURE	EVALUATION		
	1	2	3
1. Check supplies.			
a. Obtain biofeedback unit, coupling gel, and tape.			
b. Insure that batteries in unit are fresh.			
2. Question patient.			
a. Verify identity of patient and review previous treatment notes.			
b. Verify the absence of contraindications.			
3. Position patient.			
a. Place patient in a well-supported, comfortable position.			

b. Select and expose appropriate muscle or group to monitor.			
c. Drape patient to preserve patient's modesty, and protect clothing, but allow access to muscle or group.			
4. Select appropriate electrode.			
5. Prepare the electrode site.			
a. Clean the skin surface with alcohol or soap and water.			
6. Apply the electrodes.			
a. Secure with tape or wrap.			
7. Explain the procedure to patient.			
8. Begin the indicated procedure.			
a. Muscle reeducation			
i. Adjust unit to lowest threshold (µV) that picks up any activity (MUAPs).			
ii. Adjust audio and visual feedback.			
iii. Have patient contract target muscle to produce maximum audio and visual feedback.			
iv. Facilitate target muscle contraction as necessary by tapping, stroking, or contracting opposite like muscle.			
v. When maximum feedback is obtained for selected threshold, advance threshold and attempt again.			
vi. Advance muscle or limb to other positions.			
vii. Continue muscle contractions for 10–15 minutes per training session or until maximal muscle activation is obtained.			
b. Spasticity inhibition			
i. Adjust unit to sensitivity threshold (µV) that picks up maximal activity (MUAPs).			
ii. Adjust audio or visual feedback.			
iii. Have patient relax target muscle to produce minimum audio or visual feedback.			
iv. Facilitate target muscle relaxation as necessary by tapping, stroking, or contracting opposite like muscle.			
v. When minimum feedback is obtained for selected threshold, reduce threshold and attempt relaxation again.			
vi. Advance muscle or limb to other functional positions.			
vii. Continue muscle relaxation for 10–15 minutes per training session or until muscle relaxation is obtained.			
viii. Complete the treatment.			

9. Remove the electrodes.			
a. Thoroughly clean electrode site.			
b. Record results of session.			
c. Assess treatment efficacy.			
10. Instruct the patient in any indicated exercise.			
11. Return equipment to storage after cleaning.			

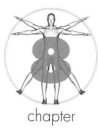

chapter

Principles of Electrophysiologic Evaluation and Testing

John Halle and David Greathouse

OBJECTIVES

Following completion of this chapter, the student will be able to:

➤ Define and describe the anatomic and physiologic basis of clinical electrophysiologic testing (neural conduction and electromyographic [EMG] studies).

➤ Given a patient with a neuromuscular dysfunction, evaluate the appropriateness of requesting clinical electrophysiologic testing (neural conduction and electromyographic studies), and describe the specific additional information that would be provided by this testing, if ordered.

➤ Describe the basic role of each of the following pieces of equipment in routine electrophysiologic testing: electrodes (needle, reference, and ground), differential amplifiers, oscilloscope, audio speakers, stimulator, electrophysiologic processing unit, and printer.

➤ Discuss why nerve conduction studies (NCS) assess both sensory and motor fibers within a nerve, the information obtained from these tests, and the reason why sensory studies are typically assessed in microvolts, while motor studies are typically assessed in millivolts.

➤ Explain the role of latency, shape, amplitude, and nerve conduction velocity (NCV) in a NCS. Within this explanation, compare and contrast the information provided by normal and abnormal findings.

➤ Describe a "central conduction study" (F-wave) physiologically and the information provided by this portion of the examination.

➤ An H-wave (**Hoffman's reflex**) can only be elicited in select sites in the upper and lower extremities. Explain why this testing procedure cannot be applied universally, identify the specific regions where this test is appropriate, and discuss the additional information that it provides to the clinical electrophysiologist.

➤ Identify the type of nerve conduction evaluation that is particularly useful with conditions affecting the neuromuscular junction, such as myasthenia gravis and Lambert–Eaton syndrome. For each of these conditions, describe the anticipated neurophysiologic results.

➤ List and describe the four basic components of the electromyographic study (needle evaluation) outlined in this chapter. Within the description, identify the type of information that can be obtained from each component.

➤ While pathologic states often represent conditions that cause some damage to both myelin and axons, the pattern of damage is often predominantly demyelinating or axonal. Compare and contrast the electrophysiologic findings demonstrated in a primarily demyelinating condition (e.g., entrapment syndrome such as carpal tunnel syndrome) with a primarily axonal condition (e.g., radiculopathy).

➤ Compare and contrast anterior primary rami (APR) and posterior primary rami (PPR). Include in your discussion the anatomic and functional differences of the APR and PPR. In addition, discuss the importance of performing needle EMG examination of the paravertebral muscles (PVM) in a patient with a suspected radiculopathy.

➤ Describe the specific electrophysiologic parameters associated with positive sharp waves (PSWs) and fibrillation potentials, and discuss what these abnormal spontaneous electrical potentials represent physiologically.

➤ Given a patient who is suspected of having a myopathic disease (e.g., dermatomyositis), describe the type of electrophysiologic findings that would be present if this muscle disease was validated.

➤ The EMG obtained from single motor units provides indirect information regarding the status of structures such as the axon, neuromuscular junction, and innervated muscle fibers. Recognizing that there is variability inherent in the shape of single motor unit EMG, describe what constitutes abnormal findings in terms of phases, the prevalence of increased phases, and the implications of other waveform alterations such as nascent potentials.

➤ List and discuss four potential limitations associated with electrophysiologic testing.

➤ Explain the purpose of somatosensory evoked potential (SEP) testing and the additional data that this form of testing can provide.

➤ Discuss the relative sensitivity and specificity for routine electrophysiologic tests for entrapment neuropathies, radiculopathies, and polyneuropathies.

➤ Given electrophysiologic test results (neural conduction and electromyographic studies), describe how this information could be used to assist in diagnosis, tailor treatment plans, and guide patient prognosis.

INTRODUCTION

Patients are referred to an electrophysiologic specialist (ES) when their signs and symptoms suggest dysfunction involving the function of nerves, the neuromuscular junction, or muscle fibers. Function is stressed since neurophysiologic testing involves the direct assessment of how this portion of the peripheral nervous system (PNS) and its component parts work. A metaphor that can be used to illustrate nerve conduction studies (NCS; a portion of the electrophysiologic examination) is the following. Everyone has had the experience of turning a faucet on at a house and then going to the other end of the hose, squeezing the nozzle, and for whatever reason, not having the appropriate amount of water, or the appropriate pressure, be expressed from the nozzle to wash the car. When that happens, the individual looks back along the hose to determine if there is a problem at the faucet, or if there is a kink or tear in the hose, or if some other problem is limiting the flow of water. In a very general way, starting an action potential (AP) at one point along a nerve, and then assessing parameters associated with its conduction such as speed (nerve conduction velocity [NCV]), or size (amplitude), permits the ES to make direct determinations about the function of the nerve and the axons that make up that nerve. If the test also involves the neuromuscular junction and muscle fibers, similar determinations can be made about the way that they are working. Other procedures, such as the use of a needle electrode during the electromyographic (EMG) portion of the examination, allow the ES to make judgments regarding the function of individual muscle fibers and align any observed abnormalities with what is known about specific diseases. Through this type of direct measurement of the function of structures such as the nerve and the axons that make up the nerve, the neuromuscular junction, and muscle fibers, information regarding the integrity of each of these components is obtained. This type of testing may be sufficient to stand alone and identify a patient's dysfunction, or it may be used in collaboration with other diagnostic procedures to make a diagnosis. Common procedures that are used in association with electrophysiologic testing are x-rays or magnetic resonance imaging (MRI), which provide a "picture" of the structures that can be identified with each of these procedures. Thus, electrophysiologic testing assesses function, and other procedures such as MRIs image the structures in the region at one moment in time. Through the collaborative use of these evaluative methodologies that look at different aspects of specific structures, precise diagnoses can often be made.

Most electrophysiologic testing is the result of a referral requesting additional information on the function of neuromuscular structures as outlined above. In these situations where additional clarification is required, electrophysiologic testing is performed in association with an excellent physical examination. The physical examination is stressed as a key element obtained prior to electrophysiologic testing because it forms the basis for the subsequent assessment performed during electrophysiologic testing for neuromuscular problems. As such, the role that electrophysiologic testing takes is somewhat analogous to an ordered MRI examination or some other procedure that assists in forming the medical diagnosis. Electrophysiologic testing potentially provides objective findings that are used to corroborate or refute the working hypothesis developed from the initial subjective and physical examination. When coupled with a good physical examination, this form of testing often permits clear identification of the specific neuromuscular problem and provides insight regarding the mechanisms associated with findings such as numbness or weakness.[1-3] Additionally, the initial physical examination and detailed history dictate the key elements that will be evaluated during the electrophysiologic examination. To an extent, each electrophysiologic evaluation is customized to the needs of the individual being evaluated, based on the findings presented during the history and physical examination.

The electrophysiologic testing referred to above typically consists of some combination of three procedures: (1) **NCS**, (2) **EMG**, and (3) somatosensory evoked potentials (**SEPs**).[2] NCS basically evaluate the function of peripheral nerves, the neuromuscular junction, and the collective muscle fibers innervated by the nerve being examined. These studies look at elements such as the speed of conduction and the size of the collective AP generated to make a determination about the health of the aforementioned structures.[4,5]

The EMG examination evaluates the electrical activity of the muscles and the muscle APs monitored from a small sample of muscle fibers through the use of a small gauge needle electrode inserted into a specific muscle. While more detail will be provided later, this portion of the electrophysiologic examination monitors the muscle at rest and during various states of voluntary contraction, and evaluates the overall function of the muscle fibers located near the tip of the needle.[6,7] From the shape, size, duration, and presence or absence of the muscle APs generated, judgments can be made on the health or dysfunction of both the nerves that innervate these muscle fibers and the muscle itself.[8,9] The combination of NCS and EMG testing provides an excellent way of directly evaluating the PNS and its constituent parts. While an excellent evaluative tool for the PNS, the two procedures listed above have limited utility for evaluating the brain and spinal cord, or central nervous system (CNS).[10] Since not all pathologies are isolated to the PNS, the third procedure of SEPs has some capability of evaluating elements of the CNS such as specific tracts within the spinal cord.[11–13] Apart from specialized electrophysiologic testing practices, however, the vast majority of electrophysiologic testing is limited to the first two procedures outlined, the NCS and the EMG. Most electrophysiologic evaluations are limited to the PNS and the constituent parts of a motor unit that include the anterior horn cell and one or more synapses located between **afferent** and **efferent** neurons, which are technically part of the CNS.[14,15]

ELECTROPHYSIOLOGIC TESTING EQUIPMENT AND SETUP

After obtaining the patient history and performing the physical evaluation, the electrophysiologic examination is constructed to evaluate any suspected areas of neuromuscular dysfunction. To perform this portion of the examination, specialized equipment is required that permits the objective evaluation of nerves, neuromuscular junctions, muscle fibers, and other elements associated with the PNS. The basic elements of this type of a system are electrodes (to couple to the patient), differential amplifiers (to boost the signal), a way to monitor the signal generated (an oscilloscope to see the signal and/or speakers to hear the signal), a processing unit of some type (typically a computer or laptop that has word processing capabilities), and a way of eliciting a response from a patient (a stimulus electrode capable of stimulating the patient or a needle electrode inserted into the muscle and monitored during insertion, at rest, and during a voluntary contraction).[16] This "system" is then combined with a printer so that reports can be generated, and if desired, examples of particular findings can be recorded and placed into the patient's records (Figure 8–1).

Electrodes

From patients' perspective, this is the part of the equipment that they actually come into contact with during a NCV study (Figure 8–2). There are three electrodes that are attached to the individual:

1. active (pickup) electrode;
2. reference electrode;
3. ground electrode—filters out background noise (Figure 8–2A).

The electrodes are typically reusable with silver/silver chloride contacts that are coupled to the patient with an electrode gel that decreases the resistance across the skin and is taped into place, or disposable electrodes that are pregelled, and self-adhesive. In either case, the skin must be clean and free of any agents that would create a barrier to the transfer of an electrical signal (such as hand lotion).

Specific types of electrodes for NCV studies are:

1. sensory ring electrodes (Figure 8–2B);
2. stimulation electrodes (Figure 8–2C);

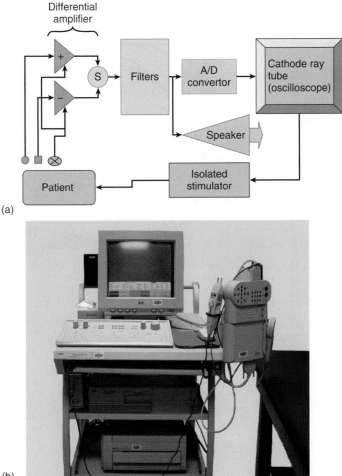

(a)

(b)

Figure 8–1. Component parts of a typical electrophysiologic evaluation system. (A) Schematic illustration. (B) Photograph of an electrophysiologic system used with patients.

3. bar electrodes (Figure 8–2D);

4. clip.

Specific types of electrodes for EMG studies are:

1. Monopolar needle electrode—a thin wire electrode, often coated with Teflon or some other material to insulate all areas except the tip that remains active (able to conduct a signal).

2. Concentric or coaxial needle electrode—this typically produces a smaller AP than a monopolar needle electrode. This type of needle is sometimes referred to as a "bipolar electrode," since the active and reference electrodes are both built into one single needle; the gauge of the needle is larger in these concentric needle electrodes than in a monopolar electrode. In this chapter, all references made will be for monopolar electrodes.

Note: There may be some mixing and matching because a monopolar electrode can be used as an active electrode for a deep muscle or as a stimulation electrode for a deeply placed nerve. Thus, the electrodes should not be thought of as having only one function by design—rather, their description should be based on the way they are being used.

Amplifier

The electrodes are plugged into amplifiers that take a very small signal and magnify it. The first amplifier is called a preamplifier, and it is the unit that the electrode leads are plugged into. This signal is then sent to the main amplifier that is part of the basic unit (used to convert

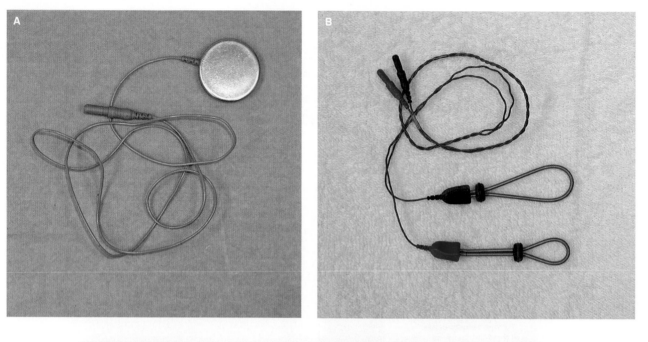

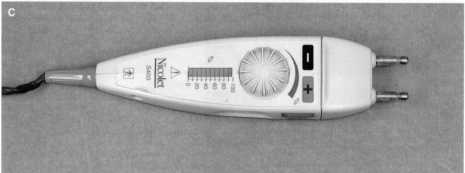

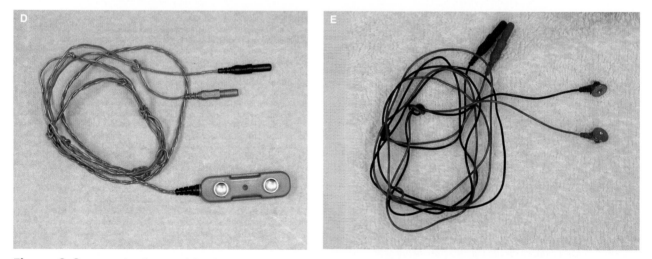

Figure 8–2. Example of some of the electrode types used during electrophysiologic testing. (A) Ground electrode. (B) Sensory ring electrode. (C) Stimulation electrode (probe). (D) Bar electrode. (E) Disk electrode.

a low voltage potential to a higher voltage signal). The preamplifier is functionally a "differential amplifier," which will subtract out the portions of the signal that are common to both the active and reference electrodes.

Visual Feedback (Oscilloscope)

The signal is monitored (viewed) through the use of an oscilloscope. This displays the evoked potentials (a form either of AP moving across the surface of the muscle or of a segment of a nerve), or the motor unit action potentials (MUAP) generated from individually contracting muscle fibers. Since the signals generated vary in size depending on the type of test being performed, the oscilloscope has the capability of changing its gain (sensitivity setting) and also altering the sweep speed of the signal. This ability to adjust the vertical and horizontal aspects of the signal allows the evaluator to optimally view whatever type of signal is elicited. In addition to displaying the signal, modern oscilloscopes (linked with the base unit) are also capable of storing the signal for a more detailed examination, or computing a given characteristic associated with the signal such as summing and averaging small signals to create a more defined response.

Auditory Feedback (Speakers)

During the EMG portion of the examination, speakers are also used to monitor the signal for the benefit of both the patient and the evaluator. For patients, the sound emitted from the speakers provides direct feedback on whether they are relaxed or not. There are times during the examination when patients need to relax completely, and they can "hear" if this is being accomplished by noting when the speakers go quiet. There are other times when they are asked to contract mildly or strongly, and again, the magnitude of the sound generated gives patients direct "biofeedback" on their performance of these tasks. The evaluator, on the other hand, uses the sound in all the ways mentioned above plus uses it to identify particular findings. While intended to only illustrate an example or two and not provide a complete summary, sound can be used to identify spontaneous electrophysiologic potentials at rest such as **positive sharp waves** (PSWs; an indicator of muscle fiber irritability and suggestive of denervation),[17] or document that not all of the motor units are firing during a maximal volitional contraction (suggesting loss of motor units in that particular muscle). Thus, the addition of this form of acoustic monitoring to the evaluation provides a much better characterization of the signal and enhances the ability to identify abnormal findings.

Testing Units

The items listed above (electrodes, amplifiers, oscilloscope, speakers) are all interfaced with some type of primary unit that has the hardware and software needed to perform the specific tests performed. While there are many variations on this theme, the two basic types of units are standalone workstations on wheels that are used in one facility or portable laptop units that can easily travel to many locations. In both cases, the computer screen functions as the oscilloscope during the examination and then serves as a word processor screen for report generation. Regardless of the size of the unit and whether it is relatively fixed or portable, it will remain capable of performing the majority of evaluations required for this type of testing. As is the case with any piece of equipment, the more expensive, dedicated workstations may have some additional options that are useful in a specialized practice or speed the ability to collect data for a given type of electrophysiologic test. Having said that, all of these units integrate the operation of the electrode signals, amplifiers, filters, etc., to provide a means of monitoring the signal generated from the patient.

Eliciting an Action Potential

With all the equipment in place and attached to the patient, a response needs to be elicited on which a judgment can be rendered. For the nerve conduction portion of the evaluation, an AP is initiated by a stimulus electrode with a trigger (on–off switch). The stimulus electrode also has two probes: one that is the active probe or cathode and one that is the passive probe or anode. The cathode is the negative pole that is placed over the course of the nerve. The anode is the positive pole of the stimulator and with a stimulus, also placed along the nerve's course but away from the active electrode. Electrical current flows between the two poles. Functionally, the cathode depolarizes the nerve while the tissue in the region of the anode becomes hyperpolarized.[18-20]

This handheld stimulus electrode is placed along the course of the nerve with the cathode located toward the previously attached active pickup electrode, and the trigger is activated that creates a monophasic square wave stimulus. The goal of this stimulation is to create a sudden and rapid alteration in the resting membrane potential of the nerve being evaluated, and bring all axons of that nerve to threshold (e.g., generate an AP).[21] For most procedures, the intensity of the stimulus is adjusted until it is clear that a supramaximal stimulus has been delivered. A supramaximal stimulus is needed to ensure that all the axons contained within a given peripheral nerve are being stimulated, so that the obtained results are both reproducible and representative of the capabilities of that peripheral nerve.[21]

It should be noted at this point that when an external electrical stimulus is introduced to a patient, the manner by which APs are generated is not the same as those APs occurring volitionally. Normally, when the CNS activates a voluntary contraction, we recruit motor units and their associated axons from small to large. This has come to be known as the **Henneman size principle**[22-25] and basically is the application of Ohm's law of *electromotive force = current multiplied by resistance*. Simply stated, smaller cell bodies and their smaller-diameter axons have higher resistance than large axons. A crude analogy is looking at the diameter of two straws and the resistance generated in sucking a thick fluid through the straws. A small-diameter straw will generate much more resistance (harder to suck the fluid) than a larger-diameter straw. Applying this crude analogy to nerve diameters, current flows most easily (least resistance) through large-diameter axons.[26] Thus, the smaller cell bodies with smaller-diameter axons and higher resistance will experience a greater change in electromotive force (voltage) and reach threshold easier. This is due to the equation above that illustrates that current multiplied by a relatively higher resistance (than a large cell body and axon with less resistance) will have a greater voltage change. As a result, small motor neurons such as those associated with type I muscle fibers, or slow twitch muscle fibers, are activated first during voluntary contraction.[22]

This is not what occurs when electricity is applied externally, such as with a handheld stimulus electrode used in nerve conduction testing. In this case, current simply flows down the paths of least resistance, which are the larger-diameter axons assuming that all axons are at the same depth. While this is not completely accurate since an axon located on the periphery of a nerve may be exposed to a slightly greater level of current, the principle holds for the most part.[21,26] Thus, with external stimulation, current flows to the largest axons first causing them to depolarize, and the overall recruitment is now from the largest axons to the smallest. The only way to fully activate the peripheral nerve and achieve stimulation of all the axons associated with a given nerve is to supramaximally stimulate the nerve. This is verified by increasing the stimulus intensity until the compound AP does not get larger with higher levels of stimulus. The signal thus generated should be both reproducible and representative of the collective ability of that nerve to conduct. This level of stimulation is known as supramaximal stimulation, and it is the level used for most procedures where stimulation is required. Additionally, it should be noted that this level will vary from individual to individual based on issues such as intervening adipose tissue, connective tissue, musculature, and so on. Thus, the stimulation electrode needs to be adjusted to the appropriate level for each patient evaluated.

When monitoring the response from a patient during the EMG portion of the examination, electrical stimulation is not used. This is because the purpose of the EMG examination is to assess muscle fibers individually, and later collectively, during states of rest and during voluntary contraction from mild to maximal. Due to this focus, no external stimulation is required. Instead, a reference pad electrode is placed on or near the muscle of interest, and a small gauge needle is inserted into the muscle. The differential amplifier detects any APs traveling across the muscle fibers in the immediate vicinity of the tip of the needle and conveys that signal to the oscilloscope and acoustic speakers. This permits evaluation of the status of the muscle while the needle is being inserted, at rest, and during varying states of voluntary contraction. To ensure a representative sample, because this area of muscle evaluated is very small around the tip of the needle, the needle is gently moved approximately a dozen times to collect information from a variety of muscle fibers during the state of rest, or complete muscle relaxation. A normal response at rest is a brief change in potential associated with the needle movement that resolves back to the rest state within 230 milliseconds.[27–29] Failure of rapid reestablishment of a normal rest state, or unexpected activity during insertion or during the voluntary contraction part of the examination, is an indicator that some type of dysfunction may be present. Further elaboration on what is expected within each of phase of the typical EMG evaluation (insertion, rest, and voluntary activation) is provided in the section "The Electromyographic Examination."

Generating a Record

The final piece of equipment associated with this type of system is a printer. All the printer does is provide a means by which the report generated can be recorded on paper and placed in the patient's records. Depending on the algorithms used by various manufacturers, some of the reports generated simply provide numerical summaries of the data collected, while others output representative waveforms to the printer that are integrated into the report. Regardless of the form generated by a given manufacturer, the printer provides a mechanism for a hard copy that can be placed in the patient's records and is the primary means of communicating back to the referring health care provider.

EVALUATION OF THE PERIPHERAL NERVOUS SYSTEM

The two primary examination procedures of NCS and EMG are designed to evaluate the component parts of the PNS. To provide a common reference point, a typical spinal nerve will be used as a model to discuss the PNS (Figure 8–3).

The entire nervous system is artificially divided into two primary components: (1) the CNS that consists of the brain and spinal cord and (2) the PNS that consists of everything else.[14] This is an artificial designation since the two portions work seamlessly together to provide overall neural function for an individual. While useful both conceptually and descriptively, the fact that this is a classification scheme without a clear border between these two systems is seen when examining the motor component of peripheral nerves. The cell bodies

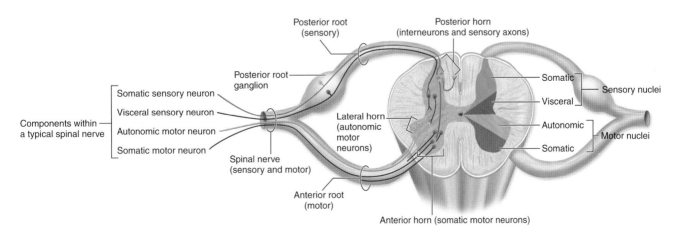

Figure 8–3. Spinal cord cross-section with roots and primary rami identified.

for these motor axons lie within the ventral horn of the spinal cord and are technically part of the CNS[30] (Figure 8–3A). This alpha motor neuron cell body directly influences the generation of APs that travel along motor axons of the PNS. Two examples illustrate how this specific portion of the CNS (the anterior horn cell) can be evaluated by NCS and EMG testing. First, if the anterior horn cell is diseased and dies, the motor axon associated with it also dies. In this case, that axon will not be able to conduct a signal, and if this has occurred to a large number of anterior horn cells, the size (amplitude) of the compound motor AP assessed following an externally applied stimulus will be decreased. Second, the EMG evaluation will also be able to identify anterior horn cell loss by abnormal spontaneous potentials associated with muscle fibers that have lost their normal nerve innervation. The presence of these abnormal spontaneous potentials can occur with the loss of fewer anterior horn cells than are needed to see a drop in the size of the compound motor unit action potential (CMAP), so the EMG is a more sensitive procedure for this type of problem. In any case, these two examples illustrate that while the NCS and EMG procedures most commonly used are described as capable of testing only the PNS, there are select elements of the CNS such as the alpha motor neurons that can also be evaluated.

Two other terms need to be introduced because they relate directly to the ability of peripheral nerves to function as these nerves are assessed with electrodiagnostic testing.[118] The first is **demyelination**, and it is related to some type of damage to the myelin sheath that is synthesized by Schwann cells. Myelinated nerves conduct an AP via saltatory (node to node) conduction at a faster rate than nonmyelinated nerves. When myelin is damaged, regardless of the causative agent, the speed by which an AP can travel down an axon is reduced. Therefore, demyelinating conditions result in a slowed conduction velocity, in both afferent and efferent axons. Two conditions that may have a significant demyelinating component are longstanding diabetes mellitus and carpal tunnel syndrome. The second major type of problem is an **axonopathy**. An axonopathy is found when a portion of the potential pools of axons available no longer functions. In this case, the speed of conduction is largely preserved, since the remaining axons conduct normally. What is affected is the amplitude of the summed synchronous depolarization of the muscle fibers innervated by the depolarized nerve and the stability of the sarcolemma of the muscle fibers. The decreased stability of the muscle membrane is the earliest finding, with abnormal spontaneous electrical activity to needle EMG that was described in the preceding paragraph. After significant axonal loss has occurred, a smaller sensory nerve action potential (SNAP) or CMAP amplitude will be observed in the response to stimulation of a motor or sensory nerve. The previously mentioned loss of anterior horn cells with the subsequent loss of axons is one example of an axonopathy. As will be seen in the subsequent sections, many of the dysfunctions encountered will have demyelinating components, characteristics of axonopathy, or some combination of both.

ANATOMY OF THE SPINAL NERVE AND NEUROMUSCULAR JUNCTION

Starting at the periphery and working proximally, the typical spinal nerve consists of the following elements (Figure 8–4): (1) specialized sensory receptor that functions as a transducer to transform one type of energy (e.g., touch, temperature, pain, etc.) into a sensory AP, (2) at least one synapse within the CNS that links the afferent neuron to efferent neurons, (3) the alpha motor neurons located in the anterior (ventral) horn of the spinal cord and their respective axons in the PNS, (4) the neuromuscular junction, and (5) the muscle fibers innervated by the nerve being investigated.[30]

The sensory neuron is functionally a combination of the specialized sensory receptor and the afferent axon or first-order neuron with its cell body located in the posterior (dorsal) root ganglion—as such, they will be considered together.[31] The cell body type is a pseudounipolar neuron, and it projects into the CNS where the first synapse occurs. A key point to be made here is that this afferent neuron is one cell, often with an axon over a meter in length, with the cell body representing the metabolic center of the cell. If there is any problem with the nerve

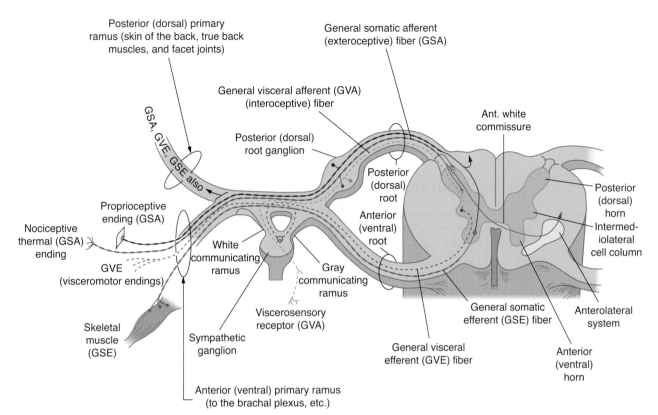

Figure 8–4. Typical spinal nerve.

anywhere along its length, the most distal aspects of the afferent neuron will normally manifest signs of the problem first.

Sensory Receptor and Size of the Axon

The specific sensory receptor associated with this receptor neuron is not really important for the NCS/EMG evaluations, apart from the fact that some receptors are linked with large-diameter axons (e.g., muscle spindles have Ia and group II fibers, both of which are large and fast conducting), and the loss of a given modality (e.g., light touch) is often what brings the patient into the clinic. The size of the afferent axon is important, however, because when an electrical signal is evoked by an external stimulus, the time measured from one point to another is only representative of the fastest conducting fibers. The large-diameter axons are the ones that are preferentially affecting this time measurement, and the speed by which impulses are conducted in humans varies tremendously, from a slow speed of approximately 0.3 m/s for unmyelinated fibers to 60–70 m/s for large, myelinated fibers.[32-34] Additionally, there are some nerves, such as the superficial radial nerve in the forearm and sural nerve in the leg, that are predominantly sensory nerves (they may also contain a few visceral motor fibers [autonomic nervous system—specifically sympathetic nervous system (SNS) fibers], but these are functionally ignored). Thus, the integrity of these afferent axons can be directly assessed through electrophysiologic testing.

Synapse

The second part needed for a reflex arc is at least one synapse that occurs within the CNS to link the afferent AP to the generation of an AP by the alpha motor neuron. The functioning of this synapse can be assessed by a procedure known as an H-reflex (to be discussed in more detail later).

Alpha Motor Neuron

The alpha motor neuron with its axon is responsible for the motor signal projected from the spinal cord to the periphery. Alpha motor neurons vary in size, with the largest neurons going to extrafusal (skeletal) muscle fibers associated with group II or fast twitch fibers. Conversely, the smallest alpha motor neurons are those that go to the group I or slow twitch fibers.[23,35] As was the case with the afferent axons, any time measurements taken due to an external stimulus are measuring only the fastest conducting fibers and thus are preferentially biased toward the axons supplying the fast twitch fibers.

Neuromuscular Junction

The neuromuscular junction is the space that links the efferent AP with the muscle fibers that it innervates. This is a chemically gated channel that has many receptors sensitive to the release of acetylcholine (ACh) embedded within a membrane with numerous folds to increase its surface area.[36] With conduction of an AP down an efferent neuron, ACh is released into the neuromuscular junction, and if sufficient in quantity, the neurotransmitter will bind with the receptor and gates will open to begin the conduction of an AP along a muscle fiber. Normally, the "quantal" release of ACh in response to an efferent AP is more than sufficient to achieve this opening of the gates on the muscle fiber and the conduction of a motor AP. However, there are conditions such as myasthenia gravis (postsynaptic problem) and Lambert–Eaton syndrome (presynaptic problem), where the neuromuscular junction can be implicated as the cause of the weakness that a patient is experiencing.[37,38]

Muscle Fiber

The muscle fibers themselves are the effector organs that the efferent fibers are acting on. When individuals volitionally contract a muscle, they are sending a signal from the CNS and activating a population of alpha motor neurons that transmit APs down the efferent axons, across the neuromuscular junction, resulting in contraction of skeletal muscle. When done through external stimulation, the process is the same except that the AP begins at the point along the nerve where stimulation is provided, and an AP travels away from that site in both directions (**orthodromic** conduction if in the direction that the axon normally conducts, and antidromic conduction if in the direction opposite that of normal AP conduction).[39,40] As mentioned earlier, because electrical current follows the path of least resistance, the largest axons are preferentially activated first and the first muscle fibers to respond to electrical stimulation are the fast twitch fibers.[23] Normally, the external activation of a nerve is done supramaximally, to attempt to activate all the muscle fibers innervated by that peripheral nerve. When supramaximal stimulation is achieved, judgments can be made regarding the entire population of muscle fibers activated.

The Elements of the Spinal Nerve

While the typical spinal nerve and its associated elements provide a good starting point to examine what can and cannot be reasonably evaluated through electrophysiologic testing, a few comments are needed. First, the typical spinal nerve represented in Figure 8–4 appears to have both afferent and efferent fibers that pass directly from or directly to the periphery, without mixing with other nerves. This may roughly be the case for the simple segmental nerves represented by the intercostal nerves of the thorax. For virtually all other afferent and efferent fibers, they are integrated through a plexus (or mixing), as is the case with the brachial, cervical, lumbar, or sacral plexuses. The examiner needs to be aware of the actual course taken by the axons being evaluated in order to be able to make potential judgments about where a problem may be occurring. Additionally, the typical spinal nerve shows two major branches traveling to the periphery, the anterior (ventral) primary rami and the posterior (dorsal) primary rami. The anterior primary rami (APR) are what supply the vast majority of the muscles and areas of cutaneous sensation for the limbs and anterior body wall, and the axons contained within them are what merge together in the various plexuses. The posterior primary rami (PPR), on the other hand, supply three structures: (1) skin of the back, (2) the true back muscles (erector spinae, transversospinalis, interspinalis, intertransversarii, and levator costarum), and (3) the facet (zygapophyseal) joints.[15] To evaluate both the APR and PPR and some of the structures innervated, muscles representative of both these regions need to be assessed. Second, the typical spinal nerve as has been drawn in Figure 8–3B has been taken from the thoracic level of the spinal cord. As such, the cell bodies associated with the presynaptic sympathetic neurons are evident in the intermediolateral cell column of the spinal cord, and the sympathetic chain ganglia are also included adjacent to the APR. This serves as a reminder that peripheral nerves contain some autonomic (e.g., SNS fibers) components, and many injuries reflect this contribution through physical manifestations such as altered sweating or skin color changes.[41,42] There are no parasympathetic nervous system fibers found in peripheral nerves of the extremities.[15] While these autonomic fibers are part of virtually every peripheral nerve, there is currently not a good way to selectively evaluate the function of these specific fibers. Therefore, the autonomic nervous system is not currently evaluated in the typical electrophysiologic test. This is an area of investigation, and in the future, it may be possible to quantify function of portions of the autonomic nervous system.[43–46]

Structurally, there are other elements of the typical spinal nerve that need to be considered that are not readily apparent from Figure 8–3. All nerves are located below the skin, either in the subcutaneous tissue (some of the cutaneous nerves) or at a deeper level. Because of the nerve's physical location, any stimulation or detection of the AP traveling across the nerve has to pass through both the skin and any fat in the region.[15] Since fat is a reasonably good insulator, this creates a potential barrier to easy stimulation or identification of the evoked response. Additionally, the collection of axons that make up a peripheral nerve is organized in a bundle. Starting at the level of the axon, the connective tissue surrounding a given axon is termed the endoneurium. A collection of axons grouped together makes up a fasciculus, the next larger layer, with the connective tissue enclosing this bundle termed the perineurium.[47] Finally, the collection of fasciculi is grouped together and surrounded by more connective tissue, termed the epineurium. Each of these connective tissue layers assists in giving the peripheral nerve strength, but they also create additional barriers to the direct electrical evaluation of the axons of interest.

TESTING PROCEDURES

Once the clinician has an understanding of the equipment and pertinent anatomy, electrophysiologic evaluation may begin. There is no particular order for this portion of the examination, with some clinicians preferring to collect NCS data prior to proceeding with the EMG evaluation that requires inserting needle electrodes into select muscles. Other clinicians prefer to determine what they can from the EMG first and use this to assist them in designing the rest of the examination. In reality, different disorders lend themselves to suggesting one element as particularly advantageous to perform first, so given clinicians may adjust the order of testing to optimize the evaluation in terms of time and the number of elements of each test that the patient is exposed to. Recognizing that the order of testing is an arbitrary choice, this overview of the basic procedures will begin with the NCS and then cover the EMG evaluation. Following this, a brief overview of the much less frequently used SEP test will be provided.

Limb Temperature and Age Considerations

The examiner performing these electrophysiologic tests additionally needs to be aware of other factors that will impact on the results obtained. Two of the most important are temperature of the limb being examined and age. Numerous studies have demonstrated that there is an inverse correlation between temperature of the region being studied and the speed of the AP.[48,49] A cold limb will conduct electrical impulses slower than a limb of normal temperature. To control for this variable, skin temperature is monitored during the examination, and if the temperature drops too low, it is warmed prior to continuing with the examination. For the upper extremities, the surface temperature of the hand should be at least 30°C, with 32°C preferred.[50] For the feet, the temperature should be at least 30°C, although these values do vary between electrophysiologic laboratories.[21,51] To promote an optimal environment for this type of testing, the room should also be maintained at a temperature of at least 25°C.[51] Due to the importance of temperature in obtaining valid results, the temperature of the limb being evaluated should be indicated on any report published. Additionally, individuals that are young (under 16) or are over 50 years of age may have APs that conduct at a speed different than adults between the ages of 18 and 50.[21,51] Most nerves mature by the age of 4, but this varies and some elements of the PNS may not be fully mature until approximately 14–16 years of age. A nerve that is not fully mature typically conducts slower than would be expected, and the normative tables that have been constructed for this younger age group take this factor into consideration. On the other end of the spectrum, individuals older than 40 years of age begin to see slight slowing in NCV. By the age of 50, this 1 or 2 m/s per decade slowing that begins over the age of 40 is enough that a separate set of normative values is available for individuals over the age of 50.[21,51] After the age of 70, the slowing becomes much more significant.[21,51] Due to the inverse correlation between aging and NCV, the aging process also needs to be factored in when performing this type of testing.

Nerve Conduction Study

The family of tests commonly performed and grouped under the label of NCS includes the following: (1) sensory nerve studies, (2) motor nerve studies, (3) reflex studies (Hoffman's reflex and central conduction studies), and (4) repetitive stimulation testing. Each of these tests has a common characteristic of stimulating a nerve with an evoked (or generated) potential, and then picking up the response at some other location. By providing a known stimulus, and knowing other factors such as the distance between the point of stimulation and the time required for the response to occur, factors such as speed of conduction and the size of the sensory or motor nerve AP can be measured.

Sensory Nerve Studies

The general premise of a sensory NCS is that the examiner is introducing an AP along a peripheral nerve and picking up that AP at a second site. APs travel in both directions from the point of stimulation. In sensory testing, if the active recording electrode is placed proximal to the point of stimulation, the conduction is orthodromic (in the direction that sensory fibers normally conduct an AP, with afferent fibers conducting toward the CNS). Conversely, if the active recording electrode is placed along the nerve distal to the point of stimulation, then the conduction is antidromic (opposite the direction that sensory fibers normally conduct an AP). In some cases an antidromically generated AP will be larger or easier to elicit than one obtained orthodromically. An orthodromic latency may be slightly shorter than one obtained antidromically; however, Dumitru and Zwarts state that antidromic and orthodromic latencies are equivalent if the distance between the active and directive electrodes is 4 cm apart.[51,52] Because there are advantages to both methods, both are options commonly used by clinical electrophysiologists, with the direction used usually noted in the written report.

The setup for a typical sensory NCS is illustrated in Figure 8–5 for an orthodromically generated AP of the two-digit-(index finger) wrist segment of the median nerve. In this case, stimulating ring electrodes have been placed on the index finger spanning the course of the nerve, with the cathode (negative pole that is responsible for depolarization of the nerve) placed proximally and the anode placed distally. At a given distance proximal to the cathode, typically 14 cm for this type of study, the active electrode is positioned on the skin of the wrist over the course of the nerve. The reference electrode is similarly placed along the course of the nerve, several centimeters proximal to the active electrode. The ground electrode is positioned on the same extremity, typically on the opposite side of the limb between the point of stimulation and point of pickup. Recall that the skin has to be clean prior to the positioning of the electrodes, and conduction gel is used to maximize conduction at the site of the stimulation.

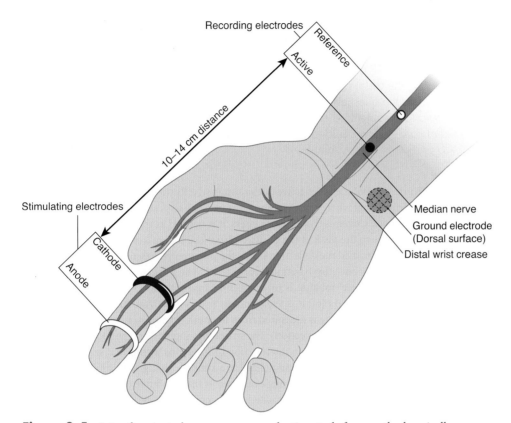

Figure 8–5. Setup for a typical sensory nerve conduction study for an orthodromically generated action potential of the two-digit-wrist segment of the median nerve. (*Source*: Ref.[53])

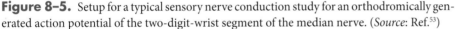

Conduction gel is also used for the other electrodes if they are reusable metal electrodes and they are taped into place. If disposable electrodes are used, then the self-adhering gel fixes the electrodes onto the extremity being tested. Recall also that other probes may also be placed on the limb, such as the surface temperature probe discussed earlier, to monitor and record the temperature of the limb at the time of testing.

When the examiner triggers or activates the stimulating electrode, a single brief monophasic square wave is created. This "electrical shock" results in a sudden and rapid alteration of the axons contained within the collective peripheral nerve being examined, resulting in some or all of those fibers being depolarized past the point of threshold. If the stimulus intensity is not sufficient to activate all of the axons, then a submaximal SNAP has been generated. Because factors such as the size of the potential are reflective of the number of axons activated, a submaximal SNAP is not what is sought. With adequate stimulus intensity, all of the axons within the nerve being investigated will be activated and a supramaximal SNAP will be obtained. Because each individual AP is "all or none," the summed responses of all the APs traveling down the peripheral nerve create a representative picture of the function of this nerve. The signal being monitored along the course of the nerve does not involve either the neuromuscular junction or the innervated muscle, so the SNAP is primarily reflective of the contribution of sensory axons because they are the largest and fastest conducting fibers.[44]

Specific parameters measured in association with a SNAP are the following (see Figure 8–6): (1) amplitude or the size of the potential, measured in microvolts, (2) shape of the AP, which is usually biphasic with a phase on each side of the baseline, (3) latency, or the time that it takes from stimulus to the response over a predetermined distance, measured in milliseconds, and (4) NCV, the speed by which a nerve conducts an AP, measured in meters per second. (Note that latency and NCV are both based on the same information, with latency reflecting a measure of time over a given distance, and NCV reflecting speed. If one is known, the other can be calculated.)

Clinical Decision-Making *Exercise 8–1*

Decreased SNAP amplitudes and slightly prolonged latencies are noted when evaluating the distal aspect of the ulnar nerve. The student observing this testing asks the question, "Does this finding solely implicate the ulnar nerve, or could the problem be originating from a more proximal location like the medial cord?" How could this be addressed electrophysiologically, using the NCS portion of the examination?

Amplitude. Amplitude is reflective of the summed APs within the peripheral nerve assessed in an environment where there is some resistance due to skin, subcutaneous tissue (fat), and connective tissue elements. For sensory fibers, it is defined as the distance from the peak of the negative phase to the peak of the positive phase (see Figure 8–6). By convention, electrophysiologists have named the deflection below the isopotential baseline as a positive deflection, while a deflection above this baseline is considered to be a negative deflection. While this positive and negative phase notation is reversed compared with the construction of a typical *y*-axis on a two-dimensional plot, it is the standard that is used. Another way of saying the same thing is that the amplitude is measured from the peak (top of the negative deflection) to the trough (peak of the positive deflection). The size of the amplitude of the SNAP provides the examiner with information regarding the function of the axons within that segment. A relatively large-amplitude SNAP is good, and charts are available that give minimum normative values for a variety of sensory nerves being evaluated. If the amplitude of the SNAP is smaller than these values, or a SNAP cannot be elicited, this suggests some type of compromise of the axons within that segment of the nerve. These amplitude values are obtained with the oscilloscope using a fairly large gain and measured in microvolts, since the size of the potential obtained from a SNAP is small when compared with the CMAP that is measured in millivolts. (For conversion, 1000 μV = 1 mV.)

Shape. Prior to discussing latency, it is necessary to clarify what is meant in the paragraph above by a waveform that is described as having one or more positive and negative phases. For a SNAP, the phase simply means that as the collective depolarizing waveform travels down the nerve, the individual axons that have been brought to threshold are conducting

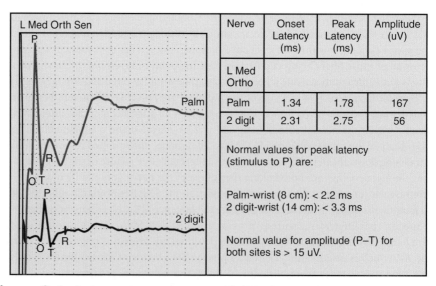

Nerve	Onset Latency (ms)	Peak Latency (ms)	Amplitude (uV)
L Med Ortho			
Palm	1.34	1.78	167
2 digit	2.31	2.75	56

Normal values for peak latency (stimulus to P) are:

Palm-wrist (8 cm): < 2.2 ms
2 digit-wrist (14 cm): < 3.3 ms

Normal value for amplitude (P–T) for both sites is > 15 uV.

Figure 8–6. Sensory nerve action potential (SNAP)—associated parameters include (a) amplitude: measured in microvolts, from peak to trough, (b) latency: measured from stimulus onset to peak of the negative potential, and (c) shape: biphasic potential with initial negative and then positive phase (small positive phase in this case) is typical.

an AP along their length. Since these axons vary in both type (myelinated and unmyelinated) and size (large axons conduct faster than similarly structured smaller-diameter axons), the cumulative waveform represents the contribution of all of the axons contained within the peripheral nerve. Recall that the site where the AP is being picked up has two electrodes in place, an active electrode (sometimes referred to as electrode-1 [E1]) and a reference electrode (sometimes referred to as electrode-2 [E2]). The reference electrode is plugged into an inverting port on the differential amplifier, so that any signal that it receives will be inverted and then added to the signal detected by the active electrode.[54] This functional subtraction of one electrode potential from the other (inverting and adding is the same as subtraction) provides a flat baseline at rest and a potential that is typically biphasic when stimulated. Prior to any stimulation, both the active and reference electrodes are measuring the nerve at rest and are at essentially the same voltage level, producing a baseline of zero volts. Immediately after the stimulus has been delivered, the resting potential of the nerve under the active and reference electrodes remains unaffected, and the isopotential line remains flat, or unchanged. With time, however, this elicited waveform will travel down the nerve, and the leading edge (fastest conducting axons) will begin to depolarize in the vicinity of the active electrode. At this moment in time, a potential difference will be observed between the electrical potentials recorded by the active and reference electrodes. As the collective waveform continues to progress down the length of the nerve, more axons will have their APs reach the active electrode and contribute to this potential electrical difference. Since the obtained SNAP measured on the oscilloscope is the difference between the active and reference electrodes (differential amplifier amplifies the difference in potential), and the reference electrode measures this collective waveform with a slight temporal delay because it is further along the nerve, a biphasic potential is generated. This biphasic potential simply reflects the potential difference between the active and reference electrodes as the collective waveform is moving under them along the course of the nerve. Normally, the initial deflection associated with a SNAP is a negative deflection, followed by a positive deflection—these two phases thus create a biphasic potential. Once the evoked waveform has moved past the two electrodes assessing any potential difference, the resting baseline of zero potential difference is reestablished. Since a given nerve's AP is approximately 0.5 millisecond in duration within the nerve and approximately 2.0–3.0 milliseconds at the surface of the skin, this is the typical duration of a SNAP.[54]

Since this SNAP is assessing simultaneously what is measured at the active and reference electrodes, the waveform could be inverted by reversing the electrode leads into the differential amplifier. While this would break with convention since measurements are typically made to the peak of the negative deflection of a SNAP (see the section "Latency"), it has been mentioned here to illustrate that the deflections are not fixed and are simply reflective of potential differences between two electrode sites. For completeness, it should also be noted that the changes in potential at any one site (either the active or reference electrode) are really physiologically triphasic within the nerve. The observed biphasic potential is a product of the differential amplifier measuring equivalent voltage changes separated temporally.[54] Thus, there may be some SNAP waveforms that have triphasic morphology, typically positive–negative–positive phase, if the reference electrode is not placed directly along the path of the nerve being assessed and the two electrodes are not measuring equivalent voltage changes.

Latency. The latency measurement associated with a SNAP is the time that it takes from a stimulus to the peak of the negative response, over a predetermined distance, measured in milliseconds (see Figure 8–6). For a number of common clinical conditions, such as a distal median neuropathy with slowing at or distal to the wrist (carpal tunnel syndrome), this may be the most sensitive and earliest indicator of a clinically significant problem.[44,55] Since the latency measurement is a given time, irrespective of the size of the individual, it is based on known distances and the normative values are available in tables.

The latency value obtained is reflective only of the function of the fastest conducting fibers (e.g., the large-diameter, myelinated fibers). Recall from the discussion above that the collective waveform contains some contribution from all of the axons that make up the nerve being examined. Since the latency is from the point of the stimulation to the peak of the negative phase of the waveform, the fastest conducting axons will be the ones that are responsible for the latency assessed. In a condition that is typified by demyelination of a nerve, such as carpal tunnel syndrome, a prolonged latency (slowing) would be observed because the large, myelinated axons will be involved. On the other hand, in a condition such as a cervical radiculopathy where select axons have been damaged somewhere along their course, but most axons have remained intact, the latency value will remain unchanged. The reason that the latency value will remain unchanged is that the intact axons still present in the nerve are conducting as fast as they ever have and this preserves the overall speed of the nerve.

These **distal sensory latencies** (DSLs) are typically obtained on the most peripheral (or distal) aspect of the nerve under investigation. The DSL may involve several segments of a sensory nerve, such as a palm to wrist segment and a digit to wrist segment of a nerve such as the median. Or, the DSL may involve simply one segment of the nerve, such as with the sural in the leg or the lateral cutaneous nerve of the forearm (lateral antebrachial cutaneous nerve). In either case, since the distal aspect of the nerve is located farthest from the cell body that lives in the posterior (dorsal) root ganglion, this segment is sensitive to either a proximal problem affecting overall neuron functioning of multiple axons or a distal problem such as peripheral compression or microcirculation ischemia. A five-digit-(little finger) wrist orthodromic stimulation setup is shown in Figure 8–7A, while an antidromic stimulation setup for the superficial branch of the radial nerve is shown in Figure 8–7B.

Nerve conduction velocity. While the most common procedure performed with sensory nerve fibers is that of DSL determination just described, there are occasionally times when a sensory NCV will be sought. An example of where this might be employed is if the examiner wanted to test the speed of conduction over a particular segment of a nerve, such as where the ulnar nerve passes under the medial epicondyle of the humerus (normally done with a motor nerve study but can be done with a sensory latency). The procedure here is similar to the setup described previously, with a stimulating electrode, active electrode, and reference electrode located along the course of the nerve, and a ground electrode located on the extremity. Stimulation is identical to what has been discussed previously. The only functional difference here is that rather than using predetermined distances for which normative latencies have been developed, the examiner creates an appropriate setup and then measures the distances between the stimulation and pickup sites. This distance is then used as the numerator, and the time from the stimulation to the peak of the negative potential is the value used in the denominator. This creates a speed (in meters per second) that can be compared against known values for peripheral nerves. Normally, nerves in the upper extremities conduct at a speed of at least 50 m/s, and nerves in the lower extremities conduct at a speed of 40 m/s or more.[50,56,57] Tables are available for more specific nerve conduction velocities for a given nerve, if desired.[57]

For illustrative purposes, a typical set of sensory nerve studies performed on a screening examination of the upper extremity might include the following: (1) palm–wrist segment and two-digit-wrist of the median nerve (orthodromic), (2) palm–wrist and five-digit-wrist of the ulnar nerve (orthodromic), and (3) forearm to wrist of the superficial radial nerve (antidromic). The two segments assessed with the median and ulnar nerve permit examination of potential entrapment at sites such as where the median nerve passes under the transverse carpal ligament, or the ulnar nerve transverses Guyon's canal, as well as note any other differences that one segment may reveal. With a single problem, such as carpal tunnel syndrome, only one nerve would be expected to be affected, in this case the median. If all of the SNAPs had prolonged latencies, however, then a more systemic problem might be suspected such as **polyneuropathy**. It should be noted that diagnostic labels such as carpal tunnel syndrome and polyneuropathy are included here as illustrative examples of what might be found in a patient that presented one of these conditions. By its nature, the neurophysiologic examination provides collaborative information that is used by the health care provider coordinating a patient's care to make a diagnosis, but by itself this type of evaluation is not diagnostic. The examples provided above of the median, ulnar, and superficial radial nerve SNAPs are just that, select examples. As has been stressed throughout this discussion, the evaluators will use their expertise and experience to select the appropriate SNAPs and other portions of the examination based on the patient's condition.

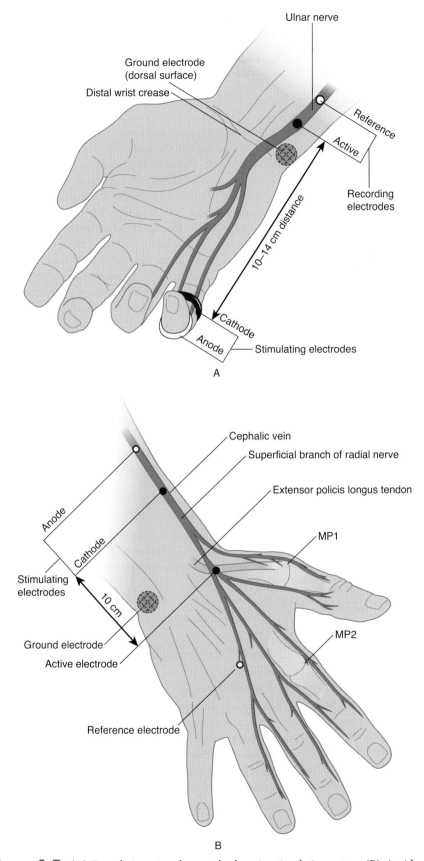

Figure 8–7. (A) Five-digit-wrist ulnar orthodromic stimulation setup. (B) Antidromic stimulation setup for the superficial branch of the radial nerve. (*Source*: Ref.[53])

CASE STUDY 8–1
ELECTROPHYSIOLOGIC TESTING

Diagnosis and Reason for Referral: Distal median neuropathy at or distal to the wrist (carpal tunnel syndrome).

Background: During the clinical examination, patients with this condition will often present with altered sensation over the palmar aspect of the thumb, index, middle, and half of the ring finger (median nerve sensory distribution) with symptoms often increasing at night. They may also have some weakness and/or atrophy of the muscles of the thenar eminence (median innervated muscles). During the NCS, both sensory and motor latencies are often slowed for the segment of the nerve distal or across the wrist (median nerve). The slowing is typically due to compression of the median nerve as it passes under the transverse carpal ligament. The compression is multifactorial in its impact, causing changes in microcirculation of the axons that collectively make up the nerve, inflammation, as well as demyelination of a segment of many of these axons.[28,42,73,87] Therefore, the slowed NCV across this segment is largely due to the loss of myelin and an interruption of the normal salutory conduction. From an electrophysiologic standpoint, this is a condition that is characterized primarily by demyelination. This demyelination mechanism will typically be reflected in the interpretation provided by the clinical electrophysiologists in their write-up.

While nerve conduction slowing across the region of compression is the typical finding in a patient with carpal tunnel syndrome, the segment of the median nerve from the wrist to the elbow is usually normal in terms of speed and size of the APs conducted. This suggests that the more proximal segment of the median nerve is unaffected. Thus, by identifying where the change in NCV is occurring and demonstrating that other segments of the nerve conduct normally, the clinical electrophysiologist has provided information that is valuable in localizing the lesion. Amplitude decrements may also be noted in association with a moderate to severe compression.

Testing Procedures and Findings: The EMG examination might find positive findings (fibrillation potentials, PSWs, dropped units, etc.) in muscles such as the APB (C8–T1, median innervated) and the opponens pollicis (C8–T1, median innervated). On further evaluation, normal EMG would be noted in the first dorsal interossei (also C8–T1), the pronator teres (C6–7, median innervated), and the other muscles innervated by the median nerve proximal to the wrist or any other terminal nerve root. The fact that changes in select muscles innervated by only the median nerve distal to the wrist are observed suggests that some axons within the median nerve have been damaged to the point where APs are no longer being conducted along their length. These findings are consistent with an axonopathy, and it is suggestive of a more severe compression than one limited to only changes in the speed of nerve

conduction. Since the physical examination, NCS findings, and EMG findings are all limited to the segment of the median nerve at or distal to the wrist, and the muscles that this segment supplies, a strong case can be made that this is the source of the patient's problem. This is further supported by other findings, such as the normal EMG with the first dorsal interossei that contains C8–T1 nerve roots similar to the thenar muscles, yet is normal because it is derived from the ulnar nerve that does not pass under the transverse carpal retinaculum. Other findings are the normal median NCV in the forearm and the normal EMG found in the pronator teres. These findings help delineate the problem and rule out alternative possibilities that could be compatible with the patient's presentation. An electrophysiologic description of these findings might be something like "moderate median neuropathy with slowing at or distal to the wrist (demyelination > axonopathy), consistent with the referring consult of carpal tunnel syndrome." The demyelination is emphasized since slowing is the primary finding in this case, with no or minimal EMG changes often encountered. Additionally, the findings are typically written in a way that is not diagnostic, but rather provides the health care professional who is responsible for coordinating the patient's care with the information that he or she needs to make a diagnosis, when viewed in light of any other special tests or procedures ordered.

Discussion Questions

- In a patient with a distal median neuropathy at or distal to the wrist (carpal tunnel syndrome), what alterations would be expected in the following parameters? Why would these be observed physiologically?
  - (a) DSL
  - (b) amplitude of the SNAP
  - (c) DML
  - (d) amplitude of the compound motor unit action potential (CMAP)
  - (e) EMG alterations
- When reading the report of this same patient, the central conduction study (F-wave) for the median nerve is slightly prolonged. What does this mean in the context of this patient and what are factors that might affect this reflex value?
- Would a Hoffman's reflex (H-wave) be appropriate for the APB muscle? Why or why not?
- What is the impact of temperature of a limb on the nerve conduction latency and NCV values obtained?
- Carpal tunnel syndrome is often described as a compression neuropathy. From a physiologic standpoint, what structure

(continued)

CASE STUDY 8-1   (continued)
ELECTROPHYSIOLOGIC TESTING

or structures are affected by this compression and how does this impact nerve function?

- Will the compression associated with a typical case of carpal tunnel syndrome have electrophysiologic findings most consistent with a demyelinating condition or an axonopathy? Why?

- The flexor pollicis longus, pronator teres, and APB are innervated by the median nerve. Assuming a moderate-to-severe case of carpal tunnel syndrome, which of these median innervated muscles would demonstrate EMG changes? Why?

- Would repetitive nerve stimulation procedures typically be used as part of the assessment of an individual with a distal median neuropathy (carpal tunnel syndrome)? Why or why not, and if not appropriate, when would this particular type of testing procedure be appropriate?

- For the patient with a distal median neuropathy (carpal tunnel syndrome) that has documented neural slowing (prolonged latencies), what additional information is provided by the finding of fibrillation potentials and PSWs in both the APB and opponens pollicis?

Other variations to sensory nerve studies

Comparison studies. The purpose of performing comparison studies in determining the presence of mononeuropathies, for example, median mononeuropathy at or distal to the wrist or carpal tunnel syndrome, is to improve the sensitivity of the NCS study while maintaining the specificity. In evaluating a patient with a suspected median mononeuropathy at or distal to the wrist, the history and physical examination findings may direct you to a compromise of the median nerve at or distal to the carpal tunnel. However, when performing the motor and sensory NCS studies, specifically distal motor latencies (DMLs) and DSLs, the values are normal. To improve on the sensitivity of the NCS examination, one would then perform comparison studies. Abnormal comparison studies would in this case be suggestive of median nerve compromise.

Clinical Decision-Making   *Exercise 8-2*

When conducting the NCS portion of the electrophysiologic examination, the first several DSLs are noted to be borderline or marginally prolonged. What parameter of testing is essential to assess, and if necessary correct, prior to coming to a conclusion that there is some type of dysfunction of the nerves being examined?

Comparison studies for determining median mononeuropathy at or distal to the wrist might include:

1. Comparing the digit 4 (D4) median DSL and the D4 ulnar DSL in the same hand. The normal difference between the D4 median and ulnar DSLs is <0.6 millisecond when the distance is equivalent for both measurements. The sensitivity for this comparison study is 77–82%.[1]

2. Comparing the digit 1 (D1) median DSL and the D1 radial DSL in the same hand. The normal difference between the D1 median and radial DSLs is <0.5 millisecond when distance is equivalent for both measurements. The sensitivity for this comparison study is 69–74%.[1]

3. Comparing the median palmar DSL and the ulnar palmar DSL in the same hand. The normal difference between the median and ulnar palmar DSLs is <0.5 millisecond when distance is equivalent for both measurements, usually 8 cm. The sensitivity for this comparison study is 61%.[1]

4. Comparing the median digit (D2) DSL and the ulnar digit (D5) DSL in the same hand. The normal difference between the median and ulnar digit DSLs is <0.5 millisecond when the distance is equivalent for both measurements, usually 14 cm.[1]

While the above demonstrated strictly comparison studies for sensory nerve studies (typically DSLs) that would implicate the median nerve, other comparison studies can be done for other nerves or with techniques that involve DMLs. An example of a comparison study involving a DML is comparing the median DML to the ulnar DML in the same hand (see the section "Motor Nerve Studies"). The normal difference between the median and ulnar DMLs is <1.0 millisecond, when the distance is equivalent for both measurements, usually 8 cm.[1] Comparison studies may also be performed comparing the DML or DSL values of the involved hand and the uninvolved hand (e.g., right median DML compared with the left median DML). Van Dijk et al state that two or more comparison studies must be abnormal to determine an early mononeuropathy.[58]

Clinical Decision-Making   *Exercise 8–3*

The electrophysiologist is attempting to assess the DSL of the lateral cutaneous nerve of the thigh (LCNT; old name: lateral femoral cutaneous nerve). One common antidromic technique is to stimulate the nerve as it crosses under the inguinal ligament, 1–2 cm medial to the anterior iliac spine. Pickup and reference electrodes are typically located along the course of the nerve 12–14 cm distal to the stimulation site. It is not uncommon, particularly in an overweight individual, to not be able to achieve adequate stimulation of this rather deeply situated nerve. What can the electrophysiologist do to increase his or her chance of eliciting this sensory nerve?

Near-nerve stimulation techniques. As is the case with any evaluative technique, for those cases that are not technically easy to obtain, there are additional ways to obtain the information provided by SNAPs. For example, some nerves are located more deeply in the body (e.g., lateral cutaneous nerve of the thigh [LCNT]) and may need to be stimulated through a needle electrode placed in the vicinity of the nerve. This is called a "near-nerve" stimulation technique. When this is done, other factors may be taken into consideration, such as the rise time of the SNAP, which is defined as the time from the deviation of the waveform from baseline to the peak of the negative potential. The slope of this line is used to determine how close the needle is to the deeply situated nerve, with the steepest slope possible desired.[57] While the basic premise of the obtained SNAP is similar to what has been described previously, a full description of this and other more specialized techniques that can be used when performing more advanced studies is beyond the scope of this text. For further information on these specialized procedures, the interested reader is referred to the excellent electrodiagnostic texts of Oh,[59] Kimura,[2] and Dumitru et al.[1]

Motor Nerve Studies

A second major piece of the NCS is to assess the combined function of the nerve, neuromuscular junction, and the muscle fibers innervated by the available axons. The latencies for these motor NCS are typically a little longer than those for a SNAP, given the same distance, due to several factors. First, the AP recorded here has to cross the neuromuscular junction and this takes a small amount of time, on the order of 0.5–1.0 millisecond.[60] Then, the AP has to spread across the muscle fiber and this is relatively slow, on the order of 3–5 m/s.[61,62] This is added to the fact that the absolutely fastest conducting axons are sensory (e.g., Ia axons associated with muscle spindles), and while the large motor axons conduct functionally at a high speed, they are not quite as fast as the largest sensory fibers.[63,64] Consequently, while a typical DSL latency at a distance of 8 cm would be 2.2 milliseconds (median nerve), the same DML at a distance of 8 cm would be approximately 4.2 milliseconds.[50]

Another clear difference between a sensory potential and a motor potential is the size of the obtained response. As was alluded to earlier, the motor response obtained from the motor nerve studies is relatively large, measured in millivolts. Compare this with the typical SNAP response, measured in microvolts, where a normal response might be only 5 or 10 µV in amplitude. Thus, the motor response may easily be 1000 times larger than that obtained with a SNAP, requiring different sensitivity settings on the oscilloscope when the motor nerve studies are being performed. The size difference is due to the summed APs moving across the surface of all the muscle fibers activated by the triggered response, known as the CMAP.[17]

A third basic difference is the variety of structures that can be either directly or indirectly assessed. While sensory nerve studies permitted evaluation of a segment of the afferent fibers of a nerve to be evaluated, motor nerve studies can be used to assess efferent fiber function in a nerve, the neuromuscular junction, innervated muscle fibers, and the overall status of the full length of the nerve or of the typical reflex arc (abridged list). The last two items of examining the entire length of the nerve or the reflex arc are tested by central conduction studies (F-waves) and the Hoffman's reflex, respectively. These two procedures will be covered at the end of this section, after discussing the main elements sought in the basic motor nerve study.

The premise for obtaining a CMAP is analogous to what was done when eliciting a SNAP. Stimulation will still occur with a stimulating electrode placed along the course of the nerve, with the cathode and anode located along the course of the nerve and the cathode located distally (e.g., closest to the muscle being stimulated). A ground electrode is also used when performing motor nerve studies, and it is placed on the same limb to minimize background noise. The key difference here is that the active (pickup) electrode is ideally placed on the skin over the motor point, the site where the nerve enters the muscle and usually located near the center of the muscle. The reference electrode is placed several centimeters away from it in an area that typically will not conduct as well as at the active site.[17] This setup, demonstrated in Figure 8–7, has the cathode of the hand stimulator and the active electrode located in line with each other and the respective anode and reference electrodes away from the middle of the assembly.[57] As was the case with the SNAP, the active electrode is coupled with the noninverting port of the differential amplifier and the reference electrode is attached to the inverting port. Due to the differential amplifier, the obtained CMAP (Figure 8–8) observed on the oscilloscope following an adequate stimulation is the difference in voltage between the two electrodes (e.g., active—reference).[57]

With a supramaximal stimulus similar to that used with the SNAP, all of the muscle fibers innervated by the nerve under investigation should be activated, and a muscle contraction should occur under the active electrode. The CMAP thus obtained will provide on the oscilloscope a representative picture of the synchronous depolarization of the muscle fibers innervated by the depolarized nerve. Additionally, this CMAP is reflective of the collective state of the motor axons contained in the nerve under investigation, the neuromuscular junction, and the collective muscle fibers innervated. Specific elements that are examined in relation to the evoked motor potential are: (1) latency, measured in milliseconds from the time of the stimulus to the initial onset of the AP; (2) amplitude, measured in millivolts and representing the sum of all the muscle fibers recruited assessed from onset to peak; (3) rise time, measured in milliseconds, representing the time that it takes to "rise" from the initial deflection to the negative peak; (4) duration, measured in milliseconds and reflecting the time that it takes from initial departure from baseline to reestablishment of baseline; (5) shape, which is usually biphasic; and (6) the calculation of NCV along the length of the nerve under investigation.

Clinical Decision-Making   *Exercise 8–4*

During the motor portion of the NCS, it is expected that the compound motor unit action potential (CMAP) will have a "negative" initial deflection. If the observed deflection is in the "positive" direction, what can be done?

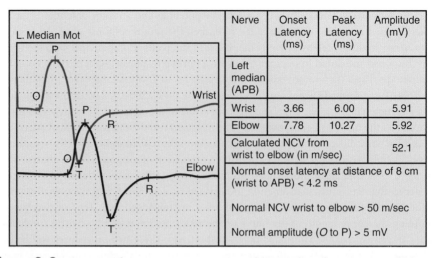

Nerve	Onset Latency (ms)	Peak Latency (ms)	Amplitude (mV)
Left median (APB)			
Wrist	3.66	6.00	5.91
Elbow	7.78	10.27	5.92
Calculated NCV from wrist to elbow (in m/sec)			52.1
Normal onset latency at distance of 8 cm (wrist to APB) < 4.2 ms			
Normal NCV wrist to elbow > 50 m/sec			
Normal amplitude (O to P) > 5 mV			

Figure 8–8. Compound motor unit action potential (CMAP), with parameters of (a) onset latency: from stimulus to take-off of negative phase of the CMAP, (b) amplitude: measured in millivolts from onset (O) to peak of negative phase of the CMAP (P), and (c) shape: typical biphasic shape with initial negative phase (reflected here). (*Source*: Ref.[53])

Latency. The latency is a particularly valuable variable because it provides information on the speed of conduction of the efferent axons innervating the muscle under the active electrode. It is defined as the time from the stimulus to the initial departure from baseline over a known distance, which should be in the direction of a negative phase if the electrodes are properly positioned. Because this is typically done with muscles located at the distal extent of the nerve under investigation, these latencies are referred to as DML. For each nerve investigated, there are normative charts available with predetermined distances and maximal normal DML values. For example, the setup for a median nerve DML is shown in Figure 8–10. In this case, the distance between the active electrode and the cathode of the hand stimulator is 8 cm, measured anatomically along the course of the nerve along a direct straight line linking the two points. The normal DML for the median nerve is less than 4.2 milliseconds measured at a distance of 8 cm.[54] If the latency is longer than this value, and assuming that the temperature of the hand is appropriate, this suggests that the nerve is conducting slower than normal. This type of prolonged latency is often found across regions where some demyelination has occurred.

Amplitude. The amplitude for a CMAP is measured conventionally from the baseline to the peak of the negative deflection and is measured in millivolts. As mentioned earlier, this is a much larger deflection than the SNAP, enabling a relatively clear identification of the point of departure from baseline. This fact will become important when discussing latency and the calculation of NCV, because the true onset of the CMAP (this departure from baseline) is the point used when calculating these values, rather than the peak of the negative potential that was used with SNAP calculations. For many of the motor nerve studies performed in the upper extremity, amplitude values of 5 mV or greater are expected.[10] In the lower extremity, the amplitude of the CMAPs are typically a little smaller, with normal amplitude values expected to exceed 2 mV.[10] A value less than those referenced above suggests either poor technique (e.g., the active electrode not properly positioned over the motor point of the muscle) or a loss of axons supplying the muscle and consequently the recruitment of fewer muscle fibers. (*Note*: There is an alternate method of determining the amplitude used by some practitioners that calculates the amplitude from peak to peak.[57])

Rise time. If the active electrode is ideally positioned over the motor point of the muscle, the initial deflection from baseline will be negative.[57] Rise time is then the time that it takes from this initial deflection to the peak of the negative phase. The slope of this rise time is felt to be reflective of the distance between the active electrode and the source of the AP.[57]

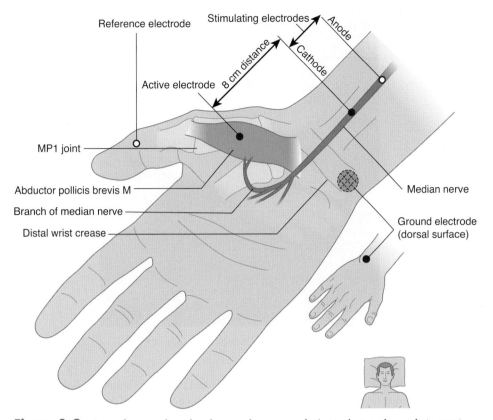

Figure 8–9. Setup for a median distal motor latency study (stimulating electrode is proximal at the wrist, with the cathode located distally). The active pickup electrode is positioned over the belly of the abductor pollicis brevis, with the reference electrode positioned at the interphalangeal joint. Ground electrode is positioned on the ulnar side of the wrist.

A steep slope is ideal and is indicative of good electrode positioning. If the active electrode is not optimally positioned, then the initial deflection may be in a positive direction. In this case, the rise time is measured from the peak of the positive deflection to the peak of the negative deflection or the practitioner may reposition the active recording electrode. This initial positive deflection is indicative of the CMAP reaching the reference electrode prior to reaching the active electrode and is suggestive of less-than-optimal technique. The rise time assists the clinicians in assessing their technique and working toward optimal electrode positioning.

Duration. Duration is the length of time that the CMAP persists, measured in milliseconds. Since the typical CMAP has two phases, a negative and a positive phase (see Figure 8–9), there is the potential for two duration measurements. The first and the one most commonly used is the time from the onset of the CMAP, through the negative peak, until baseline is reached again.[57] An excessively prolonged duration may be suggestive of a demyelinating condition that increases the normal temporal dispersion of the axons making up the peripheral nerve. The second way that duration can be calculated is from the initial onset, through both the positive and negative phases, until reestablishment of baseline. This value is used less frequently, but when excessively prolonged, can be suggestive of some demyelinating conditions.[57]

Shape. The shape of the CMAP is typically biphasic, as is illustrated in Figure 8–9. As has been mentioned earlier, the obtained shape provides information that assists the examiner in ensuring that good technique is being employed. If the shape of the potential obtained has an initial positive deflection, then the electrodes should be rearranged prior to conducting the motor nerve study.

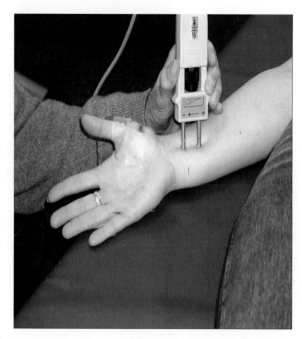

Figure 8–10. Setup for a median nerve DML at a distance of 8 cm.

Nerve conduction velocity. While the DML values provide information about one predetermined segment of a nerve, they do not provide information about the state of the entire nerve. For example, if a prolonged DML is noted for the median nerve with an active electrode over the muscle belly of the abductor pollicis brevis (APB) and the cathode stimulating 8 cm proximal to that point (Figure 8–10), it only indicates that this portion of the nerve is not conducting normally. It does not provide the examiner with the information needed to make judgments about the median nerve proximal to the point of stimulation.

To make judgments about more proximal portions of the nerve, the active electrode is left in place and the stimulating electrode is moved proximally. The illustration in Figure 8–11 shows the setup for the median nerve being stimulated in the cubital fossa of the elbow. This second stimulation at the cubital fossa (the first was the initial DML obtained) provides a biphasic potential that represents the time that it took for the CMAP to travel down the median nerve to the site of the stimulation for the DML, *plus* the time that it took to travel down the distal 8 cm of the nerve, cross the neuromuscular junction, and cause the synchronous depolarization of the muscle fibers of the APB (the initial DML time). By measuring the distance from the cathode during initial point of stimulation used when obtaining the DML to the point of the cathode for this second stimulation, a known distance is obtained. (This technique of motor nerve conduction velocity [MNCV] assessment has to be done for each individual, because depending on one's body size and morphologic characteristics, the length of the forearm will vary considerably.) Subtracting the initial DML from the newly obtained latency provides the time that was required for the CMAP to travel from the cubital fossa to the DML stimulation site. This provides the examiner with a known distance and a known time, which permit calculation of the NCV over the second segment of the nerve, which in this case is the forearm. Since NCV is measured in meters per second, the ratio of the two obtained variables of distance and time is calculated as follows: NCV = distance (in millimeters)/time (in milliseconds). Note that by subtracting out the time and distance of the preceding stimulation, in this case the DML, the nerve conduction value thus obtained reflects the NCV of the specific segment of the nerve last examined. Thus, the NCV value recorded reflects the speed of conduction from the cubital fossa to the wrist. Note also that as was the case with the SNAPs, the obtained NCV values are reflective only of the fastest conducting motor axons contained within the nerve. Using the current EMG equipment, the calculation of MNCV is determined by the computer program.

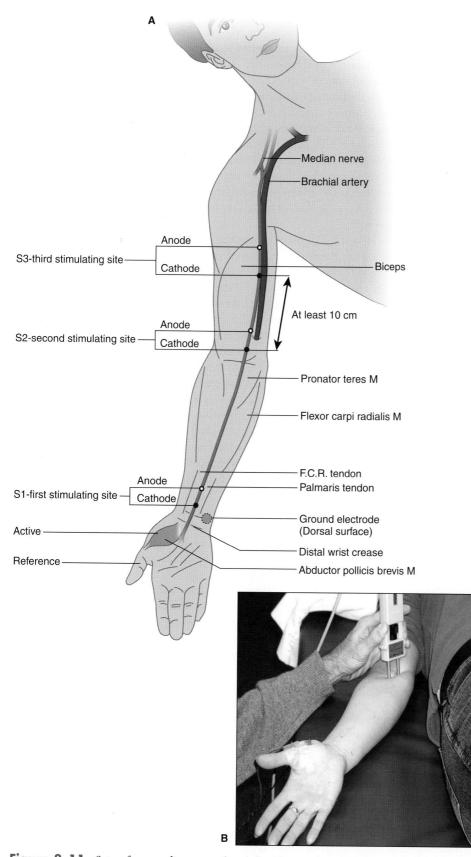

A

Median nerve

Brachial artery

Anode

S3-third stimulating site

Cathode

Biceps

At least 10 cm

Anode

S2-second stimulating site

Cathode

Pronator teres M

Flexor carpi radialis M

F.C.R. tendon

Palmaris tendon

Anode

S1-first stimulating site

Cathode

Ground electrode
(Dorsal surface)

Active

Distal wrist crease

Reference

Abductor pollicis brevis M

B

Figure 8–11. Setup for a median nerve (motor) with stimulation at the cubital fossa. (a) Photograph of the procedure. (b) Line illustration with stimulation sites identified. (*Source*: Ref.[53])

While Figure 8–10 illustrates how the NCV can be computed for the segment of the nerve from the cubital fossa to the wrist, the NCV of other segments can also be obtained. For example, if a third stimulation were desired along the course of the median nerve in the arm, a third CMAP latency would be obtained. By subtracting the cubital fossa CMAP latency (second stimulation) from this arm CMAP (third latency), a new time in milliseconds is obtained that reflects the time that it took for the CMAP to travel from the site of stimulation to the cubital fossa. By measuring this distance, the NCV of this segment can be calculated. This can be done again with stimulation at the axilla, and done again with stimulation at *Erb's* point or supraclavicularly. Erb's point is located posterior to midportion of the clavicle and is the site of a rather strong, supramaximal stimulus designed to activate the brachial plexus. The Erb's point or supraclavicular stimulation site is also used in more advanced techniques with other nerves that do not otherwise lend themselves to direct stimulation, such as the long thoracic nerve, suprascapular nerve, axillary nerve, musculocutaneous nerve, and the proximal radial nerve.[65]

This ability to obtain NCVs from incremental segments of a given nerve is quite valuable in several ways. First, the overall speed of efferent (motor) axons in the upper extremity is faster than that in the lower extremity, with values typically exceeding 50 m/s in the upper extremity and 40 m/s in the lower extremity.[10,50] The reasons for these differences between the upper and lower extremities include slightly lower temperatures in the lower extremities, an inverse relationship between nerve length and conduction velocity, and possibly more abrupt distal axonal tapering.[21] By comparing an obtained NCV to these general values, the overall state of that segment of the nerve can be assessed. In the case of a severe compression at a given point, the NCV could be normal distal to this point, slowed across the segment that includes this compression, and then resume a normal NCV for the more proximally assessed segment.[116] This could occur with the median nerve, for example, if there was a significant compression/restriction where the median nerve passes through the two heads of the pronator teres. By identifying this segment with an abnormal conduction velocity, information is provided that provides an understanding of the mechanism of the problem that the patient is experiencing. This segment-by-segment assessment is often used to evaluate the function of the ulnar nerve as it passes under the medial epicondyle in the cubital tunnel and is prone to compression. Second, the normal changes in NCV that occur from distal to proximal can be clinically observed. Nerves tend to have a larger diameter proximally and become smaller as they pass distally. In addition, the temperature of the arm is normally higher than the temperature measured at the wrist. Theoretically, therefore, it would be expected that the NCV observed would generally increase as the nerve is assessed more proximally. This is what is typically found, with all segments in the upper extremity conducting at least 50 m/s, but the more proximal segments conduct an AP at an even faster speed.

Latency compared with NCV. Latency and NCV are directly related to each other, even though the desirable characteristics with each on first pass appear to be different. The desired latency is one that is short (time measurement), while the desired NCV is one that is fast (speed). As has been discussed previously, latencies are used for known distances, typically the distal segment of the motor nerve being investigated (DML) and compared with a chart of normative values (e.g., DMLs and amplitudes). Metaphorically, a latency can be compared with an automobile driver who encounters "mile marker one" on the road, and times how long it takes to reach "mile marker two." Since this is a known distance, if we expect that cars will travel down the freeway at a speed of at least 60 mph, the expected "latency" time value for this distance would be 60 seconds. Any time measurement less than 60 seconds would be good, indicating a fast car. Any latency measurement greater than 60 seconds would suggest a slow car, which for the sake of this discussion would be considered abnormal. Similarly, when measuring the time that an AP takes to pass from one point to a second point, at a known distance, normal latencies have been obtained and are part of a "table of normal values" used by an electrophysiologic laboratory. Latency values shorter than those found in the table of normal values are good, since they indicate that the speed of the AP traveling down the composite bundle of axons is appropriately fast. It is noteworthy, however, to point out that DMLs are typically much longer than DSLs, since in addition to the AP traveling down axons (all that is assessed with DSLs), the DML also reflects the time for transmission across the neuromuscular junction and the time for the AP to travel down muscle fibers. Since the release of ACh across the neuromuscular junction takes approximately 1 millisecond, and the speed of an AP along muscle fibers is slower than along axons, the obtained DML is longer than a similar-length DSL.

Conduction velocities are used typically for segments of the nerve proximal to the point of the initial stimulation obtained with the DML, and are compared with the known normal conduction speeds for the upper and lower extremities as identified in a table of normal values. Nerve conduction velocities are computed for several reasons. The first is that the lengths of extremities vary, so by determining a "speed" regardless of limb length, comparisons can be made across individuals. Second, since they are obtained by subtracting out the DML, the contribution of the neuromuscular junction and AP along muscle fibers is eliminated. Third, this type of evaluation permits examination of segments of a nerve that are proximal to the distal part of an extremity, permitting the site of potential conduction blocks or other abnormalities to be identified. Collectively, this type of assessment permits an accurate representation of the speed that the AP is traveling across all segments of the motor nerve of interest.

To complete this discussion contrasting latency and NCV, it should be noted that one is not necessarily more accurate than the other, but rather that they both use basically the same information to look at the issue of nerve function in slightly different ways. While it is theoretically possible that NCV could be calculated for the segment measured with a DML, it is not routinely done since inaccuracies would be inherent due to the contribution of the neuromuscular junction and the slowed speed of muscle fiber AP conduction. Conversely, while latencies are automatically calculated for each segment of the nerve stimulated when obtaining the NCV, because limbs are of different lengths, the latencies obtained are not directly comparable. Rather, the DMLs are subtracted from one another to obtain the time measurement used in the NCV calculation. The key points to recognize are that the desired states are a short latency and a fast conduction velocity, and the two variables are measuring the same entity but are expressed in different units to facilitate communication.

Other Motor Nerve Conduction Procedures

Central conduction studies. A central conduction study in NCS testing is also known as an F-wave.[66-68] Functionally, this is an AP that is transmitted proximally (antidromically) via efferent axons to the level of the anterior horn cell, which then "bounces back" along the same efferent axons to result in a secondary contraction of the innervated muscle fibers. The term secondary contraction is used because, when the stimulation at a distal site is generated, there is initially a direct activation of the muscle fibers from the distal segment of the efferent axons that directly activate the muscle fibers, creating a CMAP. This CMAP is known as an "M-wave." While the M-wave occurs in close association with the stimulus, the F-wave occurs significantly later in time, because the AP has to pass antidromically up the efferent axons to the level of the alpha motor neuron, and travel back down the efferent axons orthodromically to elicit a CMAP. Thus, one of the strengths of the F-wave is that it is representative of the overall conduction status of the entire nerve under investigation.

The technique of generating an F-wave is largely the same as that used to generate a DML, except that the cathode and anode of the handheld stimulator are reversed in their position. In this case, the cathode is placed proximally along the nerve being investigated, so that the evoked potential proceeds directly to the level of the spinal cord without passing under the anode (which is now placed distal to the cathode). The amplitude of the F-wave is generally small, only about 1–5% the size of the M-wave generated by direct stimulation.[69] Additionally, the F-wave has significant variability, and while it can be elicited from many muscles in the upper and lower extremities, it may not be present universally. Typically, still using supramaximal stimulation, a reasonable number of F-waves (e.g., 10–12) are elicited, and the shortest latency obtained is recorded as the F-wave latency value. Normal values are less than 32 milliseconds for the upper extremity and less than 58 milliseconds for the lower extremity,[67] in an individual with a height of no more than 6 ft (72 in). For individuals taller than 6 ft, normative values and/or methods for calculating F-wave latencies are available.[70] In addition to being a way to examine the conduction status over the entire length of the nerve, a prolonged F-wave is often collaborative to other findings of decreased NCV over a segment that may be indicative of a demyelinating condition.[71-73] Additionally, this technique may be useful in the identification of plexus problems (plexopathy) or proximal neuropraxic dysfunction.

Hoffman's reflex. The Hoffman's reflex, or H-wave, is a physiologic example of the normal reflex arc that is present in only a few select muscles. The evoked AP for this reflex travels proximally via afferent axons (orthodromic conduction) into the segmental level of the spinal cord. The compound AP results in neurotransmitters passing between one or more synapses to ultimately reach anterior horn cells, eliciting an orthodromic conduction that results in a CMAP. The H-wave follows the same course that would be used with a muscle stretch reflex (MSR), traveling proximally via afferent axons to the spinal cord, traversing the spinal cord to the alpha motor neurons, and then traveling distally via efferent neurons to depolarize muscle fibers. This is a very stable reflex and can be a sensitive indicator of a problem along the nerve, such as an S1 radiculopathy.[74] As was the case with the F-wave, there is an initial M-wave that occurs temporally close to the time of stimulation, with the H-wave occurring later in time due to its much longer course. Compared with the maximum amplitude of the M-wave of the same muscle (e.g., soleus), the H-wave has a smaller amplitude, a longer latency, and a lower optimal stimulus intensity.[75] The magnitude of the H-reflex usually peaks at or just prior to the observation of a direct CMAP or M-response, from the soleus muscle. Further increases in the current intensity result in a continually increasing M-response but a steadily declining H-reflex amplitude.[76] It has been determined that 24–100% of the motor neuron pool may participate in the H-reflex. This suggests that the H-reflex amplitude is quite variable and subject to multiple factors including a mild voluntary contraction of the muscle under investigation and/or suprasegmental influence of central facilitation.[76] The H-wave has a much smaller amplitude than the M-wave and a much lower optimal stimulus intensity. The biggest drawback to the H-wave is that it can only be elicited reliably in a limited group of muscles, primarily the calf muscles[69] and more rarely with the flexor carpi radialis.[77] This procedure is not used routinely except with muscles in the leg, but it can provide valuable collaborative information with select conditions such as the aforementioned S1 radiculopathy.

CASE STUDY 8–2
ELECTROPHYSIOLOGIC TESTING

Diagnosis and Reason For Referral: Radiculopathy involving the C5 nerve root.

Testing Procedures and Findings: In this case, it would be expected that the clinical examination and EMG will be the most informative portions of the examination. Slowing of nerve conduction will probably not be observed, since the segments of the nerve that can be readily measured will not be affected by a restriction at the C4–5 intervertebral foramina. The clinical examination, however, may demonstrate weakness, a dermatome pattern of sensory alteration, or an altered reflex (e.g., biceps brachii reflex is predominantly C5). Additionally, the EMG examination will sample a number of muscles with C5 contributions that span a number of different nerves. If positive EMG findings are noted in the biceps brachii (musculocutaneous nerve: C5–6), deltoid muscle (axillary nerve: C5–6), clavicular portion of the pecto-

ralis major (lateral pectoral nerve: C5–7), supraspinatus muscle (suprascapular nerve: C5–6), and the midcervical paraspinals (dorsal primary rami), then either the C5 or C6 root level is strongly implicated. When this is combined with normal findings in the pronator teres (median nerve: C6–7), extensor carpi radialis longus (radial nerve: C6–7), and other muscles with C6 but not C5 contributions, the C5 nerve root level emerges as the most likely cause of the patient's problem. The positive findings in the cervical paraspinals indicate that the pathologic process is proximal and also involves the posterior (dorsal) primary rami. Normal nerve conduction velocities suggest that there is not a compression along one of the named peripheral nerves that is responsible for what is being observed. Taken collectively, these findings strongly implicate a nerve root compression, specifically the C5 root level, as the cause of the symptoms noted by

(continued)

CASE STUDY 8–2 *(continued)*
ELECTROPHYSIOLOGIC TESTING

the patient. In this case, the electrophysiologic description of the findings might be something like axonopathy affecting cervical muscles sharing C5 nerve root contributions, consistent with referring consult of cervical radiculopathy. Note that in this case, the potential demyelination has not been addressed since there was nothing in the electrophysiologic workup that suggested a demyelinating contribution.

Discussion Questions

- In a patient with a cervical radiculopathy, what NCV alterations, if any, would typically be found?
- Since the electrophysiologic examination is based on an excellent physical examination, what motor, sensory, reflex, and special test findings might be evident in an individual with a C6 radiculopathy?
- In the absence of any physical examination findings (such as those alluded to in question #2 above), would it still be expected that the electrophysiologic examination will demonstrate pathology?
- If a C5 cervical radiculopathy were suspected, which of the following muscles might be expected to demonstrate positive findings? (For each positive or negative response, be able to provide a rationale for your answer.)

  1. midcervical paraspinals
  2. low cervical paraspinals

  3. supraspinatus
  4. deltoid
  5. brachioradialis
  6. extensor digitorum
  7. pronator teres
  8. flexor carpi ulnaris
  9. opponens pollicis
  10. first dorsal interossei

- What information do positive EMG findings in the paraspinals provide that was not available by doing the EMG examination on an extremity muscle?
- If motor units at a low level of contraction were observed that were very small (e.g., <300 µV) and of very short duration (e.g., =3 milliseconds), what generic pathology might be implicated? Why?
- What is the clinical significance of 1+ PSWs being reported, versus 4+ PSWs being reported?
- How can the clinical findings from a NCS/EMG examination be helpful in confirming a diagnosis, assisting with development of an appropriate treatment plan, and guiding the patient prognosis?
- Why would a SEP examination ever be included as part of the electrophysiologic testing performed?

Repetitive nerve stimulation. The repetitive nerve stimulation procedure is used to assess conditions potentially affecting the neuromuscular junction, such as myasthenia gravis and Lambert–Eaton syndrome. Myasthenia gravis is a problem with the postsynaptic receptors, limiting the ability of ACh to bind. When ACh is released by the distal aspect of the efferent axon and does not interact with the postsynaptic receptors, most of this neurotransmitter is reabsorbed prior to being able to bind with the few existing receptors that would normally cause depolarization. With repetitive nerve stimulation, the quantal content decreases by approximately 50% from the initial stimulus.[78] This drop in available ACh coupled with the decreased number of receptors to bind with results in a decreased amplitude of the CMAP response with repetitive nerve stimulation. There are strict protocols that need to be followed with this procedure,[78] such as rate of stimulation and stimulation performed after exercise and over time. For Lambert–Eaton syndrome, a presynaptic problem with the calcium channels, the repetitive stimulation tends to result in increasing CMAP amplitude responses. The observed incrementing response is due to more calcium entering the distal aspect of the neuron following repetitive stimulation, resulting in a larger quantal release of ACh, creating improved CMAPs. While simplified greatly, these two examples illustrate how repetitive stimulation can be used to help determine the nature of a suspected problem at the neuromuscular junction.

Additional neural conduction techniques. There are a number of other techniques or procedures that can be used when performing NCS, such as the previously mentioned near-nerve stimulation technique, or an "inching" technique where a stimulating electrode is moved small distances over a peripheral nerve in an attempt to identify the specific location of a problem. These techniques and other more advanced procedures are beyond the scope of this overview description of NCS. The interested reader is referred to the excellent texts on this topic written by Oh,[59] Kimura,[2] and Dumitru et al.[1]

An Example of One Upper Quarter Examination Using Sensory and Motor Nerve Conduction Procedures

Prior to discussing the next major component of the examination, an example is provided of a generic NCS for one upper extremity. The following NCS might be incorporated as a part of the complete electrophysiologic testing of patients with suspected carpal tunnel syndrome or cubital tunnel syndrome. The following might be the types of tests that would be selected:

1. Sensory nerve studies:
    (a) DSL of the median nerve (both palm–wrist and two-digit-wrist);
    (b) DSL of the ulnar nerve (both palm–wrist and five-digit-wrist);
    (c) DSL of the superficial radial nerve (forearm-wrist).

2. Motor nerve studies:
    (a) median nerve:
      - DML of the median nerve (wrist–APB),
      - NCV of the median nerve (elbow–wrist segment) (e.g., forearm),
      - F-wave of the median nerve;
    (b) ulnar nerve:
      - DML of the ulnar nerve,
      - NCV of the ulnar nerve (both below elbow–wrist and above elbow–below elbow segment) (e.g., forearm and across the elbow).

3. F-wave of the ulnar nerve.

The sensory and motor nerve studies outlined above provide the examiner with some information about the function of the three major nerves of the upper extremity: the median, ulnar, and radial. The DSL studies, often more sensitive than the motor studies for early problems, provide data about the ability of the distal afferent axons to conduct.[2,55,59] The DML studies provide equivalent information about the status of the distal efferent axons to conduct and additionally test the neuromuscular junction and the innervated muscle fibers. Nerve conduction velocities of specific segments of both the median and ulnar nerves are assessed, as is the total length of the nerve through the use of the F-wave. All of the data collected need to be compared against normative values, known conduction velocities, expected amplitudes, and so forth. Tables of normal values for NCS measurements should be developed for each clinical electrophysiologic laboratory. Based on this evaluation, the examiner performing the examination can add other specialized tests to look at a given area in more detail, or proceed to the EMG portion of the examination. (Several case studies have been provided to illustrate how the data obtained with the above NCS testing can be used to formulate clinical conclusions.)

THE ELECTROMYOGRAPHIC EXAMINATION

The EMG portion of the examination involves inserting a sterile needle electrode into a muscle to provide the examiner with information regarding the spontaneous and voluntary electrical activity of the muscular tissue.[115] The general setup for this procedure is diagrammed in Figure 8–12 and contains the same basic elements used to monitor APs during the neural conduction studies. A ground electrode is used on the limb being examined, and there is an active electrode and a reference electrode. The two key differences with this setup are that the active electrode is a needle electrode placed within the muscle, and there is no externally supplied electrical stimulus. All activity monitored is from the muscle at rest, or due to the insertion of the needle, movement of the needle, or the patient's prompted voluntary activity. The needle electrode is typically coated with a material such as Teflon to both insulate all portions of the needle except

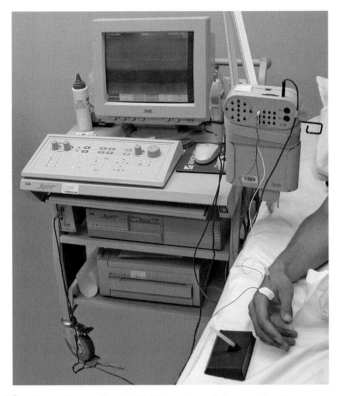

Figure 8–12. General setup for the EMG portion of the examination.

the very tip and minimize discomfort during insertion. The active tip monitors the few muscle fibers located within approximately 0.5 mm of the noninsulated region.[76] It has been estimated that at any one time, the electrical activity of 1–12 muscle fibers is being evaluated by this small active region on the needle electrode.[76] It is therefore necessary to move the needle slightly over the course of the examination of a muscle to increase the pool of potential muscle fibers that are observed. Due to the combination of potential discomfort associated with inserting the needle, moving the needle slightly, and asking the patient to contract the muscle while the needle electrode remains in the muscle, this portion of the examination is typically, but not always, performed following neural conduction studies. Good communication with patients is essential to prepare them for this portion of the examination and to solicit their cooperation during the course of the evaluation.

Prior to providing an overview of a basic EMG examination, it may be beneficial to provide a rationale for why this portion of the examination is performed. Direct observation of the spontaneous and voluntary activity of muscle fibers can provide a great deal of information regarding the efferent portion of the neuromuscular system, from the anterior horn cell to the muscle fibers themselves. For example, if an anterior horn cell has become diseased, then the axon associated with that structure dies and the muscle fibers associated with that axon become denervated. This creates a situation where the muscle fibers and muscle fiber membrane are "irritable" and prone to abnormal spontaneous electrical activity (e.g., PSWs and fibrillation potentials) during needle movement and at rest. A second potential site of entrapment is where a nerve root exits the intervertebral foramina. If the root is compromised at this site, the axons passing through this space can become damaged, again resulting in abnormal spontaneous electrical activity. Identification of a nerve root compression at a specific level is done by sampling a variety of muscles, noting which ones have evidence of abnormal electrical activity, and correlating this with the root levels that supply the muscles sampled. For example, a patient with findings in the right pronator teres (median nerve, C6–7), extensor carpi radialis brevis (posterior interosseous nerve of radial, C7–8), triceps brachii (radial nerve, C6–8), and the flexor carpi ulnaris (ulnar nerve, C7–8) have common findings in the C7 nerve root contributions to all of these different nerves. If this is coupled with normal hand intrinsics (median and ulnar nerves, C8–T1), normal biceps brachii (musculocutaneous, C5–6), normal deltoid (axillary, C5–6), and normal supraspinatus (suprascapular nerve, C5–6), the examination suggests that the C5, C6, C8, and T1 root levels are not involved. The single most probable site for this type of a finding is at the C7 intervertebral foramina where the nerve root could be compressed as it exits this space. The final piece of the puzzle is to test the lower cervical paraspinals, thus sampling the muscles supplied by the posterior (dorsal) primary rami of the C7 nerve root (review the section "Anatomy of the spinal nerve and neuromuscular junction"– Figure 8–3 and 8–4). If the cervical paravertebral muscles (PVM) also demonstrate abnormal electrical findings and these findings correlate with the patient's physical examination, the implication is quite strong that the problem is occurring proximal to the point where the posterior (dorsal) and anterior (ventral) primary rami split and contribute to the brachial plexus and the true muscles of the back. This would be strong evidence in support of a C7 cervical radiculopathy. Practically, the EMG examination is the most useful aspect of the electrophysiologic examination to detect radiculopathies, and it is a valuable adjunct to collaborate the findings of MRI or other specialized imaging tests. A third potential site of a neuromuscular problem is within the muscle itself, with myopathic diseases such as Duchenne muscular dystrophy. With diseases affecting the muscle fibers themselves, the electrical potentials generated are unusual in aspects such as their size and duration. This information in the hands of an experienced clinician can be used to aid in the diagnosis of the underlying pathology.

The three examples provided in the paragraph above were not meant to suggest that this is the range of disorders that can be identified with EMG testing, but rather provide illustrative examples of locations within the efferent neuromuscular chain where problems can be identified. While three simple examples were provided here, there are literally hundreds of conditions that manifest themselves in different ways with signs evident during an EMG examination. It takes significant skill, experience, as well as an excellent understanding of anatomy and the pathophysiology of disease to provide a linkage between the patient's problem and the mechanism underlying the condition. The range of problems that can be evaluated with EMG testing is very broad and beyond the scope of what can be provided in this chapter. As has been referenced previously, the specific approach used for any one patient will be customized by the practitioner based on the patient's particular findings during the physical examination and history. Recognizing this need to customize examinations and the range of specific pathologies, there are common elements to the basic approach to this portion of the examination used during most EMG examinations. The generic EMG information provided below deals with the elements commonly examined during the evaluation of one muscle. For the interested reader desiring more detail on specialized techniques or ways of modifying this type of examination, see some of the excellent texts on this topic written by Oh, Kimura, and Dumitru.

Clinical EMG Procedures

The routine EMG examination does not have a set format, nor is there a set number of muscles that needs to be examined. The judgment regarding which distal and proximal muscles to test, the number of muscles that should be examined, and whether or not the paraspinals (innervated by posterior [dorsal] primary rami) should be evaluated is based on the clinician's experience and to some extent on the insurance companies' willingness to reimburse.[117] The four steps of the evaluation typically performed on each muscle examined are as follows. The first step comprises insertion activity, the spontaneous electrical activity due to the insertion of the EMG needle electrode.[79] Additionally, the needle electrode is moved slightly to sample different regions and different depths of the muscle, assess muscle membrane irritability, and look for abnormal spontaneous electrical activity. The second step includes identifying any abnormal spontaneous electrical potentials while the muscle is at rest. The normal muscle is electrically silent at rest. If any spontaneous electrical activity is observed, it is recorded. The third step of the EMG examination includes observation of the muscle fibers during voluntary contraction. The patient is asked to contract the muscle, first at a very low level to allow the observation of single motor units, and then with increasing intensity to examine for an orderly recruitment from the smaller, type I muscle fibers to the larger, type II muscle fibers. Ultimately, with a full contraction the oscilloscope screen should be completely "filled" when examining a normal muscle. Synthesis of the information obtained in steps 1–3 provides a summary of the EMG testing and is the fourth and final step. A more detailed explanation of each of these four steps is provided below.

Clinical Decision-Making   *Exercise 8–5*

A clinician has completed the EMG portion of the electrophysiologic examination and plans to report that the identified problem has a location at the level of a nerve root. What EMG finding is needed to positively assert that the location is as proximal as a nerve root?

Insertion

The insertion activity assesses the electrical response of a sample of muscle fibers to the insertion and moving of the needle electrode within a resting muscle. When a needle electrode is placed within a muscle or is moved, it is normal for electrical activity to be observed on the oscilloscope screen lasting from 50 to 230 milliseconds.[27,79] Since the tip of the needle typically samples the muscle AP of less than 12 muscle fibers, it needs to be moved to provide a representative sample of the muscle under investigation. One recommended scheme is to move the needle to "the four corners of a small box," and repeat this three times assessing a different depth of the muscle with each series of sampling.[76] After each needle movement, the electrical activity of the muscle is assessed. This provides data from 12 samples of the muscle and increases the likelihood of identifying any abnormal electrical activity, if it exists. When abnormal spontaneous electrical activity is observed that persists longer than 230 milliseconds following cessation of needle movement, this is abnormal and the particular characteristics of that activity are described. Additionally, if no electrical activity is observed with the needle movement, this is also considered to be abnormal. The increased abnormal electrical activity associated with insertion and needle movement is associated with conditions such as denervation, myotonic disorders, and some myogenic disorders (myositis).[79,80] When reduced electrical activity is observed, this is suggestive of chronic muscle changes and a muscle that is subject to fatty or fibrotic degeneration. In this case, there may be an abnormal feel or resistance to movement of the needle, such as if the needle were being moved through a bag of sand. These examples are intended to illustrate that with insertion of a needle, increased or decreased electrical activity can be observed in addition to normal insertional activity. Additionally, with movement of the needle in the relaxed muscle, other abnormal spontaneous electrical activities can be observed beyond the 230 milliseconds reflective of normal muscle fiber activity.

Several of the more common examples of abnormal spontaneous electrical activity at rest are provided below.

Fibrillation potentials. This represents the electrical activity associated with the spontaneous contraction of a single muscle fiber. Since the contraction of a single muscle fiber is too small to be either felt or observed visually, the only way to assess for this condition is through EMG needle electrode examination. The origin of fibrillation potentials is from membrane instability due to loss of axonal innervation of the individual muscle fibers that collectively make up a motor unit. These denervated fibers become irritable and, in a response to encourage reinnervation by another axon, begin to have their resting membrane potential oscillate toward the level of threshold.[54] As this threshold level is reached, the single muscle fiber will spontaneously fire, or fibrillate. These fibrillation potentials have a characteristic shape, with an initial positive deflection, typically two to three phases, and are of a very short duration of a few milliseconds (less than 5 milliseconds). Additionally, they emit a characteristic high-pitched sound that has been described as "rain on a tin roof" when heard through a loudspeaker.[54]

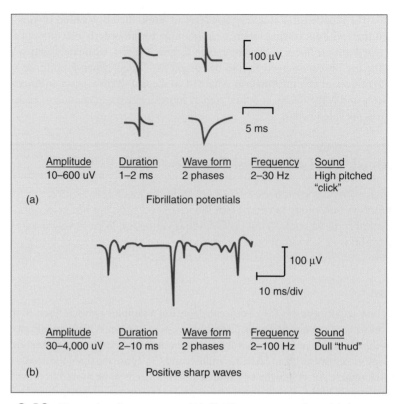

Figure 8–13. Figure that demonstrates: (A) fibrillation potentials and (B) positive sharp waves. (*Source*: Ref.[53])

The amplitude of these potentials can vary from a few hundred microvolts to over 1 mV, with fibrillation potential amplitude more prominent in acute denervation compared with chronic denervation.[69] Figure 8–13A is an illustration of a typical fibrillation potential.

Positive sharp waves. PSWs are biphasic, positive and then negative, potentials recorded in response to needle movement with a muscle at rest. These potentials, like the previously described fibrillation potentials, are representative of muscle denervation. The basic etiology of these PSWs is believed to be similar to fibrillation potentials, in that they indicate membrane instability secondary to the loss of axonal innervation.[69] The true origin of these PSWs has not been clearly identified, but it is clear that these potentials represent an unstable muscle fiber membrane. The shape of these potentials is characteristic, with an initial positive deflection and two phases, a regular firing rate of between 1 and 50 Hz, amplitudes that range from 100 to 1000 μV, and a duration that can vary from several to 100 milliseconds.[54] When amplified on a speaker system, these potentials sound like a dull thud or plop. These potentials are often seen mixed in with fibrillation potentials, and are found with a variety of pathologic conditions ranging from denervation to polymyositis, progressive muscular dystrophy, and motor neuron diseases. Figure 8–13B provides an example of PSWs mixed in with fibrillation potentials.

Grading fibrillation potentials and PSWs. In a patient's records, the presence of fibrillation potentials and/or PSWs will be quantified through the use of the following notations used by the Mayo Clinic[81,82]: (1) 0 indicates the absence of either of these two potentials, (2) 1+ indicates that the potential being quantified persisted for over 1 second in at least 2 of the 12 areas examined, (3) 2+ indicates one or both of these potentials persisted over 1 second in many but not all areas, (4) 3+ indicates observation of one or both of these potentials in all areas, but the potentials were intermittent, and (5) 4+ indicates continuous abnormal electrical activity observed in all areas examined. From a prognostic standpoint, 1+ findings are less severe than 3+ or 4+ fibrillation potentials and/or PSWs, which are indicative of a more widespread or severe pathology.

Myotonic discharges. These are variations on the theme discussed above with fibrillation potentials and PSWs, with myotonic discharges representing a sustained run of potentials that resemble PSWs. A difference here is that the potentials wax and wane, sounding over a loudspeaker such as a motorcycle, dive bomber, or chainsaw.[82,83] Potentials of this type are observed in conditions such as myotonia congenita, myotonia dystrophia, paramyotonia congenital, and hyperkalemic periodic paralysis.[82,83] Myotonic discharges have an initial positive deflection and two phases, fire at a rate of 20–100 Hz, have an amplitude of 10–1000 μV, and have a very short duration of approximately 2–5 milliseconds.[82,83]

Other potentials. The three types of potentials noted above (fibrillation potentials, PSWs, and myotonic discharges) are not the only types of abnormal electrical activity observed with needle insertion and movement, but they are the most common. Other types of abnormal potentials such as complex repetitive discharges and myokymic discharges can be seen across a variety of patient conditions. The above potentials are illustrative of the more common abnormal findings that might be observed in a patient's records with significant EMG results. For additional information, see the excellent EMG texts on this topic by Oh,[59] Kimura,[11,21] and Dumitru et al.[1]

Rest. With a needle electrode inserted into a muscle and the muscle at rest, the isoelectric line should remain stable and the loudspeaker should be silent. There are exceptions to this electrical silence that occur in normal muscle, such as the detection of the random release of a quanta of ACh at the neuromuscular junction (miniature end-plate potential) or the detection of a spontaneous nonpropagated potential occurring at the neuromuscular junction (end-plate potential). While these are exceptions found in normal muscle, they are relatively easily identified by their size, shape, and sound, and are eliminated by moving the needle to a new site. Exceptions to electrical silence that can occur within a muscle at rest include all of the previously discussed potentials in the section "Insertion" (fibrillation potentials, PSWs, myotonic discharges, complex repetitive discharges, etc.), as well as fasciculations.

A fasciculation potential is the potential associated with the random and spontaneous activation of a group of muscle fibers or all of the muscle fibers originating from a motor unit. Everyone has experienced fasciculation potentials, such as when the eyelid "twitches" at the end of the day when an individual is fatigued. This is generally thought to be due to the abnormal discharge of an alpha motor neuron, resulting in contraction of all the muscle fibers innervated by the motor unit. Because a single alpha motor neuron innervates up to several thousand muscle fibers in muscles such as the soleus in the leg,[75,82] these contractions can be both felt by the individual and observed by a clinician. In a pathologic state, their etiology is not as clear, and it has been shown that the fasciculation potential can originate from the anterior horn cell, the peripheral nerve, or the terminal nerve membrane.[84] A general rule of thumb is that fasciculations are known by the company that they keep. In other words, since everyone experiences fasciculations on occasion when particularly fatigued or stressed, they are not in and of themselves pathognomic of a neuromuscular problem. Fasciculations occurring in normal muscle and those associated with disease visually appear to be identical. However, when they occur in the presence of clinical findings such as atrophy and unexplained loss of strength, the "company" that they are associated with is less than ideal and the importance of noting their regular appearance is greatly increased. The clinician looking for fasciculation potentials will normally observe a muscle at rest from one to several minutes and count the number of fasciculation potentials observed. Abnormal fasciculation potentials are graded on a scale from 1+ to 4+. A 1+ finding indicates that fasciculations were observed in two samples, occurring at a rate of between 2 and 10/min. A 4+ finding means that these potentials were observed in all areas sampled, and the fasciculations were occurring at a rate of over 60/min.[85] The 2+ and 3+ grades are simply levels expressing findings between these two ends of the grading scale. This provides one more bit of information that may assist in making a diagnosis, because abnormal fasciculation potentials are associated with anterior horn cell disease, metabolic disturbances, and other disorders such as primary muscular atrophy and syringomyelia.[76]

Voluntary activity. The next step in the evaluation is to have the patient initiate a voluntary contraction. Initially, a very slight contraction is sought that will cause the activation of only a few motor units. This type of slight contraction provides the examiner with the information needed to examine the summated activity of the muscle fibers from a single motor unit that are volitionally activated. Recall from the previous discussion of normal recruitment patterns of motor neurons that the smallest motor neurons innervating slow twitch (type I) fibers will be recruited initially.[65] With increasing levels of voluntary activation, larger motor units will be recruited. The examiner is looking for an orderly recruitment of motor units suggesting this small-to-large pattern, and also identifying at least 12 motor units to characterize in each muscle examined. The elements typically used to characterize a motor unit are the following: (1) shape, which typically has two to three phases (areas above and below the isoelectric baseline); (2) amplitude, which normally ranges from 300 to 5000 µV (5 mV, with the amplitude of some normal intrinsic hand muscles in the 10,000-µV range), with the motor units associated with the earlier recruited type I fibers having the smaller amplitudes; (3) duration, representing the time involved from the departure of the potential from the baseline until the baseline is reestablished and that normally varies between 3 and 15 milliseconds; and (4) sound of the motor unit. A healthy motor unit with the needle electrode positioned near it will have a sharp, crisp sound. The first three of these traits are often characterized by the acronym SAD (shape, amplitude, and duration).

Shape. A normal MUAP and a MUAP with too many phases (polyphasic potential) are both presented in Figure 8–14. A normal MUAP has two to three phases typically. A polyphasic potential has five or more phases. A phase is that portion of the AP that occurs on one side of the baseline. Thus, a biphasic potential may have an initial positive deflection that ends when the potential returns to the baseline, and a negative deflection that is the continuation of the upward sweep of the waveform to a peak, returning again to the baseline that completes the second phase.

Polyphasic potentials are often found in tissue that has been denervated and is in the process of regeneration.[82] While the presence of polyphasic potentials can be collaborative of denervation, interpretation solely on the basis of observing these potentials is problematic, because it has been shown that normal muscle can have polyphasic potentials that range from 12% to 35%.[54] Having said that, low-amplitude and long-duration polyphasic potentials may be suggestive of nascent (from Latin, meaning *to be born*) potentials that are observed during early states of reinnervation of muscle.[69] Identification of potentials with an abnormal number of phases may assist in understanding what is occurring in the muscle tissue.

A related issue associated with the topic of phases is turns. Turns are the change in direction of a portion of the MUAP (in either a positive or negative direction) that does not continue to the point where the baseline is encountered (see Figure 8–14). The typical normal MUAP does not have turns, but these small changes in direction of the waveform increase with age.[86] A few turns without other findings are not indicative of pathology. If they are noted in a patient's record, then the minimal excursion required to be classified as a turn should be specified.[69]

Amplitude. The amplitude is the size of the MUAP, measured from peak to peak[87] (see Figure 8–14). Normal MUAPs range from 300 to 5000 µV (5 mV),[88-92] with distal muscles occasionally normally exhibiting larger amplitudes that may range up to 10 mV. The type I (slow twitch) MUAPs should have an amplitude that ranges from 300 to 1000 µV, while the type II (fast twitch) MUAPs normally range from 1000 to 5000 µV. Deviations of amplitude size from this range of normal values may be a clue in a pathologic process. For example, many MUAPs that are reduced below normal values (300 µV or less) are often observed in patients with myopathies.[89,90,93] Additionally, small-amplitude motor units may be present during early axonal regeneration, indicating ongoing recovery from a nerve injury. On the other hand, extremely large-amplitude MUAPs are indicative of a neuropathic process where axonal sprouting has occurred. For example, in a patient with anterior horn cell disease, axons are dying and muscle fibers are losing their innervation. Early in this cycle, the denervated muscle fibers will attract axonal sprouts from neurons that are still relatively healthy, creating a motor unit with more than its typical contingent of muscle fibers. This "giant motor unit" will have an amplitude that exceeds the normal range, thus providing collaborative information that a neuropathic process is present. The amplitude of a MUAP will often provide the examiner with important information regarding the underlying state of aspects of the motor unit.

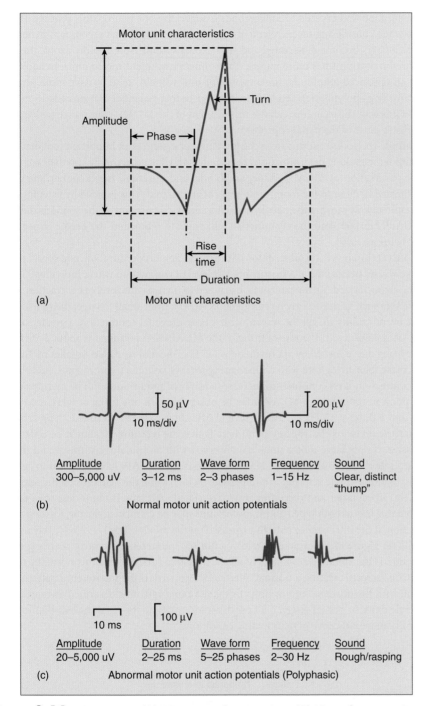

Figure 8–14. Motor units. (A) Motor unit characteristics. (B) Normal motor unit action potentials. (C) Abnormal motor unit action potentials (polyphasic). (*Source*: Ref.[53])

Duration. The duration of a MUAP is the length of time, expressed in milliseconds, from the onset of the potential until a normal baseline is reestablished (see Figure 8–14). Normal MUAP durations range from 3 to 15 milliseconds. Duration deviations from this range of normal values provide additional important information regarding the status of the motor unit. A duration of less than 3 milliseconds is suggestive of a myopathic process and is the most consistent motor unit morphologic parameter[94] (recall from the paragraph above that a myopathic process will also typically have a small amplitude of less than 300 μV). On the other hand, a duration that exceeds 15 milliseconds is suggestive of a neuropathic process. This can be seen when considering several elements discussed previously that accompany axonal loss. As muscle fibers become denervated and seek axonal sprouts from healthy axons, the newly configured motor unit has more muscle fibers innervated (giant motor unit). In addition to having an enhanced amplitude, this new motor unit will also tend to have more phases to the MUAP (e.g., polyphasic), resulting in a longer lasting potential that exceeds 15 milliseconds. In this way, the examiner can use this element of the MUAPs appearance to deduce the mechanistic cause of the patient's problem.

Sound. The sound emitted from the loudspeaker system is an important tool that assists the examiner in making determinations regarding both what is occurring and their technique. For the observation of MUAPs' shape, amplitude, and duration, the examiner attempts to locate the needle close to the motor unit being characterized. This is aided by listening to the sound emitted and moving the needle to elicit a sharp, crisp sound. If the sound is dull, then the MUAP is distant, and the examiner should work to reposition the needle closer to the MUAP being assessed.

Contraction level. The description of the shape, amplitude, duration, and sound provided above was all performed at a reasonably low level of contraction where individual MUAPs could be characterized. As the patient is instructed to increase the level of contraction, due to other factors such as the orderly recruitment of MUAPs from small to large, the rate of firing, and the overall ability to "fill the screen" with a near-maximal contraction, a greater number of MUAPs are observed. The rate of firing of the MUAPs first recruited is about 2–3 Hz with a stable firing rate achieved by approximately 5–7 Hz. The first recruited, smaller motor units will increase their firing rate with an increasing level of voluntary contraction. Additionally, as the contraction level continues to increase, additional motor units will be recruited. Thus, at one point in time, several MUAPs may be observed, with one firing at 5 Hz, a second at 10 Hz, and a third at 15 Hz.[82,84] When several MUAPs have been recruited, their firing rate may increase up to 20 Hz. The key point here is that the recruitment should be orderly and progressive. If only large motor units are observed with an initial recruitment and they are firing at a rate clearly in excess of 10 Hz, this suggests that MUAPs have been lost to denervation and that the muscle is trying to compensate by increasing the demands on the remaining fibers (e.g., firing faster and recruiting units associated with type II fibers described earlier). This potential loss of both type I and II motor units may be confirmed during a strong muscle contraction, if the interference pattern expressed on the oscilloscope is not relatively uniform and full (see Figure 8–15 for an example of a normal interference pattern). A strong muscle contraction is the summed responses of all the available MUAPs, and this normally fills the oscilloscope screen, creating a normal interference pattern. If the interference pattern is less than full with the observed motor units firing at a rapid rate, it is described as representing only single units, or partial screen fill. Loss of motor units and the resulting less-than-optimal screen fill can be indicative of neuropathic conditions.[93]

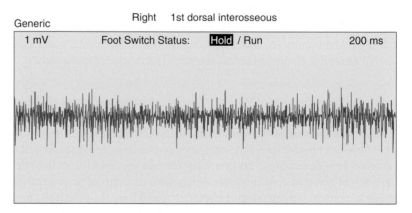

Figure 8–15. Interference pattern with normal motor units.

Summarizing the voluntary contraction part of the examination, the patient will be asked to contract minimally, increase the level of contraction from mild to strong, and then relax the muscle. The minimal contraction permits identification of the MUAP characteristics outlined above. The increase in level of contraction permits examination of recruitment order, the overall amplitude of the largest units, and the ability to achieve a full, smooth contraction (e.g., complete screen fill or normal interference pattern). Finally, the patient needs to relax, and the muscle should be monitored until the normal rest state is reestablished.

The number of muscles that should be assessed in a given examination is the prerogative of the examiner. While in some cases this is limited due to reimbursement issues, the examiner is tasked with ensuring that enough muscles have been sampled with EMG that the question that brought the patient into the clinic can be answered and reasonable alternative explanations can be addressed. This typically entails selecting a sample of muscles that span both the nerve levels of interest (e.g., C5–T1 for an upper extremity problem where some element of the brachial plexus or its derivative elements may be suspected—this includes the nerve roots, the trunks, the divisions, and the cords) and the terminal elements of the named nerve branches. Additionally, if a nerve root impingement is suspected, the examination should include a sample of the posterior (dorsal) primary rami that supply the true muscles of the back (e.g., erector spinae, transversospinalis muscles, and others).[15] See the introduction of this section for one example of a possible screen for the upper extremity.

CASE STUDY 8–3
CLINICAL ELECTROPHYSIOLOGIC TESTING

Background: A 43-year-old automobile manufacturing plant worker noted the sudden onset of left shoulder pain and weakness 6 weeks ago. His job involves a great deal of overhead work. He has been treated for impingement syndrome over the past 3 weeks without relief of the symptoms, and the industrial medicine physician has requested a study to rule out a suprascapular nerve injury.

Physical Examination: The patient has full cervical range of motion although he does note some left midcervical pain with rotation to the left. He has a slight decrease in light touch perception on the thumb, and profound weakness in shoulder abduction. His left biceps brachialis reflex is absent, and all other upper limb reflexes are 2+/4.

Results of Study: The left median DML was prolonged, and the left median sensory NCV across the wrist was slowed. The left median MNCV in the forearm as well as the left median sensory nerve conduction velocity in the palmar segment was within established normal limits, as were all ulnar motor and sensory values. The median and ulnar F-wave latencies were within established normal limits. With needle EMG, evidence of acute denervation (increased insertional activity with 3+/4 fibrillations and PSWs) was observed in the deltoid, biceps brachialis, brachioradialis, serratus anterior, and the midcervical paraspinal muscles. The rhomboid major, triceps brachialis,

extensor indicis proprius, flexor carpi ulnaris, first dorsal interosseus, and opponens pollicis muscles demonstrated normal electrical activity.

Impression: Acute axonopathy of the C6 nerve root with distal (L) median neuropathy at or distal to the wrist.

Follow-up Care: The patient was referred to a neurosurgeon who obtained an MRI of the cervical spine. The MRI demonstrated a large herniation of the C5–6 intervertebral disc, with compression of the C6 nerve root. The patient underwent a discectomy with fusion, and returned to work 12 weeks later. However, the patient was unable to tolerate the constant overhead work on the line he worked on prior to the injury, so he was transferred to another area of the assembly line.

Discussion Questions

- Of what significance are the median nerve abnormalities?
- What would the study have revealed if the referring physician's initial impression (suprascapular neuropathy) had been correct?
- What additional muscles would be denervated?
- How did the study of the rhomboid major help localize the lesion to the C6 nerve root? What would you expect to find on a repeat EMG 16 weeks after the surgery?

Drawing information from the EMG examination (information synthesis). As stated earlier, conclusions are drawn based on the collaborative findings from all the clinical electrophysiologic testings performed. Beginning with the physical examination and any clinical abnormal finding of weakness, sensory alteration, reflex change, atrophy, or any other unusual presentation, the findings from the NCS and EMG examination are analyzed and synthesized. Two examples are provided below that may be illustrative of how this information can be pulled together.

Sensitivity and Specificity of the NCS/EMG Examination

Given a patient with either a positive or negative finding from the collective NCS/EMG examination, what is the likelihood that he or she actually has the problem identified or ruled out by this examination? As is the case with virtually all diagnostic tests, there is the potential for some false positives or false negatives to occur with this type of testing. Sensitivity and specificity values are often used for interpreting the results of diagnostic tests. Test sensitivity is representative of the proportion of patients with the condition that have a positive test result, so a sensitive test is one that recognizes a problem when a problem is actually present. Test specificity, on the other hand, is the ability to recognize when the condition is absent.[95] Each of these measures can have values up to 100%, and higher values are better than lower values. Thus, the ideal is to have a test that has a high level of both sensitivity and specificity. Unfortunately, few tests possess both high sensitivity and specificity.[95]

Sensitivity and specificity values will also depend on the region of the body being investigated and the type of test being performed. These values vary by region and type of test, because the electrophysiologic techniques work better in some areas than in others and are more specific and/or sensitive, with specific conditions. As an example, for the distal median nerve, sensitivity of composite electrophysiologic measures has ranged between 49% and 84%.[2,96–98] Specificity values associated with the median nerve have typically been even better, yielding values of 95% or higher,[55,93,98] for a variety of electrodiagnostic tests. When looking at other pathologies that are more readily identified by the EMG portion of the examination (e.g., radiculopathies), studies have shown that the sensitivity of EMG alone is limited, although the specificity remains relatively high.[6,77,99] For lumbar radiculopathies and plexopathies, specificity ranges of 77–100% were obtained, depending on the diagnostic criteria employed.[100] For other conditions such a chronic inflammatory demyelinating polyneuropathies (CIDP), sensitivity and specificity values are relatively good. For example, in a study by Koski et al[85] that examined 117 patients, a combination of clinical criteria such as time since onset and weakness in one or more extremity, combined with some abnormal motor and sensory latencies and/or nerve conduction velocities, resulted in a sensitivity of 83% (95% confidence interval of 69–93%), and a specificity of 97% (95% confidence interval of 89–99%). Numerous other studies using a variety of criteria for CIDPs have demonstrated sensitivities that range from 54% to 100%, and specificities that range from 48% to 100%.[101–104]

Note that values like those reported above are not based on only one finding, but on the collaborative picture that emerges from the complete electrophysiologic examination. The range of findings is not surprising because sensitivity and specificity are examined across a wide variety of conditions, and the criteria used to make a clinical judgment can be markedly different. Recognizing that electrophysiologic testing is based on a strong physical examination, when there are more clinical findings (e.g., abnormal history, weakness, sensory changes, changes in MSRs), the percentage of patients with abnormal findings also increases. In a recent study, abnormal EMG was found in 90% of subjects with three clinical signs, 59% with two signs, and only 10% with one sign.[105] In another report examining the sensitivity and specificity of 19 separate parameters for carpal tunnel syndrome, the collective presence of 9 parameters permitted a specificity of 97% in the electrodiagnosis of this problem.[106] While these are excellent sensitivity and specificity values, they are not perfect and false-positive electrophysiologic findings have been reported.[3] If individual parts rather than collaborative findings of the electrophysiologic examination are examined, the results in terms of sensitivity and specificity may appear to be markedly different. For example, in patients with carpal tunnel syndrome, the sensory NCS are more frequently abnormal than the motor NCS.[106] Or, some aspects of the examination such as the central conduction study (**F-wave**), by itself, can have a high sensitivity yet low specificity and be of little value when considered alone.[106] Thus, the above findings underscore two key elements associated with electrophysiologic testing: (1) these procedures can yield high sensitivity and specificity based on collaborative findings across the physical examination, NCS, and EMG studies and (2) the findings identified by electrophysiologic testing will be higher in patients with abnormal findings on the physical examination.[107] At the risk of being redundant, it is important to realize that this type of testing is based on an accurate and complete physical examination.

Limitations Associated with the NCS/EMG Process

Electrophysiologic testing has an advantage over some forms of medical testing, in that the methodology employed permits direct evaluation of the functional status of nerves, and to a degree neuromuscular synapses and muscle fibers. This is in contrast to other procedures such as MRIs and x-rays that identify structure rather than function. While the functional approach of electrophysiologic testing is an important adjunctive procedure to delineate a problem suggested by clinical examination or other testing procedures such as MRI, this procedure like all tests has clear limitations. The following abridged list identifies some of the limitations that health care practitioners sending patients for electrodiagnostic testing or interpreting the obtained results should take into consideration:

1. By itself, the electrophysiologic examination is not diagnostic, but provides information that the health care practitioner who is overseeing the patient's care can consider when making a medical diagnosis.

2. Not all nerves and muscles lend themselves to electrophysiologic testing. Significant technical difficulties are present when attempting to obtain nerve conduction values from nerves that are not superficially situated or found in individuals with a significant amount of fat. Thus, not all procedures will be obtainable on all individuals. This also holds true for select muscles, where the risk of performing an EMG might outweigh the potential benefit. For example, obtaining an EMG of an internal intercostal muscle might be technically possible, but the risk of having the needle pierce the parietal pleura and creating a pneumothorax is too great. Therefore, these procedures are not routinely performed.

3. As mentioned in the section "Sensitivity and Specificity of the NCS/EMG Examination", the findings from a NCS/EMG examination are not perfect. Rather, they are reflective of the functional state of the structures sampled at a moment in time and the skill of the individual both performing and interpreting the examination. Therefore, the findings need to be considered in light of all the medical examination procedures performed to form an appropriate picture of the patient's condition.

4. As alluded to in the point above, there are a number of technical pitfalls that can be confusing to an inexperienced electrophysiologic examiner. Dumitru and Zwarts in their excellent text state: "Lack of medical training, lack of expertise in the operation of electrophysiologic instruments, and inability to collect electrodiagnostic data accurately are a prescription for potential misdiagnoses and hence possible patient harm. This is likely the most common pitfall in electrodiagnostic medicine consultations."[52]

5. All the procedures that have been discussed thus far are limited to basically evaluating the PNS, synapses directly involved with the PNS (including some at the segmental level of the spinal cord in the case of an H-reflex), and muscle fibers. Thus, the electrophysiologic testing typically performed provides collaborative information that aids in making a diagnosis, and the information obtained is largely limited to the PNS. There are special tests, such as the SEPs discussed below, that can be used to evaluate some elements of the CNS. Additionally, the use of electrophysiologic testing has expanded in recent years to include intraoperative monitoring (IOM).[108,109]

Somatosensory Evoked Potentials

In the procedures outlined thus far, the only nerve elements that could be examined directly with stimulation at one site and picking up a signal at a second site were either the efferent (motor) or afferent (sensory) fibers distal to the spinal cord. The obtained latencies and amplitudes formed the basis of the motor and sensory NCS described previously. SEPs, on the other hand, expand the structures that can be assessed by this form of stimulation and pickup. With pickup sites at various locations along the spinal cord (lumbosacral region and cervical region), portions of the brainstem (e.g., medulla), and also for cortical structures (e.g., thalamus and central sulcus of the cortex), these other structures can also be evaluated. It should be noted here that the tracts in the spinal cord and brainstem leading up to the cortex that are assessed with this technique are sensory tracts. Therefore, SEPs are reflective of only sensory neurons and the APs traveling along them. The two major pathways that carry sensory information in the CNS are (1) the anterolateral system (a composite reference to the individual tracts of the spinothalamic, spinomesencephalic, and spinoreticular tracts) carrying the modalities of pain, temperature, and crude touch and (2) the dorsal column system, carrying the modalities of two-point discrimination, light touch, vibration, and proprioception.[110,111]

While the equipment and specific setups are beyond the scope of this text, the basic premise of SEPs is the following. A stimulator is used to generate an AP that involves the largest, myelinated axons within a peripheral sensory nerve.[11] This stimulation intensity is typically adjusted by increasing the intensity until a twitch response is noted in the adjacent musculature and using an intensity slightly greater than the onset of the observed twitch. It is believed that this intensity of stimulation will be picked up by these large, myelinated axons since the externally applied current will flow to them preferentially due to their decreased internal resistance (e.g., current will flow along the path of least resistance in accordance with Ohm's law, as described earlier in the chapter). With an elicited SNAP, the AP is carried into the spinal cord and transmitted up to the thalamus via either the anterolateral system or the dorsal column system. From the thalamus, the information being conveyed by a later-generation neuron of the original AP is conveyed to the cortex. If the multiple neuron pathway from the periphery to the cortex is healthy, there will be characteristic positive or negative deflection potentials that can be obtained. This information can then be used to assert that the sensory neurons within the CNS (spinal cord and brain) are conducting normally. If, however, there is a problem in a specific tract in the spinal cord, brainstem, or cortex, the expected deflection potential may be smaller than normal or not obtainable, may have a prolonged latency (e.g., be slowed), or may demonstrate some other type of unusual characteristic. This basic type of assessment can be used to examine the anterolateral system with conditions such as syringomyelia and the dorsal columns in disease states such as multiple sclerosis.[35] In these and a host of other conditions, the obtained information can be used in association with other medical tests performed (e.g., MRIs, laboratory tests, etc.) to attempt to localize the lesion and provide an explanation for the patient's symptoms.

Several other points need to be made in this very brief overview. First, because only sensory fiber tracts are involved and the collective APs are typically being picked up by surface electrodes (epidural needle electrodes can be used in the lumbosacral region), the size of any one obtained potential is too small to be observed. To correct this potential limitation, numerous stimuli are given and averaged together. The theory here is that time-locked phenomena will build on themselves while random noise will cancel out during the averaging process. Depending on the latency component of the potential under investigation, the number of stimuli may vary from 200 to 4000 that are averaged together. The rate of stimulation typically varies from once to four times per second. With modern computers, the averaging and subsequent processing can be done to provide a set of positive and negative potentials that can be interpreted by an expert in these types of studies. Second, there can be numerous pickup electrodes positioned over the scalp, brainstem, cervical region, or other area, and they can record simultaneously. When mapping of the cortex is desired, electrodes are placed on 16–32 sites for monitoring.[11] For most clinical procedures, two to four electrodes at preestablished scalp sites will usually suffice. Clinicians that perform these procedures have a universal system that adapts to skulls of varying size and permits evaluation of areas of suspected pathology. As the above description implies, the nomenclature used to describe the many types and locations of potentials and their associated latencies and amplitudes is confusing. This is an area where consultation with an expert in the field is warranted. Third, because the sensory systems cross the neuraxis prior to reaching the cortex, if unilateral monitoring is done, the stimulation of an extremity will be contralateral to the skull site being evaluated. With today's modern computer systems, bilateral stimulation and monitoring can be done, in addition to unilateral evaluation. Fourth, the most common sites of stimulation are the median nerve at the wrist for the upper extremities and the tibial nerve at the ankle for the lower extremities. Other nerves that are frequently used include the ulnar nerve, fibular nerve, and the pudendal nerve. Fifth, the stability of the obtained SEPs is related to the stimulation site, with APs evoked from the upper extremities providing a more stable response than those obtained from the lower extremities. There is also a strong correlation of obtained latencies with the height of the individual. This is to be expected, because taller individuals have a longer tract pathway from the periphery to the cortex and this creates a longer latency response. Additionally, body temperature affects latency, because nerves conduct faster as temperature increases. The examiner performing these tests needs to consider these and other factors when making judgments regarding the obtained findings.

Electrophysiologic Testing Within The Operating Room

While being a clear specialty practice, the use of electrophysiologic testing in the operating room has grown in recent years as the need for the data provided by the testing procedures has been established and the technology for obtaining the data has improved (e.g., computers have become faster and the signal quality more refined). The examination of somatosensory pathways was first introduced into the operating room in the early 1970s, in an effort to minimize the incidence of paralysis during surgery of the spine.[109] Expansion of IOM grew exponentially with the refinement of motor evoked potential in the 1990s that allowed assessment of motor spinal pathways and related structures.[108] Monitoring is now used for multiple procedures including craniotomies, spinal cord tumor resection, surgery involving structures intimately associated with nerves such as the recurrent laryngeal nerve, tethered cord, pedicle screw placement, and deep brain stimulation for movement disorders such as Parkinson's disease.[108,109] The intent of this type of IOM is to quickly identify problems during surgery so that the severity of any potential neural insult can be minimized or eliminated. The utility of this type of intraoperative testing was demonstrated in a cervical spine case study, where free-running EMG during the surgery demonstrated that with the planned surgery, an observed irritation at C5–6 did not subside. This information was used to extend the surgery to a decompression with foraminotomy, which did eliminate the observed irritation and resulted in a normal neurological examination immediately after surgery and at 3 months follow-up.[112]

This brief description of SEPs and IOM has been provided to make the point that while the most commonly used NCS/EMG procedures described earlier in the chapter evaluate predominantly the PNS, there are methodologies that permit examination of the less accessible areas of the spinal cord, brainstem, thalamus, and cortex. SEPs do this for sensory fibers, and motor evoked potentials can be used to evaluate portions of the voluntary motor system and during IOM. These techniques are not performed in all electrophysiologic laboratories, and they require a practitioner with significant experience with this type of testing. Having said that, these adjunctive techniques are used with patient categories ranging from bowel, bladder, and sexual dysfunction to the impact of diabetes within the CNS, Charcot–Marie–Tooth, subacute combined degeneration, and select surgical interventions.[11] Thus, techniques such as SEPs and IOM are electrophysiologic testing procedures that may be employed as part of the evaluation and care that a patient receives.

Other Electrophysiologic Testing Procedures

Electrophysiologic testing is a specialty area. The NCS/EMG examinations outlined in this chapter are routinely performed and with some education and experience, readily interpreted. The aforementioned SEPs and many other forms of testing that can be done in an electrophysiologic laboratory do not lend themselves to interpretation without significant time, education, and experience in this field. Therefore, while there are many other procedures such as single fiber techniques, motor evoked potentials, IOM,[113,114] and magnetic stimulation of the CNS and PNS, to name just a few, they are beyond the scope of this chapter. (The interested reader is referred to the excellent texts by Dumitru et al,[1] Oh,[59] and Kimura.[75] The intent of the description provided in this chapter was to simply provide general information regarding basic NCS and EMG procedures, along with the type of clinical information that they provide.)

REQUESTING NCS/EMG EXAMINATIONS

If requesting an NCS/EMG examination, the following is suggested:

1. It is based on a good physical examination.
2. Specific clinical findings are highlighted and a working hypothesis put forth.

NCS and EMG examinations are appropriate for patients who require information beyond that regularly available from a clinical examination or imaging studies, regarding the status of their neuromuscular system. Since the information that will be provided from the NCS/EMG examination will be collaborative with the clinical examination and imaging studies, this information should be provided along with the consult. A key point stressed throughout this chapter is that the NCS/EMG examination is based on a good physical examination. Therefore, the referring clinician should ideally obtain a good subjective (history) and complete a thorough objective (physical) examination. A working hypothesis should be formulated based on the specific findings of the history and physical examinations. This working hypothesis or referring diagnosis will assist the clinical electrophysiologist in developing and implementing the NCS and EMG examinations. In the presence of a completely normal physical examination, it is the exception rather than the rule that electrophysiologic testing will reveal any additional information.

It is not appropriate to send patients for NCS/EMG examinations as a method of screening the neuromuscular system when the physical examination is completely normal. This is because the tests are relatively expensive, involve some discomfort and risk due to the insertion of needle electrodes and electrical shocks, and have a relatively low yield in patients without physical findings. However, with signs and symptoms such as sensory changes, weakness, atrophy, reflex changes, and easy fatigability, the likelihood of identifying abnormal electrophysiologic parameters increases dramatically. This collaborative information is then used along with the previously obtained information to make a clear diagnosis and provide the basis from which a logical treatment program can be developed. Thus, a consult for this type of evaluation should be based on a good physical examination and be as specific as is reasonable.

CONCLUSION

NCS and the EMG examination provide a great deal of information regarding the functional status of nerves, neuromuscular junctions, and muscle. As such, they are excellent adjunctive procedures to complement the findings by either a clinical physical examination or other special tests such as MRIs or x-rays. Strengths associated with this form of testing include the fact that they are minimally invasive, very safe, and provide information that is a direct assessment of the functional status of the structures under examination. Limitations include the fact that some aspects of the examination are technically difficult, significant skill and sophisticated equipment need to be possessed by the examiner, and the primary region that is investigated with the typical NCS/EMG examination is the PNS, synapse, and muscle. While other regions of the nervous system such as the brain and spinal cord can be examined, this is beyond the scope of all but the most specialized practitioners, and these tests are consequently not as frequently performed. The findings from these tests are typically provided back to the referral source in language that describes what was observed electrophysiologically. This information then gives the health care practitioner additional information on which a diagnosis can be developed.

It is hoped that the information provided on basic neurophysiology and an overview of the generic NCS/EMG procedures used has shed some insight on the application of these procedures. While the chapter has been written to provide a basic understanding of the process, it is not intended to provide the information needed to perform these procedures. The electrophysiologic testing is an area of specialization that requires advanced didactic and clinical experience.

SUMMARY

1. Electrophysiologic testing is an extension of a good physical examination and normally consists of:
   (a) nerve function evaluation (integrity, speed, and the size of obtained potentials);
   (b) EMG (use of a needle assessing muscle APs); and less frequently
   (c) SEPs that are capable of evaluating some CNS components.

2. Specialized equipment is needed to perform an electrophysiologic evaluation. The basic components involved include the following:
   (a) electrodes to couple the equipment to the patient to obtain an electrical signal;
   (b) an amplifier to boost the normally small natural change in voltage potentials;
   (c) an oscilloscope to observe the response;
   (d) a computer to quantify the response;
   (e) a stimulator to provide an electrical current to elicit a response;
   (f) speakers to permit audio assessment of the response;
   (g) a printer to document findings.

   Depending on the testing performed, these and potentially other equipment will be used to test the integrity of specific portions of the nervous system.

3. The typical NCS and EMG evaluation primarily focuses on evaluating the PNS, the neuromuscular synapse, and function of muscle fibers. In addition to these peripheral structures, the function of anterior horn cells located in the gray matter of the anterior horn of the spinal cord, and thus technically part of the CNS, can also be evaluated. (As stated in #1, specialized testing with additional techniques such as SEPs is needed if more CNS evaluation is required.)

4. Not all nerves conduct with equal speed and the environment that they exist in can affect their function. NCV tests evaluate the fastest conducting fibers, and generally these fibers conduct faster in the upper extremity than in the lower extremity. Additionally, the speed of nerve function is influenced by other factors such as temperature (nerves that are cold conduct slower) and age (the nerves of young and old individuals typically conduct slower than those of young adults).

5. The typical elements of a NCS are:
   (a) Sensory nerve studies that assess the time it takes for a signal to pass over a known distance or latency. This is evaluating the fastest conducting sensory fibers of a segment of a nerve, and the small signal is typically measured in microvolts. In addition to the latency, the size (amplitude), shape, and NCV of the SNAP are assessed.
   (b) Motor nerve studies, assessing the ability of the fastest conducting motor axons to conduct to the neuromuscular junction, cross the junction, and activate the innervated muscle fibers. Because this is the combined signal of numerous muscle fibers, the assessed response is much larger than a sensory potential and is measured in microvolts. Some of the factors evaluated in these studies include latency, amplitude, rise time, duration, shape, and NCV.
      • Other complementary tests can also be performed, such as central conduction studies and H-waves that assess the integrity of the nerve along its entire length, up to the level of the spinal cord and back.

6. The EMG evaluation consists of placing some type of small-diameter, sterile needle electrode (these vary) into a muscle and obtaining a signal. Abnormal responses during the insertion, examination of the muscle at rest, or during voluntary contraction are noted and correlated with the patient's complaint and physical examination. This portion of the examination is very useful for a wide variety of conditions, including those that result in abnormal axon function (axonopathy) or in diseases affecting muscle function (myopathies).

7. A NCS/EMG evaluation is a reasonably sensitive and specific test for problems involving anterior horn cells, the PNS, the neuromuscular junction, and innervated muscle fibers. The sensitivity and specificity improve when the physical examination provides more than

one clinical finding. While being reasonable tests, these evaluation procedures are not perfect and false-positive electrophysiologic findings have been reported.

8. Electrophysiologic testing is a valuable adjunct to the physical examination, but it does not lend itself to all nerves and muscles. Some nerves and muscles are too technically difficult to assess routinely (e.g., the intercostal nerves and muscles in close proximity to the lungs). The electrophysiologic examination, by itself, is not diagnostic. The electrophysiologic examination confirms the information assessed during the subjective physical examination and provides information the health care provider overseeing an individual's care can consider when making a medical diagnosis.

9. Electrophysiologic testing is a specialty area that requires considerable training, anatomic and physiologic knowledge, and experience.

REVIEW QUESTIONS

1. What are the characteristics of patients that make them prime referral candidates for a NCS/EMG evaluation?

2. In examining the portions of the typical electrophysiologic evaluation (NCS/EMG), what portion of the examination and findings suggests a problem that is predominantly due to the loss of myelin?

3. In examining the portions of the typical electrophysiologic evaluation (NCS/EMG), what portion of the examination and findings suggests a problem that is predominantly due to damage or loss of axons (axonopathy)?

4. Within the context of a NCS, what is the general principle behind a sensory nerve study compared with a motor nerve study?

5. Two measurements of speed of conduction are latency and NCV. How are these two variables related, how do they differ, and on what are they based?

6. If a patient has a suspected problem with the neuromuscular junction, how will the NCS/EMG examination be modified to address this particular area of the neuromuscular system?

7. How does the duration, shape, and size of MUAPs compare between an individual with normally innervated muscle and an individual with a myopathy?

8. What do the following findings suggest, in terms of both altered function and potential disease processes?
   (a) PSWs
   (b) fibrillations
   (c) fasciculations
   (d) interference pattern that is not uniform and full (dropped motor units)
   (e) myotonic discharges

9. During voluntary contraction of muscle, what is the normally expected order of recruitment of motor units? Why?

10. What are five limitations associated with electrophysiologic testing, as outlined in the chapter?

SELF-TEST QUESTIONS

True or False

1. Both myasthenia gravis and Lambert–Eaton are examples of postsynaptic dysfunction.

2. A fibrillation potential is defined as the "spontaneous firing of a motor neuron and all of the muscle fibers innervated by that motor neuron."

3. An H-reflex is physiologically equivalent to a MSR. Following stimulation, an AP is carried proximally via afferent axons to the spinal cord, where the combined potential enters

the dorsal horn of the spinal cord, passes through at least one synapse, and then is carried via efferent axons to the appropriate distal muscle.

Multiple Choice

4. Which of the following *best* represents the role of a patient history and physical examination, in relation to electrophysiologic testing?
   a. Electrophysiologic testing stands by itself as an objective assessment of nerve function (no history or physical examination is needed).
   b. A history can assist with items such as the potential for inherited traits, but there is no compelling need to perform a physical examination.
   c. If laboratory tests and preceding assessment measures such as MRIs have been obtained, it is redundant to take the time to perform a history and/or physical examination.
   d. Electrophysiologic testing is based on a sound history and physical examination.

5. With a compression of the superficial branch of the ulnar nerve at Guyon's canal, which of the following would be expected?
   a. prolonged distal latency to D5
   b. faster conduction velocity of the motor fibers
   c. increased amplitude of the ulnar SNAP
   d. decreased recruitment of the ADM and first DI

6. What is the typical minimum NCV speed of a normal mixed nerve (motor and sensory) in the upper extremity?
   a. 40 m/s
   b. 50 m/s
   c. 60 m/s
   d. 70 m/s

7. When comparing DSLs to DMLs, taken over the same distance (e.g., 8 cm), what would be expected?
   a. DSL > DML
   b. DML > DSL
   c. DSL = DML
   d. It is variable throughout various regions of the body—there is not one consistent relationship as expressed above.

8. When examining a patient with a potential neuromuscular junction disorder, which of the following repetitive stimulation findings would be most likely?
   a. Repetitive stimulation amplitude would equal single-stimulation amplitude in myasthenia gravis.
   b. NCV in Lambert–Eaton would be expected to decrease following repetitive stimulation.
   c. NCV in myasthenia gravis would be expected to increase following repetitive stimulation.
   d. Repetitive stimulation amplitude would increase compared with single-stimulation amplitude in Eaton–Lambert.

9. The time lapse from the stimulation (stimulus artifact) to the onset of the compound motor unit action potential (CMAP) is referred to as the
   a. amplitude
   b. rise time
   c. DML
   d. neural conduction velocity

10. EMG is the recording and study of the electrical activity of muscle. The first procedure typically performed during an EMG evaluation is the study of
    a. voluntary activity—minimal contraction
    b. insertional activity
    c. muscle at rest
    d. spontaneous activity

11. A polyphasic MUAP is defined as having how many phases?
 a. >3
 b. >5
 c. >7
 d. >9

SOLUTIONS TO CLINICAL DECISION-MAKING EXERCISES

8-1

The findings that are listed above may be isolated solely to the ulnar nerve, but this finding may also be a piece of a larger involvement. Electrophysiologic testing permits a number of nerves to be assessed, beyond the ones that are typically done in an upper extremity or lower extremity screen. In this case, the electrophysiologist could add in the assessment of one or more additional nerves. An ideal one to assess in this case would be the medial cutaneous nerve of the forearm, which arises off of the medial cord. If it also demonstrated a diminished SNAP amplitude and/or prolonged latency, this would provide additional evidence implicating a medial cord (a plexopathy) or some other proximally located problem. The EMG portion of the assessment could then also explore additional muscles with innervation off of the medial cord, such as the sternocostal portion of the pectoralis major muscle (medial pectoral nerve, C8–T1), APB (median nerve, C8–T1), or flexor pollicis longus (AIN, C8–T1), for additional data that would assist with the diagnosis.

8-2

It is essential to assess skin temperature of the distal portion of an extremity being evaluated, since temperature of the nerve bed under the skin is inversely related to NCV. If the skin temperature is below optimal (e.g., less than 32°C in the hands), the assessed nerves will conduct slower and the obtained latencies will be longer. In the presence of obtained temperatures less than optimal, the clinician needs to warm the distal extremity up using an appropriate heating method, or at a minimum, employ a correction factor (see reference texts by Dumitru, Kimura, Oh), to adjust for the impact of suboptimal temperatures on nerve conduction parameters.

8-3

There are several things that can be done to increase the chance of eliciting a nerve such as the LCNT, which is technically a challenge to elicit. First, with the stimulating electrode, ensure that the area being stimulated is clean and any resistance created by oil or lotions on the skin is removed. This is easily done with an alcohol swap. Then, ensure firm pressure with the stimulating electrode, and following obtaining maximum stimulation intensity without a good result, it may be necessary to increase the pulse width of the stimulation used. The increase in pulse width functionally allows more current to flow into the area being stimulated that can assist in having the axons reach threshold. If all of these measures are unsuccessful, a lead from a needle can be attached to the stimulator, and a needle inserted through the skin in the immediate vicinity of the LCNT. This is using a needle electrode as an active electrode (near-nerve stimulation), and as the needle is slowly advanced while triggering the stimulator, the electrophysiologist can assess the response and work to find the ideal depth of the needle electrode for an optimal response.

Two things should be noted from the previous discussion. First, even with employment of a needle stimulating electrode, there will be some individuals where a clear SNAP is not obtained. This is particularly true of overweight or obese individuals. Second, this near-nerve needle stimulation technique can be used at other locations in the body where it is challenging to stimulate the nerve directly using a surface stimulator. In addition, if the symptoms are unilateral, testing of the contralateral (nonsymptomatic) LCNT must be performed.

8–4

Normally, a positive deflection or less-than-optimal "rise time" of the initial deflection suggests that the pickup electrode is not positioned over the motor point of the muscle. Taking the electrode off and repositioning the pickup and/or the reference electrode will often resolve the problem. This can be somewhat of a "trial and error" process, but an acceptable CMAP initial deflection is typically found within a trial or two. It should also be noted that some conditions, such as the normal variant expressed in a Martin-Gruber anastomosis, can cause an initial positive deflection. In this case, repositioning the active and/or reference electrode will not resolve the initial positive deflection.

8–5

The level of a radiculopathy is typically identified by examining the nerve root contributions of all muscles with identified denervation or other altered EMG activity, and seeking a common root level or two that is consistent with the identified findings. For all of the extremity muscles and the majority of muscles originating from the axial skeleton, the branch of the typical spinal nerve that contributes to those named nerves is the anterior (ventral) primary rami. To assert that the location is as proximal as a nerve root, there will ideally also be EMG findings in the paraspinals that are supplied by the posterior (dorsal) primary rami. When muscles innervated by both APR and PPR show the same types of abnormal EMG, this implicates the nerve root since this branching occurs as the nerve root exits the intervertebral foramina.

REFERENCES

1. Dumitru D, Amato A, Zwarts M. *Electrodiagnostic Medicine*. 2nd ed. Philadelphia, PA: Hanley & Belfus; 2002.

2. Kimura J. *Electrodiagnosis in Diseases of Nerve and Muscle*. 2nd ed. Philadelphia, PA: FA Davis; 1989.

3. Redmond M, Rivner M. False positive electrodiagnostic tests in carpal tunnel syndrome. *Muscle Nerve*. 1988;11:511–518.

4. Bahrami M, Rayegani S, Zare A. Studying nerve conduction velocity and latency of accessory nerve motor potential in normal persons. *Electromyogr Clin Neurophysiol*. 2004;44:11–14.

5. Shakir A, Micklesen P, Robinson L. Which motor nerve conduction study is best in ulnar neuropathy at the elbow? *Muscle Nerve*. 2004;29:585–590.

6. Blijham P, Hengstman G, Ter Laak H, Van Engelen B, Zwarts M. Muscle-fiber conduction velocity and electromyography as diagnostic tools in patients with suspected inflammatory myopathy: a prospective study. *Muscle Nerve*. 2004;29:46–50.

7. Dobner J, Nitz A. Postmeniscectomy tourniquet palsy and functional sequelae. *Am J Sports Med*. 1982;10:211–214.

8. Boon A, Harper C. Needle EMG of abductor hallucis and peroneus tertius in normal subjects. *Muscle Nerve*. 2003;27:752–756.

9. Ulas U, Cengiz B, Alanoglu E, Ozdag M, Odabasi Z, Vural O. Comparison of sensitivities of macro EMG and concentric needle EMG in L4 radiculopathy. *Neurol Sci*. 203;24:258–260.

10. Dumitru D, Amato A, Zwarts M. Nerve conduction studies. In: Dumitru D, Amato A, Zwarts M, eds. *Electrodiagnostic Medicine*. 2nd ed. Philadelphia, PA: Hanley & Belfus; 2002:159–223.

11. Kimura J, ed. Somatosensory and motor evoked potentials. In: *Electrodiagnosis in Diseases of Nerve and Muscle*. 2nd ed. Philadelphia, PA: FA Davis; 1989:375–426.

12. Oh S, ed. Somatosensory evoked potentials in peripheral nerve lesions. In: *Clinical Electromyograph—Nerve Conduction Studies*. 2nd ed. Baltimore, MD: Williams & Wilkins; 1993:447–478.

13. Storm S, Kraft G. The clinical use of dermatomal somatosensory evoked potentials in lumbosacral spinal stenosis. *Phys Med Rehabil Clin N Am*. 2004;15:107–115.

14. Amaral D. The anatomical organization of the central nervous system. In: Kandel E, Schwartz J, Jessell T, eds. *Principles of Neural Science*. 4th ed. New York: McGraw-Hill; 2000:317–336.

15. Moore K, Dalley A. *Clinically Oriented Anatomy*. Philadelphia, PA: Lippincott Williams & Wilkins; 1999.

16. Dumitru D. Instrumentation. In: Dumitru D, Amato A, Zwarts M, eds. *Electrodiagnostic Medicine*. 2nd ed. Philadelphia, PA: Hanley & Belfus; 2002:69–97.

17. Dumitru D, Stegeman D, Zwarts M. Electrical sources and volume conduction. In: Dumitru D, Amato A, Zwarts M, eds. *Electrodiagnostic Medicine*. 2nd ed. Philadelphia, PA: Hanley & Belfus; 2002:27–53.

18. Howard FJ. The electromyogram and conduction velocity studies in peripheral nerve trauma. *Clin Neurosurg*. 1970;17:63–75.

19. Stevens J. AAEM minimonograph #26: the electrodiagnosis of carpal tunnel syndrome. *Muscle Nerve*. 1887;20:1477–1486.

20. Wilbourn A. Sensory nerve conduction studies. *J Clin Neurophysiol*. 1994;11:584–601.

21. Kimura J, ed. Principles of nerve conduction studies. In: *Electrodiagnosis in Diseases of Nerve and Muscle*. Philadelphia, PA: FA Davis; 1989:78–102.

22. Bawa P, Binder M, Ruenzel P, Henneman E. Recruitment order of motoneurons in stretch reflexes is highly correlated with their axonal conduction velocity. *J Neurophysiol*. 1984;52:410–420.

23. Clamann H, Henneman E. Electrical measurement of axon diameter and its use in relating motoneuron size to critical firing level. *J Neurophysiol*. 1976;39:844–851.

24. Davidoff R. Skeletal muscle tone and the misunderstood stretch reflex. *Neurology*. 1992;42:951–963.

25. Knaflitz M, Merletti R, De Luca C. Inference of motor unit recruitment order in voluntary and electrically elicited contractions. *J Appl Physiol*. 1990;68:1657–1667.

26. Tasaki I. Electric stimulation and the excitatory process in the nerve fiber. *Am J Physiol*. 1838;125:385.

27. Dumitru D, King J, Stegeman D. Normal needle electromyographic insertional activity morphology: a clinical and simulation study. *Muscle Nerve*. 1998;21:910–920.

28. Preston D, Shapiro B. Needle electromyography: fundamentals, normal and abnormal patterns. *Neurol Clin*. 2002;20:361–396.

29. Wiechers D, Stow R, Johnson E. Electromyographic insertional activity mechanically provoked in the biceps brachii. *Arch Phys Med Rehabil*. 1977;58:573–578.

30. Haines D, Mihailoff G, Yezierski R. The spinal cord. In: Haines D, ed. *Fundamental Neuroscience*. New York: Churchill Livingstone; 1997:129–141.

31. Aidley D, ed. The organization of sensory receptors. In: *The Physiology of Excitable Cells*. New York: Cambridge University Press; 1998:346–365.

32. Aidley D, ed. Electrical properties of the nerve axon. In: *The Physiology of Excitable Cells*. New York: Cambridge University Press; 1989:30–53.

33. Dumitru D, ed. Nerve and muscle anatomy and physiology. In: *Electrodiagnostic Medicine*. Philadelphia, PA: Hanley & Belfus; 1995:3–28.

34. Waxman SG, Foster RE. Ionic channel distribution and heterogeneity of the axon membrane in myelinated fibers. *Brain Res Rev*. 1980;2:205–234.

35. Kawamura Y, Okazaki H, O'Brien P, Dych P. Lumbar motoneurons of man: I) number and diameter histogram of alpha and gamma axons of ventral root. *J Neuropathol Exp Neurol*. 1977;36:853–860.

36. Kandel E, Siegelbaum S. Signaling at the nerve–muscle synapse: directly gated transmission. In: Kandel E, Schwartz J, Jessell T, eds. *Principles of Neural Science*. 4th ed. New York: McGraw-Hill; 2000:187–206.

37. Richman D, Agius M. Treatment of autoimmune myasthenia gravis. *Neurology*. 2003;61:1652–1661.

38. Takamori M, Komai K, Iwasa K. Antibodies to calcium channel and synaptotagmin in Lambert–Eaton myasthenic syndrome. *Am J Med Sci*. 2000;318:204–208.

39. Ellenberg M, Gardin H, Hyman S, Chodoroff G. Orthodromic vs. antidromic latencies. *Arch Phys Med Rehabil*. 1991;72:431–432.

40. Seror P. The medial antebrachial cutaneous nerve: antidromic and orthodromic conduction studies. *Muscle Nerve*. 2002;26:421–423.

41. Hassantash S, Afrakhteh M, Maier R. Causalgia: a meta-analysis of the literature. *Arch Surg*. 2003;138:1226–1231.

42. Naftel J, Hardy S. Visceral motor pathways. In: Haines D, ed. *Fundamental Neuroscience*. New York: Churchill Livingstone; 1997:417–430.

43. Burke D. Microneurography, impulse conduction, and paresthesias. *Muscle Nerve*. 1993;16:1025–1032.

44. Hanson P, Deltombe T. Preliminary study of large and small peripheral nerve fibers in Charcot–Marie–Tooth disease, type I. *Am J Phys Med Rehabil*. 1998;77:45–48.

45. Prout B. Independence of the galvanic skin reflex from the vasoconstrictor reflex in man. *J Neurol Neurosurg Psychiatr*. 1967;30:319–324.

46. Torebjork E. Human microneurography and intraneural microstimulation in the study of neuropathic pain. *Muscle Nerve*. 1883;18:1483.

47. Ross M, Kaye G, Pawlina W, eds. Nerve tissue. In: *Histology: A Text and Atlas*. 4th ed. Baltimore, MD: Lippincott Williams & Wilkins; 2003:282–325.

48. Halle J, Scoville C, Greathouse D. Ultrasound's effect on the conduction latency of the superficial radial nerve in man. *Phys Ther*. 1981;61:345–350.

49. Rutkove S. Effects of temperature on neuromuscular electro-physiology. *Muscle Nerve*. 2001;24:867–882.

50. Greathouse DG, Halle JS. *Neural Conduction Study Guidelines—Laboratory Values*. Fort Campbell, Clarksville, TN, Electrophysiology Laboratory, Blanchfield Army Community Hospital; 2004.

51. Oh S, ed. Physiological factors affecting nerve conduction. In: *Clinical Electromyography—Nerve Conduction Studies*. 2nd ed. Baltimore, MD: Williams & Wilkins; 1993:297–313.

52. Dumitru D, Zwarts M. Electrodiagnostic medicine pitfalls. In: Dumitru D, Amato A, Zwarts M, eds. *Electrodiagnostic Medicine*. 2nd ed. Philadelphia, PA: Hanley & Belfus; 2002:541–577.

53. Nestor DE, Nelson RM. *Performing Motor and Sensory Neuronal Conduction Studies in Adult Humans—A NIOSH Technical Manual*. DHHS (NIOSH) publication no. 89-XXX. Morgantown, WV: Division of Safety Research, National Institute for Occupational Safety and Health; 1987.

54. Dumitru D, ed. Volume conduction. In: *Electrodiagnostic Medicine*. Philadelphia, PA: Hanley & Belfus; 1995:29–64.

55. Dumitru D, Zwarts M. Focal peripheral neuropathies. In: Dumitru D, Amato A, Zwarts M, eds. *Electrodiagnostic Medicine*. 2nd ed. Philadelphia, PA: Hanley & Belfus; 2002:1043–1126.

56. Ayotte K, Boswell L, Hansen D. A comparison of orthodromic and antidromic sensory neural conduction latencies and amplitudes for the palmar branch of the median and ulnar nerves in healthy subjects. *J Clin Electrophysiol.* 1992;4:12–18.

57. Dumitru D, ed. Nerve conduction studies. In: *Electrodiagnostic Medicine.* Philadelphia, PA: Hanley & Belfus; 1995:111–176.

58. Van Dijk JG, Tjon-a-Tsien A, van der Kamp W. CMAP variability as a function of electrode site and size. *Muscle Nerve.* 1995;18(1):68–73.

59. Oh S. *Clinical Electromyography—Nerve Conduction Studies.* 2nd ed. Baltimore, MD: Williams & Wilkins; 1993.

60. Aidley D, ed. Neuromuscular transmission. In: *The Physiology of Excitable Cells.* 3rd ed. New York: Cambridge University Press; 1989:110–138.

61. Dumitru D, Gitter A. Nerve and muscle anatomy and physiology. In: Dumitru D, Amato A, Zwarts M, eds. *Electrodiagnostic Medicine.* 2nd ed. Philadelphia, PA: Hanley & Belfus; 2002:3–26.

62. Guyton A. *Textbook of Medical Physiology.* 8th ed. Philadelphia, PA: WB Saunders; 1991:38–50.

63. Brown P. The electrochemical basis of neuronal integration. In: Haines D, ed. *Fundamental Neuroscience.* New York: Churchill Livingstone; 1997:31–50.

64. Dumitru D, Robinson L, Zwarts M. Somatosensory evoked potentials. In: Dumitru D, Amato A, Zwarts M, eds. *Electrodiagnostic Medicine.* 2nd ed. Philadelphia, PA: Hanley & Belfus; 2002:357–414.

65. Dumitru D, ed. Special nerve conduction techniques. In: *Electrodiagnostic Medicine.* Philadelphia, PA: Hanley & Belfus; 1995:177–209.

66. Dumitru D, ed. Special nerve conduction techniques. In: *Electrodiagnostic Medicine.* Philadelphia, PA: Hanley & Belfus; 2002:225–256.

67. Kimura J, ed. The F wave. In: *Electrodiagnosis in Diseases of Nerve and Muscle: Principles and Practice.* 2nd ed. Philadelphia, PA: FA Davis; 1989:332–355.

68. Magladery J, McDougal DJ. Electrophysiological studies of nerve and reflex activity in normal man. *Bull Johns Hopkins Hosp.* 1950;86:265–290.

69. Dumitru D, ed. AAEM glossary of terms. In: *Electrodiagnostic Medicine.* Philadelphia, PA: Hanley & Belfus; 1995:1172–1208.

70. Fisher M. F response latency determination. *Muscle Nerve.* 1982;5:730–734.

71. Kimura J, Butzer J. F-wave conduction velocity in Guillain Barre syndrome: assessment of nerve segment between axilla and spinal cord. *Arch Neurol.* 1975;32:524–529.

72. Kimura J, Yamada T, Stevland N. Distal slowing of motor nerve conduction velocity in diabetic polyneuropathy. *J Neurol Sci.* 1979;42:291–302.

73. Kimura J. Proximal versus distal slowing of motor nerve conduction velocity in the Guillain–Barre syndrome. *Ann Neurol.* 1978;3:344–350.

74. Troni W. The value and limits of the H reflex as a diagnostic tool in S1 root compression. *Electromyogr Clin Neurophysiol.* 1883;23:471–480.

75. Kimura J. *Electrodiagnosis in Diseases of Nerve and Muscle: Principles and Practice.* 3rd ed. New York, NY: Oxford University Press; 2001.

76. Dumitru D. Needle electromyography. In: *Electrodiagnostic Medicine.* Philadelphia, PA: Hanley & Belfus; 1995: 211–248.

77. Wainner R, Fritz J, Irrgang J, Boninger M, Delitto A, Allison S. Reliability and diagnostic accuracy of the clinical examination and patient self-report measures for cervical radiculopathy. *Spine.* 2003;28:52–62.

78. Dumitru D, ed. Neuromuscular junction disorders. In: *Electrodiagnostic Medicine.* Philadelphia, PA: Hanley & Belfus; 1995:929–1030.

79. Kimura J, ed. Techniques and normal findings. In: *Electrodiagnosis in Diseases of Nerve and Muscle: Principles and Practice.* 2nd ed. Philadelphia, PA: FA Davis; 1989: 227–248.

80. Wiechers D. Mechanically provoked insertional activity before and after nerve section in rats. *Arch Phys Med Rehabil.* 1977;58:402–405.

81. Daube JA. *AAEM Minimonograph #11: Needle Examination in Electromyography.* Rochester, MN: AAEM; 1979.

82. Dumitru D, ed. Needle electromyography. In: Dumitru D, Amato A, Zwarts M, eds. *Electrodiagnostic Medicine.* Philadelphia, PA: Hanley & Belfus; 2002:257–291.

83. Brumlik J, Drechsler B, Vannin T. The myotonic discharge in various neurological syndromes: a neurophysiologic analysis. *Electromyography.* 1970;10:369–383.

84. Dorfman L, Howard J, McGill K. Motor unit firing rates and firing variability in the detection of neuromuscular disorders. *Electroencephalogr Clin Neurophysiol.* 1989;73: 215–224.

85. Koski CL, Baumgarten M, Magder LS, et al. Derivation and validation of diagnostic criteria for chronic inflammatory demyelinating polyneuropathy. *J Neurol Sci.* 2009;15;277(1–2):1–8.

86. Howard J, McGill K, Dorfman L. Age effects on properties of motor unit action potentials: ADEMG analysis. *Ann Neurol.* 1988;24:207–213.

87. Nandedkar S, Stalberg E, Sanders D. Quantitative EMG. In: Dumitru D, Amato A, Zwarts M, eds. *Electrodiagnostic Medicine.* 2nd ed. Philadelphia, PA: Hanley & Belfus; 2002:293–356.

88. Finsterer J, Fuglsang-Frederiksen A. Concentric-needle versus macro EMG. II. Detection of neuromuscular disorders. *Clin Neurophysiol.* 2001;112:853–860.

89. Goodgold J, Eberstein A. Myopathy. In: Goodgold J, Eberstein A, eds. *Electrodiagnosis of Neuromuscular Diseases.* Baltimore, MD: Williams & Wilkins; 1972:116–138.

90. LaHoda F, Russ A, Issel W, eds. Electromyography. In: *EMG Primer.* Berlin, GE: Springer-Verlag; 1974:16.

91. Nelson R, Nestor D. Electrophysiological evaluation: an overview. In: Nelson R, Currier D, eds. *Clinical Electrotherapy*. Norwalk, CT: Appleton & Lange; 1991:331–384.

92. Nelson R, Shedlock M, Kaczmarek C, Gahrs J, MacLaughlin H. Comparison of motor unit action potentials using monopolar vs. concentric needle electrodes in the middle deltoid and abductor digiti minimi muscles. *Electromyogr Clin Neurophysiol*. 2003;43:459–464.

93. Kimura J, ed. Types of abnormality. In: *Electrodiagnosis in Diseases of Nerve and Muscle: Principles and Practice*. 2nd ed. Philadelphia, PA: FA Davis; 1989:249–274.

94. Dumitru D, Amato A. Introduction to myopathies and muscle tissue's reaction to injury. In: Dumitru D, Amato A, Zwarts M, eds. *Electrodiagnostic Medicine*. 3rd ed. Philadelphia, PA: Hanley & Belfus; 2002:1229–1264.

95. Fritz J, Wainner R. Examining diagnostic tests: an evidence-based perspective. *Phys Ther*. 2001;81:1546–1564.

96. American Association of Electrodiagnostic Medicine. Practice parameter for electrodiagnostic studies in carpal tunnel syndrome: summary statement. *Muscle Nerve*. 1993;16:1390–1391.

97. Jablecki C, Andary M, So Y. Literature review of the usefulness of nerve conduction studies and electromyography for the evaluation of patients with carpal tunnel syndrome. *Muscle Nerve*. 1993;16:1392–1414.

98. Robinson LR, Micklesen PJ, Wang L. Strategies for analyzing nerve conduction data: superiority of a summary index over single tests. *Muscle Nerve*. 1998;21:1166–1171.

99. Dillingham T. Electrodiagnostic approach to patients with suspected radiculopathy. *Phys Med Rehabil Clin N Am*. 2003;14:567–588.

100. Tong HC, Haig AJ, Yamakawa KS, Miner JA. Specificity of needle electromyography for lumbar radiculopathy and plexopathy in 55 to 79-year-old asymptomatic subjects. *Am J Phys Med Rehabil*. 2006;85(11):908–912.

101. De Sousa EA, Chin RL, Sander HW, Latov N, Brannagan TH 3rd. Demyelinating findings in typical and atypical chronic inflammatory demyelinating polyneuropathy: sensitivity and specificity. *J Clin Neuromuscul Dis*. 2009;10(4):163–169.

102. Isose S, Kiwabara S, Kokubun N, et al. Utility of the distal compound muscle action potential duration for diagnosis of demyelinating neuropathies. *J Peripher Nerv Syst*. 2009;14(3):151–158.

103. Rajabally YA, Narasimhan M. The value of sensory electrophysiology in chronic inflammatory demyelinating polyneuropathy. *Clin Neurophysiol*. 2007;118(9):1999–2004.

104. Rajabally YA, Nicholas G, Pieret F, Bouche P, Van den Bergh PY. Validity of diagnostic criteria for chronic inflammatory demyelinating polyneuropathy: a multicentre European study. *J Neurol Neurosurg Psychiatry*. 2009;80(12):1364–1368.

105. Miller T, Pardo R, Yaworski R. Clinical utility of reflex studies in assessing cervical radiculopathy. *Muscle Nerve*. 1999;22:1075–1079.

106. Kuntzer T. Carpal tunnel syndrome in 100 patients: sensitivity, specificity on multi-neurophysiological procedures and estimation of axonal loss of motor, sensory and sympathetic median nerve fibers. *J Neurol Sci*. 1994;20:221–229.

107. Nardin R, Patel M, Gudas T, Rutkove S, Raynor E. Electromyography and magnetic resonance imaging in the evaluation of radiculopathy. *Muscle Nerve*. 1999;22:149–150.

108. Erwin CW, Erwin AC. Up and down the spinal cord: intraoperative monitoring of sensory and motor spinal cord pathways. *J Clin Neurophysiol*. 1993;10(4):425–436.

109. Toleikis JR. Intraoperative monitoring using somatosensory evoked potentials: a position statement by the American Society of Neurophysiological Monitoring. *J Clin Monit Comput*. 2005;19(3): 241–258.

110. Warren S, Capra N, Yezierski R. The somatosensory system II: nondiscriminative touch, temperature, and nociception. In: Haines D, ed. *Fundamental Neuroscience*. New York: Churchill Livingstone; 1997:237–254.

111. Warren S, Yezierski R, Capra N. The somatosensory system I: discriminative touch and position sense. In: Haines D, ed. *Fundamental Neuroscience*. New York: Churchill Livingstone; 1997:219–236.

112. Chappuis JL, Johnson G. Using intraoperative electrophysiologic monitoring as a diagnostic tool for determining levels to decompress in the cervical spine: a case report. *J Spinal Disord Tech*. 2007;20(5):403–407.

113. Lopez J. The use of evoked potentials in intraoperative neurophysiologic monitoring. *Phys Med Rehabil Clin N Am*. 2004;15:63–84.

114. Slimp J. Electrophysiologic intraoperative monitoring for spine procedures. *Phys Med Rehabil Clin N Am*. 2004;15:85–105.

115. Goodgold J, Eberstein A. The normal electromyogram. In: Goodgold J, Eberstein A, eds. *Electrodiagnosis of Neuromuscular Diseases*. Baltimore, MD: Williams & Wilkins; 1972:60–73.

116. Lundborg G, Dahlin L. Pathophysiology of nerve compression. In: Szabo R, ed. *Nerve Compression Syndromes: Diagnosis and Treatment*. Thorofare, NJ: Slack Incorporated; 1989:15–39.

117. Mayo Clinic. *Mayo Clinic EMG Laboratory Procedure Manual*. Rochester, MN: Mayo Clinic; 1992.

118. Seddon H. Three types of nerve injury. *Brain*. 1943;66: 237–288.

GLOSSARY

afferent   Axons from neurons carrying a signal toward the spinal cord (a sensory fiber).

amplitude   The size of the potential. In a sensory nerve assessment, this represents the summed action potential traveling across one point of that nerve. In a motor nerve assessment, this represents the summed action potentials traveling across the collective muscle fibers under the pickup electrode. Motor amplitudes are typically much larger than sensory action potentials.

anterior (ventral) primary rami   A branch of a mixed spinal nerve emanating from the spinal cord that carries both motor and sensory axons. The anterior primary rami are the origin of the fibers that make up the various plexi and named peripheral nerves.

antidromic   An electrical signal conducted in a direction that is opposite of normal. For example, for sensory neurons, an antidromic conduction would be toward the periphery.

axonopathy   Disease or pathology involving an axon.

biphasic   A nerve potential with two phases.

compound motor unit action potential (CMAP)   The action potential generated by stimulating a nerve that innervates the muscle under investigation. This CMAP represents the collective action potentials passing across all of the muscle fibers under the pickup electrode.

demyelination   Damage or removal of the myelin sheath that covers myelinated nerves. This results in slowed or blocked conduction of an electrical signal along individual axons and the collective nerve.

differential amplifier   The action potentials passing across nerves or over muscle fibers are small and need to be amplified to be seen, heard, and measured. A differential amplifier boosts the signal strength and subtracts out the portions of the signal that are common to both the active and reference electrodes.

distal motor latency (DML)   The time that it takes from stimulation of a motor nerve to pickup of the action potentials traveling across the appropriately innervated muscle fibers. Note that this action potential travels down to the distal end of the nerve, crosses the neuromuscular junction, and elicits a contraction of the muscle under investigation. Since this is a latency value, the time is compared with a table of normal values, for that known measured distance.

distal sensory latency (DSL)   The time that it takes from stimulation to pickup of a peripheral sensory nerve, measured in milliseconds. Since this is a latency value, the time is compared with a table of normal values for that known measured distance.

duration   The length of time that the compound motor unit action potential persists, measured in milliseconds.

efferent   Axons from neurons carrying a signal away from the spinal cord (a motor fiber).

electromyographic studies   The needle electrode portion of the examination that typically involves four steps: needle insertion, observation of electrical activity at rest, observation of electrical activity during voluntary contraction ranging from minimal to maximal, and information synthesis.

Erb's point   A stimulation point where the brachial plexus can be activated. The point of stimulation is located supraclavicularly at the midportion of the clavicle.

F-wave (central conduction study)   An electrically stimulated action potential that travels antidromically to the spinal cord (anterior horn cells) and then is bounced back orthodromically to elicit a secondary contraction of the muscle under investigation. This central conduction study provides a way of looking at the entire loop from the point of stimulation to the spinal cord, and back again. Through the obtained latency values, clinical judgments can be made.

fasciculation potential   The potential associated with the random and spontaneous activation of a group of muscle fibers or all of the muscle fibers originating from a motor unit. These are large enough to be felt, such as an "eyelid twitch" when an individual is tired. Cause can be something as innocent as fatigue, or it may be indicative of a serious problem.

fibrillation potential   Represents the electrical activity associated with the spontaneous contraction of a single muscle fiber.

Henneman size principle   A skeletal muscle consists of potentially hundreds of motor units of different sizes. Voluntary recruitment in the central nervous system of the spinal cord occurs in an orderly manner, recruiting the different size units from small to large. Functionally, this recruits the smaller neurons associated with slow twitch, high endurance muscle fibers prior to recruiting the larger motor neurons associated with the more easily fatigable fast twitch muscle fibers.

Hoffman's reflex (H-wave)   An electrically stimulated reflex that is a physiologic example of the normal reflex arc (entering the spinal cord by way of afferent neurons and exiting via efferent motor neurons). This reflex can only be elicited in a few muscles (such as the calf muscles) but has clinical utility in conditions such as an S1 radiculopathy.

latency   The time that it takes from the stimulus to the response over a predetermined distance, measured in milliseconds.

myopathic   An acquired or congenital disease that clinically presents with either focal or diffuse muscular weakness. A myopathic process is characterized electrophysiologically by short-duration and low-amplitude motor action potentials.

myotonic discharges   A sustained run of potentials that wax and wane, sounding over a loudspeaker such as a "dive bomber." Visually, these resemble either or both fibrillation potentials and positive sharp waves. These discharges are found in conditions such as myotonic dystrophy.

nerve conduction studies   Studies that evaluate the ability of a nerve to conduct an electrical signal. These are performed in ways that assess the sensory fibers within a nerve, specific segments of a nerve (either sensory or motor fibers), or the combined contribution of the neuromuscular junction and the innervated muscle fibers of the nerve under investigation.

nerve conduction velocity (NCV)   The speed by which an action potential travels down a peripheral nerve, measured in meters per second (distance/latency = NCV). This measures only the fastest conducting fibers, because the measured response is the first detected arrival of the action potential at the pickup electrode.

neuromuscular junction   The junction between the distal end of a nerve fiber and the muscle fibers that it innervates. Communication at this junction site is done via the neurotransmitter acetylcholine.

normative values   Tables of nerve conduction values (latency, amplitude, duration, nerve conduction velocity, etc.) considered to be normal. Because techniques can vary slightly between electrophysiologic laboratories, the normal values should be developed for each clinical electrophysiologic laboratory.

orthodromic   An electrical signal conducted in the normal direction. For example, for sensory neurons, this is toward the spinal cord.

polyneuropathy   Any disease that affects multiple peripheral nerves (e.g., diabetes myelitis).

positive sharp wave   Potentials that are typically biphasic, with a positive and then negative potential, often seen mixed with positive sharp waves. These potentials are representative of muscle denervation.

posterior (dorsal) primary rami   A branch of a mixed spinal nerve emanating from the spinal cord that carries both motor and sensory axons. The posterior primary rami supply three structures: (1) facet joints of the vertebral column, (2) deep (true) muscles of the back, and (3) the overlying skin of the back.

radiculopathy   Compression of a nerve root. This most frequently occurs as it exits the intervertebral foramina, but there are many potential causes of compression ranging from arthritic changes to vertebral disk herniations.

repetitive stimulation testing   A procedure used to assess the impact of various conditions on the neuromuscular junction. The two most commonly assessed conditions with this technique are myasthenia gravis and Lambert–Eaton syndrome.

sensitivity   The proportion of patients with the condition that have a positive test result. Sensitive tests recognize when a problem is actually present.

sensory nerve action potential (SNAP)   The action potential obtained by a pickup electrode placed over a segment of a nerve, in response to external electrical stimulation of that nerve at another site. The obtained potential represents the collective response of all of the nerve axons stimulated.

specificity   The ability of a test to recognize when a condition is absent.

spontaneous activity   Electrical activity that occurs at rest during needle electrode investigation, without any voluntary contribution on the part of the patient. Since the normal response at rest is electrical silence, spontaneous activity is usually indicative of pathology.

voluntary activity   The electrical activity generated by a patient intentionally contracting the muscle under needle electrode investigation. This may range from a minimal contraction where individual motor units can be assessed to a strong contraction with subsequent oscilloscope screen fill.

LAB ACTIVITY

CLINICAL ELECTROPHYSIOLOGIC TESTING

DESCRIPTION

Clinical electrophysiologic testing (CEPT) involves both NCS and EMG. NCS includes both motor and sensory studies and late responses (F-wave and H-reflexes). The EMG requires the use of needle electrodes, as surface electrodes (as are used for biofeedback and kinesiologic studies) are not capable of examining individual muscle fibers, nor even isolated motor units.

INDICATIONS

Indications for CEPT include weakness, numbness, diminished or absent muscle stretch responses, and pain. CEPT often complements imaging studies (e.g., MRI, myelogram) to assess function of the peripheral neuromuscular system.

CONTRAINDICATIONS

- There are no specific contraindications for CEPT.

CLINICAL ELECTROPHYSIOLOGIC TESTING

PROCEDURE FOR MEDIAN MOTOR NCS	EVALUATION		
	1	2	3
1. Gather equipment (electromyography machine, tape measure, alcohol wipes, pen to mark skin, electrodes, tape, paper towels).			
2. Prepare the subject.			
a. Position the subject supine on a treatment table, with the limb to be tested in the anatomic position.			
b. Using the alcohol pad, vigorously rub the area over the abductor pollicis brevis, the radial aspect of the first MCP joint, and the dorsum of the hand.			
c. Dry the areas prepared with the alcohol pad.			
d. Using the pen, mark the skin over the belly of the abductor pollicis brevis (midway between the base of the first metacarpal and the first MCP joint); this will be the location of the active recording electrode, Ra.			
e. Using the tape measure, measure 8 cm proximal to the Ra following the course of the median nerve, and mark this location (between the tendons of the flexor carpi radialis and the palmaris longus).			
f. Secure the ground electrode to the posterior aspect of the hand, the Ra over the abductor pollicis brevis, and the reference recording electrode (Rr) over the radial aspect of the first MCP joint. If using reusable electrodes, use conductant gel between the skin and the electrode, and tape to secure the electrode. If using disposable electrodes, do not use conductant gel or tape.			
3. Prepare equipment.			
a. Turn electromyography machine on; wait for warm-up.			
b. If available, select the protocol for a motor nerve conduction study. If protocols are not available, set the gain to 5000 µV per division, the sweep speed to 2 or 5 milliseconds per division, the low-pass filter to 10 Hz, the high-pass filter to 10,000 Hz, and the stimulus and pulse width to 100 microseconds.			
4. Obtain the distal response.			
a. Verify that the stimulation amplitude is at zero.			
b. Apply conductant gel to the stimulator.			
c. Place the stimulator with the cathode on the mark 8 cm proximal to the Ra, and the anode oriented proximal to the cathode. It is not necessary to have the anode off the median nerve.			
d. Turn the stimulator intensity up slightly, and stimulate the nerve. Continue to increase the intensity in small increments until the subject reports perception of the stimulation, and a motor response is visualized.			

e. Continue to stimulate the nerve with increasing stimulus amplitude until the M-wave (CMAP) observed on the screen no longer increases in amplitude. Store this response (typically done by depressing a footswitch).			
5. Obtain the proximal response.			
a. Identify the location of the median nerve at the elbow (just medial to the tendon of the biceps brachialis).			
b. Stimulate the median nerve at the elbow using the same stimulus intensity as for the final stimulus at the wrist. Increase the amplitude slightly, and observe for any further increase in CMAP amplitude. The cathode should remain distal to the anode.			
c. Store the proximal response.			
6. Calculate the NCV in the forearm.			
a. Measure the distance between the wrist and elbow stimulation sites in millimeters.			
b. Subtract the latency from the wrist to the APB from the latency from the elbow to the APB.			
c. Divide the distance in millimeters by the latency difference in milliseconds to obtain the velocity in meters per second.			
7. Assess the F-wave.			
a. Change the gain to 200 μV per division and the sweep speed to 5 milliseconds per division (all other settings remain the same).			
b. Decrease the stimulus amplitude to zero, and place the cathode of the stimulator over the stimulation site at the wrist, with the anode distal.			
c. Slowly increase the stimulus amplitude as before, observing the response on the screen for a second response with a latency of about 25 milliseconds. This late response is the F-wave, and it follows the M-wave.			
d. Store the response.			
e. Keeping the stimulus amplitude constant, stimulate the nerve at least 10 more times, recording each response.			
f. Measure the latency from the stimulus to the beginning of the F-wave with the shortest latency. This minimum latency is the value used for the F-wave.			
8. Complete the activity.			
a. Remove all electrodes; remove any conductant gel on the subject.			
b. Compare the distal latency, CMAP amplitude, forearm NCV, and F-wave latency to normal values.			
c. Interpret the results.			

CLINICAL ELECTROPHYSIOLOGIC TESTING

PROCEDURE FOR MEDIAN MOTOR NCS	EVALUATION		
	1	2	3
1. Gather equipment (electromyography machine, tape measure, alcohol wipes, pen to mark skin, electrodes, tape, paper towels).			
2. Prepare the subject.			
a. Position the subject supine on a treatment table, with the limb to be tested in the anatomic position.			
b. Using the alcohol pad, vigorously rub the palmar surface of the third digit (D3, the long finger) and the midpalm area.			
c. Dry the areas prepared with the alcohol pad.			
d. Using the pen, mark the skin of the palmar aspect of D3 just distal to the skin crease at the MP joint. This will be the location of the active recording electrode, Ra.			
e. Using the tape measure, measure 7 cm proximal to the Ra following the course of the median nerve, and mark this location (the midpalmar area). Continue another 7 cm proximal along the median nerve, and mark this location (proximal to the carpal tunnel).			
f. Secure the ground electrode to the posterior aspect of the hand, the Ra on D3, and the reference recording electrode (Rr) 3 cm distal to the Ra. If using reusable electrodes, use conductant gel between the skin and the electrode, and tape to secure the electrode. If using disposable electrodes, do not use conductant gel or tape.			
3. Prepare equipment.			
a. Turn electromyography machine on; wait for warm-up.			
b. If available, select the protocol for a sensory nerve conduction study. If protocols are not available, set the gain to 20 μV per division, the sweep speed to 2 milliseconds per division, the low-pass filter to 10 Hz, the high-pass filter to 2000 Hz, and the stimulus pulse width to 100 microseconds.			
4. Obtain the distal response.			
a. Verify that the stimulation amplitude is at zero.			
b. Apply conductant gel to the stimulator.			
c. Place the stimulator with the cathode on the mark 7 cm proximal to the Ra, and the anode oriented proximal to the cathode. It is not necessary to have the anode off the median nerve.			
d. Turn the stimulator intensity up slightly, and stimulate the nerve. Continue to increase the intensity in small increments until a response (SNAP) is observed on the screen.			
e. Continue to stimulate the nerve with increasing stimulus amplitude until the SNAP observed on the screen no longer increases in amplitude, or until the stimulus artifact begins to obscure the response. Rotation of the anode around the cathode may help decrease the stimulus artifact. Store this response (typically done by depressing a footswitch).			

5. Obtain the proximal response.			
a. Identify the location of the median nerve at the wrist (between the flexor carpi radialis and palmaris longus tendons).			
b. Stimulate the median nerve at the wrist using the same stimulus intensity as for the final stimulus at the wrist. Increase the amplitude slightly, and observe for any further increase in SNAP amplitude. The cathode should remain distal to the anode.			
c. Store the proximal response.			
6. Calculate the NCV in the palmar segment and across the wrist.			
a. Divide 70 mm by the latency measured to the peak of the negative component of the SNAP; this gives the NCV in meters per second in the palmar segment of the median nerve.			
b. Divide 70 mm by the difference in latency between the stimulation sites. This gives the NCV in meters per second in the wrist segment of the median nerve.			
c. Divide the distance in millimeters by the latency difference in milliseconds to obtain the velocity in meters per second.			
7. Complete the activity.			
a. Remove all electrodes; remove any conductant gel on the subject.			
b. Compare the NCV and SNAP amplitude values to normal values.			
c. Interpret the results.			

PART **THREE**

Thermal Energy
Modalities

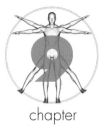

chapter

Cryotherapy and Thermotherapy

William E. Prentice

OBJECTIVES

Following completion of this chapter, the student will be able to:

➤ Explain why cryotherapy and thermotherapy are best classified as thermal energy modalities.

➤ Differentiate between the physiologic effects of therapeutic heat and cold.

➤ Describe thermotherapy and cryotherapy techniques.

➤ Categorize the indications and contraindications for both cryotherapy and thermotherapy.

➤ Select the most effective conductive energy modalities for a given clinical diagnosis.

➤ Explain how the clinician can use the conductive energy modalities to reduce pain.

Of the therapeutic modalities discussed in this chapter, perhaps none are more commonly used than heat and cold modalities. As indicated in Chapter 1, the infrared region of the electromagnetic spectrum falls between the diathermy and the visible light portions of the spectrum in terms of wavelength and frequency. There is confusion over the relationship between electromagnetic energy and conductive thermal energy associated with the infrared region. Traditionally, it has been correct to think of the **infrared** modalities as being those modalities whose primary mechanism of action is the emission of infrared radiation for increasing tissue temperatures.[1,2] Warm objects emit infrared radiation. But the amount of infrared energy that is radiated from these objects is negligible. These modalities operate by conduction of heat energy, so they are better described as **conductive thermal energy modalities.** The conductive thermal energy modalities are used to produce a local and occasionally a generalized heating or cooling of the superficial tissues.

Conductive thermal energy modalities are generally classified into those that produce a tissue temperature decrease, which we refer to as **cryotherapy**, and those that produce a tissue temperature increase, which we call **thermotherapy**. Cryotherapy treatment techniques include ice massage, cold hydrocollator packs, ice packs, cold whirlpools, ice immersion, cold spray, contrast baths, cold compression, and cryokinetics. Thermotherapy treatment techniques include warm whirlpool, warm hydrocollator packs, paraffin baths, Fluidotherapy, and ThermaCare wraps.

Luminous infrared and nonluminous infrared lamps are classified as electromagnetic energy modalities. While the wavelength and frequency of the energy emitted by these modalities are similar to the other thermotherapy and cryotherpy modalities, the mechanism by which the infrared lamps produce a tissue temperature increase has nothing to do with conduction. Their mechanism of energy transfer is through electromagnetic radiation, thus explaining why they are classified as electromagnetic energy modalities. However, since they are used for increasing superficial temperature and have wavelengths and frequencies similar to the other cryotherapy and thermotherapy techniques, they will also be discussed in this chapter.

MECHANISMS OF HEAT TRANSFER

Easy application and convenience of use of cryotherapy and thermotherapy modalities provide the clinician with the necessary tools for primary care of injuries. Heat is defined as the internal vibration of the molecules within a body. The transmission of heat occurs by three mechanisms: **conduction**, **convection**, and **radiation**. A fourth mechanism of heat transfer, **conversion**, is discussed in Chapter 10, the chapter on ultrasound. Conduction occurs when the body is in direct contact with the heat or cold source. Convection occurs when particles (air or water) move across the body, creating a temperature variation. Radiation is the transfer of heat from a warmer source to a cooler source through a conducting medium, such as air (e.g., infrared lamps). The body may either gain or lose heat through any of these three processes of heat transfer. The cryotherapy and thermotherapy modalities discussed in this chapter use these three methods of heat transfer to effect a tissue temperature increase or decrease. Table 9–1 summarizes the mechanisms of heat transfer for the various modalities.

APPROPRIATE USE OF CRYOTHERAPY AND THERMOTHERAPY MODALITIES

As indicated previously, heating techniques used for therapeutic purposes are referred to as *thermotherapy*. Thermotherapy is used when a rise in tissue temperature is the goal of treatment. The use of cold, or *cryotherapy*, is most effective in the acute stages of the healing process immediately following injury when a loss of tissue temperature is the goal

Table 9–1 Mechanisms of Heat Transfer of the Various Modalities

CONDUCTION	CONVECTION	RADIATION	CONVERSION
Ice massage	Hot whirlpool	Infrared lamps	Ultrasound
Cold packs	Cold whirlpool	Laser	Diathermy
Hydrocollator packs	Fluidotherapy	Ultraviolet light*	
Cold spray			
Ice immersion			
Contrast baths**			
Cryo-Cuff			
Cryokinetics			
Paraffin bath			

* Ultraviolet therapy does not involve a tissue temperature change, but the energy from the ultraviolet source radiates to the skin surface.

** Contrast baths could also involve convection if hot or cold whirlpools are being used.

of therapy. Cold applications can be continued into the reconditioning stage of injury management.[3] Thermotherapy and cryotherapy are included in this section based on their classification in the electromagnetic spectrum. The term "**hydrotherapy**" can be applied to any cryotherapy or thermotherapy technique that uses water as the medium for tissue temperature exchange.

Although this chapter is concerned primarily with application of the cryotherapy and thermotherapy modalities and their physiologic effects, several other modalities discussed in this text (e.g., diathermy and ultrasound) cause similar physiologic responses. Specifically, the effects of heat and cold therapy discussed in this chapter may be applied to any modality that alters tissue temperature.

Cryotherapy and thermotherapy can be used successfully to treat injuries and trauma.[4] The clinician must know the injury mechanism and specific pathology, as well as the physiologic effects of the heating and cooling agents, to establish a consistent treatment schedule. Conductive energy modalities transmit thermal energy to or from the patient. In most cases, they are simple, efficient, and inexpensive. Clinicians who choose to compare modalities and use the most appropriate technique for their patients will be providing quality care for that patient. A haphazard approach to the use of infrared modalities will only reflect a disregard for the health care of the patient.

CLINICAL USE OF THE CONDUCTIVE ENERGY MODALITIES

The physiologic effects of heat and cold discussed previously are rarely the result of direct absorption of infrared energy. There is general agreement that no form of infrared energy can have a depth of penetration greater than 1 cm.[5] Thus, the effects of the conductive energy modalities are primarily superficial and directly affect the cutaneous blood vessels and the cutaneous nerve receptors.[6]

Absorption of energy cutaneously increases and decreases circulation subcutaneously in both the muscle and fat layers. If the energy is absorbed cutaneously over a long enough period to raise the temperature of the circulating blood, the hypothalamus will reflexively increase blood flow to the underlying tissue. Likewise, absorption of cold cutaneously can decrease blood flow via a similar mechanism in the area of treatment.[5]

Thus, if the primary treatment goal is a tissue temperature increase with a corresponding increase in blood flow to the deeper tissues, it is wiser perhaps to choose a modality—such as diathermy or ultrasound—that produces energy that can penetrate the cutaneous tissues and be directly absorbed by the deep tissues. If the primary treatment goal is to reduce tissue temperature and decrease blood flow to an injured area, the superficial application of ice or cold is the only modality capable of producing such a response.

Perhaps the most effective use of the conductive energy modalities should be to provide analgesia or reduce the sensation of pain associated with injury. These modalities stimulate primarily the cutaneous nerve receptors. Through one of the mechanisms of pain modulation discussed in Chapter 4 (most likely the gate control theory), hyperstimulation of these nerve Aβ receptors by heating or cooling reduces pain. Within the philosophy of an aggressive program of rehabilitation, the reduction of pain as a means of facilitating therapeutic exercise is a common practice. As emphasized in the preface to this chapter, therapeutic modalities are perhaps best used as an adjunct to therapeutic exercise. Certainly, this should be a prime consideration when selecting an infrared modality for use in any treatment program.

Continued investigation and research into the use of heat and cold is warranted to provide useful data for the clinician. Heat and cold applications, when used properly and efficiently, will provide the clinician with the tools to enhance recovery and provide the patient with optimal health care management. Thermotherapy and cryotherapy are only two of the tools available to assist in the well-being and reconditioning of the injured patient.

Effects of Tissue Temperature Change on Circulation

Local application of heat or cold is indicated for *thermal* physiologic effects. The main physiologic effect is on superficial circulation because of the response of the temperature receptors in the skin and the sympathetic nervous system.

Circulation through the skin serves two major functions: nutrition of the skin tissues and conduction of heat from internal structures of the body to the skin so that heat can be removed from the body.[7] The circulatory apparatus is composed of *two major vessel types:* arteries, capillaries, and veins; and vascular structures for heating the skin. Two types of vascular structures are the subcutaneous venous plexus, which holds large quantities of blood that heat the surface of the skin, and the arteriovenous anastomosis, which provides vascular communication between arteries and venous plexuses.[8] The walls of the plexuses have strong muscular coats innervated by sympathetic vasoconstrictor nerve fibers that secrete norepinephrine. When constricted, blood flow is reduced to almost nothing in the venous plexus. When maximally dilated, there is an extremely rapid flow of blood into the plexuses. The arteriovenous anastomoses are found principally in the volar or palmar surfaces of the hands and feet, lips, nose, and ears.

When cold is applied directly to the skin, the skin vessels progressively constrict to a temperature of about 10°C (50°F), at which point they reach their maximum constrictions. This constriction results primarily from increased sensitivity of the vessels to nerve stimulation, but it probably also results at least partly from a reflex that passes to the spinal cord and then back to the vessels. At temperatures below 10°C (50°F), the vessels begin to dilate. This dilation is caused by a direct local effect of the cold on the vessels themselves, producing paralysis of the contractile mechanism of the vessel wall or blockage of the nerve impulses coming to the vessels. At temperatures approaching 0°C (32°F), the skin vessels frequently reach maximum vasodilation.

Skin plexuses are supplied with sympathetic vasoconstrictor innervation. In times of circulatory stress, such as exercise, hemorrhage, or anxiety, sympathetic stimulation of these skin plexuses forces large quantities of blood into internal vessels. Thus, the subcutaneous veins of the skin act as an important blood reservoir, often providing blood to serve other circulatory functions when needed.[7]

Three types of sensory receptors are found in the subepithelial tissue: cold, warm, and pain. The pain receptors are free nerve endings. Temperature and pain are transmitted to the brain via the lateral spinothalamic tract (see Chapter 4). The nerve fibers respond differently at different temperatures. Both cold and warm receptors discharge minimally at 33°C (91.4°F). Cold receptors discharge between 10°C and 41°C (50–105.8°F), with a maximum discharge in the 37.5–40°C (99.5–104°F) range. Above 45°C (113°F), cold receptors begin to discharge again, and pain receptors are stimulated. Nerve fibers transmitting sensations of pain respond to the temperature extremes. Both warm and cold receptors adapt rapidly to temperature change; the more rapid the temperature change, the more rapid the receptor adaptation. The number of warm and cold receptors in any given small surface area is thought to be few. Therefore, small temperature changes are difficult to perceive in localized areas. Larger surface areas stimulate summation of thermal signals. These larger patterns of excitation activate the vasomotor centers and the hypothalamic center.[1,2] Stimulation of the anterior hypothalamus causes cutaneous vasodilation, whereas stimulation of the posterior hypothalamus causes cutaneous vasoconstriction.[7,9]

The cutaneous blood flow depends on the discharge of the sympathetic nervous system. These sympathetic impulses are transmitted simultaneously to the blood vessels for cutaneous vasoconstriction and to the adrenal medulla. Both norepinephrine and epinephrine are secreted into the blood vessels and induce vessel constriction.[7] Most of the sympathetic constriction influences are mediated chemically through these neural transmitters. General exposure to cold elicits cutaneous vasoconstriction, shivering, piloerection, and an increase in epinephrine-secretion; therefore, vascular contraction occurs. Simultaneously, metabolism and heat production are increased to maintain the body temperature.[7]

Increased blood flow supplies additional oxygen to the area, explaining the analgesic and relaxation effects on muscle spasm. An increased proprioceptive reflex mechanism may explain these effects. Receptor end organs located in the muscle spindle are inhibited by heat temporarily, whereas sudden cooling tends to excite the receptor end organ.[1,2]

Effects of Tissue Temperature Change on Muscle Spasm

Cold may be better for reducing muscle spasm.

Numerous studies deal with the effects of heat and cold in the treatment of many musculoskeletal conditions. Although it is true that the use of heat as a therapeutic modality has long been accepted and documented in the literature, it is apparent that most recent research has been directed toward the use of cold. There seems to be general agreement that the physiologic mechanisms underlying the effectiveness of heat and cold treatments in reducing muscle spasm lie at the level of the muscle spindle, Golgi tendon organs, and the gamma system.[10]

Heat is believed to have a relaxing effect on skeletal muscle tone.[11] Local application of heat relaxes muscles throughout the skeletal system by simultaneously lessening the stimulus threshold of muscle spindles and decreasing the gamma efferent firing rate. This suggests that the muscle spindles are easily excited. Consequently, the muscles may be electromyographically silent while at rest during the application of heat, but the slightest amount of voluntary or passive movement may cause the efferents to fire, thus increasing muscular resistance to stretch. If this is indeed the case, then it seems logical that decreasing the afferent impulses by raising the threshold of the muscle spindles might be effective in facilitating muscle relaxation, as long as there is no movement.

The rate of firing of both primary and secondary endings is directly proportional to temperature. Local applications of cold decrease local neural activity. Annulospiral, flower-spray (small fibers located in the muscle spindle that detect changes in muscle position), and Golgi tendon organ endings all fire more slowly when cooled. Cooling actually decreases the rate of afferent activity even more, with an increase in the amount of tension on the muscle. Thus, cold appears to raise the threshold stimulus of muscle spindles, and heat tends to lower it.[12] Although firing of the primary spindle afferents increases abruptly with the application of cold, a subsequent decrease in spindle afferent activity occurs and persists as the temperature is lowered.[13]

Simultaneous use of heat and cold in the treatment of muscle spasm has also been studied.[8,14] Local cooling with ice, although maintaining body temperature to prevent shivering, results in a significant reduction of muscle spasm, greater than that which occurs with the use of heat or cold independently. This effect was attributed to maintenance of body temperature, which decreases efferent activity, whereas local cooling decreases afferent activity. If the core temperature of the body is not maintained, the reflex shivering results in increased muscle tone, thus inhibiting relaxation.

There is a substantial reduction in the frequency of action potential (stimulus intensity necessary for firing muscle fibers) firing of the motor unit when the muscle temperature is reduced. Muscle spindle activity is most significantly reduced when the muscle is cooled, whereas normal body temperature is maintained.[15]

Miglietta[15] presented a slightly different perspective on the effect of cold in reducing muscle spasm. He performed an electromyographic analysis of the effects of cold on the reduction of clonus (increased muscle tone) or spasticity in a group of 15 patients. After immersion of the spastic extremity in a cold whirlpool for 15 minutes, it was observed that electromyographic activity dropped significantly and in some cases disappeared altogether. The cold was thought to induce an afferent bombardment of cold impulses, which modify the cortical excitatory state and block the stream of painful impulses from the muscle. Thus, relaxation of skeletal muscle is assumed to occur with the disappearance of pain.[16] It is not certain whether it is the excitability of the motor neurons or the hyperactivity of the gamma system, which is changed either at the muscle spindle level or at the spinal cord level, that is responsible for the reduction of spasticity. However, it is certain that cold is effective in reducing spasticity by reducing or modifying the highly sensitive stretch-reflex mechanism in muscle.

Another factor that may be important to the reduction of spasticity is reduction in the nerve conduction velocity because of the application of cold.[17] These changes may result from a slowing of motor and sensory nerve conduction velocity and a decrease of the afferent discharges from cutaneous receptors.

Several studies investigated the use of cold followed by some type of exercise in the treatment of various injuries to the musculotendinous unit.[18–20] Each of these studies indicated that the use of cold and exercise were extremely effective in the treatment of acute pathologies of the musculoskeletal system that produced restrictions of muscle action. However, if stretching was indicated, it has been stressed that stretching is more important for increasing flexibility than using either heat or cold.[21,22]

Effects of Temperature Change on Performance

Several studies have examined the effects of altering tissue temperature on physical performance capabilities.[23–25]

Changes in the ability to produce torque during isokinetic testing following the application of heat and cold have been demonstrated, although there appears to be some disagreement relative to the degree of change in concentric and eccentric torque capabilities.[26,27,28] One study observed that the strength of an eccentric contraction was improved with the application of ice, whereas another indicated the ice helped to facilitate concentric but not eccentric strength.[29,30] This may be due to an increase in the ability to recruit additional motor neurons during and after cooling.[31] It also appears that higher torque values can be produced following the application of cold packs than hot packs.[32] The use of cryotherapy does not seem to effect peak torque but may increase endurance.[33] Cold appears to have some effect on muscular power; also, it has been shown that performance in vertical jumping is decreased following the application of cold.[34,35] Cold water immersion does not seem to affect range of motion.[36] Joint cryotherapy negated movement deficiencies represented by peak knee torque and power decreases.[37]

It seems that heating or cooling of an extremity has minimal or no effects on proprioception, joint position sense, and balance.[30,38–49] Thus, it follows that tissue temperature changes have no effect on agility or the ability to change direction.[12,50,51] The application of ice prior to a warm-up has been shown to negatively affect functional performance but an active warm-up period decreases detrimental effects.[52,53]

CRYOTHERAPY

Cold should be used to decrease temperature and thermal metabolic rate.

Cryotherapy is the use of cold in the treatment of acute trauma and subacute injury and for the decrease of discomfort after reconditioning and rehabilitation.[54,55]

Physiologic Effects of Tissue Cooling

The physiologic effects of cold are the opposite of those of heat for the most part, the primary effect being a local decrease in temperature. Cold has its greatest benefit in acute injury.[26,56–60] There is general agreement that the use of cold is the initial treatment for most conditions in the musculoskeletal system. See Table 9–2 for a summary of indications and contraindications for the use of cryotherapy.

The primary reason for using cold in acute injury is to lower the temperature in the injured area, thus reducing the metabolic rate with a corresponding decrease in production of metabolites and metabolic heat.[61] This helps the injured tissue survive the hypoxia and limits further tissue injury.[59,62] Cold has been demonstrated to be more effective when applied along with compression than using ice alone for reducing metabolism in injured tissue.[60,63] It is also used immediately after injury to decrease pain and promote local **vasoconstriction**, thus controlling hemorrhage and edema.[64,65] However, preexercise cooling does not affect the magnitude of muscle damage in response to eccentric exercise.[66] Cold is also used in the acute phase of inflammatory conditions, such as bursitis, tenosynovitis, and tendinitis, in which heat may cause additional pain and swelling.[2]

Cold is also used to reduce pain and the reflex muscle spasm and spastic conditions that accompany it.[60] Its analgesic effect is probably one of its greatest benefits.[10,13,67,68] Although ice

Table 9–2 Indications and Contraindications for Cryotherapy

INDICATIONS   (during acute or subacute inflammation)
Acute pain
Chronic pain
Acute swelling (controlling hemorrhage and edema)
Myofascial trigger points
Muscle guarding
Muscle spasm
Acute muscle strain
Acute ligament sprain
Acute contusion
Bursitis
Tenosynovitis
Tendinitis
Delayed onset muscle soreness

CONTRAINDICATIONS
Impaired circulation (i.e., Raynaud's phenomenon)
Peripheral vascular disease
Hypersensitivity to cold
Skin anesthesia
Open wounds or skin conditions (cold whirlpools and contrast baths)
Infection

seems to be effective in treating pain there is little evidence-based material to support the use of ice in treating other musculoskeletal conditions.[69] One explanation of the analgesic effect is that cold decreases the velocity of nerve conduction, although it does not entirely eliminate it.[13,17,60] It is also possible that cold bombards central pain receptor areas with so many cold impulses that pain impulses are lost through the gate control theory of pain modulation. With ice treatments, the patient usually reports an uncomfortable sensation of cold followed by stinging or burning, then an aching sensation, and finally complete numbness.[71]

Cold also has been demonstrated to be effective in the treatment of **myofascial pain**.[16] This type of pain is referred from active myofascial trigger points with various symptoms, including pain on active movement and decreased range of motion. Trigger points may result from muscle strain or tension, which sensitizes nerves in a localized area. A trigger point may be palpated as a small nodule or as a strip of tense muscle tissue.[72]

It appears that cold is more effective in treating acute muscle pain as opposed to de-layed-onset muscle soreness (DOMS), which occurs following exercise.[73] Ultrasound has been shown to be more effective than ice for treating DOMS.[74]

Cold depresses the excitability of free nerve endings and peripheral nerve fibers, and this increases the pain threshold.[75] This is of great value in short-term treatment. Cold applications can also enhance voluntary control in spastic conditions, and in acute traumatic conditions they may decrease painful spasms that result from local muscle irritability.[76]

Reduction in muscle-guarding relative to acute trauma has been observed by all active clinicians. The literature reviewed indicates various reasons behind reduced muscle guarding, with the common thought of decreased muscle spindle activity.[77]

The initial reaction to cold is local vasoconstriction of all smooth muscle by the central nervous system to conserve heat.[65] Localized vasoconstriction is responsible for the decrease in the tendency toward formation and accumulation of edema, probably as a result of a decrease in local hydrostatic pressure.[78] There is also a decrease in the amount of nutrients and phagocytes delivered to the area, thus reducing phagocytic activity.[78]

It has been hypothesized that when local temperature is lowered considerably for a period of about 30 minutes, intermittent periods of vasodilation occur, lasting 4–6 minutes. Then vasoconstriction of the blood vessels in the superficial tissues recurs for a 15- to 30-minute cycle, followed again by vasodilation. This phenomenon has come to be known as the **hunting response** and is said to be necessary to prevent local tissue injury caused by cold.[79–81] The hunting response has been accepted for a number of years as fact; in reality, however, these investigations have studied measured temperature changes rather than circulatory changes. Some clinicians have taken the liberty of inferring that temperature changes produce circulatory changes and this is simply not what the hunting response is. The hunting response is more likely a measurement artifact than an actual change in blood flow in response to cold.[71,81] Even if some cold-induced vasodilation does occur, the effects are negligible.[26]

If a large area is cooled, the hypothalamus (the temperature-regulating center in the brain) will reflexively induce shivering, which raises the core temperature as a result of increased production of heat. Cooling of a large area might also cause arterial vasoconstriction in other remote parts of the body, resulting in an increased blood pressure.[78] Because of the low thermal conductivity of underlying subcutaneous fat tissue, applications of cold for short periods of time probably are ineffective in cooling deeper tissues.[65] It has been shown also that using cold for too long may be detrimental to the healing process.[58]

Cold treatments do not necessarily have as much of an effect in the deeper tissues' relation to blood flow. Positron emission tomography is an imaging technique that can be used to quantify directly local blood flow in response to cold application. Using this technology, it has been shown that muscle tissue blood flow is reduced after a 20-minute ice treatment. However, this reduction only occurs in the most superficial layer, which may suggest that the therapeutic effects of ice application diminish with tissue depth.[83]

The length of treatment time needed to cool tissue effectively depends on differences in subcutaneous tissue thickness.[84] Patients with thick subcutaneous tissue should be treated with cold applications for longer than 5 minutes to produce a significant drop in intramuscular temperature.[85] Grant treated acute and chronic conditions of the musculoskeletal system and found that thin people require shorter icing periods and that response was more successful.[18] McMaster supported these findings.[64] Fifteen minutes of cooling increase knee joint stiffness and lessen the sensitivity of position sense.[86] Recommended treatment times range from direct contact of 5–45 minutes to obtain adequate cooling.

In general, it has been recommended that treatments last for 20 minutes.[87] It has also been recommended that in patients with differing subcutaneous adipose thickness the duration of cryotherapy treatment needed to produce a standard cooling effect must vary. To produce similar intramuscular temperature changes, treatment duration should be adjusted based on the subject's subcutaneous adipose thickness as determined through skinfold measurements.[88] A 25-minute treatment may be adequate for a patient with a skin-fold of 20 mm or less; however, a 40-minute application is required to produce similar results in a patient whose skin-fold is between 20 and 30 mm. A 60-minute treatment is required to produce similar results in a patient whose skin-fold is between 30 and 40 mm.[89]

It is generally believed that cold treatments are more effective in reaching deep tissue than most forms of heat. Cold applied to the skin is capable of significantly lowering the temperature of tissue at a considerable depth. The extent of this lowered tissue temperature is dependent on the type of cold applied to the skin, the duration of its application, the thickness of the subcutaneous fat, and the region of the body on which it is applied.[90] A 20-minute cryotherapy

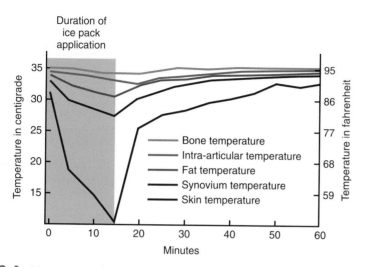

Figure 9-1. Temperature changes in various tissues during ice application.

treatment applied to the ankle does not alter core temperature.[91] Figure 9-1 shows the temperature changes in various tissues associated with an ice pack treatment.

The application of cold decreases cell permeability, decreases cellular metabolism, and decreases accumulation of edema and should be continued in 5- to 45-minute applications for at least 72 hours after initial trauma.[26] Care should be taken to avoid aggressive cold treatment to prevent disruption of the healing sequence.

The physiologic effects of cold are summarized in Table 9-3.

Frostbite

Frostbite is defined as freezing of a body part and occurs when tissue temperatures fall below 0°C (32°F). Symptoms of frostbite initially include tingling and redness from hyperemia, which indicate blood is still circulating to the superficial tissues, followed by pallor (a lack of color in the skin) and numbness, which indicate that vasoconstriction has occurred and blood is no longer circulating to the superficial tissues.

When using a cryotherapy technique the chances of frostbite are minimal if the recommended procedures are followed. However, if treatment time exceeds recommendations, or if the temperature of the modality is below what is recommended, the chances of frostbite will be increased. Certainly if there is circulatory insufficiency the chances of frostbite are also increased.

If frostbite is suspected, the body part should be immediately removed from the cold source and immersed in water at 38–40°C (100–104°F). It is also advisable to refer the patient to a physician.

Cryotherapy Treatment Techniques

Tools of cryotherapy include ice packs, cold whirlpool, ice whirlpool, ice massage, commercial chemical cold spray, and contrast baths. Application of cryotherapy produces a three- to four-stage sensation. First, there is an uncomfortable sensation of cold followed by a stinging, then a burning or aching feeling, and finally numbness. Each stage is related to the nerve endings as they temporarily cease to function because of decreased blood flow and decreased nerve conduction velocity. The time required for this sequence varies, but several authors indicate that it occurs within 5–15 minutes.[18,65,71,76,92–96] After 12–15 minutes the hunting response is sometimes demonstrated with intense cold (10°C [50°F]).[64,79,95,97] Thus, a minimum of 15 minutes are necessary to achieve extreme analgesic effects.

Application of ice is safe, simple, and inexpensive. Cryotherapy is contraindicated in patients with cold allergies (hives, joint pain, nausea), Raynaud's phenomenon (arterial spasm), and some rheumatoid conditions.[4,7,18,98,99]

Table 9–3 Physiologic Effects of Cold and Heat

EFFECTS OF HEAT
Increased local temperature superficially
Increased local metabolism
Vasodilation of arterioles and capillaries
Increased blood flow to part heated
Increased leukocytes and phagocytosis
Increased capillary permeability
Increased lymphatic and venous drainage
Increased metabolic wastes
Increased axon reflex activity
Increased elasticity of muscles, ligaments, and capsule fibers
Analgesia
Increased formation of edema
Decreased muscle tone
Decreased muscle spasm

EFFECTS OF COLD
Decreased local temperature, in some cases to a considerable depth
Decreased metabolism
Vasoconstriction of arterioles and capillaries (at first)
Decreased blood flow (at first)
Decreased nerve conduction velocity
Decreased delivery of leukocytes and phagocytes
Decreased lymphatic and venous drainage
Decreased muscle excitability
Decreased muscle spindle depolarization
Decreased formation and accumulation of edema
Extreme anesthetic effects

Depth of penetration depends on the amount of cold and the length of the treatment time because the body is well equipped to maintain skin and subcutaneous tissue viability through the capillary bed by reflex vasodilation of up to four times normal blood flow. The body has the ability to decrease blood flow to the body segment that is supposedly losing too much body heat by shunting the blood flow. Depth of penetration is also related to intensity and duration of cold application and the circulatory response to the body segment exposed. If the person has normal circulatory responses, frostbite should not be a concern. Even so, caution should be exercised when applying intense cold directly to the skin. If deeper penetration is desired, ice therapy is most effective using ice towels, ice packs, ice massage, and ice whirlpools.[100] The patient should be advised of the four stages of cryotherapy and the discomfort he or she will experience. The clinician should explain this sequence and advise the patient of the expected outcome, which may include a rapid decrease in pain.[17,18,82,101] It has been recommended that patients not engage in activity requiring power performance immediately after cryotherapy. However, the use of cold is not contraindicated for use as an analgesic before submaximal exercise focusing on restoring neuromuscular control to injured tissues.[102]

Ice Massage

Ice massage can be applied by the clinician or the patient if the patient can reach the area of application to administer self-treatment. It is best for the first three treatments to be administered by the clinician to give the patient the full benefit of the treatment. When positioning the patient's body segment to be treated, it should be relaxed, and the patient should be made comfortable. If possible, the body part to be treated should be elevated. Appropriate seating and positioning should be taken into consideration with the application of ice. Administration must be thorough to get maximal treatment. Ice massage is perhaps best indicated in conditions in which some type of stretching activity is to be used. It appears that ice massage cools muscle more rapidly than an ice bag.[103]

Equipment Needed. (Figures 9–2 and 9–3)

1. Styrofoam cups: A regular 6- to 8-ounce styrofoam cup should be filled with water and placed in the freezer. After it is frozen, all the styrofoam on the sides should be removed down to 1 inch from the bottom. A frozen cup of ice with a tongue depressor inserted is preferred because it has a handle with which to hold the block of ice.

2. Ice cups: A cup is filled with water, and a wooden tongue blade is placed in the cup. The cup is then placed in the freezer. After it is frozen the paper cup is torn off. A block of ice on a stick is now ready to be used for massage.

3. Paper cups: Utilize the same technique as the Styrofoam cups, except toweling may be needed to insulate the clinician's hand holding the paper cup.

4. Cryocup: A commercially available reusable plastic cup that is ideal for ice massage.

5. Towels: These are used for positioning and absorbing the melting water in the area of the ice massage application.

Treatment. Preferred positions are side lying, prone, supine, hook lying, or sitting, depending on the area to be treated. Self-treatment should be used when patients can comfortably reach the area to be treated by themselves. Apply ice massage in a circular pattern, with each succeeding stroke covering half the previous stroke, or in a longitudinal motion, with each stroke overlapping half the previous stroke. Ice should be applied for 15–20 minutes; consistent patterning of circular and longitudinal strokes includes the sequence described in the clinical uses section.

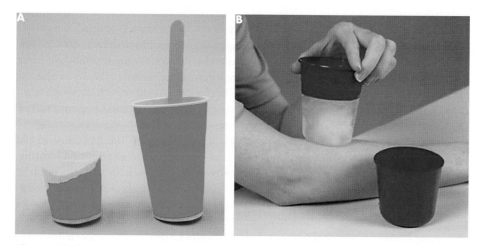

Figure 9–2. (a) Water may be frozen in a paper cup, styrofoam cup, or on a tongue depressor for the purpose of ice massage. (b) Cyrocup is a commercially produced product for ice massage.

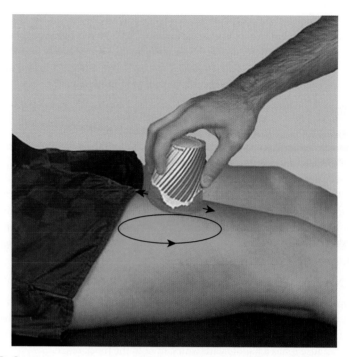

Figure 9–3. Ice massage may be applied using either circular or longitudinal strokes.

Physiologic Responses. Cold progression proceeds through the four stages: cold, stinging, burning, and numbness. Reddening of the skin **(erythema)** occurs as a result of blanching or lack of blood in the capillary bed. A common example occurs when one works outside in the cold without gloves or appropriate footwear and returns inside to find the toes beet red. This is an example of the body attempting to pool blood in the area to prevent further temperature loss. Ice applications of 5–15 minutes at greater than 10°C (50°F) will not stimulate the hunting response and do not stimulate the reflex vasodilation that creates the body's own physically induced heat or increased blood flow.

Considerations. The time necessary for the surface area to be numbed will depend on the body area to be massaged. Approximate time will depend on how fast the ice melts and what thermopane develops between the skin and ice massage. Patient comfort should be considered at all times. If adequate circulation is present, frostbite should not be a concern. However, if the patient has diabetes, the extremities, especially the toes, may require reduced temperature and adjustment of the intensity and duration of the cold.

Application. After the type of cold applicator for ice massage is selected, the patient should be positioned comfortably, and clothing should be removed from the area to be treated. The area should be set up before positioning the patient. Remove the top two-thirds of paper from the ice-filled paper or Styrofoam cup, leaving 1 inch on the bottom of the cup as a handle for the clinician or patient to use as a handgrip. The clinician should smooth the rough edges of the ice cup by gently rubbing along the edges. Ice should be applied to the patient's exposed skin in circular or longitudinal strokes, with each stroke overlapping the previous stroke. Firm pressure during stroking increases numbness following ice massage.[104] The application should be continued until the patient goes through the cold progression sequence of cold, stinging, burning or aching, and numbness. Once the skin is numb to fine touch, ice application can be terminated. The cold progression is the response of the sensory nerve fibers in the skin. The difference between cold and burning is primarily between the dropping out (sensory deficit) of the cold and warm nerve endings. Standard treatments allow the patient to place cold applications every other 20 minutes, thus facilitating the hunting response. Some thermobarrier is developed during the ice massage in the layer of water directly on the skin, but this allows the ice cup to move smoothly over the skin. The time from application to numbing of the body segment depends on the size of the segment, but progression to numbing should be around 7–10 minutes.

Treatment Protocols: Ice Massage

1. Expose block of ice.
2. Rub ice on hand to smooth rough edges.
3. Warn the patient that you are going to put your cold hand on the body part to be treated, then do so.
4. Remove your hand after 2 or 3 seconds, and warn the patient that you are going to put the ice on the body part to be treated, then do so.
5. Begin rubbing the ice block in a circular motion on the body part being treated. Do not put additional pressure on the ice. Move the ice at about 5–7 cm/sec. Do not let melted water run onto areas of the body that are not being treated.

CASE STUDY 9–1
CRYOTHERAPY: ICE MASSAGE

Background: A 35-year-old man sustained a Colles fracture of the right wrist during a fall 13 weeks ago. He was treated with a closed reduction and plaster for 12 weeks; the cast was removed 1 week ago. The fracture is well healed with good position. In addition to active and passive exercise, you begin joint mobilization on an every other-day schedule. In spite of the fact that the tissues are strong enough to tolerate grades II and III mobilization, the patient experiences so much pain that you are limited to grade I mobilization. To increase the patient's tolerance for mobilization, you decide to perform an ice massage prior to mobilization.

Impression: Limitation of motion secondary to fracture and immobilization.

Treatment Plan: A cup of ice was applied to the anterior and posterior aspects of the wrist until the patient experienced numbness. The duration of the treatment was approximately 9 minutes. Immediately following the ice massage, joint mobilization techniques were used to increase the range of motion of the wrist.

Response: The patient's tolerance for more aggressive mobilization was increased for approximately 5 minutes following the ice massage. As the accessory motions were restored, the active range of motion also improved. After six sessions, joint mobilization was discontinued, the patient continued with active and passive range of motion exercise, and strengthening exercise was added to the program. Ten weeks after removal of the cast, the patient's range of motion in all planes was approximately 90 percent of normal, and the patient was discharged to a home program.

Discussion Questions

- What tissues were injured/affected?
- What symptoms were present?
- What phase of the injury-healing continuum did the patient present for care in?
- What are the physical agent modality's biophysical effects (direct/indirect/depth/tissue affinity)?
- What are the physical agent modality's indications/contraindications?
- What are the parameters of the physical agent modality's application/dosage/duration/frequency in this case study?
- What other physical agent modalities could be utilized to treat this injury or condition? Why? How?
- What other techniques could have been used to provide pain management for the joint mobilization?
- What are the physiologic mechanisms for the pain relief?
- Why was it necessary to begin the joint mobilization immediately following the ice massage?
- What effect might the ice massage have on the properties of the tissues being mobilized? Is there another treatment that would have the opposite effect?

The rehabilitation professional employs physical agent modalities to create an optimum environment for tissue healing while minimizing the symptoms associated with the trauma or condition.

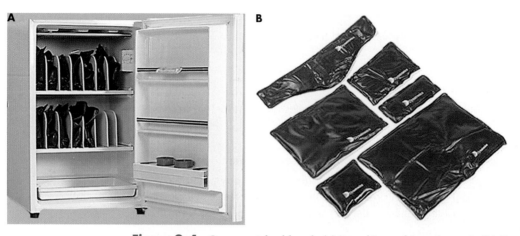

Figure 9–4. Commercial cold pack. (a) Stored in a refrigeration unit. (b) Come in a variety of sizes.

Commercial (Cold) Hydrocollator Packs

Cold hydrocollator packs (Figure 9–4) are indicated in any acute injury to a musculoskeletal structure.

Equipment Needed

1. Hydrocollator cold pack: This must be cooled to 8°F (15°C). It needs plastic liners or protective toweling for placement on a body segment. Petroleum distillate gel is the substance contained in the plastic pouch design.
2. Moist cold towels: Towels may be immersed in ice water and molded to the skin surface, or they can be packed in ice and allowed to remain in place. The commercial cold pack should be placed on top of a moist towel.
3. Plastic bag: The hydrocollator should be placed in the bag. Air should be removed from the bag. The plastic bag may then be molded around the body segment.
4. Dry towel: To prevent the cold hydrocollator from losing heat rapidly, the towel is used as a covering to insulate the cold pack.

   Treatment. Preferred positions are side lying, prone, supine, hook lying, or sitting, depending on the area to be treated. The patient must remain still during the treatment to maintain appropriate positioning of the cold pack. The cold pack must be molded onto the skin. The pack should be covered with a towel to limit loss of cold. A timer should be set, or time should otherwise be noted. Treatment time should be 20 minutes.

   Physiologic Responses. Erythema occurs. Cold progression proceeds through the four stages.

Considerations

   Body area should be covered to prevent unnecessary exposure.

   The physiologic response to cold treatment is immediate.

   Patient comfort should be considered at all times.

   Frostbite should not be a concern unless circulation is inadequate.

   The patient should not lie on top of the cold pack.

   Application. The patient should be positioned with the treatment area exposed and a towel draped to protect clothing. The commercial cold pack should be placed against wet toweling to enhance transfer of cold to the body segment. If the injury is acute or subacute, the body segment should be elevated to reduce gravity-dependent swelling.[105] Pack the cold pack around the joint in a manner designed to remove all air and ensure placement directly against wet toweling. Cold progression will be the same as with ice massage but not as quick because of the toweling between the skin and cold pack.[72] General treatment time required for numbing is about 20 minutes. The importance of a comfortable, properly positioned patient is evident. Checking the sensory area after application is important. Again, frostbite should not be a concern if circulation is intact. If swelling is a concern, a wet compression (elastic) wrap could be applied under the cold pack. A sequence of 20 minutes on and 20 minutes off should be repeated for 2 hours; the same sequence can be used in home treatment. Elevation is a key adjunct therapy during the sleeping hours.

Treatment Protocols: Cold Hydrocollator

1. Wrap cold pack in towels to provide six to eight layers of towel between the cold pack and the patient. If using a commercial cold pack cover, use at least one layer of towel to keep the cover clean.
2. Inform the patient that you are going to put the cold pack on the body part to be treated then do so.
3. Set a timer for the appropriate treatment time and give the patient a signaling device. Make sure the patient understands how to use the signaling device.
4. Check the patient's response after the first 5 minutes by asking the patient how it feels as well as visually checking the area under the cold pack. If the area is blotchy, additional toweling may be needed. Recheck verbally about every 5 minutes. A visual inspection every 5 minutes is not inappropriate.

Ice Packs

Like cold hydrocollator packs, ice packs are indicated in acute stages of injury, as well as for prevention of additional swelling after exercise of the injured part (Figure 9–5). It appears that ice packs may lower intermuscular temperatures more than commercial gel packs.[90,106]

Equipment Needed

1. Small plastic bags: Vegetable or bread bags may be used.
2. Ice flaker machine: Flaked or crushed ice is easier to mold than cubed ice.
3. Moist towels: These are used to facilitate cold transmission and should be placed directly on the skin.
4. Elastic bandaging: Bandaging holds the plastic ice pack in place and applies compression. The body segment to be treated may be elevated.

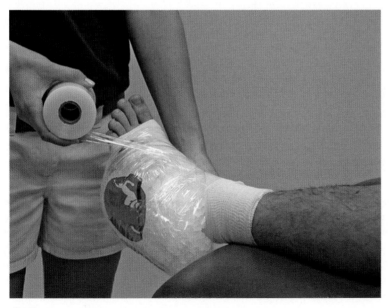

Figure 9–5. Ice pack molded to fit the injured part.

Treatment. The patient's position depends on the part to be treated. The patient must remain still during the treatment. A pack must be placed on the skin. The pack should be secured in place with toweling or an elastic bandage. The pack should be covered with a towel to limit cold loss. A timer should be set, or time should otherwise be noted. The treatment time should be 20 minutes.

Physiologic Responses. Cold progression proceeds through the four stages. Erythema occurs.

Considerations. The body area to be treated should be covered to prevent unnecessary exposure.

The physiologic response to cold is immediate.

Patient comfort should be considered at all times.

Frostbite should not be a concern unless circulation is inadequate.

The patient should not lie on top of the ice pack.

Application. The application of ice packs is similar to the use of commercial cold hydrocollator packs; the equipment to be set up in the treatment area consists of flaked or cubed ice in a plastic bag large enough for the area to be treated. The plastic bag can be applied directly to the skin and held in place by a moist or dry elastic wrap. It has been shown that wrapping a cold pack tightly in place produces a significantly greater decrease in intramuscular temperature.[107,108] However, patient comfort is of the utmost importance during this application to facilitate patient relaxation. The clinician may want to add salt to the ice to facilitate melting of the ice to create a colder slush mixture. Melting ice gives off more energy because of its less stable state, and therefore it is colder. It has been shown that regular ice contained in an ice pack that undergoes a phase change causes lower skin and 1-cm intramuscular temperatures than cold modality in commercial ice packs (Wet-Ice, Flexi-i-Cold) that do not possess these properties.[81] A towel should be placed over the ice pack to decrease the warming effect of the environmental air, thus facilitating the cold application. The normal physiologic response progression is cold, stinging, burning, and finally numbness, at which time the setup can be terminated. Because of the pliability of the flaked ice pack, it can be molded to the body segment treated. If cubed ice is used instead of flaked ice, it can still be molded, but it will not readily hold its position and will need to be secured via elastic wrap or toweling.

Treatment Protocols: Ice Pack

1. Wrap cold pack in wet towel.
2. Warn the patient that you are going to put the cold pack on the body part to be treated then do so.
3. Set a timer for the appropriate treatment time (generally about 20 minutes), and give the patient a signaling device. Make sure the patient understands how to use the signaling device.
4. Check the patient's response verbally after the first 2 minutes, then about every 5 minutes. Perform a visual check of the area if the patient reports any unusual sensation. If wheals or welts appear, or if the skin color changes to absolute white within the first 4 minutes of treatment, stop the treatment.

Clinical Decision-Making   *Exercise 9–1*

The clinician is treating an acute inversion ankle sprain and has placed an elastic wrap around the ankle for compression. Crushed ice bags have been applied to both sides of the ankle and it has been elevated. How long should the ice bags be left in place?

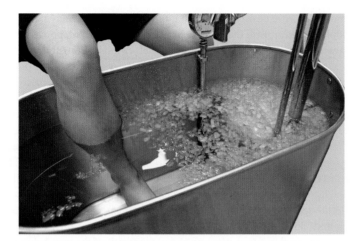

Figure 9–6. The ice should be melted in a cold whirlpool before it is turned on.

Cold Whirlpool

The cold whirlpool is indicated in acute and subacute conditions in which exercise of the injured part during a cold treatment is desired (Figure 9–6).

Equipment Needed

1. Whirlpool: The appropriate size whirlpool must be filled with cold water or ice to lower the temperature to 50–60°F. The clinician should use flaked ice and make sure the ice melts completely because pieces of ice could become projectiles if a body segment is in the pool.
2. Ice machine: Flaked ice acts faster than cubed to lower the water temperature.
3. Toweling: Sufficient toweling is needed for padding the body segment on the whirlpool and for drying off after treatment.
4. Appropriate setup in area: A chair, whirlpool, and a bench in the whirlpool must be arranged before treatment.

   Treatment. The temperature should be set at 50–60°F. The body segment to be treated must be immersed. For total body immersion, the water temperature should be set at 65–80°F. The treatment time should be 5–15 minutes.

Physiologic Responses

Cold progression proceeds through the four stages.

Erythema occurs.

   Considerations. *Caution*: Even though the immediate application of cold will help to control edema if applied immediately following injury, the gravity-dependent positions should be avoided with acute and subacute injuries.[80,109–111] It has been shown that treatment in the dependent position causes a significant increase in ankle volume over a 20-minute period. However, if high-voltage pulsed electrical currents of sufficient intensity to produce muscle contraction are used simultaneously, increases in ankle volume are minimized.[112] Cold wet compression or elastic wrap should be put in place before treatment. The body area to be treated should be completely immersed. A cold whirlpool allows exercises to be done during treatment. Patient comfort should be considered at all times. Frostbite should not be a concern unless circulation is inadequate. A toecap made of neoprene can be used to make the patient more comfortable in the cold whirlpool.[113]

   Application and Precautions. The unit should be turned on after it has been established that the ground fault interrupter (GFI) is functioning. The patient should be cautioned to use care when standing or walking on slippery floors and particularly when getting in and out of the whirlpool. The patient should be positioned in the whirlpool area, and appropriate padding should be provided for the patient's comfort. The timer should be set for the amount of time desired, depending on the size of the body part to be treated. Treatment should continue until the body segment becomes numb (approximately 15 minutes). Numbness is the cutaneous (skin or superficial) response. Frostbite should not be a concern unless the individual has a history of circulatory deficiencies or has diabetes. Treatment time will be between 7 and 15 minutes to allow the complete circulatory response. Caution is indicated in the gravity-dependent position because of the likelihood of additional swelling if the body segment is already swollen.[80] This is the most intense application of cold of the cryotherapy techniques listed. Therefore, the first two or three treatments should be administered with the clinician remaining in the area. One of several reasons for the intensity of cold is that the body cannot develop a **thermopane** (insulating layer of water) on the skin because of the convection effect of the whirlpool. Cold whirlpools have been shown to be more effective than ice packs at maintaining prolonged significant temperature reduction for at least 30 minutes post-treatment.[114] Additional benefits include the massaging and vibrating effect of the water flow. A review of the skin surface and an assessment of edema in the extremities will require removal of the part being treated from the whirlpool. If total body immersion is used, care should be taken for the intensity and duration of the whirlpool and for protection of the genitals from direct water flow. Applications can be repeated following rewarming of the body segment after sensation has returned. If the cold application is administered before practice, it should be done before the application of preventive strapping. Enough time should also be allowed for sensation to return before taping. Studies have indicated that the reflex vasodilation lasts up to 2 hours. A patient could exercise then return to the clinic and receive additional treatment without additional edema created by **congestion** as a result of vascular and capillary insufficiency occurring during the healing process. Increased heart rate and blood pressure are associated with cold application. Conditioned patients should not have a problem with dizziness after cold applications, but care should be taken when transferring the patient from the whirlpool area. Whirlpool cultures of the tank and jet should be taken weekly to keep bacterial growth under control.

Whirlpool Maintenance. Safety considerations for using both cold and hot whirlpools have been discussed previously. It is equally important to mention the importance of maintaining the cleanliness of the whirlpools in a clinical setting. It is not uncommon for several individuals to use a whirlpool between cleanings. This practice is certainly not recommended and in fact is contrary to the standards of most health regulatory agencies in many states.

It is recommended that the whirlpool be drained and cleaned after each treatment to minimize the potential risks of spreading fungal, viral, or bacterial infections, especially in those individuals who have open lesions. Whirlpools should be cleaned by filling the basin above the level of the turbine, adding a commercial antibiotic solution, disinfecting agent, or chlorine bleach, and then running the turbine for at least 1 minute. The turbine and drain filter should be scrubbed and the tub thoroughly rinsed. The outside surface of the whirlpool should be cleaned daily. To keep bacterial and fungal growth in check, whirlpool cultures should be taken monthly.

Treatment Protocols: Cold Whirlpool

1. Pad edge of tank with toweling, warn patient that the water is cold, then place body part in water.
2. Instruct patient to keep away from all parts of the turbine.
3. Turn on the turbine, adjust the aeration, agitation, and direction of the water being pumped.
4. Check the patient's response verbally and visually about every 2 minutes. Remind the patient to tell you if the area starts hurting or if sensation is lost.

Clinical Decision-Making *Exercise 9–2*

On day 2 following an ankle sprain, the clinician decides to put a patient in a cold whirlpool to have her do exercises. At this point in a rehabilitation program is this really the best course of action?

CASE STUDY 9–2
HYDROTHERAPY: COLD WHIRLPOOL

Background: A 32-year-old woman fell onto her outstretched left hand 12 weeks ago and sustained a comminuted fracture of the distal radius as well as a non-comminuted fracture of the scaphoid. She was treated with a closed reduction and external fixation (fiberglass cast) for 8 weeks, then a splint for 4 weeks. She has been referred for rehabilitation, to include mobilization, strengthening, and range-of-motion exercise. The radius demonstrates radiographic healing, and there is no evidence of aseptic necrosis. Her distal forearm, wrist, hand, and fingers remain markedly swollen, and she is experiencing significant pain at rest. She is unable to tolerate more than mild pressure on the wrist, making joint mobilization extremely difficult, and has severe pain with attempted active range of motion.

Impression: Posttraumatic pain and swelling, postimmobilization pain and loss of motion.

Treatment Plan: A small extremity hydrotherapy tank was filled with ice and water to achieve a water temperature of 17°C (63°F). The patient's left upper member was immersed in the water up to the level of the mid-forearm, and the turbine was used to direct water onto the wrist and hand. For the initial 5 minutes, the patient was instructed to gently move the wrist and hand actively. For the next 5 minutes, passive range of motion was conducted by the therapist; 5 minutes of joint mobilization followed the passive range of motion. The total treatment time in the cold whirlpool was 15 minutes. She was instructed in a home exercise program to gain motion and strength.

Response: The patient was treated with the cold whirlpool 3 days per week for 3 weeks, at which time the swelling had subsided to a minimal amount. Her range of motion was approximately 50 percent that of the right wrist and hand. The cold whirlpool was discontinued after 9 sessions, and other physical agents were used to facilitate a return to function. After an additional 12 sessions, the patient was discharged to a home program, with her left wrist and hand motion and strength approximately 80 percent that of the right wrist and hand.

Discussion Questions

- What tissues were injured or affected?
- What symptoms were present?
- What phase of the injury-healing continuum did the patient present for care in?
- What are the physical agent modality's biophysical effects (direct, indirect, depth, and tissue affinity)?
- What are the physical agent modality's indications and contraindications?
- What are the parameters of the physical agent modality's application, dosage, duration, and frequency in this case study?
- What other physical agent modalities could be used to treat this injury or condition? Why? How?
- What is aseptic necrosis? Are particular areas more vulnerable? What areas? What is the mechanism of the disorder?
- What does the abbreviation "FOOSH" stand for? What types of injuries would you anticipate in a patient who had experienced a "FOOSH"?
- If the cold whirlpool was helpful in achieving the therapeutic goals, why was the cold whirlpool discontinued after nine sessions? Why was a cold whirlpool selected for this patient?
- What disadvantages are there in using a whirlpool to assist in the resolution of the soft-tissue swelling? Advantages?
- If the patient had coexisting cardiovascular pathology (e.g., heart failure, peripheral vascular disease), would the ideal treatment have been different? Why or why not?
- What effect does the water driven by the turbine have on the ability of the patient to tolerate the aggressive stretching? What is the mechanism for this effect?

The rehabilitation professional employs physical agent modalities to create an optimum environment for tissue healing while minimizing the symptoms associated with the trauma or condition.

Cold Spray

Cold sprays, such as Flouri-Methane, do not provide adequate deep penetration, but they do provide adjunctive therapy for techniques to reduce muscle spasm. Physiologically this is accomplished by stimulating the Aβ fibers involved in the gate control theory. The primary action of a cold spray is reduction of the pain spasm sequence secondary to direct trauma. However, it will not reduce hemorrhage because it works on the superficial nerve endings to reduce the spasm via the stimulation of Aβ fibers to reduce the so-called painful arc. Cold spray is an extremely effective technique in the treatment of myofascial trigger points. Precautions concerning the use of cold spray include protecting the patient's face from the fumes and spraying the skin at an acute rather than a perpendicular angle.[115] Cold spray is indicated when stretching of an injured part is desired along with cold treatment.

Equipment Needed

1. Fluori-Methane
2. Toweling
3. Padding

Treatment

The area to be treated should be sprayed and then stretched.

Spasm should be reduced.

Treatment should be distal to proximal.

A quick jetstream spray or stroking motion should be used.

Cooling should be superficial; no frosting should occur.

Cold sprays may be used in conjunction with acupressure.

Treatment time should be set according to body segment.

Physiologic Responses

Muscle spasm is reduced.

Golgi tendon organ response is facilitated.

Muscle spindle response is inhibited.

Musculoskeletal structures may be stimulated.

Considerations

Both the acute and the subacute response should be positive.

The room should be well ventilated to avoid the accumulation of fumes.

Patient comfort should be considered at all times.

Application. The application of Fluori-Methane is typical of the application of other cold sprays (Figure 9–7). The following application procedures apply specifically to Fluori-Methane, but they provide an outline of the procedures, indications, and precautions applicable to all cold sprays. The clinician should follow the manufacturer's instructions in the use of any cold spray.

Fluori-Methane is a topical vapocoolant that acts as a counterirritant to block pain impulses of muscles in spasm. When used in conjunction with the "spray-and-stretch" technique, Fluori-Methane can break the pain cycle, allowing the muscle to be stretched to its normal length (pain-free state). The application of the "spray-and-stretch" technique is a therapeutic modality that involves three stages: evaluation, spraying, and stretching. The therapeutic value of "spray-and-stretch" becomes most effective when the practitioner has mastered all stages and applies them in the proper sequence.

Evaluation. During the evaluation phase the cause of pain is determined as local spasm of an irritated trigger point. The method of applying "spray-and-stretch" to a muscle spasm differs slightly from application to a trigger point. The trigger point is a deep hypersensitive localized spot in a muscle that causes a referred pain pattern. With trigger points the source of pain is seldom the site of the pain. A trigger point may be detected by a snapping palpation over the muscle, causing the muscle in which the irritated trigger point

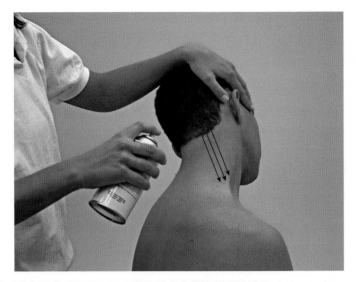

Figure 9–7. Spray-and-stretch technique using Fluori-Methane.

is situated to "jump." In the case of muscle spasm, the source and site of pain are identical. A trigger point may also be effectively treated using ultrasound and electrical stimulation.[116]

Spraying

The following steps should be followed to apply Fluori-Methane.

1. The patient should assume a comfortable position.
2. Take precautions to cover the patient's eyes, nose, and mouth if spraying near the face.
3. Hold the spray can or spray bottle (upside down) 12–18 inches away from the treatment surface, allowing the jetstream of vapocoolant to meet the skin at an acute angle.
4. Apply the spray in one direction only—not back and forth—at a rate of 4 inches (10 cm) per second. Three or four sweeps of the spray in one direction only are sufficient to treat the trigger point or to overcome painful muscle spasms. The skin must not be frosted. It is possible but not very likely that the intense cold (15°C) of the Fluori-Methane can freeze the skin, causing frostbite, and result in superficial tissue necrosis. The chances of this occurring are not nearly as likely as when using ethyl chloride. In the case of trigger point, spray should be applied from the trigger point to the area of referred pain. If there is no trigger point, the spray should be applied from the affected muscle to its insertion. The spray should be applied in an even sweep. About two to four parallel, but not overlapping, sweeps of spray should be enough to cover this skin representation of the affected muscle.

    Stretching. The static stretch should begin as you start spraying from the origin to the insertion (simple muscle spasm pain) or from the trigger point to the referred pain when the trigger point is present. Spray and stretch until the muscle reaches its maximal or normal resting length. You will usually feel a gradual increase in range of motion. The spraying and stretching may require two to four spray applications to achieve the therapeutic results in any treatment session. A patient may have multiple treatment sessions in any 1 day.

    The spray-and-stretch technique outlined in the preceding must be considered a therapeutic system. The practitioner should spend some time each day practicing until the technique is mastered.

    Composition. Fluori-Methane is a combination of two chlorofluorocarbons—15% dichlorodifluoromethane and 85% trichloromonofluoromethane. The combination is not flammable and at room temperature is only volatile enough to expel the contents from the inverted container. Fluori-Methane is supplied in amber Dispenseal bottles that emit a jetstream from a calibrated nozzle.

    Indications. Fluori-Methane is a vapocoolant intended for topical application in the management of myofascial pain, restricted motion, and muscle spasm. Clinical conditions that may respond to the spray-and-stretch technique include low back pain (caused by muscle spasm), acute stiff neck, torticollis, acute bursitis of shoulder, muscle spasm associated with osteoarthritis, ankle sprain, tight hamstring, masseter muscle spasm, certain types of headache, and referred pain from trigger points.

Precautions. Federal law prohibits dispensing without a prescription. Although Fluori-Methane is safe for topical application to the skin, care should be taken to minimize inhalation of vapors, especially when it is being applied to the head or neck. Fluori-Methane is not intended for production of local anesthesia and should not be applied to the point of frost formation. Freezing can occasionally alter pigmentation.

Clinical Decision-Making   *Exercise 9–3*

An assembly-line worker is diagnosed with a myofascial trigger point in her middle trapezius. What conductive thermal energy therapeutic modality would likely be a good choice for treating this condition?

Treatment Protocols: Vapocoolant Spray

1. Position body part such that the area to be treated is on a stretch.
2. Protect the patient's eyes and ensure that the patient does not inhale fumes.
3. Holding the vapocoolant upside down, with the nozzle at about a 30-degree angle from the perpendicular with the skin, and about 45 cm from the skin, spray the skin from distal to proximal.
4. Spray in one direction only three to four times, then apply direct pressure or increased stretch as indicated and tolerated by the patient. Repeat the procedure as needed after the skin has rewarmed.
5. Check the patient's response frequently during the treatment.

Contrast Bath

Contrast baths are used to treat subacute swelling, gravity-dependent swelling, and vasodilation–vasoconstriction response. Both contrast baths and cold whirlpools have been demonstrated to be effective in treating delayed-onset muscle soreness.[96] A contrast-therapy technique using hot and cold packs has been shown to have little or no effect on deep muscle -temperatures.[117,118]

Equipment Needed. (Figure 9–8)

1. Two containers. One container is used to hold cold water (50–60°), and the other is used to hold warm water (104–106°F). Whirlpools may be used for one or both containers.
2. Ice machine
3. Towels
4. Chair

Treatment. Hot and cold immersions are alternated. Treatment time should be at least 20 minutes. Treatments should consist of five 1-minute cold immersions and five 3-minute warm immersions, although the exact ratio of cold to hot treatment is highly variable.

Treatment Tip. Contrast baths produce little or no "pumping action" and are not very effective in treating swelling. A better alternative is to use cryokinetics, which involves cold followed by active muscle contractions and relaxation to help eliminate swelling.

Physiologic Responses. Vasoconstriction and vasodilation occur.

Necrotic cells are reduced at the cellular level.

Edema is decreased.

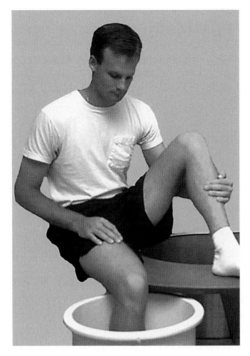

Figure 9–8. Contrast bath using a warm whirlpool and ice immersion cylinder.

Considerations

The temperatures of the baths must be maintained.

A large area is required for treatment.

Patient comfort must be considered at all times.

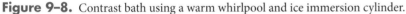

Application. After the area is set up, a whirlpool can be used for either hot or cold application, with the opposite method of treatment contained in a bucket or sterile container. The temperatures of these immersion baths must be maintained (cold at 50–60°F, hot at 98–110°F) by adding ice or warm water. It is generally easier to use a large whirlpool for the warm water application and a bucket for the cold water application. There has been considerable controversy regarding the use of contrast baths to control swelling. Contrast baths are most often indicated when changing the treatment modality from cold to hot to facilitate a mild tissue temperature increase. The use of a contrast bath allows for a transitional period during which a slight rise in tissue temperature may be effective for increasing blood flow to an injured area without causing the accumulation of additional edema. The theory that contrast baths induce a type of pumping action by alternating vasoconstriction with vasodilation has little or no credibility. Contrast baths probably cause only a superficial capillary response, resulting from inability of the larger deep blood vessels to constrict and dilate in response to superficial heating.[119,120]

Thus, it is recommended that during the initial stages of contrast bath treatment the ratio of hot to cold treatment begins with a relatively brief period in the hot bath, gradually increasing the length of time in the hot bath during subsequent treatments. Recommendations as to specific lengths of time are extremely variable. However, it would appear that a 3:1 ratio (3 minutes in hot, 1 minute in cold) or 4:1 ratio for 19–20 minutes is fairly well accepted. Whether the treatment is ended with cold or hot depends to some extent on the degree of tissue temperature increase desired. Other clinicians prefer to use the same ratios of 3:1 or 4:1, beginning with cold. The technique may be modified to meet specific needs. Since the extremity is in the gravity-dependent position, once the injured part is removed from the contrast bath, skin sensation and the amount of edema accumulation should be assessed to make sure that the treatment has not actually increased the amount of edema.[92]

Clinical Decision-Making *Exercise 9–4*

The clinician is treating a patient with a grade 2 MCL sprain. After the first week, there is still considerable swelling on the medial side of the knee just below the joint line. He decides to use a contrast bath to take advantage of the "pumping action" of vasoconstriction/vasodilation. Is this technique likely to be effective?

CASE STUDY 9–3
HYDROTHERAPY: CONTRAST BATH

Background: A 29-year-old police officer sustained a laceration of the right posterior forearm as a result of a struggle with an individual using a knife. There was a partial laceration of the extensor carpi radialis longus and brevis, and the extensor digitorum (communis), no arterial damage, no motor nerve damage, but a complete transection of the superficial radial nerve. The laceration was sutured primarily, and a splint applied to prevent stress on the repair. The patient is now 12 weeks postinjury, and has full wrist and hand motion and near-normal strength. However, he has developed extreme sensitivity to any stimulus over the dorsal-radial aspect of the wrist and hand, which is disabling. The patient guards the area by holding the right forearm with his left hand, and experiences severe pain when anything touches the area (including a breeze). The area innervated by the superficial radial nerve is glossy in appearance, and is now hairless (as compared to the left forearm and hand). He has been referred for pain management and desensitization.

Impression: Complex regional pain syndrome (CRPS) type II (also known as causalgia).

Treatment Plan: Two basins large enough to immerse the entire forearm were filled with water, one at 40°C (104°F) and the other at 14°C (57°F). The patient's forearm was immersed in the warm water for 2 minutes, then removed and immersed in the cold water for 1 minute. The sequence was repeated six times, for a total treatment duration of 18 minutes. Immediately after the final immersion, the patient was encouraged to brush the painful area with his left hand, and to tap over the mid- and distal-radius, along the course of the superficial radial nerve.

Response: After the initial treatment, the patient noted little improvement, and was unable to tolerate the desensitization. The treatment was repeated the next day, and he was able to tolerate a few seconds of desensitization. He was treated in the clinic daily for a total of four sessions, and, he was then instructed to continue the contrast bath treatment on a home

program, with weekly rechecks. He completed twice-daily sessions at home, and noted very gradual increases in the duration of the increased tolerance to touch and tapping, as well as an ability to tolerate more vigorous touch. Two months later, there was no hypersensitivity in the superficial radial nerve distribution, and the skin had returned to a normal appearance.

Discussion Questions

- What tissues were injured or affected?
- What symptoms were present?
- What phase of the injury-healing continuum did the patient present for care in?
- What are the physical agent modality's biophysical effects (direct, indirect, depth, and tissue affinity)?
- What are the physical agent modality's indications and contraindications?
- What are the parameters of the physical agent modality's application, dosage, duration, and frequency in this case study?
- What other physical agent modalities could be used to treat this injury or condition? Why? How?
- What is CRPS type II?
- What is the difference between CRPS type I and CRPS type II?
- Is it likely that CRPS could have been prevented in this patient? How?
- If the patient's fingertips had become very pale during the immersion in the cold water, and the patient had complained of severe pain in the fingertips, what would have been your response? What pathology would you suspect?

The rehabilitation professional employs physical agent modalities to create an optium environment for tissue healing while minimizing the symptoms associated with the trauma or condition.

Cold-Compression Units

The Cryo-Cuff is a device that uses both cold and compression simultaneously. The Cryo-Cuff is used both acutely following injury and postsurgically (Figure 9–9).

Equipment Needed. Originally developed by Aircast, the Cryo-Cuff is made of a nylon sleeve that connects via a tube to a 1-gallon cooler/jug.

Application. Cold water flows into the sleeve from the cooler. As the cooler is raised, the pressure in the cuff is increased. During the treatment, the water warms and can be rechilled by lowering the cooler to drain the cuff, mixing the warmer water with the colder water, and then again raising the jug to increase pressure in the cuff.

CASE STUDY 9–4
CRYO-CUFF

Background: A 28-year-old woman sustained blunt trauma to her right forefoot when she dropped a full box of copy paper on it while attempting to remove the box from a shelf. She reported to an occupational health clinic and after having an x-ray taken to rule out fracture, she was referred to you for emergent care. The forefoot was noted to be visibly swollen and discolored. Circumferential measure taken at MTI heads was increased by 1 cm over the uninvolved side measure. You quickly repositioned the patient with her foot elevated above heart level and continued your examination. Both PD and TP were intact, and there was no medial or lateral ankle ligament tenderness. Attempts at assessing AROM/PROM were abandoned secondary to the patient's complaints of forefoot pain.

Impression: Soft tissue contusion with acute soft-tissue edema formation right forefoot.

Treatment Plan: You apply a moistened cotton stock-ing-nette to the right foot and ankle followed by the application of a Cryo-Cuff ankle sleeve. The sleeve was filled from the ice water reservoir until full. Treatment with the cold, mild compression and elevation lasted approximately 20 minutes. Immediately following the completion of the initial cold, compression, and elevation treatment, the patient was instructed in crutch walking, nonweight-bearing right lower extremity, and the use of the Cryo-Cuff once each waking hour along with attention to maintaining the limb in an elevated position. The patient was advised to return to the clinic first thing the next morning.

Response: The patient tolerated cold compression and elevation very well and reported immediate pain relief in the forefoot. Upon return to the clinic the next morning, the patient was noted to have no further increase in forefoot edema. Gentle passive- and active-assistive range of motion exercise for digits and ankle were initiated. Weight-bearing as tolerated with crutches was attempted. By treatment day 5

strengthening exercises were added to the program. Between treatments, the patient was placed in a compression stocking and walker boot. One week after the injury, the patient was able to wear a shoe without discomfort and return to full work status.

Discussion Questions

- What tissues were injured/affected?
- What symptoms were present?
- What phase of the injury-healing continuum did the patient present for care in?
- What are the physical agent modailty's biophysical effects (direct/indirect/depth/tissue affinity)?
- What are the physical agent modality's indications/contraindications?
- What are the parameters of the physical agent modality's application/dosage/duration/frequency in this case study?

The rehabilitation professional employs physical agent modalities to create an optimum environment for tissue healing while minimizing the symptoms associated with the trauma or condition.

- What other physical agent modalities could be utilized to treat this injury or condition? Why? How?

Further Discussion Questions

- What other techniques could have been used to provide pain management/acute edema control?
- What are the physiologic mechanisms for the pain relief/acute edema control?
- Why was it necessary to elevate the foot above the level of the heart?
- What effect might the Cryo-Cuff have on the properties of the forefoot soft tissues?

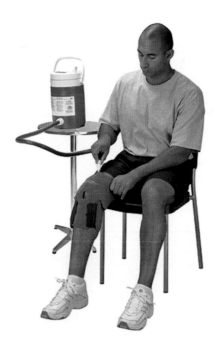

Figure 9–9. Cyro-Cuff combines cold and pressure.

Considerations. The only drawback to this simple yet effective piece of equipment is that the water in the cuff must be continually rechilled. However, the Cryo-Cuff is portable, easy to use, and inexpensive.[26]

Cryokinetics

Cryokinetics is a technique that combines cryotherapy or the application of cold with exercise.[26,62] The goal of cryokinetics is to numb the injured part to the point of analgesia and then work toward achieving normal range of motion through progressive active exercise. Using cryokinetics does not seem to delay the onset of fatigue.[121]

Equipment Needed. The technique uses ice immersion, cold packs, or ice massage.

Application. The technique begins by numbing the body part via ice immersion, cold packs, or ice massage. Most patients will report a feeling of numbness within 12–20 minutes. If numbness is not perceived within 20 minutes, the clinician should proceed with exercise regardless. The numbness usually will last for 3–5 minutes, at which point ice should be reapplied for an additional 3–5 minutes until numbness returns. This sequence should be repeated five times.

Considerations. Exercises are performed during the periods of numbness. The exercises selected should be pain-free and progressive in intensity, concentrating on both flexibility and strength.[122] Changes in the intensity of the activity should be limited by both the nature of the healing process and individual patient differences in perception of pain. However, progression always should be encouraged.

Ice Immersion

Equipment Needed. Ice buckets allow ease of application for the clinician.

Application. Again, a wet area should be selected (where spilled water is not a concern), with the patient positioned for comfort. Water should be at 50–60°F and treatment should last for 20 minutes. The immersion, like the contrast bath, should be maintained until desired results are reached. If cryokinetics are part of the treatment, then the container should be large enough to allow for the movement of the body segment.

Considerations. Although ice immersion has been shown to be effective in controlling posttraumatic edema,[123] ice immersion is similar to cold whirlpool in that the body segment may be subject to gravity-dependent positions. Cold pain may be worse during ice immersion than during cold pack application.[124]

THERMOTHERAPY

Physiologic Effects of Tissue Heating

Local superficial heating (infrared heat) is recommended in subacute conditions for reducing pain and **inflammation** through analgesic effects. Superficial heating produces lower tissue temperatures at the site of the pathology (injury) relative to the higher temperatures in the superficial tissues, resulting in **analgesia**. During the later stages of injury healing, a deeper heating effect is usually desirable; it can be achieved by using the diathermies or ultrasound. Heat dilates blood vessels, causing the patent capillaries to open up and increase circulation. The skin is supplied with sympathetic vasoconstrictor fibers that secrete norepinephrine at their endings (especially evident in feet, hands, lips, nose, and ears). At normal body temperature, the sympathetic vasoconstrictor nerves keep vascular anastomoses almost totally closed, but when the superficial tissue is heated, the number of sympathetic impulses is greatly reduced so that the anastomoses dilate and allow large quantities of blood to flow into the venous plexuses. This increases blood flow about twofold, which can promote heat loss from the body.[7]

The **hyperemia** created by heat has a beneficial effect on injury. This is based on increases of blood flow and pooling of blood during the metabolic processes. Recent hematomas (blood clots) should never be treated with heat until resolution of bleeding is completed. Some clinicians have advocated never using heat during any therapeutic modality application.[26,61,97,99]

Clinical Decision-Making   *Exercise 9–5*

A patient is about 1 week post–quadriceps contusion. To this point, the patient has had only cryotherapy and some mild stretching exercises. At what point should the clinician choose to switch to heat?

The rate of metabolism of tissues depends partly on temperature. The metabolic rate increases approximately 13% for each 1°C (1.8°F) increase in temperature.[99] A similar decrease in metabolism has been demonstrated when temperatures are lowered.

A primary effect of local heating is an increase in the local metabolic rate with a resulting increase in the production of **metabolites** and additional heat. These two factors lead to an increased intravascular hydrostatic pressure, causing arteriolar **vasodilation** and increased capillary blood flow.[78] However, increased hydrostatic pressure involves a tendency toward formation of edema, which may increase the time required for rehabilitation of a particular injury.[125] Increased capillary blood flow is important with many types of injury in which mild or moderate inflammation occurs because it causes an increase in the supply of oxygen, antibodies, leukocytes, and other necessary **nutrients** and enzymes, along with an increased clearing of metabolites. With higher heat intensities, vasodilation and increased blood flow will spread to remote areas, causing increased metabolism in the unheated area. This is known as **consensual heat vasodilation** and may be useful in many conditions where local heating is contraindicated.[1]

The application of heat can produce an analgesic effect, resulting in a reduction in the intensity of pain. The analgesic effect is the most frequent **indication** for its use.[78] Although the mechanisms underlying this phenomenon are not well understood, it is related in some way to the gate control theory of pain modulation. Heat has been shown to reduce pain associated with delayed-onset muscle soreness following a 30-minute treatment.[27]

Heat is applied in musculoskeletal and neuromuscular disorders, such as sprains, strains, articular (joint-related) problems, and muscle spasms, which all describe various types of muscle pain.[11] Heat generally is considered to produce a relaxation effect and a reduction in guarding in skeletal muscle. It also increases the elasticity and decreases the viscosity of connective tissue, which is an important consideration in postacute joint injuries or after long periods of immobilization. This may also be important during a warm-up activity prior to exercise for increasing intramuscular temperatures.[126] However, it has also been demonstrated that heat alone without stretching has little or no effect in improving flexibility.[129–130] It appears that a deep heating treatment using ultrasound may be more effective for increasing range of motion than using a more superficial heating technique.[131]

Many clinicians empirically believe that heat has little effect on the injury itself but serves rather to facilitate further treatment by producing relaxation in these types of disorders.[11] This is accomplished by relieving pain, lessening hypertonicity of muscles, producing sedation (which decreases spasticity, tenderness, and spasm), and decreasing tightness in muscles and related structures.

Thermotherapy Treatment Techniques

Heat is still used as a universal treatment for pain and discomfort. See Table 9–4 for a summary of uses of thermotherapy. Much of the benefit is derived from the treatment simply feeling good. However, in the early stages after injury, heat causes increased capillary blood pressure and increased cellular permeability; this results in additional swelling or **edema** accumulation.[11,71,82,132,133] *No patient with edema should be treated with any heat modality until the reasons for the edema are determined.* It is in the best interest of the clinician to use cryotherapy techniques to reduce the edema before applying heat. Superficial heat applications seem to feel more comfortable for complaints of the neck, back, low back, and pelvic areas and may be most appropriate for the patient who exhibits some allergic response to cold applications. However, the tissues in these areas are absolutely no different from those in the extremities. Thus, the same physiologic responses to the use of heat or cold will be elicited in all areas of the body.

Table 9–4 Indications and Contraindications for Thermotherapy
INDICATIONS
Subacute and chronic inflammatory conditions
Subacute or chronic pain
Subacute edema removal
Decreased ROM
Resolution of swelling
Myofascial trigger points
Muscle guarding
Muscle spasm
Subacute muscle strain
Subacute ligament sprain
Subacute contusion
Infection
CONTRAINDICATIONS
Acute musculoskeletal conditions
Impaired circulation
Peripheral vascular disease
Skin anesthesia
Open wounds or skin conditions (cold whirlpools and contrast baths)

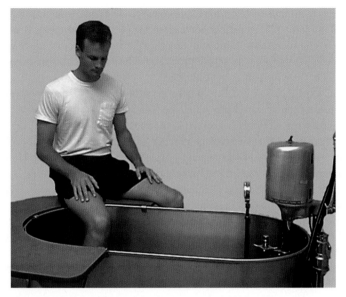

Figure 9–10. Warm whirlpool.

Primary goals of thermotherapy include increased blood flow and increased muscle temperature to stimulate analgesia, increased nutrition to the cellular level, reduction of edema, and removal of metabolites and other products of the inflammatory process.[134,135]

Warm Whirlpool

Equipment Needed. (Figure 9–10)

1. Whirlpool: The whirlpool must be the correct size for the body segment to be treated.
2. Towels: These are to be used for padding and drying off.
3. Chair
4. Padding: This is to be placed on the side of the whirlpool.

Treatment. The patient should be positioned comfortably, allowing the injured part to be immersed in the whirlpool. Direct flow should be 6–8 inches from the body segment. Temperature should be 98–110°F (37–45°C) for treatment of the arm and hand. For treatment of the leg, the temperature should be 98–104°F (37–40°C), and for full body treatment, the temperature should be 98–102°F (37–39°C). Time of application should be 15–20 minutes.

Considerations. Patient positioning should allow for exercise of the injured part. The size of the body segment to be treated will determine whether an upper extremity, lower extremity, or full body whirlpool should be used.

Application. The temperature range of a warm whirlpool is 100–110°F (39–45°C). It is similar in setup to a cold whirlpool. The patient must be positioned in the whirlpool with appropriate padding provided for the patient's comfort. The unit should be turned on after it has been ascertained that the GFI is functioning. The timer should be set for the amount of time desired, depending on the size of the body part to be treated (10–30 minutes). Treatment time should be long enough to stimulate vasodilatation and reduce muscle spasm (approximately 20 minutes). Again, caution is indicated in the gravity-dependent position in subacute injuries.[136] If some pitting edema exists (i.e., finger pressure on the skin leaves an indentation), cold or contrast baths are better indicated. In addition to increased circulation and reduction of spasm, benefits of the warm whirlpool include the massaging and vibrating effects of the water movement. On removal of the body segment from the whirlpool, it is necessary to review the skin surface and limb girth to see if the warm whirlpool increased swelling; this step is indicated even if the patient is past the subacute stage. After allowing the body segment to cool down, appropriate preventive strapping or padding can be placed on the body segment. If the patient receives the treatment before exercising, it is recommended that he or she gently do range-of-motion exercises to reduce congestion and increase proprioception (sense of position) in all joints. If the patient is complaining of muscle soreness, it would be more appropriate to recommend swimming pool exercises. The whirlpool provides a sedative effect. It is recommended that the patient shower or clean the body surface before using a whirlpool. Random access to the whirlpool is not warranted.

The warm whirlpool is an excellent postsurgical modality to increase systemic blood flow and mobilization of the affected body part. The appropriateness of whirlpool therapy needs to be addressed by the clinician because it is the most commonly abused physical therapy modality. An example of this abuse is the practice of placing an individual in the whirlpool without taking the time to assess the specific physiologic responses desired. However, it is an excellent adjunctive modality when used appropriately in the clinical setting.

Whirlpools should be cleaned frequently to prevent bacterial growth. When a patient with any open or infected lesion uses the whirlpool, it must be drained and cleaned immediately. Cleaning should be done using both a disinfecting and antibacterial agent. Particular attention should be paid to cleaning the turbine by placing the intake valves in a bucket

---

CASE STUDY 9–5
HYDROTHERAPY: WARM WHIRLPOOL

Background: An 82-year-old man underwent bilateral total knee arthroplasty 6 weeks ago. He was treated in the hospital postoperatively with strengthening and range-of-motion exercise, and gait and ADL training. His range of motion at hospital discharge was 5/90 bilaterally, and he was independent in ambulation with a walker. Arrangements for home health visits were completed prior to discharge; however, due to an administrative error, no visits were made. Two days ago, the patient returned to the orthopaedic surgeon, who noted that the patient had bilateral flexion contractures, limiting his knee motion to 45/70 bilaterally. The patient was referred to you for aggressive range-of-motion and strengthening exercise. He is ambulating independently with a walker, although he walks with both hips and knees flexed. His incisions are completely healed, and there is no joint effusion. He has no significant cardiovascular or pulmonary disorders.

Impression: Severe postoperative limitation of motion of both knees.

Treatment Plan: Active, active-assistive, and passive (stretching) range of motion in a "lowboy" whirlpool, with water temperature at 38°C (100°F) for 30 minutes, 3 days per week. For the initial 10 minutes, the patient was instructed to actively flex and extend the knees, using the buoyancy of the water to help extend the knees. The next 10 minutes consisted of gentle overpressure at the end of the available range of motion (active-assistive), and the final 10 minutes consisted of more forceful static stretching into both flexion and extension. In addition, generalized and specific strengthening exercises were performed, as well as additional gait training.

Response: There was a gradual increase in knee range-of-motion over the course of 8 weeks; after 24 visits, the patient was discharged to a home program. His knee range-of-motion was 0/110 bilaterally, and he was ambulating independently with a single cane.

Discussion Questions

- What tissues were injured or affected?
- What symptoms were present?
- What phase of the injury-healing continuum did the patient present for care in?
- What are the physical agent modality's biophysical effects (direct, indirect, depth, and tissue affinity)?
- What are the physical agent modality's indications and contraindications?
- What are the parameters of the physical agent modality's application, dosage, duration, and frequency in this case study?
- What other physical agent modalities could be used to treat this injury or condition? Why? How?
- If the patient had significant effusion of the knee joints, would the warm whirlpool have been the optimal physical agent of choice? Why or why not? What would the effect of the exposure to warm water have been on the physiologic mechanisms of the effusion?
- If the patient's incisions were not fully healed, would his treatment have been altered? Why or why not? What unique features of the whirlpool need to be considered in the case of open wounds?
- Why was a "lowboy" chosen? What advantages and disadvantages are there to a "lowboy" versus a "large extremity" whirlpool for this patient?
- If the patient had coexisting cardiovascular pathology (e.g., heart failure, peripheral vascular disease), would the ideal treatment have been different? Why or why not?
- What effect does the water driven by the turbine have on the ability of the patient to tolerate the aggressive stretching? What is the mechanism for this effect?

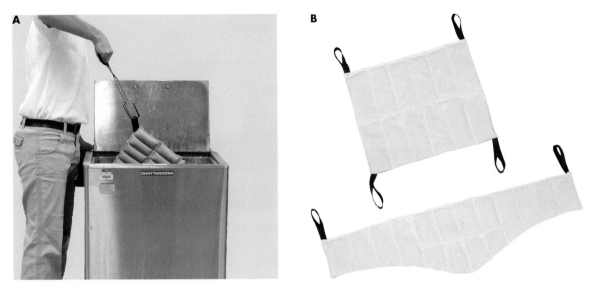

Figure 9–11. A. Hydrocollator packs stored in a tank. B. Come in a variety of sizes.

containing the disinfecting solution and turning the power on. Bacterial cultures should be monitored periodically from the tank, drain, and jets.

Commercial (Warm) Hydrocollator Packs

Equipment Needed. (Figure 9–11)

1. Unit heat packs: These are canvas pouches of petroleum distillate. A thermostat maintains the high temperature (170°F) and helps prevent burns. Unit heat packs come in three sizes: (1) regular size is 12 inch × 12 inch for most body segments; (2) double size is 24 inch × 24 inch for the back, low back, and buttocks; and (3) cervical is 6 inch × 18 inch for the cervical spine. Packs are removed by tongs or scissor handles.

2. Towels: Regular bath towels and commercial double pad towels are required. Commercial double pad toweling has a pouch for pack placement and 1-inch thick toweling to be placed in cross fashion, tags on the edge of packs folded in, toweling overlapped on one side and four layers on the opposite side. Six layers equal 1 inch of toweling. Additional toweling may be needed depending on total body surface covered.

   Treatment. Position six layers of toweling as shown in Figure 9–12. Sufficient toweling should be provided to protect the patient from burns. Patient position should be comfortable. Treatment time should be 15–20 minutes.

Physiologic Responses

   Circulation is increased.

   Muscle temperature is increased.

   Tissue temperature is increased.

   Spasms are relaxed.

   Considerations. The size of the body segment to be treated should determine how many packs are needed. Patient comfort is always a consideration. Time of application should be 15–20 minutes. Also, after use rewarming of the pack requires about 20 minutes.[137]

   Application. Appropriate toweling and positioning of the patient is necessary for a comfortable treatment. The moist heat pack tends to stimulate the circulatory response. Dry heat, as discussed in the infrared section, has a tendency to force blood away from the cutaneous capillary bed, thus increasing the possibility of a burn with the skin's inability to dissipate heat.[138] The patient must not be allowed to lie on the packs because this will increase the risk of burn. Also, it may force the silicate gel out through the seams of the fabric sleeves. If the patient cannot tolerate the weight of the moist heat pack, alternate methods can be used. For example, the patient can be placed lying on his or her side, with the majority of the weight of

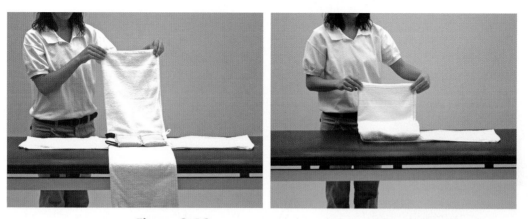

Figure 9–12. Techniques of wrapping hydrocollator packs.

the hot pack on the side of the pack and the pack held in place by additional towels or sheets wrapped around the patient. The most common indications are for muscular spasm, back pain, or as a preliminary treatment to other modalities. Hot packs have been shown to attenuate delayed-onset muscle soreness 30 minutes after treatment.[27]

CASE STUDY 9–6
THERMOTHERAPY: HYDROCOLLATOR PACK

Background: A 15-year-old boy sustained a non-comminuted, transverse fracture of the left patella during a football game 6 weeks ago. He was treated with plaster immobilization for 6 weeks; the cast was removed yesterday. He has full knee extension (the knee was immobilized in full extension) and has only 20 degrees of flexion. The patella is well healed and nontender, and patellar mobility is severely limited. As an adjunct to active and passive exercise, you begin joint mobilization of the patellofemoral joint every day. To enhance the response of the connective tissue, you decide to increase the tissue temperature prior to mobilization.

Impression: Limitation of motion secondary to fracture and immobilization.

Treatment Plan: Because the target tissues are immediately subcutaneous, you elect to use a hydrocollator pack. Using a cervical pack, heat was applied to the circumference of the knee for 12 minutes. Immediately after removal of the hot pack, joint mobilization was initiated. Following joint mobilization, active range of motion and strengthening exercises were performed.

Response: The patient was treated 3 days per week for 4 weeks, then discharged to a home program. He had full active and passive range of motion, patellar mobility was normal, and strength was 80% of the unaffected limb.

Discussion Questions

- What tissues were injured or affected?
- What symptoms were present?
- What phase of the injury-healing continuum did the patient present for care in?
- What are the therapeutic agent modality's biophysical effects (direct, indirect, depth, and tissue affinity)?
- What are the therapeutic agent modality's indications and contraindications?
- What are the parameters of the therapeutic agent modality's application, dosage, duration, and frequency in this case study?
- What other therapeutic agent modalities could be used to treat this injury or condition? Why?

The rehabilitation professional employs therapeutic agent modality to create an optimum environment for tissue healing while minimizing the symptoms associated with the trauma or condition.

Paraffin Baths

A **paraffin bath** is a simple and efficient, although somewhat messy, technique for applying a fairly high degree of localized heat. Paraffin treatments provide six times the amount of heat available in water because the mineral oil in the paraffin lowers the melting point of the paraffin.

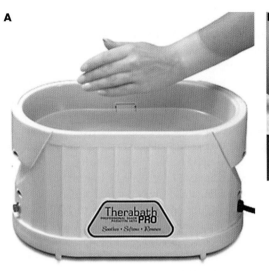

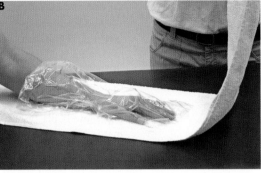

Figure 9–13. (a) Hand being dipped in paraffin bath. (b) After being dipped in paraffin, the hand should be wrapped in plastic bags and toweling.

The combination of paraffin and mineral oil has a low specific heat, which enhances the patient's ability to tolerate heat from paraffin better than from water of the same temperature.

The risk of a burn with paraffin is substantial. The clinician should weigh heavily the considerations between a paraffin bath and warm whirlpool bath in the athletic setting. The majority of paraffin baths are used for chronic arthritis in the hands and feet. If the patient has a chronic hand or foot problem, the use of paraffin instead of water usually gives longer lasting pain relief.

Equipment Needed

1. Paraffin bath (Figure 9–13)
2. Plastic bags and paper towels
3. Towels

Treatment

Dipping. The extremity should be dipped into the paraffin for a couple of seconds, then removed to allow the paraffin to harden slightly for a few seconds. This procedure is repeated until six layers have accumulated on the part to be treated.

Wrapping. The paraffin-coated extremity should be wrapped in a plastic bag with several layers of toweling around it to act as insulation (Figure 9–13). Treatment time should be 20–30 minutes.

Physiologic Responses

Tissue temperature increases.

Pain relief occurs.

Thermal hyperthermia occurs.

Considerations. Some units are equipped with thermostats that may elevate the temperature to 212°F, thus killing any bacteria that may grow in the paraffin. Otherwise the temperature should be set at 126°F.

If the paraffin becomes soiled, it should be dumped and replaced at no longer than 6-month intervals.

Application. A paraffin bath purchased for the clinic should have a built-in thermostat. Before treatment, the patient's body segment should be cleaned thoroughly with soap, water, and finally alcohol to remove any soap residue. This will prevent bacterial buildup in the bottom of the paraffin bath, which is an excellent medium for culture growth.

The mixture ratio of paraffin to mineral oil is 1 gallon of mineral oil to 2 pounds of paraffin. The mineral oil reduces the ambient temperature of the paraffin, which is 126°F (at which temperature a burn could occur). It is important to build six layers of paraffin, with the first layer highest on the body segment and each successive layer lower than the previous one. This is important because when dipping the extremity in the paraffin, if the second layer of paraffin is allowed to get between the skin and the first layer of paraffin, the heat will not dissipate and the patient could be burned. Because heat is retained in the body and is also radiated from the paraffin, capillary dilation and blood supply in the treated segment increase. The clinician should place the patient in a comfortable position and enclose the paraffin in paper towels, plastic bags, and toweling to maintain the heat. Treatment is applied for approximately 20–30 minutes. Removing the paraffin calls for extra care not to contaminate the used portion so that it does not affect the entire bath when it is returned.

Removal of paraffin involves removing towels, plastic bag, and paper towels, then using a tongue depressor to split the paraffin to allow easy removal. If the paraffin has not touched the floor, remove the paraffin cast over the open paraffin bath. It will dissolve on returning to the remaining liquid paraffin. Clean the body segment with soap and water. If a postsurgical patient is being treated, give a massage because the mineral oil will make the skin moist and supple. When cleaning the skin, the clinician must examine the surface for burns or mottling.

A less safe but likely more effective technique for increasing tissue temperature is to immerse the body part in the paraffin bath. The treatment begins by repeatedly dipping the body part in the paraffin as described above until at least six layers have accumulated. Next the body part is placed in the paraffin for the remainder of the treatment time. The patient should be instructed not to move the body part to keep the paraffin from cracking and to avoid touching the bottom or sides of the paraffin unit.

The thermostat will raise the temperature of the paraffin to 212°F, destroy any bacteria, and maintain a sterile contact medium. Paraffin baths require supervision to prevent contamination, but they do provide a special type of treatment that is well adapted to the patient with injuries of the hands and feet.

Treatment Protocols: Paraffin Bath

1. Guide the body part into the paraffin, making sure the patient does not contact the bottom of the cabinet or the heating coils.
2. After 2 or 3 seconds, remove the body part and keep it above the paraffin so that none of the paraffin drips onto the floor. Reimmerse the body part, and repeat until the appropriate number of dips have been completed, or reimmerse for the duration of the treatment.
3. Set a timer for the appropriate treatment time and give the patient a signaling device. Make sure the patient understands how to use the signaling device.
4. Check the patient's response after the first 5 minutes by asking the patient how it feels. Recheck verbally about every 5 minutes.

Fluidotherapy

Fluidotherapy is a unique, multifunctional physical medicine modality. The fluidotherapy unit is a dry heat modality that uses a suspended air stream, which has the properties of a liquid (Figure 9–14). Its therapeutic effectiveness in rehabilitation and healing is based on its ability to apply simultaneously heat, massage, sensory stimulation for desensitization, levitation, and pressure oscillations. Fluidotherapy is capable of significantly elevating superficial skin temperature.[139] Unlike water, the dry, natural medium does not irritate the skin or produce thermal shocks.[140] This allows for much higher treatment temperatures than with aqueous or paraffin heat transfer. The pressure oscillations may actually minimize edema, even at very high treatment temperatures. Clinical success has been reported in treatment of pain, range of motion, wounds, acute injuries, swelling, and blood flow insufficiency. Fluidotherapy treatment of the hand at 115°F (46.2°C) results in a sixfold increase in blood flow and a four-

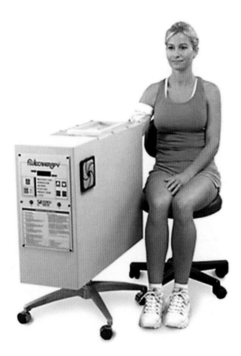

Figure 9–14. Upper Extremity Fluidotherapy unit.

fold increase in metabolic rates in a normal adult. These properties will increase blood flow, sedate, decrease blood pressure, and promote healing by accelerating biochemical reactions.

Counterirritation, through mechanoreceptor and thermoreceptor stimulation, reduces pain sensitivity, thus permitting high temperatures without painful heat sensations. Pronounced hyperthermia accelerates the chemical metabolic processes and stimulates the normal healing process. The high temperatures enhance tissue elasticity and reduce tissue viscosity, which improves musculoskeletal mobility. Vascular responses are stimulated by long-lasting hyperthermia and pressure fluctuations, resulting in increased blood flow to the injured area.

Equipment Needed

1. Choose the appropriate fluidotherapy unit.
2. Toweling

Treatment

The patient must be positioned for comfort.

The patient should place the body segment to be treated (hand or foot) in the fluidotherapy unit.

Protective toweling must be placed at the unit interface and body segment.

Treatment time should be 15–20 minutes.

Physiologic Responses

Tissue temperature increases.

Pain relief occurs.

Thermal hyperthermia occurs.

Considerations

Fluidotherapy unit must be kept clean.

All knobs must be returned to zero after treatment.

Application. The patient should be positioned comfortably. The treated body segment should be submerged in the medium before the unit is turned on. There is no thermal shock when heat is applied. Treatments are approximately 20 minutes. Recommended temperature varies by body part and patient tolerance, with a range of 110–125°F (43–53°C). Maximum temperature rise in the treated part occurs after 15 minutes of treatment. Unless contraindicated, active and passive exercise are encouraged during treatment.

In case of open lesions or infections, a protective dressing is recommended to prevent soiling or contaminating the cloth entry ports. Patients with splints, bandages, tape, orthopedic pins, plastic joint replacement, and artificial tendons may be treated with fluidotherapy. The medium is clean and will not soil clothing. It is not necessary to disrobe to get the full benefit of heat and massage; however, direct contact between skin and the medium is desirable to maximize heat transfer.

In treating the hands, muscles, ankles, and conditions that manifest themselves relatively near the surface of the skin, appreciably higher body temperatures can be achieved using superficial heating modalities. Further, the superficial modalities treat a larger area of the body than ultrasound or microwave diathermies, thus the total amount of heat absorbed will be much higher. Fluidotherapy, hydrotherapy, and paraffin cause about the same amount of temperature increase.[4]

Treatment Protocols: Fluidotherapy

1. With the agitation off, open the sleeved portion of the unit.
2. Instruct patient to insert body part into the cellulose particles, reminding her to tell you if the temperature is too hot.
3. Fasten the sleeve around the body part to prevent the cellulose particles from being blown out of the unit, and start the agitation.
4. Check the patient's response verbally after about 5 minutes. Remind the patient to tell you if the heating sensation becomes uncomfortable.

ThermaCare Wraps

ThermaCare Heatwraps are made of a clothlike material that conforms to the body's shape to provide therapeutic heat (Figure 9-15). Each wrap contains small discs containing iron, charcoal, table salt, and water that heat up when exposed to oxygen in the air providing at least 8 hours of continuous, low-level heat. Once opened the ThermaCare wrap begins to warm immediately and reaches its therapeutic temperature within approximately 30 minutes.[117,141,142] Wraps are made for the neck, back, and lower abdomen.[143-145] The ThermaCare wrap has been shown to effectively increase intramuscular temperature at a depth of 2 cm.[146,147]

Infrared Lamps

As mentioned earlier in this chapter, unlike all of the other modalities discussed previously, infrared lamps are considered an electromagnetic energy modality rather than a conductive energy modality. When talking about infrared modalities, the clinician most typically thinks of the infrared lamp. The biggest advantage of an infrared lamp is that superficial tissue temperature can be increased, even though the unit does not touch the patient. However, radiant heat is seldom used because it is limited in depth of skin penetration to less than 1 mm. Dry heat from an infrared lamp tends to elevate superficial skin temperatures more than moist heat; however, moist heat probably has a greater depth of penetration.

Superficial skin burns occasionally occur because of intense infrared radiation and the reflector becoming extremely hot (4000°F). It is recommended that a warm moist towel be placed over the body segment to be treated to enhance the heating effects. Dry towels should cover the remainder of the body not being treated. This will allow a greater blood to tissue exchange by trapping the heat buildup in the moist towel and reducing the stagnant air over the body segment. Caution should be used, and the skin should be checked every few minutes for mottling.

Infrared generators may be divided into two categories: (i) luminous and (ii) nonluminous. Nonluminous generators consist of a spiral coil of resistant metal wire wound around a cone-shaped piece of nonconducting material. The resistance of the wire to the electric flow produces heat and a dull red glow. A properly shaped reflector then radiates the heat to the

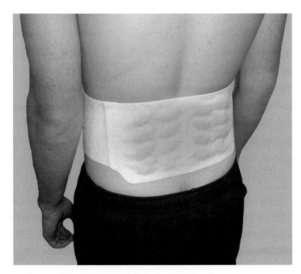

Figure 9–15. ThermaCare wrap applied to low back.

body. All incandescent bodies and tungsten and carbon filament lamps are in the category of luminous generators. No nonluminous lamps are currently being manufactured because infrared at a wavelength of 12,000 A will penetrate slightly more deeply than either longer or shorter waves, owing to a certain unique characteristic of human skin. Tungsten filament and special quartz red sources produce significant amounts of infrared heat at 12,000 A. Flare because of reflection off the skin can be a serious problem.

Equipment Needed
1. Infrared lamp (Figure 9–16)
2. Dry toweling: This is to be used for draping the parts of the body not being treated.
3. Moist toweling: Moist towels are used to cover the area to be treated.
4. A GFI should be used with an infrared lamp.

   Treatment. The patient should be positioned 20 inches from the source.
   Protective toweling should be put in place.
   Treatment time should be 15–20 minutes.

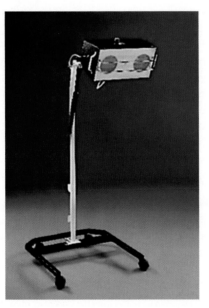

Figure 9–16. Infrared heating lamp. (Courtesy NOMEQ, Ltd.)

Skin should be checked every few minutes for mottling.

Areas that are not to be treated must be protected.

Physiologic Responses. A superficial rise in tissue temperature occurs. There is some decrease in pain.

Moisture and sweat appear on the skin surface.

Considerations. To avoid a generalized temperature rise, only the portion that is injured should be treated. The infrared lamp should be used primarily when a patient cannot tolerate pressure from another type of modality (e.g., hydrocollator packs). Caution must be exercised to avoid burns.

Application. The patient should be placed in a comfortable position. Moist heat should be used to stimulate blood flow without forcing blood away from the area as with dry heat. A moist, warm towel should be applied to the area to be treated. A squirt bottle should be used to keep the towel moist. All areas not to be treated should be draped. The distance from the area to be treated to the lamp should be adjusted according to treatment time: The standard formula is 20 inches distanceequals 20 minutes treatment time. After treatment, the skin surface should be checked. This type of treatment tends to force the blood away from the capillary bed and should be used only in superficial skin complaints related to dry heat requirements.

Treatment Protocols: Infrared Lamps

1. Position lamp such that the bulb is parallel to the body part being treated (such that the energy will strike the body at a 90° angle) and is 20 inches away from the patient. Measure and record the distance from the lamp to the closest part of the body being treated.
2. Inform the patient that he should feel only a mild warmth; if it is hot, he should inform you. Start the lamp.
3. Set a timer for the appropriate treatment time and give the patient a signaling device. Make sure the patient understands how to use the signaling device.
4. Check the patient's response after the first 5 minutes by asking the patient how it feels as well as visually checking the area being treated. Recheck visually and verbally about every 5 minutes.

Clinical Decision-Making *Exercise 9–6*

A volleyball player has an acute strain of the erector spinae muscles in the low back. The clinician feels that using ice on the low back will cause the patient to be uncomfortable and perhaps induce muscle guarding in the injured muscle. Thus, the clinician chooses to use a hot hydrocollator pack instead of an ice pack. Is this the appropriate clinical decision?

COUNTERIRRITANTS[1]

Although counterirritants are not an infrared modality, they are often associated with ice and heat because of their common sensations. Counterirritants are topically applied ointments that chemically stimulate sensory receptors in the skin.[148] Four major active ingredients are found in counterirritants. Menthol and methyl salicylate, which are found in peppermint and wintergreen

---

[1] The authors would like to thank Dr. Brian G. Ragan from the University of Northern Iowa for his contribution of this section to the chapter.

oils, respectively, are the two most common and they are often combined. Camphor is another irritant that is usually combined with the other two, producing a chemical irritant. Perhaps the most promising irritant is capsaicin, which is derived from hot peppers. Capsaicin, the most researched, has been shown to be effective in reducing chronic pain.[149] Application of either menthol analgesic balm or capsaicin on the skin has analgesic effects on signals from receptors located in muscles.[150,151] Capsaicin and menthyl salicylate have been used in combination to help reduce pain.[152] Allied health professionals along with an increasing active population use skin counterirritants to relieve some pain from the strains and sprains of jobs and recreational activities.

The mechanism of pain relief from the counterirritants is not exactly known. It is very probable that multiple methods of pain control could be at work. Some speculate that the rubbing application stimulates the large myelinated mechanoreceptors and works by the gate control theory. Because the irritants produce a noxious stimulus and a cool/warming sensation, they are also thought to stimulate both noxious and thermal receptors. By applying a noxious stimulus and superficial thermal response, the thin $A\delta$ and C afferent fibers are stimulated and inhibit pain in a manner similar to acupuncture. There is no evidence of tissue temperature response or a significant increase in blood flow from the application of a counterirritant. Capsaicin is thought to have a preferential action on C fibers by stimulating the release and depletion of substance P stores in the nociceptors, which are responsible for transmitting the pain signal. There is strong evidence that capsaicin affects synapses in the spinothalamic tract.[153] Counterirritants have been shown in clinical trials to decrease pain and increase range of motion[154] when compared to warm placebo ointment. Some researchers have speculated that it may act similarly to the spray-and-stretch technique. It has been suggested that they work similarly to nonsteroidal anti-inflammatory medication by limiting prostaglandin production.

Methods of application include massaging, vigorous rubbing, and combine padding. The most common method used is massaging a generous amount on the affected area until no ointment is visible. Counterirritants can be applied with vigorous rubbing or friction massage for the benefit of soft-tissue treatment. The combine padding method involves applying a generous amount of counterirritant, between 1/4 and 1/2 inch, on the pad and applying it to the affected area with a wrap. Manufactured counterirritant packs with self-adhesive are now available. Counterirritants should not be confused with other similar products containing trolamine salicylate, which has not been shown to be effective. They do not produce a chemical irritation and should be used with skeptical optimism. Because they may function like nonsteroidal anti-inflammatories, caution is indicated with people who are sensitive to such medication.

SUMMARY

1. Any modality that produces energy with wavelengths and frequencies that fall into the infrared region of the electromagnetic spectrum are referred to as infrared modalities. However energy is transferred by conduction and thus cryotherapy and thermotherapy techniques are best classified as conductive thermal energy modalities.

2. When any conductive thermal energy modalities are applied to connective tissue or muscle and soft tissue, they will cause either a tissue temperature decrease or tissue temperature increase.

3. The primary physiologic effect of heat is vasodilation of capillaries with increased blood flow, increased metabolic activity, and relaxation of muscle spasm.

4. The primary physiologic effects of cold are vasoconstriction of capillaries with decreased blood flow, decreased metabolic activity, and analgesia with reduction of muscle spasm.

5. The conductive thermal energy modalities have a depth of penetration of less than 1cm. Thus the physiologic effects are primarily superficial and directly affect the cutaneous blood vessels and nerve receptors.

6. Examples of thermotherapy are whirlpools, moist heat packs, infrared lamps, heating pads, and fluidotherapy.

7. Examples of cryotherapy are ice packs, ice massage, commercial ice packs, ice whirlpools, and cold sprays.

REVIEW QUESTIONS

1. What is the definition of a conductive energy modality?
2. What are the two basic therapeutic clinical uses for the conductive energy modalities?
3. What is the depth of penetration into the tissues of the conductive energy modalities?
4. What are the effects of changing temperatures on circulation?
5. How does changing tissue temperature affect muscle spasm?
6. What are the physiologic effects of both therapeutic heat and cold?
7. What are the differences between the terms *cryotherapy, thermotherapy,* and *hydrotherapy*?
8. What are the various cryotherapy techniques that the clinician can use?
9. What are the various thermotherapy techniques that the clinician can use?

SELF-TEST QUESTIONS

True or False

1. Applying heat or cold to an extremity will affect balance, proprioception, and performance.
2. Cold whirlpools should be set at temperatures of 50–60° F.
3. Cryokinetics is a therapeutic technique that combines cryotherapy and exercise.

Multiple Choice

4. This mechanism of heat transfer is through direct contact.
    a. radiation
    b. convection
    c. conduction
    d. conversion
5. ____ should be used on acute injuries to ____ temperature and thus slow metabolic rate.
    a. cold, decrease
    b. cold, increase
    c. heat, decrease
    d. heat, increase
6. The three to four stages of sensation following cold application, in order, are the following:
    a. sting, cold, burn/ache, numb
    b. cold, sting, numb, burn/ache
    c. burn/ache, cold, sting, numb
    d. cold, sting, burn/ache, numb
7. An insulating layer of water next to the skin is called which of the following?
    a. erythema
    b. thermopane
    c. anesthesia
    d. inflammation
8. Which of the following is *not* an effect of thermotherapy?
    a. increased circulation
    b. relaxed spasms
    c. decreased cell metabolism
    d. increased soft-tissue elasticity
9. Which of the following is a contraindication for cryotherapy?
    a. acute pain
    b. skin anesthesia
    c. muscle spasm
    d. acute ligament sprain
10. In what condition would thermotherapy be indicated?
    a. decreased range of motion
    b. skin anesthesia

c. acute musculoskeletal injury

d. acute pain

SOLUTIONS TO CLINICAL DECISION-MAKING EXERCISES

9–1

Because the elastic wrap has been placed underneath the ice bags there is an insulating layer through which the cold must penetrate. The passage of cold can be facilitated if the elastic wrap is wet. It is likely that the ice can be left in place for up to an hour as long as the patient does not have any type of sensitivity reaction to the cold.

9–2

It is likely that the combined effects of placing the ankle in a dependent position, the massaging action of the whirlpool jets, and the active exercise may cause some additional swelling, especially only 2 days postinjury when it is likely that the patient is still exhibiting signs and symptoms of inflammation. It would be more advisable to use an ice bag with elevation followed by whatever active exercises are appropriate.

9–3

A spray-and-stretch technique has been recommended as an effective technique for dealing with myofascial trigger points. Using Fluori-Methane spray, the clinician should make strokes parallel with the direction of fibers and then stretch the middle trapezius immediately following the application of the cold spray.

9–4

It is clear that a contrast bath produces little or no "pumping action" and thus would not be effective in treating swelling. A better alternative would be to use cryokinetics, which involves cold followed by active muscle contractions and relaxation to help eliminate swelling.

9–5

At day 7, the likelihood of any additional swelling is minimal. As long as the patient is not complaining of tenderness to touch it is probably safe to switch to some form of heat, but it would be recommended that either ultrasound or shortwave diathermy be used since the depth of penetration of both is greater than any infrared modality.

9–6

The clinician should have chosen to use an ice pack. Remember this is an acute injury. Muscle strains in the low back are no different than in any other muscle, and just because the patient might be a little uncomfortable is not a good reason to make an incorrect decision about which modality is the most appropriate.

REFERENCES

1. Lehman, J. *Therapeutic Heat and Cold.* 3 ed., Baltimore-Williams & Wilkins, 1982.
2. Licht, S. *Therapeutic heat and cold.* New Haven, CT: Elizabeth Licht, 1972.
3. Moore, R. Uses of cold therapy in the rehabilitation of athletes: Recent advances, Proceedings 19th American Medical Association National Conference on the Medical Aspects of Sports, San Francisco, June 1977.
4. Downey, J. Physiological effects of heat and cold. *J Am Phys Ther Assoc* 1964;44(8):713–717.
5. Abramson, D, Tuck, S, and Lee, S. Vascular basis for pain due to cold. *Arch Phys Med Rehab* 1966;47:300–305.
6. Mancuso, D, and Knight, K. Effects of prior skin surface temperature response of the ankle during and after a 30-minute ice pack application. *J Athl Training* 1992;27:242–249.
7. Guyton, A. *Medical Physiology*, 11th ed, Philadelphia: W.B. Saunders, 2005.
8. Dontigny, R, and Sheldon, K. Simultaneous use of heat and cold in treatment of muscle spasm. *Arch Phys Med Rehab* 1962;43:235–237.

9. Rocks, A. Intrinsic shoulder pain syndrome. *Phys Ther* 1979;59(2):153–159.

10. Prentice, W. An electromyographic analysis of the effectiveness of heat or cold and stretching for inducing relaxation in injured muscle. *J Orthop Sports Phys Ther* 1982;3(3):133–146.

11. Fischer, E, and Soloman, S. Physiologic responses to heat and cold. In Licht, S (ed). *Therapeutic Heat and Cold*. New Haven, CT:Elizabeth Licht, 1972.

12. Eldred, E, Lindsley, D, and Buchwald, J. The effect of cooling on mammalian muscle spindles. *Exp Neurol* 1960;2:144–157.

13. Lippold, O, Nicholls, J, and Redfearn, J. A study of the afferent discharge produced by cooling a mammalian muscle spindle. *J Physiol* 1960;153:218–231.

14. Long, B, Seiger, C, and Knight, K. Holding a moist heat pack to the chest decreases pain perception and has no effect on sensation of pressure during ankle immersion in an ice bath (Abstract). *J Athl Training* 2005;40(2) suppl:S-35.

15. Miglietta, O. Electromyographic characteristics of clonus and influence of cold. *Arch Phys Med Rehab* 1964;45:508.

16. Travell, J. Rapid relief of acute "stiff neck" by ethyl chloride spray. *Am Med Wom Assoc* 1949;4(3):89–95.

17. Dejong, R, Hershey, W, and Wagman, I. Nerve conduction velocity during hypothermia in man. *Anesthesiology* 1966;27:805–810.

18. Grant, A. Massage with ice (cryokinetics) in the treatment of painful conditions of the musculoskeletal system. *Arch Phys Med Rehab* 1964;45:233–238.

19. Knott, M, and Barufaldi, D. Treatment of whiplash injuries. *Phys Ther* 1961;41:8.

20. Long, B, Cordova, M, and Brucker, J. Exercise and quadriceps muscle cooling time. *J Athl Training* 2005;40(4):260.

21. Dufresne, T, Jarzabski, K, and Simmons, D. Comparison of superficial and deep heating agents followed by a passive stretch on increasing the flexibility of the hamstring muscle group. *Phys Ther* 1994;74(5):S70.

22. Taylor, B, Waring, C, and Brasher, T. The effects of therapeutic application of heat or cold followed by static stretch on hamstring muscle length. *J Orthop Sports Phys Ther* 1995;21(5):283–286.

23. Evans, T, Ingersoll, C, and Knight, K. Agility following the application of cold therapy. *J Athl Training* 1995;30(3):231–234.

24. Hatzel, B, Weidner, T, and Gehlsen, G. Mechanical power and velocity following cryotherapy and ankle taping. *J Athl Training* (suppl.) 2001;36(2S):S-89.

25. Rubley, M, Denegar, C, and Buckley, W. Cryotherapy, sensation and isometric-force variability. *J Athl Training* 2003;38(2):113–119.

26. Knight, K. *Cryotherapy in Sports Injury Management*, Champaign, IL: Human Kinetics, 1995.

27. Sumida, K, Greenberg, M, and Hill, J. Hot gel packs and reduction of delayed-onset muscle soreness 30 minutes after treatment. *J Sport Rehab* 2003;12(3):221–228.

28. Kimura, IF, Gulick, DT, and Thompson, GT. The effect of cryotherapy on eccentric plantar flexion peak torque and endurance, *J Athl Training* 1997;32(2):124–126.

29. Cutlaw, K, Arnold, B, and Perrin, D. Effect of cold treatment on concentric and eccentric force velocity relationship of the quads. *J Athl Training* 1995;30(2):S31.

30. Ruiz, D, Myrer, J, and Durrant, E. Cryotherapy and sequential exercise bouts following cryotherapy on concentric and eccentric strength in the quadriceps. *J Athl Training* 1993;28(4):320–323.

31. Zankel, H. Effect of physical agents on motor conduction velocity of the ulnar nerve. *Arch Phys Med Rehab* 1966;47(12):787–792.

32. Clemente, F, Frampton, R, and Temoshenka, A. The effects of hot and cold packs on peak isometric torque generated by the back extensor musculature. *Phys Ther* 1994;74(5):S70.

33. Thompson, G, Kimura, I, and Sitler, M. Effect of cryotherapy on eccentric and peak torque and endurance. *J Athl Training* 1994;29(2):180.

34. Gallant, S, Knight, K, and Ingersoll, C. Cryotherapy effects on leg press and vertical jump force production, *J Athl Training* 1996;31(2):S18.

35. Grecier, M, Kendrick, Z, and Kimura, I. Immediate and delayed effects of cryotherapy on functional power and agility. *J Athl Training* 1996;31(suppl.):S-32.

36. Comeau, MJ, and Potteiger, JA. The effects of cold water immersion on parameters of skeletal muscle damage and delayed onset muscle soreness, *J Athl Training* 2000;35(2):S-46.

37. Hopkins, J Ty. Knee joint effusion and cryotherapy alter lower chain kinetics and muscle activity. *J Athl Training* 2006;41(2):177.

38. Clarke, D. Effect of immersion in hot and cold water upon recovery of muscular strength following fatiguing isometric exercise. *Arch Phys Med Rehab* 1963;44:565–568.

39. Golestani, S, Pyle, M, and Threlkeld, AJ. Joint position sense in the knee following 30 min of cryotherapy. *J Ath Train* 1999;34(2):S-68.

40. Jameson, A, Kinzey, S, and Hallam, J. Lower-extremity-joint cryotherapy does not affect vertical ground-reaction forces during landing. *J Sport Rehab* 2001;10(2):132.

41. LaRiviere, J, and Osternig, L. The effect of ice immersion on joint position sense. *J Sport Rehab* 1994;3(1):58–67.

42. Leonard, K, Horodyski, MB, and Kaminski, T. Changes in dynamic postural stability following cryotherapy to the ankle and knee. *J Athl Training* 1999;34(2):S-68.

43. Paduano, R, and Crothers, J. The effects of whirlpool treatments and age on a one-leg balance test. *Phys Ther* 1994;74(5):S70.

44. Rivers, D, Kimura, I, and Sitler, M. The influence of cryotherapy and Aircast bracing on total body balance and proprioception. *J Athl Training* 1995;30(2):S15.

45. Schnatz, A, Kimura, I, and Sitler, M. Influence of cryotherapy thermotherapy and neoprene ankle sleeve on total body balance and proprioception. *J Athl Training* 1996;31(2):S32.

46. Thieme, H, Ingersoll, C, and Knight, K. Cooling does not affect knee proprioception. *J Athl Training* 1996;31(1):8–11.

47. Thieme, H, Ingersoll, C, and Knight, K. The effect of cooling on proprioception of the knee. *J Athl Training* 1993; 28(2):158.

48. Tremblay, F, Estaphan, L, and Legendre, M. Influence of local cooling on proprioceptive acuity in the quadriceps muscle. *J Athl Training* 2001;36(2):119–123.

49. Whittaker, T, Lander, J, and Brubaker, D. The effect of cryotherapy on selected balance parameters. *J Athl Training* 1994;29(2):180.

50. Knight, K, Ingersoll, C, and Trowbridge, C. The effects of cooling the ankle, the triceps surae or both on functional agility. *J Athl Training* 1994;29(2):165.

51. Schuler, D, Ingersoll, C, and Knight, K. Local cold application to foot and ankle, lower leg of both effects on a cutting drill. *J Athl Training* 1996;31(2):S35.

52. Nosaka, K, Sakamoto, K, and Newton, M. Influence of pre-exercise muscle temperature on responses to eccentric exercise. *J Athl Training* 2004;39(2):132.

53. Richendollar, M, Darby, L, and Brown, T. Ice bag application, active warm-up, and 3 measures of maximal functional performance. *J Athl Training* 2006;41(4):364.

54. Behnke, R. Cold therapy, *J Athl Training* 1974;9(4):178–179.

55. Knight, K. Effects of hypothermia on inflammation and swelling. *J Ath Train* 1976;11:7–10.

56. Bierman, W, and Friendiander, M. The penetrative effect of cold. *Arch Phys Med Rehab* 1940;21:585–592.

57. Chambers, R. Clinical uses of cryotherapy. *Phys Ther* 1969;49(3):145–149.

58. Griffin, J, and Karselis, T. *Physical Agents for Physical Therapists*, 2nd ed., Springfield, ILCharles C Thomas, 1988.

59. Knight, K. Ice for immediate care of injuries. *Phys Sports Med* 1982;10(2):137.

60. Merrick, MA, Knight, K, and Ingersoll C. The effects of ice and compression wraps on intramuscular temperatures at various depths. *J Athl Training* 1993;28(3):236–245.

61. Ho, S, Illgen, R, and Meyer, R. Comparison of various icing times in decreasing bone metabolism and blood in the knee. *Am J Sports Med* 1995;23(1):74–76.

62. Knight, K. *Cryotherapy: Theory, Technique and Physiology*, Chattanooga, TN: Chattanooga Corporation, 1985.

63. Merrick, MA, Knight, K, and Ingersoll, C. The effects of ice and elastic wraps on intratissue temperatures at various depths. *J Athl Training* 1993;28(2):156.

64. McMaster, W. A literary review on ice therapy in injuries. *Am J Sports Med* 1977;5(3):124–126.

65. Olson, J, and Stravino, V. A review of cryotherapy. *Phys Ther* 1972;62(8):840–853.

66. Nosaka, K, Sakamoto, K, and Newton, M. Influence of pre-exercise muscle temperature on responses to eccentric exercise. *J Athl Training* 2004;39(2):132–137.

67. Downer, A, and Oestmann, E. *Physical Therapy Procedures*, 6th ed, Springfield, IL:Charles C Thomas, 2003.

68. Galvan, H, Tritsch, A, and Tandy, R. Pain perception during repeated ice-bath immersion of the ankle at varied temperatures. *J Sport Rehab* 2006;15(2):105.

69. Hubbard, T, and Denegar, C. Does cryotherapy improve outcomes with soft tissue injury? *J Athl Training* 2004; 39(3):278–279.

70. Lowden, B, and Moore, R. Determinants and nature of intramuscular temperature changes during cold therapy. *Am J Phys Med* 1975;54(5):223–233.

71. Knight, K, Aquino, J, and Johannes S. A reexamination of Lewis' cold induced vasodilation in the finger and the ankle. *J Ath Train* 1980;15:248–250.

72. Travell, J, and Simons, D. *Myofascial Pain and Dysfunction: The Trigger Point Manual*. Baltimore: Williams & Wilkins, 1998.

73. Clark, R, Lephardt, S, and Baker, C. Cryotherapy and compression treatment protocols in the prevention of delayed onset muscle soreness, *J Athl Training* 1996;31(2):S33.

74. Mickey, C, Bernier, J, and Perrin, D. Ice and ice with nonthermal ultrasound effects on delayed onset muscle soreness. *J Athl Training* 1996;31(2):S19.

75. Knutsson, E, and Mattson, E. Effects of local cooling on monosynaptic reflexes in man. *Scand Rehab Med* 1969;1:126–132.

76. Basset, S, and Lake, B. Use of cold applications in management of spasticity. *Phys Ther* 1958;38(5):333–334.

77. Knutsson, E. Topical cryotherapy in spasticity. *Scand Rehab Med* 1970;2:159–163.

78. Stillwell, K. Therapeutic heat and cold. In Krusen F, Kootke F, and Ellwood P (eds). *Handbook of Physical Medicine and Rehabilitation*. Philadelphia: WB Saunders, 1990.

79. Clarke, R, Hellon, R, and Lind, A. Vascular reactions of the human forearm to cold. *Clin Sci* 1958;17:165–179.

80. Cote, D, Prentice, W, and Hooker, D. A comparison of three treatment procedures for minimizing ankle edema. *Phys Ther* 1988;68(7):1072–1076.

81. Lewis, T. Observations upon the reactions of the vessels of the human skin to cold, *Heart* 1930;15:177–208.

82. Baker, R, and Bell, G. The effect of therapeutic modalities on blood flow in the human calf. *J Orthop Sports Ther* 1991;13:23.

83. Coulombe, B, Swanik, C, and Raylman, R. Quantification of musculoskeletal blood flow changes in response to cryotherapy using positron emission tomography. *J Athl Training* (suppl) 2001;36(2S):S-49.

84. Myrer, JW, Myrer, K, and Measom, G. Muscle temperature is affected by overlying adipose when cryotherapy is administered. *J Athl Training* 2001;36(1):32–36.

85. Myrer, KA, Myrer, JW, and Measom, GJ. Overlying adipose significantly effects intramuscular temperature change during crushed ice pack therapy. *J Athl Training* 1999;34(2):S-69.

86. Uchio, Y, Ochi, M, and Fujihara, A. Cryotherapy influences joint laxity and position sense of the healthy knee joint. *Arch Phys Med Rehab* 2003;84(1):131–135.

87. Holcomb, W. Duration of cryotherapy application, *Athlet Ther Today* 2005;10(1):60–62.

88. Merrick, MA, Jutte, LS, and Smith, ME. Intramuscular temperatures during cryotherapy with three different cold modalities. *J Athl Training* 2000;35(2):S-45.

89. Otte, J, Merrick, M, and Ingersoll, C. Subcutaneous adipose tissue thickness changes cooling time during cryotherapy. *J Athl Training* (suppl) 2001;36(2S):S-91.

90. Merrick, MA, Jutte, L, and Smith, M. Cold modalities with different thermodynamic properties produce different surface and intramuscular temperatures. *J Athl Training* 2003;38(1):28–33.

91. Palmieri, R, Garrison, C, and Leonard, J. Peripheral ankle cooling and core body temperature. *J Athl Training* 2006;41(2):185.

92. Bibi, KW, Dolan, MG, and Harrington, K. Effects of hot, cold, contrast therapy whirlpools on non-traumatized ankle volumes. *J Athl Training* 1999;34(2):S-17.

93. Braswell, S, Frazzini, M, and Knuth, A. Optimal duration of ice massage for skin anesthesia. *Phys Ther* 1994;74(5):S156.

94. Hayden, C. Cryokinetics in an early treatment program. *J Am Phys Ther Assoc* 1964;44:11.

95. Moore, R, Nicolette, R, and Behnke, R. The therapeutic use of cold (cryotherapy) in the care of athletic injuries. *J Athl Training* 1967;2:613.

96. Murphy, A. The physiological effects of cold application. *Phys Ther* 1960;40(2):112–115.

97. Knight, K, and Londeree, B. Comparison of blood flow in the ankle of uninjured subjects during therapeutic applications of heat, cold, and exercise. *Med Sci Sports Exerc* 1980;12(1):76–80.

98. Curl, WW, Smith, BP, Marr, A, et al. The effect of contusion and cryotherapy on skeletal muscle microcirculation. *J Sports Med Phys Fitness* 1997;37(4):279–286.

99. Hocutt, J, Jaffe, R, and Rylander, C. Cryotherapy in ankle sprains. *Am J Sports Med* 1992;10(3):316–319.

100. Tsang, KKW, Buxton, BP, Guion, WK, et al. The effects of cryotherapy applied through various barriers. *J Sport Rehab* 1997;6(4):343–354.

101. Hedenberg, L. Functional improvement of the spastic hemiplegic arm after cooling, *Scand J Rehab Med* 1970;2:154–158.

102. Rubley, M, Denegar, C, and Buckley, W. Cryotherapy, sensation, and isometric-force variability. *J Athl Training* 2003; 38(2):113.

103. Zemke, JE, Andersen, JC, and Guion, K. Intramuscular temperature responses in the human leg to two forms of cryotherapy: Ice massage and icebag, *J Orthop Sports Phys Ther* 1998;27(4):301–307.

104. Rogers, J, Knight, K, and Draper, D. Increased pressure of application during ice massage results in an increase in calf skin numbing. *J Athl Training* (suppl.) 2001;36(2S): S-90.

105. Weston, M, Taber, C, and Casagranda, L. Changes in local blood volume during cold gel pack application to traumatized ankles. *J Orthop Sports Phys Ther* 1994;19(4):197–199.

106. Bender, A, Kramer, E, and Brucker, J. Local ice-bag application and triceps surae muscle temperature during treadmill walking. *J Athl Training* 2005;40(4):271.

107. Dervin, GF, Taylor, DE, and Keene, GC. Effects of cold and compression dressings on early postoperative outcomes for the athroscopic ACL reconstruction patient. *J Orthop Sports Phys Ther* 1998;27(6):403–411.

108. Serwa, J, Rancourt, L, and Merrick, M. Effect of varying application pressures on skin surface and intramuscular temperatures during cryotherapy. *J Athl Train* (suppl.) 2001; 36(2S):S-90.

109. Dolan, MG, Mendel, FM, and Teprovich, JM. Effects of dependent positioning and cold water immersions on non-traumatized ankle volumes. *J Ath Train* 1999;34(2):S-17.

110. Dolan, MG, Thornton, RM, and Fish, DR. Effects of cold water immersion on edema formation after blunt injury to the hind limbs of rats, *J Ath Train* 1997;32(3):233–237.

111. Tsang, KH, Hertel, J, and Denegar, C. The effects of gravity dependent positioning following elevation on the volume of the uninjured ankle. *J Athl Training* 2000;35(2):S-50.

112. McKeon, P, Dolan, M, and Gandloph, J. Effects of dependent positioning cool water immersion CWI and high-voltage electrical stimulation HVES on nontraumatized limb volumes. *J Athl Training* (suppl.) 2003;38(2S): S-35.

113. Misasi, S, Morin, G, and Kemler, D. The effect of a toe cap and bias on perceived pain during cold water immersion. *J Athl Training* 1995;30(1):149–156.

114. Myer, JW, Measom, G, and Fellingham, GW. Temperature changes in the human leg during and after two methods of cryotherapy. *J Athl Training* 1998;33(1):25–29.

115. Travell, J. Ethyl chloride spray for painful muscle spasm. *Arch Phys Med Rehab* 1952;32:291–298.

116. Lee, JC, Lin, DT, and Hong C. The effectiveness of simultaneous thermotherapy with ultrasound and electrotherapy with combined AC and DC current on the immediate pain relief of myofascial trigger points. *J Musculoskeletal Pain* 1997;5(1):81–90.

117. Mitra, A, Draper, D, and Hopkins, T. Application of the Thermacare knee wrap results in significant increases in muscle and intracapsular temperature (Abstract). *J Athl Training* 2005;40(2) suppl:S-35.

118. Myer, JW, Measom, G, Durrant, E, and Fellingham, GW. Cold- and hot-pack contrast therapy: subcutaneous and intramuscular temperature change. *J Athl Training* 1997;32(3): 238–241.

119. Myer, JW, Draper, D, and Durrant, E. The effect of contrast therapy on intramuscular temperature in the human lower leg. *J Athl Training* 1994;29(4):318–322.

120. Smith, K, and Newton, R. The immediate effect of contrast baths on edema. temperature and pain in postsurgical hand injuries. *Phys Ther* 1994;74(5):S157.

121. Campbell, H, Cordova, M, and Ingersoll, C. A cryokinetics protocol does not affect quadriceps muscle fatigue, *J Athl Training* (suppl) 2003;38 (2S):S-48.

122. Pincivero, D, Gieck, J, and Saliba, E. Rehabilitation of a lateral ankle sprain with cryokinetic and functional progressive exercise. *J Sport Rehab* 1993;2(3):200–207.

123. Dolan, M, Thornton, R, and Mendel, F. Cold water immersion effects on edema formation following impact injury to hind limbs of rats. *J Athl Training* 1996;31(2):S48.

124. Knight, KL, Rubley, MD, and Ingersoll, CD. Pain perception is greater during ankle ice immersion than during ice pack application. *J Athl Training* 2000;35(2):S-45.

125. Kolb, P, and Denegar, C. Traumatic edema and the lymphatic system. *J Athl Training* 1983;18:339–341.

126. Sreniawski, S, Cordova, M, and Ingeroll, C. A comparison of hot packs and light or moderate exercise on rectus femoris temperature. *J Athl Training* (suppl.) 2002;37(2S):S-104.

127. Achkar, M, Caschetta, E, and Brucker, J. Hamstring flexibility acute gains and retention are not affected by passive or active tissue warming methods (Abstract). *J Athl Training* 2005;40(2) suppl:S-90.

128. Burke, D, Holt, L, and Rasmussen, R. The effect of hot or cold water immersion and proprioceptive neuromuscular facilitation on hip joint range of motion. *J Athl Training* 2001;36(1):16–19.

129. Cosgray, N, Lawrance, S, and Mestrich, J. Effect of heat modalities on hamstring length: a comparison of Pneumatherm, moist heat pack, and a control. *J Orthop Sports Phys Ther* 2004;34(7):377–384.

130. Sawyer, P, Uhl, T, and Yates, J. Effects of muscle temperature on hamstring flexibility. *J Athl Training* (suppl.) 2002;37(2S):S-103.

131. Knight, CA, Rutledge, CR, Cox, ME, et al. Effect of superficial heat, deep heat, and active exercise warm-up on the extensibility of the plantar flexors. *Phys Ther* 2001;81:1206–1214.

132. Clarke, D, and Stelmach, G. Muscle fatigue and recovery curve parameters at various temperatures. *Res Quart* 1966;37(4):468–479.

133. Krause, BA, Hopkins, JT, and Ingersoll, CD. The relationship of ankle temperature during cooling and rewarming to the human soleus H reflex. *J Sport Rehab*, 2000;9(3):253–262.

134. Taeymans, J, Clijsen, R, and Clarys, P. Physiological effects of local heat application (Abstract). *Isokinet Exerc Sci* 2004;12(1):29–30.

135. Kuligowski, LA, Lephart, SM, and Frank, P. Effect of whirlpool therapy on the signs and symptoms of delayed-onset muscle soreness. *J Athl Training* 1998;33(3):222–228.

136. Ragan, BG, Marvar, PJ, and Dolan, MG. Effects of magnesium sulfate and warm baths on nontraumatized ankle volumes. *J Athl Training* 2000;35(2):S-43.

137. Kaiser, D, Knight, K, and Huff, J. Hot-pack warming in 4- and 8-pack hydrocollator units. *J Sport Rehab* 2004;13(2):103–113.

138. Smith, K, Draper, D, and Schulthies, S. The effect of silicate gel hot packs on human muscle temperature. *J Athl Training* 1995;30(2):S33.

139. Kelly, R, Beehn, C, and Hansford, A. Effect of fluidotherapy on superficial radial nerve conduction and skin-temperature. *J Orthop Sports Phys Ther* 2005;35(1):16.

140. Wood, C, and Knight, K. Dry and moist heat application and the subsequent rise in tissue temperatures (Poster Session). *J Athl Training* 2004;39(2) suppl:S-91.

141. Draper, D, and Trowbridge, C. The Thermacare heatwrap increases skin and paraspinal muscle temperature greater than the Cureheat Patch (Poster Session). *J Athl Training* 2004;39(2) suppl:S-93.

142. Draper, D, and Trowbridge, C. Continuous low-level heat therapy: What works, what doesn't. *Athlet Ther Today* 2003;8(5):46.

143. Nadler, S, Steiner, D, and Erasala, G. Continuous low-level heat wrap therapy provides more efficacy than ibuprofen and acetaminophen for acute low back pain (Abstract). *J Orthop Sports Phys Ther* 2002;32(12):641.

144. Nadler, S, Steiner, D, and Erasala, G. Continuous low-level heatwrap therapy for treating acute nonspecific low back pain. *Arch Phys Med Rehab* 2003;84(3):329–334.

145. Purvis, B, and Del Rossi, G. The effect of various therapeutic heating modalities on warmth perception and hamstring flexibility (Abstract). *J Ath Train* 2005;40(2) Suppl:S-89.

146. Trowbridge, C, Draper, D, and Jutte, L. A comparison of the capsicum back plaster, the ABC back plaster and the Therma-Care Heatwrap on paraspinal muscle and skin temperature. *J Athl Training* (suppl.) 2002;37(2S):S-102.

147. Trowbridge, C, Draper, D, and Feland, J. Paraspinal musculature and skin temperature changes: comparing the ThermaCare HeatWrap, the Johnson & Johnson Back Plaster, and the ABC Warme-Pflaster. *J Orthop Sports Phys Ther* 2004;34(9):549–558.

148. Hill, J, and Sumida, K. Acute effect of 2 topical counterirritant creams on pain induced by delayed-onset muscle soreness. *J Sport Rehab* 2002;11(3):202.

149. Hautkappe, M, Roizen, M, Toledano, A, et al. Review of the effectiveness of capsaicin for painful cutaneous disorders and neural dysfunction, *Clin J Pain* 1998;14(2):97–106.

150. Nelson, AJ, Ragan, BG, Bell, GW, and Iwamoto, GA. Capsaicin based analgesic balm decreases the pressor response evoked by muscle afferents. *Med Sci Sports Exerc* 2004;36(3):444–450.

151. Ragan, B, Nelson, A, and Bell, G. Menthol based analgesic balm attenuates the pressor response evoked by muscle afferents. *J Athl Training* (suppl.) 2003;38(2S):S-34.

152. Ichiyama, RM, Ragan, BG, Bell, GW, and Iwamoto, GA. Effects of topical analgesics on the pressor response evoked by group III and IV muscle afferents. *Med Sci Sports Exerc* 2002;34(9):1440–1445.

153. Chung, JM, Lee, KH, Hori, Y, and Willis, WD. Effects of capsaicin applied to a peripheral nerve on the responses of primate spinothalamic tract cells. *Brain Res* 1985;329(1–2):27–38.

154. Haynes, SC, and Perrin, DH. Effects of a counterirritant on pain and restricted range of motion associated with delayed onset muscle soreness. *J Sport Rehab* 1992;1(1):13–18.

SUGGESTED READINGS

Abraham, E. Whirlpool therapy for treatment of soft tissue wounds complicated by extremity fractures. *J Trauma* 1974;4.222.

Abraham, W. Heat vs. cold therapy for the treatment of muscle injuries. *J Athl Training* 1974;9(4):177.

Abramson, D, Bell, B, and Tuck, S. Changes in blood flow, oxygen uptake and tissue temperatures produced by therapeutic physical agents: Effect of indirect or reflex vasodilation. *Am J Phys Med* 1961;40:5–13.

Abramson, D, Chu, L, and Tuck, S. Effect of tissue temperatures and blood flow on motor nerve conduction velocity. *JAMA* 1966;198:1082.

Abramson, D, Mitchell, R, and Tuck, S. Changes in blood flow, oxygen uptake and tissue temperatures produced by a topical application of wet heat. *Arch Phys Med Rehab* 1961;42:305.

Abramson, D, Tuck, S, and Chu, L. Effect of paraffin bath and hot fomentation on local tissue temperature. *Arch Phys Med Rehab* 1964;45:87.

Abramson, D, Tuck, S, and Lee, S. Comparison of wet and dry heat in raising temperature of tissues. *Arch Phys Med Rehab* 1967;48:654.

Abramson, D, Tuck, S, and Zayas, A. The effect of altering limb position on blood flow, oxygen uptake and skin temperature. *J Appl Physiol* 1962;17:191.

Abramson, D, Tuck, S, and Chu, L. Indirect vasodilation in thermotherapy. *Arch Phys Med Rehab* 1965;46:412.

Abramson, D. Physiologic basis for the use of physical agents in peripheral vascular disorders. *Arch Phys Med Rehab* 1965;46:216.

Airhihenbuwa, C, St. Pierre, R, and Winchell, D. Cold vs. heat therapy: A physician's recommendations for first aid treatment of strain. *Emergency* 1987;19(1):40–43.

Anlauf, J, and Powers, M. Cryotherapy does not impair cervical spine extension strength, *J Athl Training* 2007;42(suppl):S67.

Anzivino, P, Guth, K. Delaying triceps surae ice bag application up to 10 minutes influences intramuscular temperatures during exercise. *J Athl Training* 2007;42(suppl):S66.

Ascenzi, J. *The Need for Decontamination and Disinfection of Hydrotherapy Equipment*, Vol. 1. Surgikos: Asepsis Monograph, 1980.

Austin, K. Diseases of immediate type hypersensitivity. In Fauci, A (ed). *Harrison's Principles of Internal Medicine*, 17 ed. New YorkMcGraw-Hill Professional, 2008.

Barnes, L. Cryotherapy: Putting injury on ice. *Phys Sports Med.* 1979;7(6):130–136.

Basur, R, Shephard, E, and Mouzos G. A cooling method in the treatment of ankle sprains. *Practitioner* 1976;216:708.

Beasley, R, and Kester, N. Principles of medical-surgical rehabilitation of the hand, *Med Clin North Am* 1969;53:645.

Becker, N, Demchak, T, and Brucker, J. The effects of cooling the quadriceps versus the knee joint on concentric and eccentric knee extensor torque (Abstract). *J Athl Training* (suppl.) 2005;40(2) :S-36.

Belitsky, R, Odam, S, and Humbley-Kozey, C. Evaluation of the effectiveness of wet ice, dry ice, and cryogen packs in reducing skin temperature. *Phys Ther* 1987;67:1080.

Bender, A, Kramer, E, Brucker, J. Local ice bag application does not decrease triceps surae muscle temperature during treadmill walking (Abstract). *J Athl Training* (suppl.) 2005; 40(2): S-35–S-36.

Benoit, T, Martin, D, and Perrin, D. Effect of clinical application of heat and cold on knee joint laxity. *J Athl Training* 1995; 30(2):S31.

Benson, T, and Copp, E. The effects of therapeutic forms of heat and ice on the pain threshold of the normal shoulder. *Rheumatol Rehab* 1974;13:101.

Berg, C, Hart, J, and Palmieri, R. Cryotherapy does not affect peroneal reaction following sudden inversion (Abstract). *J Athl Training* (suppl.) 2005;40(2):S-36–S-37.

Berg, C, Hart, J, and Palmieri-Smith, R. Cryotherapy does not affect peroneal reaction following sudden inversion. *J Sport Rehab* 2007;16(4):285.

Berne, R, and Levy, M. Cardiovascularphysiology. 4 ed, St. Louis: Mosby, 1981.

Bickle, R. Swimming pool management. *Physiotherapy* 1971;57: 475.

Bierman, W. Therapeutic use of cold. *JAMA* 1955;157:1189–1192.

Blum, M, and Kolasinski, S. Hydrotherapy for arthritis. *Alt Med Alert* 2007;10(12):136.

Bocobo, C. The effect of ice on intra-articular temperature in the knee of the dog. *Am J Phys Med Rehab* 1991;70:181.

Boes, M. Reduction of spasticity by cold. *J Am Phys Ther Assoc* 1962;42(1):29–32.

Bokulich, D, and Demchak, T. Comparison of a 30-degree contrast stimulator protocol to ice cup during 30-minute treatments. *J Athl Training* 2007;42(suppl):S68.

Boland, A. Rehabilitation of the injured athlete. In Strauss, RA (ed). *Physiology*, Philadelphia: WB Saunders, 1979.

Borgmeyer, J, Scott, B, and Mayhew, J. The effects of ice massage on maximum isokinetic-torque production. *J Sport Rehab* 2004;13(1)1:1–8.

Borrell, R, Henley, E, and Purvis H. Fluidotherapy: Evaluation of a new heat modality, *Arch Phys Med Rehab* 1977; 58:69.

Borrell, R, Parker, R, and Henley, E. Comparison of in vivo temperatures produced by hydrotherapy, paraffin wax treatment, and fluidotherapy. *Phys Ther* 1980;60(10):1273–1276.

Boyer, T, Fraser, R, and Doyle, A. The haemodynamic effects of cold immersion. *Clin Sci* 1980;19:539.

Boyle, R, Balisteri, F, and Osborne, F. The value of the Hubbard tank as a diuretic agent. *Arch Phys Med Rehab* 1964;45:505.

Brucker, J, Knight, K, Ricard, M. Effects of unilateral ankle ice water immersion on normal walking gait (Abstract). *J Athl Training* (suppl.) 2004;39(2):S-32–S-33.

Brucker, J, Matocha, M. Delayed quadriceps ice bag application up to 30 minutes does not influence superficial or deep tissue heat removal following exercise in uninjured trained cyclists. *J Athl Training* 2006;41(suppl):S43.

Carlson, A, Shaffer, S, and Mattacola,C. A 15-minute ice immersion is effective at reducing plantar sensation for laboratory assessment of induced neuropathy. *J Athl Training* 2008; 43(suppl):S85.

Chastain, P. The effect of deep heat on isometric strength, *Phys Ther* 1978;58:543.

Chesterton, L, Foster, N, and Ross, L. Skin temperature response to cryotherapy, *Arch Phys Med Rehab* 2002;83(4):543–549.

Clarke, K(ed). *Fundamentals of Athletic Training: Physical Therapy Procedures,* Chicago: AMA Press, 1971.

Claus-Walker, J. Physiological responses to cold stress in healthy subjects and in subjects with cervical cord injuries, *Arch Phys Med Rehab* 1974;55:485.

Clements, J, Casa, D, and Knight, JC. Ice-water immersion and cold-water immersion provide similar cooling rates in runners with exercise-induced hyperthermia. *J Athl Training* 2002;37(2):146–150.

Clendenin, M, and Szumski, A. Influence of cutaneous ice application on single motor units in humans, *Phys Ther* 1971;51(2):166–175.

Cobb, C, Devries, H, and Urban, R. Electrical activity in muscle pain, *Am J Phys Med* 1975;54:80.

Cobbold, A, and Lewis, O. Blood flow to the knee joint of the dog: effect of heating, cooling and adrenaline. *J Physiol* 1956;132:379.

Cohen, A, Martin, G, and Waldin, K. The effect of whirlpool bath with and without agitation on the circulation in normal and diseased extremities. *Arch Phys Med Rehab* 1949;30:212.

Conolly, W, Paltos, N, and Tooth, R. Cold therapy: an improved method. *Med J Aust* 1972;2:424.

Cook, D, Georgouras K. Complications of cutaneous cryotherapy. *Med J Aust* 1994;161(3):210–213.

Cordray, Y, and Krusen, E. Use of hydrocollator packs in the treatment of neck and shoulder pains. *Arch Phys Med Rehab* 1959;39:105.

Covington, D, and Bassett, F. When cryotherapy injures. *Phys Sports Med* 1993;21(3):78–79.

Crockford, G, Hellon, R, and Parkhouse, J. Thermal vasomotor response in human skin mediated by local mechanism. *J Physiol* 1962;161:10.

Crockford, G, and Hellon, R. Vascular responses of human skin to infrared radiation, *J Physiol* 1959;149:424.

Culp, R, and Taras, J. The effect of ice application versus controlled cold therapy on skin temperature when used with postoperative bulky hand and wrist dressings: a preliminary study. *J Hand Ther* 1995;8(4):249–251.

Currier, D, and Kramer, J. Sensory nerve conduction: Heating effects of ultrasound and infrared, *Physiotherapy Can* 1982;34:241.

Dawson, W, Kottke, P, and Kubicek, W. Evaluation of cardiac output, cardiac work, and metabolic rate during hydrotherapy exercise in normal subjects. *Arch Phys Med Rehab* 1965;46:605.

Day, M. Hypersensitive response to ice massage: report of a case. *Phys Ther* 1974;54:592.

DeLateur, B, and Lehmann, J. Cryotherapy. In Lehmann, J (ed). *Therapeutic Heat and Cold.* 3 ed, Baltimore: Williams & Wilkins,1982.

Devries, H. Quantitative electromyographic investigation of the spasm theory of muscle pain. *Am J Phys Med* 1966;45:119.

Draper, D, Schulthies, S, and Sorvisto, P. Temperature changes in deep muscles of humans during ice and ultrasound therapies: an in vivo study. *J Orthop Sports Phys Ther* 1995; 21(3):153–157.

Drez, D, Faust, D, and Evans, J. Cryotherapy and nerve palsy. *Am J Sports Med* 1981;9:256.

Drez, D. *Therapeutic Modalities for Sports Injuries,* Chicago: Yearbook, 1989.

Dykstra, J, Hill, H, and Miller, M. Comparisons of cubed ice, crushed ice, and wetted ice on intramuscular and surface temperature changes. *J Athl Training,* 2009;44(2):136.

Edwards, H, Harris, R, and Hultman, E. Effect of temperature on muscle energy metabolism and endurance during successive isometric contractions, sustained to fatigue, of the quadriceps muscle in man. *J Physiol* 1972;220:335.

Engle, J, and Demchak, T. The contrast stimulator can effectively raise skin interface temperatures. *J Athl Training* 2007;42(suppl):S4133.

Epstein, M. Water immersion: modern researchers discover the secrets of an old folk remedy. *Sciences* 1979;205:12.

Eyring, E, and Murray, W. The effect of joint position on the pressure of intraarticular effusion, *J Bone Joint Surg* 1964;46[A] (6):1235.

Farry, P, and Prentice, N. Ice treatment of injured ligaments: an experimental model, *NZ Med J* 1950;9:12.

Ferguson, K, Meyer, R, and Evans, T. Ice immersion of the hand does not alter vibratory sensory threshold. *J Athl Training* 2008;43(suppl):S87.

Folkow, B, Fox, R, and Krog, J. Studies on the reactions of the cutaneous vessels to cold exposure. *Acta Physiol Scand* 1963; 58:342.

Fountain, F, Gersten, J, and Senger, O. Decrease in muscle spasm produced by ultrasound, hot packs and IR. *Arch Phys Med Rehab* 1960;41:293.

Fox, R, and Wyatt, H. Cold induced vasodilation in various areas of the body surface in man. *J Physiol* 1962;162:259.

Fox, R. Local cooling in man. *Br Ed Bull* 1961;17(1):14–18.

French, D, and Thompson, K. The effects of contrast bathing and compression therapy on muscular performance. *Medic Sci Sports Exercise,* 2008;40(7):1297.

Galvan, H, and Tritsch, A. Pain perception during repeated ice-bath immersion of the ankle at varied temperatures. *J Sport Rehab* 2006;15(2):105.

Gammon, G, Starr, I. Studies on the relief of pain by counterirritation. *J Clin Invest* 1941;20:13.

Gerig, B. The effects of cryotherapy upon ankle proprioception (Abstract). *J Athl Training* 1990;25:119.

Gieck, J. Precautions for hydrotherapeutic devices. *Clin Manage* 1953;3:44.

Golland, A. Basic hydrotherapy. *Physiotherapy* 1951;67:258.

Green, G, Zachazewski, J, and Jordan, S. A case conference: peroneal nerve palsy induced by cryotherapy. *Phys Sports Med* 1989;17:63.

Greenberg, R. The effects of hot packs and exercise on local blood flow. *Phys Ther* 1972;52:273.

Guisbert K, and McVey, E. A 20-minute cryotherapy application does not increase the vastus medialis obliques H:M ratio in subjects following ACL reconstruction. *J Athl Training* 2008;43(suppl):S56.

Halkovich, I, Personius, W, and Clamann, H. Effect of fluorimethane spray on passive hip flexion, *Phys Ther* 1981; 61:185.

Halvorson, G. Therapeutic heat and cold for athletic injuries. *Phys Sports Med* 1990;18:87.

Harb, G. The effect of paraffin bath submersion on digital blood flow in patients with Raynaud's syndrome. *Phys Ther* 1993;73(6): S9.

Harrison, R. Tolerance of pool therapy by ankylosing spondylitis patients with low vital capacity. *Physiotherapy* 1981;67:296.

Hawkins, J, and Knight, K. Rate of cryotherapy temperature change- a function of adipose thickness or thermocouple depth?, *J Athl Training* 2007;42(suppl):S65.

Hayes, K. Heat and cold in the management of rheumatoid arthritis. *Arth Care Res* 1993;6(3):156–166.

Head, M, and Helms, P. Paraffin and sustained stretching in the treatment of burn contractures, *Burns* 1977;4:136.

Healy, W, Seidman, J, and Pfeifer B. Cold compressive dressing after total knee arthroplasty. *Clin Orthop Rel Res* 1994;299: 143–146.

Hellerbrand, T, Holutz, S, and Eubarik, I. Measurement of whirlpool temperature, pressure and turbulence. *Arch Phys Med Rehab* 1950;32:17.

Hendier, E, Crosbie, R, and Hardy, J. Measurement of heating of the skin during exposure to infrared radiation. *J Appl Physiol* 1958;12:177.

Henricksen, A, Fredricksson, K, and Persson, I. The effect of heat and stretching on the range of hip motion, *J Orthop Sports Phys Ther* 1984;6:110.

Hing, W, and White, S. Contrast therapy—A systematic review. *Phys Ther Sport*, 2008;9(3):148.

Ho, S, Coel, M, and Kagawa, R. The effects of ice on blood flow and bone metabolism in knees. *Am J Sports Med* 1994; 22(4):537–540.

Hocutt, J, Jaffe, R, and Rylander, R. Cryotherapy in ankle sprains. *Am J Sports Med* 1982;10:316.

Holcomb, W, Mangus, B, Tandy, R. The effect of icing with the Pro-Stim Edema Management System on cutaneous cooling. *J Athl Training* 1996;31(2):126–129.

Holmes, G. Hydrotherapy as a means of rehabilitation. *Br J Phys Med* 1942;5:93.

Hopkins, J, Adolph, J, and McCaw, S. Effects of knee joint effusion and cryotherapy on lower chain function (Abstract). *J Athl Training* 2004;(suppl.) 39(2): S-32.

Hormuth, J, Lemmer, J, and Carvassin, T. Intramuscular temperature changes in response to post-exercise application of two cold modalities. *J Athl Training* 2009;44(Suppl):S90.

Horton, B, Brown, G, and Roth, G. Hypersensitiveness to cold with local and systemic manifestations of a histamine-like character: Its amenability to treatment. *JAMA* 1936;107:1263.

Horvath, S, and Hollander, L. Intra-articular temperature as a measure of joint reaction. *J Clin Invest* 1949;28:469.

Hubbard, T, Aronson, S, and Denegar, C. Does cryotherapy hasten return to participation: A systematic review. *J Athl Training* 2004;39(1):88–94.

Huddleston, L, Walusz, H, and McLeod, M. Ice massage decreases trigger point sensitivity and pain (Abstract). *J Athl Training* 2005;(suppl.) 40(2): S-95.

Huffman, D, Pietrosimone, B, Grindstaff, T. A menthol counterirritant does not facilitate the quadricps motorneuron pool in healthy subjects. *J Athl Training* 2008;43(supplement): S55.

Hunter, J, and Mackin, E. Edema and bandaging. In Hunter, J (ed). *Rehabilitation of the Hand*, 1 ed., St. Louis:Mosby, 1978.

Ingersoll, C, Mangus, B, and Wolf, S. Cold-induced pain: habituation to cold immersion (Abstract), *J Athl Training* 1990;25:126.

Ingersoll, C, and Mangus, B. Sensations of cold reexamined: a study using the McGill Pain Questionnaire. *J Athl Training* 1991;26:240.

Jamison, C, Merrick, M, and Ingersoll, C. The effects of post cryotherapy exercise on surface and capsular temperature, *J Athl Training* (suppl.) 2001;36(2S):S-91.

Jessup, G. Muscle soreness: Temporary distress of injury? *J Athl Training* 1950;15(4):260.

Jezdirisky, J, Marek, I, and Ochonsky, P. Effects of local cold and heat therapy on traumatic oedema of the rat hind paw. 1. Effects of cooling on the course of traumatic oedema, *Acta Universitatis Palackianae Olomucensis Facultatis Medicae* 1973;66:155.

Johnson, D. Effect of cold submersion on intramuscular temperature of the gastrocnemius muscle. *Phys Ther* 1979;59: 1238.

Johnson, J, and Leider, F. Influence of cold bath on maximum handgrip strength, *Percept Mot Skills* 1977;44:323.

Kaempffe, F. Skin surface temperature after cryotherapy to a casted extremity. *J Orthop Sports Phys Ther* 1989;10(11): 448–450.

Kaul, M, Herring, S. Superficial heat and cold: How to maximize the benefits. *Phys Sports Med* 1994;22(12):65–72, 74.

Kawahara, T, Kikuchi, N, and Stone, M. Ice bag application increases threshold frequency of electrically induced muscle cramp (Abstract). *J Athl Training* 2005;(suppl.) 40(2): S-36.

Kennet, J, Hardaker, N, and Hobbs, S. Cooling efficiency of 4 common cryotherapeutic agents. *J Athl Training* 2007;42(3):343.

Kerperien, V, Coats, A, and Comeau, M. The effect of cold water immersion on mood states. (Abstract), *J Athl Training* (suppl.) 2005;40(2):S-35.

Kessler, R, and Hertling, D. Management of common musculoskeletal disorders, Philadelphia: Harper & Row, 1953.

Knight, K, Han, K, and Rubley, M. Comparison of tissue cooling and numbness during application of Cryo5 air cooling, crushed ice packs, ice massage, and ice water immersion, *J Athl Training* 2002;(suppl.) 37(2S).S-103.

Knight, K, Rubley, M, and Brucker, J: Knee surface temperature changes on uninjured subjects during and following application of three post-operative cryotherapy devices. *J Athl Training* (suppl.) 2001;36(2S).S-90.

Knight, K. Ankle rehabilitation with cryotherapy, *Phys Sports Med* 1979;7(11):133.

Kowal, M. Review of physiological effects of cryotherapy. *J Orthop Sports Phys Ther* 1953;6(2):66–73.

Kramer, J, and Mendryk, S. Cold in the initial treatment of injuries sustained in physical activity programs. *Can Assoc Health Phys Ed Rec J* 1979;45(4):27–29, 38–40.

Krause, B, Ingersoll, C, and Edwards, J. Ankle ice immersion facilitates the soleus Hoffman Reflex and muscle response. *J Athl Training* (suppl.) 2003;38(2S):S-48.

Krause, B, Ingersoll, C, and Edwards, J. Ankle joint and triceps surae muscle cooling produce similar changes in the soleus H:M ratio. *J Athl Training* 2001;(suppl.) 36(2S): S-50.

Krause, B. Ankle cryotherapy facilitates peroneus longus motoneuron activity (Abstract). *J Athl Training* 2004;(suppl.) 39(2):S-32.

Krusen, E. Effects of hot packs on peripheral circulation, *Arch Phys Med Rehab* 195031:145.

Landen, B. Heat or cold for the relief of low back pain? *Phys Ther* 1967;47:1126.

Lane, L. Localized hypothermia for the relief of pain in musculoskeletal injuries. *Phys Ther* 1971;51:182.

Lawrence, S, Cosgray, N, and Martin, S. Using heat modalities for therapeutic hamstring flexibility: a comparison of pneumatherm moist heat pack and a control, *J Athl Training* 2002;(suppl.) 37(2S).S-101.

Lee, J, Warren, M, and Mason, S. Effects of ice on nerve conduction velocity, *Physiotherapy* 1978;64:2.

Lehmann, J, Brurmer, G, and Stow, R. Pain threshold measurements after therapeutic application of ultrasound, microwaves and infrared, *Arch Phys Med Rehab* 1958;39: 560.

Lehmann, J, Silverman, J, and Baum, B. Temperature distributions in the human thigh produced by infrared, hot pack and microwave applications, *Arch Phys Med Rehab* 1966; 41:291.

Lehmann, J. Effect of therapeutic temperatures on tendon extensibility. *Arch Phys Med Rehab* 1970;51:481.

Levine, M, Kabat, H, and Knott, M. Relaxation of spasticity by physiological techniques. *Arch Phys Med Rehab* 1954; 35:214.

Levy, A, and Marmar, E. The role of cold compression dressings in the postoperative treatment of total knee arthroplasty. *Clin Orthop Rel Res* 1993;(297):174–178.

Long, B, Knight, K, and Hopkins, T. Arthrogenic muscle inhibition occurs with pain and is removed with cryotherapy. *J Athl Training* 2009;44(suppl):S57.

Long, B, and Hopkins, T. Superficial moist heat does not influence soleus function. *J Athl Training* 2006;41(suppl):S43.

Long, B, and Hopkins, T. Superficial moist heat's lack of influence on soleus function. *J Sport Rehab* 2009;18(3):438.

Long, B, Seiger, C, and Knight, K. Holding a moist heat pack to the chest decreases pain perception and has no effect on sensation of pressure during ankle immersion in an ice bath (Abstract). *J Athl Training* 2005;(suppl.)40(2):S-35.

Lundgren, C, Muren, A, and Zederfeldt, B. Effect of cold vasoconstriction on wound healing in the rabbit, *Acta Chir Scand* 1959;118:1.

Magness, J, Garrett, T, and Erickson, D. Swelling of the upper extremity during whirlpool baths, *Arch Phys Med Rehab* 1970;51:297.

Major, T, Schwingharner, J, and Winston, S. Cutaneous and skeletal muscle vascular responses to hypothermia. *Am J Physiol* 1981;240 (*Heart Circ Physiol* 9):H868.

Marek, I, Jezdinsky, J, and Ochonsky, P. Effects of local cold and heat therapy on traumatic oedema of the rat hind paw. II. Effects of various kinds of compresses on the course of traumatic oedema. *Acta Universitatis Palackianae Olomucensis Facultafis Medicae* 1973;66:203.

Matsen, F, Questad, K, and Matsen, A. The effect of local cooling on post fracture swelling, *Clin Orthop* 1975;109:201.

McDowell, J, McFarland, E, and Nalli, B. Use of cryotherapy for orthopaedic patients, *Orthop Nurs* 1994;13(5):21–30.

McGowen, H. Effects of cold application on maximal isometric contraction, *Phys Ther* 1967;47:185.

McGray, R, and Patton, N. Pain relief at trigger points: a comparison of moist heat and shortwave diathermy, *J Orthop Sports Phys Ther* 1984;5:175.

McMaster, W, Liddie, S, and Waugh, T. Laboratory evaluation of various cold therapy modalities. *Am J Sports Med* 1978;6(5): 291–294.

McMaster, W, Liddie, S. Cryotherapy influence on posttraumatic limb edema. Clin Orthop 1980;150:283–287.

McMaster, W. Cryotherapy, *Phys Sports Med* 1982;10(11): 112–119.

McVey, E, and Hertel, J. Influences of cryotherapy on motorneuron pool excitability in subjects with chronic ankle instability. *J Athl Training* 2008;43(suppl):S55.

Mense, S. Effects of temperature on the discharges of muscle spindles and tendon organs, *Pflugers Arch* 1978; 374:159.

Mermel, J. The therapeutic use of cold. *J Am Osteopath Assoc* 1975;74:1146–1157.

Meyer, R, Ferguson, K. Ice bath immersion of the hand alters continuous pressure sensory threshold. *J Athl Training* 2008; 43(suppl):S88.

Michalski, W, and Sequin, J. The effects of muscle cooling and stretch on muscle spindle secondary endings in the cat. *J Physiol* 1975;253:341–356.

Michlovitz, S. Thermal agents in rehabilitation, Philadelphia: A Davis, 1995.

Miglietta, O. Action of cold on spasticity, *Am J Phys Med* 1973; 52(4):198–205.

Miller, K, and Hawkins, J. Variations of skinfold thickness at different locations in college-aged physically active individuals and athletes. *J Athl Training* 2007;42(suppl):S68.

Miniello, S, Powers, M, and Tillman, M. Cryotherapy treatment does not impair dynamic stability in healthy females (Abstract). *J Athl Training* 2004;(suppl.)39(2):S-33.

Moore, A, Silvey, J, and Brucker, J. The effect of intramuscular tissue temperature on hamstring extensibility, *J Athl Training* 43(Supplement):S87, 2008.

Morris, A, Knight, K, and Draper, D. Moist heat pack re-warming following 10, 20, and 30 min applications (Poster Session). *J Athl Training* 2004;(suppl). 39(2):S-93–S-94.

Nelson, A, Ragan, B, and Bell, G. Capsaicin based analgesic balm decreases the pressor response evoked by muscle afferents. *J Athl Training* (suppl.) 2003;38(2S):S-34.

Newton, T, Lchnikuhi, D. Muscle spindle response to body heating and localized muscle cooling: implications for relief of spasticity, *J Am Phys Ther Assoc* 1965;45(2).91, 105.

Noonan, T, Best, T, and Seaber, A. Thermal effects on skeletal muscle tensile behavior, *Am J Sports Med* 1993;21(4):517–522.

Nylin, J. The use of water in therapeutics, *Arch Phys Med Rehab* 1932;13:261.

Oliver, R, Johnson, D, and Wheelhouse, W. Isometric muscle contraction response during recovery from reduced intramuscular temperature. *Arch Phys Med Rehab* 1979;60:126–129.

Palmeri, R, Garrison, J. Peripheral joint cooling increases spinal reflex excitability and serum norepinepherine. *J Athl Training* 2006;41(suppl):S43.

Panus, P, Carroll, J, and Gilbert, R. Gender-dependent responses in humans to dry and wet cryotherapy. *Phys Ther* 1994; 74(5):S156.

Perkins, J, Mao-Chih, L, and Nicholas, C. Cooling and contraction of smooth muscle, *Am J Physiol* 1950;163:14.

Petajan, H, and Watts, N. Effects of cooling on the triceps surae reflex. *Am J Phys Med* 1962;42:240–251.

Pietrosimone, B, Hart, J, and Ingersoll, C. Focal knee joint cooling facilitates quadriceps motorneuron pool excitability in healthy subjects. *J Athl Training* 2008;43 (Suppl):S55.

Pope, C. Physiologic action and therapeutic value of general and local whirlpool baths. *Arch Phys Med Rehab* 1929; 10:498.

Prentice, W. *Principles of Athletic Training*. 14 ed. New York: McGraw-Hill, 2011.

Preston, D, Irrgang, J, Bullock, A. Effect of cold and compression on swelling following ACL reconstruction, *J Ath Train* 1993;28(2):166.

Price, R, Lehmann, J, Boswell, S. Influence of cryotherapy on spasticity at the human ankle, *Arch Phys Med Rehab* 1993;74(3):300–304.

Price, R. Influence of muscle cooling on the vasoelastic response of the human ankle to sinusoidal displacement, *Arch Phys Med Rehab* 1990;71(10):745–748.

Randall, B, Imig, C, and Hines, H. Effects of some physical therapies on blood flow, *Arch Phys Med Rehab* 1952; 33:73.

Randt, G. Hot tub folliculitis, *Phys Sports Med* 1983;11:75.

Richendollar, M, Darby, L. Ice bag application, active warm-up, and 3 measures of maximal functional performance. *J Athl Training* 2006;41(4):364.

Ritzmann, S, and Levin, W. Cryopathies: A review, *Arch Intern Med* 1961;107:186.

Roberts, P. Hydrotherapy: Its history, theory and practice. *Occup Health* 1981;235:5.

Rubley, M, Gruenenfelder, A, and Tandy, R. Effects of cold and warm bath immersions on postural stability (Abstract), (suppl.) *J Athl Training* 2004;39(2): S-33.

Schaubel, H. Local use of ice after orthopedic procedures. *Am J Surg* 1946;72:711.

Schultz, K. The effect of active exercise during whirlpool on the hand, unpublished thesis, San Jose, CA:San Jose State University, 1982.

Shelley, W, Caro, W. Cold erythema: A new hypersensitivity syndrome, *JAMA* 1962;180:639.

Simonetti, A, Miller, R, and Gristina, J. Efficacy of povidone-iodine in the disinfection of whirlpool baths and hubbard tanks *Phys Ther* 1972;52:450.

Skurvydas, A, Kamandulis, S, and Stanislovaitis, A. Leg immersion in warm water, stretch-shortening exercise, and exercise-induced muscle damage. *J Athl Training* 2008; 43(6):592.

Steve, L, Goodhart, P, and Alexander, J. Hydrotherapy burn treatment: use of chloramine-T against resistant microorganisms, *Arch Phys Med Rehab* 1979;60:301.

Stewart, B, and Basmajian, J. Exercises in water. In Basmajian, J (ed). *Therapeutic Exercise,* 3rd ed, Baltimore: Williams & Wilkins, 1978.

Strandness, D. Vascular diseases of the extremities. In Isselbacher, K, Adams, R, and Braunwald, E (eds). *Harrison's Principles of Internal Medicine,* 9th ed., New York: McGraw-Hill, 1980.

Strang, A, Merrick, M. In vivo exploration of glenohumeral pericapsular temperature during cryotherapy (Poster Session) *J Athl Training* (suppl) 2004;39(2):S-91.

Streator, S, Ingersoll, C, and Knight, K. The effects of sensory information on the perception of cold-induced pain. *J Ath Train* 1994;29(2):166.

Taber, C, Contryman, K, and Fahrenbach, J. Measurement of reactive vasodilation during cold gel pack application to non-traumatized ankles. *Phys Ther* 1992;72:294.

Tamura, M, Brucker, J. The effect of a nylon shorts barrier on discomfort level and thigh skin temperature during a 20-minute −Kg ice bag application. *J Athl Training* 2007;42(supplement):S67.

Tomchuck, D, Rubley, M. The magnitude of tissue cooling during cryotherapy with varied types of compression. *J Athl Training* 2007;42(supplement):S66.

Travell, J, and Simons, D. *Myofascial pain and dysfunction: the trigger point manual,* Baltimore: Williams & Wilkins, 1983.

Tsang, K, Morris, L, and Hand, J. Ice bag application may negate the effects of interferential electrical stimulation. *J Athl Training* 2008;43(suppl):S84.

Urbscheit, N, Johnston, R, and Bishop, B. Effects of cooling on the ankle jerk and H-response in hemiplegic patients. *Phys Ther* 1971;51:983.

Usuba, M, and Miyanaga, Y. Effect of heat in increasing the range of knee motion after the development of a joint contracture: An experiment with an animal model. *Arch Phys Med Rehab* 2006;87(2).247–253.

Vannetta, M, Millis, D, and Levine, D. The effects of cryotherapy on in-vivo skin and muscle temperature and intramuscular bloodflow (Poster Session). *J Orthop Sports Phys Ther* 2006;36(1):A47.

Wakim, K, Porter, A, and Krusen, K. Influence of physical agents and of certain drugs on intra-articular temperature. *Arch Phys Med Rehab* 1951;32:714.

Walsh, M. Relationship of band edema to upper extremity position and water temperature during whirlpool treatments in normals. Unpublished thesis. Philadelphia: Temple University, 1983.

Warren, G, Lehmann, J, and Koblanski, N. Heat and stretch procedures: An evaluation using rat tail tendon. *Arch Phys Med Rehab* 1976;57:122.

Warren, G. The use of heat and cold in the treatment of common musculoskeletal disorders. In Hertling, D, Kessler, R (eds.) *Management of Common Musculoskeletal Disorders, Physical Therapy Principles and Methods,* Philadelphia: Lippincott, Williams & Wilkins, 2005.

Watkins, A. *A Manual of Electrotherapy,* 3rd ed., Philadelphia: Lea & Febiger, 1975.

Waylonis, G. The physiological effect of ice massage, *Arch Phys Med Rehab* 1967;48:37–42.

Weinberger, A, Lev, A. Temperature elevation of connective tissue by physical modalities. *Crit Rev Phys Rehab Med* 1991; 3:121.

Wessman, M, Kottke, F. The effect of indirect heating on peripheral blood flow, pulse rate, blood pressure and temperature. *Arch Phys Med Rehab* 1967;48:567.

Whitelaw, G, DeMuth, K, and Demos H. The use of the Cryo/Cuff versus ice and elastic wrap in the postoperative care of knee arthroscopy patients. *Am J Knee Surg* 1995:8(1): 28–30.

Whitney, S. Physical agents: heat and cold modalities. In Scully, R, Barnes, M (eds). *Physical Therapy.* Philadelphia: JB Lippincott, 1987.

Whyte, H, Reader, S. Effectiveness of different forms of heating. *Ann Rheum Dis* 1951;10:449.

Wickstrom, R, Polk, C. Effect of whirlpool on the strength endurance of the quadriceps muscle in trained male adolescents. *Am J Phys Med* 1961;40:91.

Wilkerson, G. Treatment of inversion ankle sprain through synchronous application of focal compression and cold. *Ath Train* 1991;26:220.

Wolf, S, Basmajian, J. Intramuscular temperature changes deep to localized cutaneous cold stimulation. *Phys Ther* 1973;53(12):1284–1288.

Wolf, S, Ledbetter, W. Effect of skin cooling on spontaneous EMG activity in triceps surae of the decerebrate cat, *Brain Res* 1975;91:151–155.

Wright, V, Johns, R. Physical factors concerned with the stiffness of normal and diseased joints. *Bull Johns Hopkins Hosp* 1960;106:215.

Wyper, D, McNiven, D. Effects of some physiotherapeutic agents on skeletal muscle blood flow. *Physiotherapy* 1976; 62:83.

Yackzan, L, Adams, C, and Francis, K. The effects of ice massage in delayed muscle soreness. *Am J Sports Med* 1984;12(2): 159–165.

Zankel, H. Effect of physical agents on motor conduction velocity of the ulnar nerve. *Arch Phys Med Rehab* 1966;47:787 .

Zeiter, V. Clinical application of the paraffin bath, *Arch Phys Ther* 20:469, 1939.

Zislis J. Hydrotherapy. In Krusen, F (ed). *Handbook of physical medicine and rehabilitation,* 2nd ed, Philadelphia: WB Saunders, 1990.

GLOSSARY

analgesia   Loss of sensibility to pain.

conduction   Heat loss or gain through direct contact.

conductive thermal energy modalities   Those modalities that transfer energy (either heat or cold) through direct contact.

congestion   Presence of an abnormal amount of blood in the vessels resulting from an increase in blood flow or obstructed venous return.

consensual heat vasodilation   Vasodilation and increased blood flow will spread to remote areas, causing increased metabolism in the unheated area.

convection   Heat loss or gain through the movement of water molecules across the skin.

conversion   Changing from one energy form into another.

c   The use of cold and exercise in the treatment of pathology or disease.

cryotherapy   The use of cold in the treatment of pathology or disease.

edema   Excessive fluid in cells

erythema   Redness of the skin.

fluidotherapy   A modality of dry heat using a finely divided solid suspended in a stream of air with the properties of liquid.

hunting response   A reflex increase in temperature that occurs in response to cold approximately 15 minutes into the treatment. The hunting response has nothing to do with vasoconstriction and/or vasodilation.

hydrotherapy   Cryotherapy and thermotherapy techniques that use water as the medium of heat transfer.

hyperemia   Presence of an increased amount of blood in part of the body.

indication   The reason to prescribe a remedy or procedure.

inflammation   A redness of the skin caused by -capillary dilation.

infrared   That portion of the electromagnetic spectrum associated with thermal changes; located adjacent to the red portion of the visible light spectrum. That part of the electromagnetic spectrum dealing with infrared wavelengths.

metabolites   Waste products of metabolism or -catabolism.

myofascial pain   A type of referred pain associated with trigger points.

nutrients   Essential or nonessential food substances.

paraffin bath   A combined paraffin and mineral oil immersion commonly used on the hands and feet for distal temperature gains in blood flow and temperature.

radiation   The process of emitting energy from some source in the form of waves.

thermopane   An insulating layer of water next to the skin.

thermotherapy   The use of heat in the treatment of pathology or disease.

vasoconstriction   Narrowing of the blood vessels.

vasodilation   Dilation of the blood vessels.

LAB ACTIVITY

PATIENT POSITIONING

DESCRIPTION

The positioning of a patient prior to the application of a physical agent modality is one of the most important aspects contributing to a successful treatment. Placing the patient in an aligned and supported position ensures muscular relaxation and facilitates venous flow of blood. Proper positioning allows the use of optimal body mechanics by the therapist in the application of the selected treatment.

THERAPEUTIC EFFECTS

Muscular relaxation
Facilitated venous blood flow

PATIENT POSITIONING			
PROCEDURE	EVALUATION		
	1	2	3
1. Check supplies.			
a. Pillows			
b. Towels			
c. Sheets			
2. Question patient.			
a. Verify identity.			
b. Verify treatment area.			
3. Position patient.			
a. Prone on table.			
i. Place pillow under abdomen; lumbar spine should be flat.			
ii. Place pillow under ankles.			
iii. Ensure proper body alignment.			
iv. Drape patient to maintain modesty.			
b. Supine.			
i. Place pillow under head and knees.			
ii. Ensure proper body alignment.			
iii. Drape patient to maintain modesty.			
c. Sitting.			
i. Seat patient on chair or stool leaning forward.			
ii. Support head and shoulders with pillows.			

	1	2	3
iii. Rest forearms and hands on table.			
iv. Ensure proper body alignment.			
v. Drape patient to maintain modesty.			
4. Administer the treatment.			
5. Complete the treatment.			
6. Return equipment to storage after cleaning.			

LAB ACTIVITY

ICE MASSAGE

DESCRIPTION

Ice massage is performed by rubbing a small area of the body with a block of ice until superficial anesthesia is achieved. The block of ice is produced by filling and then freezing a cup of water at a temperature of no colder than 5°C. Styrofoam cups are often recommended, but the chunks of styrofoam that are removed from the cup during the treatment tend to be messy. Freezing water in empty juice cans, with a tongue depressor for a handle, are sometimes used, but the tongue depressor may abrade the skin during the treatment. The ideal cup is a waxed paper cup; the wax provides some insulation to keep your hand warm, and half the cup can be torn away in a single piece. The bottom of the cup should be removed, not the top. This permits the cup to act as a funnel, and keeps the ice from slipping out of the cup.

PHYSIOLOGIC EFFECTS

Vasoconstriction
Anesthesia
Decreased local metabolism
Decreased connective tissue elasticity

THERAPEUTIC EFFECTS

Decreased or prevented swelling
Decreased pain
Decreased inflammation
Minimized secondary tissue damage

INDICATIONS

The primary indication for ice massage is pain of musculoskeletal origin that is preventing the effective use of therapeutic exercise; for example, an individual with restricted ankle motion who is prevented from applying sufficient force to produce remodeling of the connective tissue owing to pain. Ice massage will decrease the pain enough to permit an effective stretch. However, care must be taken to avoid stressing the connective tissue too much; the anesthesia provided by the ice may allow an overly aggressive individual to produce a sprain or strain.

Ice massage is also useful to help prevent an increase in inflammation and swelling of a joint following a therapeutic exercise session. It is probably no more effective than an ice pack, but often provides a more profound anesthesia.

CONTRAINDICATIONS

- Lack of normal temperature sensibility
- Cold hypersensitivity (urticaria or hemoglobinuria)
- Vasospastic disorders (e.g., Raynaud's disease)
- Coronary artery disease
- Hypertension

ICE MASSAGE

PROCEDURE	EVALUATION		
	1	2	3
1. Check supplies.			
a. Obtain towel to absorb water as it melts, ice cube, sheet or towels for draping.			
b. Check freezer for appropriate temperature.			

2. Question patient.

    a. Verify identity of patient (if not already verified).

    b. Verify the absence of contraindications.

    c. Ask about previous cryotherapy treatments, check treatment notes.

3. Position patient.

    a. Place patient in a well-supported, comfortable position.

    b. Expose body part to be treated.

    c. Drape patient to preserve patient's modesty, protect clothing, but allow access to body part.

4. Inspect body part to be treated.

    a. Check light touch perception.

    b. Check circulatory status (pulses, capillary refill).

    c. Verify that there are no open wounds or rashes.

    d. Assess function of body part (e.g., ROM, irritability).

5. Apply ice massage.

    a. Expose block of ice.

    b. Rub ice on hand to smooth rough edges.

    c. Warn the patient that you are going to put your cold hand on the body part to be treated, then do so.

    d. Remove your hand after 2 or 3 seconds, and warn the patient that you are going to put the ice on the body part to be treated, then do so.

    e. Begin rubbing the ice block in a circular motion on the body part being treated. Do not put additional pressure on the ice. Move the ice at about 5–7 cm/sec. Do not let melted water run onto areas of the body that are not being treated.

    f. Check the patient's response verbally about every 2 minutes. Perform a visual check of the area continuously during the treatment. If wheals or welts appear, or if the skin color changes to absolute white within the first 4 minutes of treatment, stop the treatment. Remind the patient to tell you when the area is numb.

6. Complete the treatment.

    a. When the patient tells you the area is numb, remove the ice and dry the area. Perform a test for light touch sensation to verify anesthesia.

    b. Remove material used for draping, assist the patient in dressing as needed. Place the unused ice in a sink, and the cup in the trash.

    c. Have the patient perform appropriate therapeutic exercise as indicated.

    d. Clean the treatment area and equipment according to normal protocol.

7. Assess treatment efficacy.

    a. Ask the patient how the treated area feels.

	1	2	3
b. Visually inspect the treated area for any adverse reactions (e.g., wheals, welts).			
c. Perform functional tests as indicated.			

LAB ACTIVITY

ICE PACKS

DESCRIPTION

Commercially available cold packs are usually a vinyl cover filled with a gel that does not solidify at low temperatures. Cooling units designed specifically for the cold packs are available, but they may be kept in a household-type freezer. The temperature of the freezer should be 0°C–25°C. Packs are available in various sizes, including one designed to encircle the cervical region. The packs are generally wrapped in a wet towel to increase the thermal conductivity from the patient.

PHYSIOLOGIC EFFECTS

Vasoconstriction
Superficial anesthesia
Decreased local metabolism
Decreased connective tissue elasticity

THERAPEUTIC EFFECTS

Decreased or prevented swelling
Decreased pain
Decreased inflammation
Decreased secondary tissue damage

INDICATIONS

The primary indication for the use of a cold pack is in the acute phase of a soft-tissue injury. The cooling of the injured area will help prevent the development of swelling and may assist in the resolution of swelling by altering the Starling–Landis forces at the capillary bed.

A cold pack is also useful to minimize or prevent increased inflammation or pain following a session of therapeutic exercise. The depth of anesthesia achieved with a cold pack is generally considerably less than with an ice massage.

CONTRAINDICATIONS

- Lack of normal temperature sensibility
- Cold hypersensitivity (urticaria or hemoglobinuria)
- Vasospastic disorders (e.g., Raynaud's disease)
- Coronary artery disease
- Hypertension

COLD PACKS			
PROCEDURE	**EVALUATION**		
	1	2	3
1. Check supplies.			
a. Obtain wet towel to wrap cold pack in, cold pack, sheet or towels for draping.			
b. Check freezer for appropriate temperature.			
2. Question patient.			
a. Verify identity of patient (if not already verified).			
b. Verify the absence of contraindications.			
c. Ask about previous cryotherapy treatments and check treatment notes.			

3. Position patient.

   a. Place patient in a well-supported, comfortable position.

   b. Expose body part to be treated.

   c. Drape patient to preserve patient's modesty, protect clothing, but allow access to body part.

4. Inspect body part to be treated.

   a. Check light touch perception.

   b. Check circulatory status (pulses, capillary refill).

   c. Verify that there are no open wounds or rashes.

   d. Assess function of body part (e.g., ROM, irritability).

5. Apply cold pack.

   a. Wrap cold pack in wet towel.

   b. Warn the patient that you are going to put the cold pack on the body part to be treated, then do so.

   c. Set a timer for the appropriate treatment time (generally about 20 minutes), and give the patient a signaling device. Make sure the patient understands how to use the signaling device.

   d. Check the patient's response verbally after the first 2 minutes, then about every 5 minutes. Perform a visual check of the area if the patient reports any unusual sensation. If wheals or welts appear, or if the skin color changes to absolute white within the first 4 minutes of treatment, stop the treatment.

6. Complete the treatment.

   a. When the treatment time is over, remove the cold pack and dry the area with a towel.

   b. Remove material used for draping, assist the patient in dressing as needed.

   c. Have the patient perform appropriate therapeutic exercise or apply tape or compression wrap as indicated.

   d. Clean the treatment area and equipment according to normal protocol.

7. Assess treatment efficacy.

   a. Ask the patient how the treated area feels.

   b. Visually inspect the treated area for any adverse reactions (e.g., wheals, welts).

   c. Perform functional tests as indicated.

LAB ACTIVITY

ICE PACKS

DESCRIPTION

An ice pack uses crushed ice at a temperature of 0°C–5°C. The ice may be placed in a plastic bag and wrapped in a wet towel or may be placed directly in a wet towel. The use of a plastic bag will minimize the potential mess from water dripping, but it may also decrease the conduction of thermal energy from the patient. A major advantage of an ice pack over a cold pack is that the ice pack can be almost any size and shape; therefore, an ice pack is useful for treating any body part.

PHYSIOLOGIC EFFECTS

Vasoconstriction
Superficial anesthesia
Decreased local metabolism
Decreased connective tissue elasticity

THERAPEUTIC EFFECTS

Decreased or prevented swelling
Decreased pain

Decreased inflammation
Decreased secondary tissue damage

INDICATIONS

The primary indication for the use of an ice pack is in the acute phase of a soft-tissue injury. The cooling of the injured area will help prevent the development of swelling and may assist in the resolution of swelling by altering the Starling-Landis forces at the capillary bed.

An ice pack is also useful to minimize or prevent increased inflammation or pain following a session of therapeutic exercise. The depth of anesthesia achieved with an ice pack is generally considerably less than with an ice massage.

CONTRAINDICATIONS

- Lack of normal temperature sensibility
- Cold hypersensitivity (urticaria or hemoglobinuria)
- Vasospastic disorders (e.g., Raynaud's disease)
- Coronary artery disease
- Hypertension

ICE PACKS			
PROCEDURE	EVALUATION		
	1	2	3
1. Check supplies.			
a. Obtain wet towel to wrap ice in, an appropriate amount of crushed ice, sheet or towels for draping.			
b. Check freezer for appropriate temperature.			
2. Question patient.			
a. Verify identity of patient (if not already verified).			
b. Verify the absence of contraindications.			
c. Ask about previous cryotherapy treatments, check treatment notes.			
3. Position patient.			
a. Place patient in a well-supported, comfortable position.			
b. Expose body part to be treated.			
c. Drape patient to preserve patient's modesty, protect clothing, but allow access to body part.			

4. Inspect body part to be treated.

    a. Check light touch perception.

    b. Check circulatory status (pulses, capillary refill).

    c. Verify that there are no open wounds or rashes.

    d. Assess function of body part (e.g., ROM, irritability).

5. Apply ice pack.

    a. Warn the patient that you are going to put the ice pack on the body part to be treated, then do so. Make sure the draping will catch any water that melts from the ice pack.

    b. Set a timer for the appropriate treatment time (generally about 20 minutes), and give the patient a signaling device. Make sure the patient understands how to use the signaling device.

    c. Check the patient's response verbally after the first 2 minutes, then about every 5 minutes. Perform a visual check of the area if the patient reports any unusual sensation. If wheals or welts appear, or if the skin color changes to absolute white within the first 4 minutes of treatment, stop the treatment.

6. Complete the treatment.

    a. When the treatment time is over, remove the ice pack and dry the area with a towel.

    b. Remove material used for draping, assist the patient in dressing as needed.

    c. Dispose of the unmelted ice in a sink.

    d. Have the patient perform appropriate therapeutic exercise or apply tape or compression wrap as indicated.

    e. Clean the treatment area and equipment according to normal protocol.

7. Assess treatment efficacy.

    a. Ask the patient how the treated area feels.

    b. Visually inspect the treated area for any adverse reactions (e.g., wheals, welts).

    c. Perform functional tests as indicated.

LAB ACTIVITY

COLD WHIRLPOOL

DESCRIPTION

A whirlpool is a tank filled with water of a particular temperature, depending on the desired therapeutic effect. The tank also contains a turbine or pump that creates convection currents in the water. Although water that is any temperature below the temperature of the body surface could be considered "cold," generally water at 10–16°C is used. Because water from the tap is rarely this cold, ice must be added to the tank. Crushed ice results in the most rapid cooling of the water, and all ice must be melted before the turbine is turned on. Using the turbine insures that a layer of warm water does not develop adjacent to the skin, thus providing a more effective cooling of the tissues. Because the limb is in a dependent position, any effect of the cooling on decreasing soft-tissue swelling may be negated; using a compression bandage during the treatment may help in reducing the effects of dependency. As with a warm whirlpool, the patient should not be left unattended and should be warned against touching any part of the turbine.

PHYSIOLOGIC EFFECTS

Vasoconstriction
Superficial anesthesia
Decreased local metabolism
Decreased connective tissue elasticity

THERAPEUTIC EFFECTS

Decreased or prevented swelling
Decreased pain
Decreased inflammation
Decreased secondary tissue damage

INDICATIONS

The principal indication for a cold whirlpool is to provide therapeutic cooling of a larger area of the body than can be achieved

readily with an ice or cold pack. Also, irregularly shaped areas of the body can be treated with total contact. In addition, the patient can perform active exercise during the application, or the therapist can perform joint mobilization on the injured limb while immersed in the water.

In addition, use of a cold whirlpool may minimize inflammation and swelling following a therapeutic exercise session. The advantage of a cold whirlpool over an ice or cold pack is the greater area that can be treated; a disadvantage is the possibility of increased swelling when the limb is in a dependent position.

CONTRAINDICATIONS

- Lack of normal temperature sensibility
- Cold hypersensitivity (urticaria or hemoglobinuria)
- Vasospastic disorders (e.g., Raynaud's disease)
- Coronary artery disease
- Hypertension

COLD WHIRPOOL

PROCEDURE	EVALUATION		
	1	2	3
1. Check supplies and equipment.			
a. Obtain towels for padding the edge of the whirlpool tank, as well as for drying the treated part.			
b. Check temperature of tank, ensure all ice is melted before applying treatment.			
c. Position chair of correct height next to whirlpool.			
2. Question patient.			
a. Verify identity of patient (if not already verified).			
b. Verify the absence of contraindications.			
c. Ask about previous cryotherapy or whirlpool treatments, check treatment notes.			
3. Position patient.			
a. Have patient sit on chair with body part out of water.			
b. Expose body part to be treated.			
c. Drape patient to preserve patient's modesty, protect clothing, but allow access to body part.			
4. Inspect body part to be treated.			
a. Check light touch perception.			

b. Check circulatory status (pulses, capillary refill).			
c. Verify that there are no open wounds or rashes.			
d. Assess function of body part (e.g., ROM, irritability).			
5. Administer cold whirlpool.			
a. Pad edge of tank with toweling, warn patient that the water is cold, then place body part in water.			
b. Instruct patient to keep away from all parts of the turbine.			
c. Turn on the turbine, adjust the aeration, agitation, and direction of the water being pumped.			
d. Check the patient's response verbally and visually about every 2 minutes. Remind the patient to tell you if the area starts hurting or if sensation is lost.			
6. Complete the treatment.			
a. Turn off the turbine at the completion of the treatment time.			
b. Remove the body part from the water and dry it off.			
c. Assist the patient in dressing as needed and instruct in therapeutic exercise as indicated.			
d. Clean the treatment area and equipment according to normal protocol.			
7. Assess treatment efficacy.			
a. Ask the patient how the treated area feels.			
b. Visually inspect the treated area for any adverse reactions (e.g., wheals, welts).			
c. Perform functional tests as indicated.			

LAB ACTIVITY

VAPOCOOLANT COLD SPRAY

DESCRIPTION

Vapocoolant sprays, such as Fluori-Methane are liquids that are sprayed on the skin. Thermal energy from the body is absorbed by the liquids, which have low boiling points; therefore, the liquid almost immediately evaporates. As it evaporates, thermal energy is removed from the body, resulting in a superficial cooling.

Fluori-Methane, a mixture of 85 percent trichloromonofluoromethane and 15 percent dichlorodifluoromethane, is not flammable and is nontoxic. Ethyl chloride is flammable, and therefore is not recommended for use.

PHYSIOLOGIC EFFECTS

Superficial anesthesia

THERAPEUTIC EFFECTS

Inhibition of painful trigger points
Decrease in pain with stretching musculotendinous tissue

INDICATIONS

Vapocoolant sprays are used mostly for the treatment of trigger points and for stretching of tight musculotendinous tissue. Trigger points are a poorly understood phenomenon, but many pain syndromes are ascribed to active trigger points. Two relatively common treatments for trigger points are deep friction massage (similar to vigorous acupressure) and stretching of the muscle the trigger point is located within. Because direct pressure on and stretching of the trigger points is painful, the area can be sprayed with a vapocoolant to decrease the pain during the treatment.

In a similar manner, if a musculotendinous strain has resulted in a loss of range of motion, spraying the skin over the injured muscle may decrease the pain perception while the therapist stretches the body part. Care must be taken to not overstretch the tissue and produce further injury.

CONTRAINDICATIONS

- Lack of normal temperature sensibility
- Cold hypersensitivity (urticaria or hemoglobinuria)
- Vasospastic disorders (e.g., Raynaud's disease)

VAPOCOOLANT COLD SPRAY

PROCEDURE	EVALUATION		
	1	2	3
1. Check supplies.			
a. Obtain vapocoolant.			
b. Obtain toweling or other draping materials needed.			
2. Question patient.			
a. Verify identity of patient (if not already verified).			
b. Verify the absence of contraindications.			
c. Ask about previous cryotherapy treatments, check treatment notes.			
3. Position patient.			
a. Place patient in a well-supported, comfortable position.			
b. Expose body part to be treated.			
c. Drape patient to preserve patient's modesty, protect clothing, but allow access to body part.			
4. Inspect body part to be treated.			
a. Check light touch perception.			
b. Check circulatory status (pulses, capillary refill).			
c. Verify that there are no open wounds or rashes.			
d. Assess function of body part (e.g., ROM, irritability).			
5. Apply vapocoolant.			
a. Position body part such that the area to be treated is on a stretch.			
b. Protect the patient's eyes and ensure the patient does not inhale fumes.			
c. Holding the vapocoolant upside down, with the nozzle at about a 30-degree angle from the perpendicular with the skin, and about 45 cm from the skin, spray the skin from distal to proximal.			
d. Spray in one direction only three to four times, then apply direct pressure or increased stretch as indicated and tolerated by the patient. Repeat the procedure as needed after the skin has rewarmed.			
e. Check the patient's response frequently during the treatment.			

Procedure	1	2	3
6. Complete treatment.			
a. On attainment of the desired therapeutic effect (or up to four repetitions of spray-and-stretch or pressure or to patient tolerance), inspect the treated body part for adverse reactions.			
b. Remove draping materials, assist the patient in dressing as needed.			
c. If further therapeutic exercise is indicated, instruct the patient to perform it.			
d. Clean the treatment area and equipment according to normal protocol.			
7. Assess treatment efficacy.			
a. Ask the patient how the treated area feels.			
b. Visually inspect the treated area for any adverse reactions (e.g., wheals, welts).			
c. Perform functional tests as indicated.			

LAB ACTIVITY

CONTRAST BATH

DESCRIPTION

A contrast bath involves the alternating immersion of the involved body part in warm water and cold water. Usually, the wrist and hand or foot and ankle are treated, though the entire upper or lower member could be treated using two whirlpool tanks. The duration of immersion in each temperature water is variable, as is the number of times immersed during a single treatment session. A suggested sequence is to start with 3 minutes in warm, followed by 1 minute in cold, with the sequence repeated five times (e.g., 3W-1C-3W-1C-3W-1C-3W-1C-3W-1C); however, some therapists recommend starting and ending with warm water. The warm water should be 40–41°C and the cold water 10–16°C.

PHYSIOLOGIC EFFECTS

Alternating vasodilation and vasoconstriction

THERAPEUTIC EFFECTS

Variable effects on swelling
Decreased pain

INDICATIONS

Contrast baths are often used in the subacute and chronic stages of recovery. Most of the information regarding benefits of contrast baths is anecdotal; there is little research documenting the efficacy of this treatment.

CONTRAINDICATIONS

- Lack of normal temperature sensibility
- Cold hypersensitivity (urticaria or hemoglobinuria)
- Vasospastic disorders (e.g., Raynaud's disease)

CONTRAST BATH			
PROCEDURE	EVALUATION		
	1	2	3
1. Check supplies and equipment.			
a. Obtain towels, containers, ice, timer, and so on.			
b. Check temperature of water in each container.			

2. Question patient.

   a. Verify identity of patient (if not already verified).

   b. Verify the absence of contraindications.

   c. Ask about previous cryotherapy or thermotherapy, treatments, check treatment notes.

3. Position patient.

   a. Have patient sit in a comfortable position.

   b. Expose body part to be treated.

   c. Drape patient to preserve patient's modesty, protect clothing, but allow access to body part.

4. Inspect body part to be treated.

   a. Check light touch perception.

   b. Check circulatory status (pulses, capillary refill).

   c. Verify that there are no open wounds or rashes.

   d. Assess function of body part (e.g., ROM, irritability).

5. Administer contrast bath.

   a. Set timer for appropriate interval, help patient immerse body part fully into warm water; start timer.

   b. After the timer goes off, set it for the next interval. Warn patient that the cold water will feel very cold; help patient immerse body part fully into cold water; start timer.

   c. Continue the cycles until the treatment is complete. Usually, the patients can time each immersion themselves.

   d. Check the patient's response verbally and visually about every 2 minutes. Remind the patient to tell you if the area starts hurting or if sensation is lost.

6. Complete the treatment.

   a. Remove the body part from the water and dry it off.

   b. Assist the patient in dressing as needed and instruct in therapeutic exercise as indicated.

   c. Clean the treatment area and equipment according to normal protocol.

7. Assess treatment efficacy.

   a. Ask the patient how the treated area feels.

   b. Visually inspect the treated area for any adverse reactions (e.g., wheals, welts).

   c. Perform functional tests as indicated.

LAB ACTIVITY
CRYO-CUFF

DESCRIPTION

A Cryo-Cuff has three parts: a cuff that holds chilled water, a cooler that holds water and ice, and a connecting tube. Cuffs are fabricated for numerous body joints including ankle, knee, and shoulder. A major advantage of a Cryo-Cuff is that the cuff can conform to a joint's unique shape, providing both cold and compression simultaneously.

PHYSIOLOGIC EFFECTS

Superficial anesthesia
Decreased local metabolism

THERAPEUTIC EFFECTS

Decreased swelling
Decreased pain
Decreased inflammation

INDICATIONS

The primary indication for the use of a Cryo-Cuff is in the acute phase of a soft-tissue injury or immediately following surgery of a joint. The cooling and compression of the injured area will provide analgesia and help prevent the development of edema or effusion. The Cryo-Cuff may assist in the resolution of swelling by altering the Starling-Landis forces at the capillary bed.

A Cryo-Cuff is also useful in minimizing or preventing increased inflammation or pain following a session of therapeutic exercise. The depth of anesthesia achieved with a Cryo-Cuff is generally considerably less than with an ice massage.

CONTRAINDICATIONS

- Lack of normal temperature sensibility
- Cold hypersensitivity (urticaria or hemoglobinuria)
- Vasospastic disorders (e.g., Raynaud's disease)
- Coronary artery disease
- Hypertension

CRYO-CUFF			
PROCEDURE	**EVALUATION**		
	1	2	3
1. Check supplies.			
a. Obtain wet towel to wrap joint in, an appropriate amount of ice to fill cooler, and a sheet or towels for draping.			
b. Add water and ice to cooler for appropriate mix.			
2. Question patient.			
a. Verify identity of patient (if not already verified).			
b. Verify the absence of contraindications.			
c. Ask about previous cryotherapy treatments, check treatment notes.			
3. Position patient.			
a. Place patient in a well-supported, comfortable position.			
b. Expose the joint to be treated.			
c. Drape patient to preserve patient's modesty, protect clothing, but allow access to body part.			

4. Inspect joint to be treated.			
a. Check light touch perception.			
b. Check circulatory status (pulses, capillary refill).			
c. Verify that there are no open wounds or rashes.			
d. Assess function of body part (e.g., ROM, irritability).			
5. Apply empty Cryo-Cuff to joint as indicated, close Velcro straps, and connect tubing from cooler to cuff.			
a. Warn the patient that you are going to fill the Cryo-Cuff, and then do so by opening cooler air vent and raising the cooler above the cuff until the cuff is full. Close the cooler air vent. Elevate the joint as required.			
b. Set a timer for the appropriate treatment time (generally about 15 min), and give the patient a signaling device. Make sure the patient understands how to use the signaling device.			
c. Check the patient's response verbally after the first 2 minutes, then about every 5 minutes. Perform a visual check of the area if the patient reports any unusual sensation. If wheals or welts appear, or if the skin color changes to absolute white within the first 4 minutes of treatment, stop the treatment.			
d. Rechill cuff as needed. Reconnect tube to cuff, open air vent, lower cooler to floor and completely drain water from cuff. Allow water to rechill, then repeat filling cuff.			
6. Complete the treatment.			
a. When the treatment time is over, remove the Cryo-Cuff and dry the area with a towel.			
b. Remove material used for draping, assist the patient in dressing as needed.			
c. Have the patient perform appropriate therapeutic exercise as indicated.			
d. Clean the treatment area and equipment according to normal protocol.			
7. Assess treatment efficacy.			
a. Ask the patient how the treated area feels.			
b. Visually inspect the treated area for any adverse reactions.			
c. Perform functional tests as indicated.			

LAB ACTIVITY

WARM WHIRLPOOL

DESCRIPTION

A whirlpool is a tank filled with water of a particular temperature, depending on the desired therapeutic effect. The tank also contains a turbine or pump that creates convection currents in the water. Although water that is any temperature above the temperature of the body surface could be considered "warm," generally water at 35–43°C is used. If the entire body is to be immersed, temperatures above 38°C should not be used to avoid interference with thermoregulation. The use of the turbine avoids the development of a layer of cooler water adjacent to the body part, thus producing more uniform warming. Because of the dependent position of the body part in the whirlpool and the increased temperature of the body part, a warm whirlpool may increase soft-tissue swelling; even in noninjured limbs, there may be a considerable increase in interstitial fluid following a warm whirlpool.

Because the turbine is powered by electricity, it is generally prudent to not let the patient touch any part of the turbine. Also, patients should not be left in the whirlpool unattended; this is true whether the entire body or only a limb is immersed.

PHYSIOLOGIC EFFECTS

Vasodilation
Decreased pain perception
Increased local metabolism
Increased connective tissue plasticity
Decreased isometric strength (transient)

THERAPEUTIC EFFECTS

Decreased pain
Increased soft-tissue extensibility
Sedative

INDICATIONS

The principal indication for a warm whirlpool is to provide therapeutic warming of a larger area of the body than can be achieved readily with a hot pack. The effective depth of therapeutic heating is the same at approximately 1 cm. In addition, the patient can perform active exercise during the application, or the therapist can perform joint mobilization on the injured limb while immersed in the water. Some therapists use whirlpool for cleaning a limb after removal of a cast; equally effective and at less cost is a shower.

The primary therapeutic effect of superficial heating is to increase the ability of the collagen to remodel. Therefore, heating the tissue is beneficial following a period of reduced mobility if the soft tissue has shortened. In addition, the tissue viscosity is reduced, resulting in a greater ease of motion through the available range of motion.

CONTRAINDICATIONS

- Lack of normal temperature sensibility
- Peripheral vascular disease with compromised circulation
- Over tumors
- Coronary artery disease

WARM WHIRLPOOL			
PROCEDURE	EVALUATION		
	1	2	3
1. Check supplies and equipment.			
a. Obtain towels for padding the edge of the whirlpool tank, as well as for drying the treated part.			
b. Check temperature of tank before applying treatment.			
c. Position chair of correct height next to whirlpool.			
2. Question patient.			
a. Verify identity of patient (if not already verified).			
b. Verify the absence of contraindications.			
c. Ask about previous thermotherapy or whirlpool treatments, check treatment notes.			
3. Position patient.			
a. Have patient sit on chair with body part out of water.			
b. Expose body part to be treated.			
c. Drape patient to preserve patient's modesty, protect clothing, but allow access to body part.			

4. Inspect body part to be treated.			
a. Check light touch perception.			
b. Check circulatory status (pulses, capillary refill).			
c. Verify that there are no open wounds or rashes.			
d. Assess function of body part (e.g., ROM, irritability).			
5. Administer warm whirlpool.			
a. Pad edge of tank with toweling; ask patient to tell you if the water is too hot, then place body part in water.			
b. Instruct patient to keep away from all parts of the turbine.			
c. Turn on the turbine, adjust the aeration, agitation, and direction of the water being pumped.			
d. Check the patient's response verbally and visually about every 2 minutes. Remind the patient to tell you if the area starts hurting or if sensation is lost.			
6. Complete the treatment.			
a. Turn off the turbine at the completion of the treatment time.			
b. Remove the body part from the water and dry it off.			
c. Assist the patient in dressing as needed and instruct in therapeutic exercise as indicated.			
d. Clean the treatment area and equipment according to normal protocol.			
7. Assess treatment efficacy.			
a. Ask the patient how the treated area feels.			
b. Visually inspect the treated area for any adverse reactions (e.g., wheals, welts).			
c. Perform functional tests as indicated.			

LAB ACTIVITY

HYDROCOLLATOR PACKS

DESCRIPTION

Commercially available hot packs (*hydrocollator packs*) are usually a canvas cover filled with a hydrophilic substance such as bentonite. Hot packs are kept in a commercial water-filled container that maintains a temperature of approximately 71°C. The packs are wrapped in six to eight layers of dry towels to protect the patient from burns; commercial hot pack covers provide approximately four thicknesses of toweling. After use, the hot pack should be returned to the cabinet for at least 30 minutes to insure reheating. Hot packs provide only superficial heating; the maximum depth of therapeutic heating is only about 1 cm, and occurs within 10 minutes of application.

PHYSIOLOGIC EFFECTS

Vasodilation
Decreased pain perception
Increased local metabolism
Increased connective tissue plasticity
Decreased isometric strength (transient)

THERAPEUTIC EFFECTS

Decreased pain
Increased soft-tissue extensibility

INDICATIONS

The principal indication for a hot pack is to provide therapeutic warming of superficial tissues. Tissues that are deeper than 1 cm do not reach a therapeutic temperature range of 30–40°C. Therefore, if the target tissue is deeper than 1 cm (e.g., the spinal facet joints), a hot pack will not be effective. Other joints, such as the knee, wrist, and ankle, can be effectively heated with a hot pack.

The primary therapeutic effect of superficial heating is to increase the ability of the collagen to remodel. Therefore, heating the tissue is beneficial following a period of reduced mobility if the soft tissue has shortened. In addition, the tissue viscosity is reduced, resulting in a greater ease of motion through the available range of motion. Although generally not a problem, in case of extreme pressure sensitivity, the weight of a hot pack may be more than the patient can tolerate. In these cases, Fluidotherapy or a warm whirlpool may be helpful.

CONTRAINDICATIONS

- Lack of normal temperature sensibility
- Peripheral vascular disease with compromised circulation
- Over tumors

HYDROCOLLATOR PACKS

PROCEDURE	EVALUATION		
	1	2	3
1. Check supplies.			
a. Obtain dry towels to wrap hot pack in, sheet or towels for draping, timer, signaling device.			
b. Check cabinet for appropriate temperature.			
2. Question patient.			
a. Verify identity of patient (if not already verified).			
b. Verify the absence of contraindications.			
c. Ask about previous thermotherapy treatments, check treatment notes.			
3. Position patient.			
a. Place patient in a well-supported, comfortable position.			
b. Expose body part to be treated.			
c. Drape patient to preserve patient's modesty, protect clothing, but allow access to body part.			
4. Inspect body part to be treated.			
a. Check light touch perception.			
b. Check circulatory status (pulses, capillary refill).			
c. Verify that there are no open wounds or rashes.			
d. Assess function of body part (e.g., ROM, irritability).			
5. Apply hot pack.			
a. Wrap hot pack in towels to provide six to eight layers of towel between the hot pack and the patient. If using a commercial hot pack cover, use at least one layer of towel to keep the cover clean.			

b. Inform the patient that you are going to put the hot pack on the body part to be treated, then do so.			
c. Set a timer for the appropriate treatment time and give the patient a signaling device. Make sure the patient understands how to use the signaling device.			
d. Check the patient's response after the first 5 minutes by asking the patient how it feels as well as visually checking the area under the hot pack. If the area is blotchy, additional toweling may be needed. Recheck verbally about every 5 minutes. A visual inspection every 5 minutes is not inappropriate.			
6. Complete the treatment.			
a. When the treatment time is over, remove the hot pack and dry the area with a towel.			
b. Remove material used for draping, assist the patient in dressing as needed.			
c. Have the patient perform appropriate therapeutic exercise as indicated.			
d. Clean the treatment area and equipment according to normal protocol.			
7. Assess treatment efficacy.			
a. Ask the patient how the treated area feels.			
b. Visually inspect the treated area for any adverse reactions.			
c. Perform functional tests as indicated.			

LAB ACTIVITY

PARAFFIN BATH

DESCRIPTION

Paraffin baths consist of dipping and removing or immersing the body part in a mixture of wax and mineral oil. The ratio of wax and mineral oil is about 7:1, which results in a substance with a melting point of about 47.8°C, a specific heat of about 0.65 cal/g/°C, and a therapeutic temperature range of 48–54°C. Because of the low specific heat, much higher temperatures can be tolerated than if water is used. The paraffin is kept in a thermostatically controlled cabinet.

Paraffin provides a superficial heat, with a depth of therapeutic heating of about 1 cm. However, because paraffin is generally used only for the hands and feet, the depth of penetration is adequate to warm these joints to a therapeutic range.

The two basic techniques of application of paraffin involve repeated dipping of the body part in the mixture, then covering the body part with plastic and toweling. The advantage of this method is that the body part can then be elevated, reducing the potential for swelling. The second method involves dipping body part in the paraffin once, letting it dry for a few seconds, then immersing the body part for the duration of the treatment. The advantage of this technique is that the source of heat is constant, so the therapeutic temperature can be maintained for a longer period.

PHYSIOLOGIC EFFECTS

Vasodilation
Decreased pain perception
Increased local metabolism
Increased connective tissue plasticity
Decreased isometric strength (transient)

THERAPEUTIC EFFECTS

Decreased pain
Increased soft-tissue extensibility

INDICATIONS

The principal indication for a paraffin bath is to provide therapeutic warming of superficial tissues. This is particularly effective in the hands and feet following a period of immobilization. The increased connective tissue plasticity that occurs with warming will enhance the effectiveness of therapeutic exercise.

Paraffin baths are also helpful in alleviation of pain caused by arthritic changes in the hands and feet. Caution should be exercised in using paraffin (or any heating agent) during an acute phase of arthritic pain and swelling.

CONTRAINDICATIONS

- Lack of normal temperature sensibility
- Peripheral vascular disease with compromised circulation
- Over tumors

PARAFFIN BATH

PROCEDURE	1	2	3
1. Check supplies.			
a. Obtain plastic bag and towels to wrap body part in, timer, signaling device.			
b. Check cabinet for appropriate temperature.			
2. Question patient.			
a. Verify identity of patient (if not already verified).			
b. Verify the absence of contraindications.			
c. Ask about previous thermotherapy treatments; check treatment notes.			
3. Prepare patient.			
a. Have patient remove all jewelry from body part, wash well and dry thoroughly.			
b. Explain to the patient that after dipping the body part into the paraffin, there should be no movement of the body part for the duration of the treatment.			
4. Inspect body part to be treated.			
a. Check light touch perception.			
b. Check circulatory status (pulses, capillary refill).			
c. Verify that there are no open wounds or rashes.			
d. Assess function of body part (e.g., ROM, irritability).			
5. Apply paraffin.			
a. Guide the body part into the paraffin, making sure the patient does not contact the bottom of the cabinet or the heating coils.			
b. After 2 or 3 seconds, remove the body part, and keep it above the paraffin so that none of the paraffin drips onto the floor. Reimmerse the body part, and repeat until the appropriate number of dips have been completed, or reimmerse for the duration of the treatment.			
c. Set a timer for the appropriate treatment time and give the patient a signaling device. Make sure the patient understands how to use the signaling device.			
d. Check the patient's response after the first 5 minutes by asking the patient how it feels. Recheck verbally about every 5 minutes.			

EVALUATION

		1	2	3
6.	Complete the treatment.			
	a. When the treatment time is over, remove the towel and plastic bag. Help the patient remove the paraffin, and either return the paraffin to the cabinet, or throw away according to local protocol.			
	b. Have the patient thoroughly wash and dry the body part.			
	c. Have the patient perform appropriate therapeutic exercise as indicated.			
	d. Clean the treatment area and equipment according to normal protocol.			
7.	Assess treatment efficacy.			
	a. Ask the patient how the treated area feels.			
	b. Visually inspect the treated area for any adverse reactions.			
	c. Perform functional tests as indicated.			

LAB ACTIVITY

INFRARED LAMPS

DESCRIPTION

Infrared lamps provide superficial (1 mm or less) heating. Because of the extremely limited penetration, they are not capable of elevating connective tissue temperatures to a therapeutic level. Therefore, their primary effect is one of mild analgesia, and their use is very limited.

PHYSIOLOGIC EFFECTS

Cutaneous vasodilation
Decreased pain perception

THERAPEUTIC EFFECTS

Decreased pain

INDICATIONS

The principal indication for infrared lamp heating is localized pain. Elevation of skin temperature may decrease the perception of pain for a short time.

CONTRAINDICATIONS

- Lack of normal temperature sensibility
- Peripheral vascular disease with compromised circulation
- Over tumors

INFRARED LAMPS

PROCEDURE	EVALUATION		
	1	2	3
1. Check supplies.			
a. Obtain sheet or towels for draping, timer, signaling device.			
b. Check lamp for frayed power cords, integrity of lamp and shields, and so on.			

2. Question patient.			
a. Verify identity of patient (if not already verified).			
b. Verify the absence of contraindications.			
c. Ask about previous thermotherapy treatments, check treatment notes.			
3. Position patient.			
a. Place patient in a well-supported, comfortable position.			
b. Expose body part to be treated, have patient remove all jewelry from the area.			
c. Drape patient to preserve patient's modesty, protect clothing, but allow access to body part.			
4. Inspect body part to be treated.			
a. Check light touch perception.			
b. Check circulatory status (pulses, capillary refill).			
c. Verify that there are no open wounds or rashes.			
d. Assess function of body part (e.g., ROM, irritability).			
5. Apply infrared light.			
a. Position lamp such that the bulb is parallel to the body part being angle), and is 45–60° treated (such that the energy will strike the body at a 90 cm away from the patient. Measure and record the distance from the lamp to the closest part of the body being treated.			
b. Inform the patient that they should feel only a mild warmth; if it is hot, they should inform you. Start the lamp.			
c. Set a timer for the appropriate treatment time and give the patient a signaling device. Make sure the patient understands how to use the signaling device.			
d. Check the patient's response after the first 5 minutes by asking the patient how it feels as well as visually checking the area being treated. Recheck visually and verbally about every 5 minutes.			
6. Complete the treatment.			
a. When the treatment time is over, move the lamp away from the patient; dry the area with a towel. Turn the intensity control to zero.			
b. Remove material used for draping, assist the patient in dressing as needed.			
c. Have the patient perform appropriate therapeutic exercise as indicated.			
d. Clean the treatment area and equipment according to normal protocol.			
7. Assess treatment efficacy.			
a. Ask the patient how the treated area feels.			
b. Visually inspect the treated area for any adverse reactions.			
c. Perform functional tests as indicated.			

LAB ACTIVITY

FLUIDOTHERAPY

DESCRIPTION

Fluidotherapy is a device manufactured by Henley International of Sugarland, TX. Heated air is forced through a container filled with cellulose particles; when heated, the cellulose takes on fluidlike characteristics. The body part to be treated is immersed in the cellulose particles, and the particles are circulated in the container, thus providing elevation of tissue temperature and a mechanical stimulation of the skin. The temperature of the unit is adjustable within a range of about 39–48°C.

There are several advantages to using Fluidotherapy to treat affected hands or feet. The source of heat is constant, so the tissue temperature can be maintained at a therapeutic level for the duration of the treatment. The body part can be exercised during the treatment, either actively or passively by the therapist. The mechanical stimulation of the skin with the cellulose particles may provide some analgesic effect and may help desensitize the injured area.

PHYSIOLOGIC EFFECTS

Vasodilation
Decreased pain perception
Increased local metabolism
Increased connective tissue plasticity
Decreased isometric strength (transient)

THERAPEUTIC EFFECTS

Decreased pain
Increased soft-tissue extensibility

INDICATIONS

The principal indication for Fluidotherapy is to provide therapeutic warming of a larger area of the body than can be achieved readily with a hot pack. In addition, the patient can perform active exercise during the application, or the therapist can perform joint mobilization on the injured limb while in the unit.

The primary therapeutic effect of superficial heating is to increase the ability of the collagen to remodel. Therefore, heating the tissue is beneficial following a period of reduced mobility if the soft tissue has shortened. In addition, the tissue viscosity is reduced, resulting in a greater ease of motion through the available range of motion.

CONTRAINDICATIONS

- Lack of normal temperature sensibility
- Peripheral vascular disease with compromised circulation
- Over tumors
- Coronary artery disease

FLUIDOTHERAPY			
PROCEDURE	EVALUATION		
	1	2	3
1. Check supplies and equipment.			
a. Obtain timer, signaling device, and so on.			
b. Check temperature of Fluidotherapy unit before applying treatment.			
c. Position chair of correct height next to unit.			
2. Question patient.			
a. Verify identity of patient (if not already verified).			
b. Verify the absence of contraindications.			
c. Ask about previous thermotherapy treatments, check treatment notes.			
3. Position patient.			
a. Have patient remove jewelry from area to be treated and thoroughly wash and dry area.			

b. Have patient sit on chair next to unit.			
c. Expose body part to be treated.			
d. Drape patient to preserve patient's modesty, protect clothing, but allow access to body part.			
4. Inspect body part to be treated.			
a. Check light touch perception.			
b. Check circulatory status (pulses, capillary refill).			
c. Verify that there are no open wounds or rashes.			
d. Assess function of body part (e.g., ROM, irritability).			
5. Administer Fluidotherapy.			
a. With the agitation off, open the sleeved portion of the unit.			
b. Instruct patient to insert body part into cellulose particles, reminding them to tell you if the temperature is too hot.			
c. Fasten the sleeve around the body part to prevent the cellulose particles from being blown out of the unit, and start the agitation.			
d. Check the patient's response verbally after about 5 minutes. Remind the patient to tell you if the heating sensation becomes uncomfortable.			
e. Instruct the patient in any indicated therapeutic exercise to be performed during the treatment.			
6. Complete the treatment.			
a. Turn off the agitation at the completion of the treatment time.			
b. Remove the body part from the unit, having the patient brush or shake off as much of the cellulose as possible.			
c. Assist the patient in dressing as needed and instruct in therapeutic exercise as indicated.			
d. Clean the treatment area and equipment according to normal protocol.			
7. Assess treatment efficacy.			
a. Ask the patient how the treated area feels.			
b. Visually inspect the treated area for any adverse reactions (e.g., wheals, welts).			
c. Perform functional tests as indicated.			

PART **FOUR**

Sound Energy
Modalities

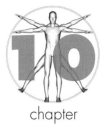

10 **Therapeutic Ultrasound**

chapter

David O. Draper and William E. Prentice

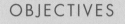

OBJECTIVES

Following completion of this chapter, the student will be able to:

➤ Analyze the transmission of acoustic energy in biologic tissues relative to waveforms, frequency, velocity, and attenuation.

➤ Break down the basic physics involved in the production of a beam of therapeutic ultrasound.

➤ Compare both the thermal and nonthermal physiologic effects of therapeutic ultrasound.

➤ Evaluate specific techniques of application of therapeutic ultrasound and how they may be modified to achieve treatment goals.

➤ Choose the most appropriate and clinically effective uses for therapeutic ultrasound. Explain the technique and clinical application of phonophoresis.

➤ Identify the contraindications and precautions that should be observed with therapeutic ultrasound.

In the medical community, ultrasound is a modality that is used for a number of different purposes including diagnosis, destruction of tissue, and as a therapeutic agent. Diagnostic ultrasound has been used for more than 50 years for the purpose of imaging internal structures. Historically, diagnostic ultrasound has been used to image the fetus during pregnancy. More recently, with a reduction of equipment costs, significant improvements in image resolution, real-time ultrasonographic imaging and detailed anatomic imaging, diagnostic ultrasound has expanded to various clinical practices that evaluate, diagnose, and treat musculoskeletal disorders. Diagnostic musculoskeletal ultrasound (MSK) can identify pathology in muscle, tendons, ligaments, bones, and joints.[1] Ultrasound has also been used to produce extreme tissue hyperthermia that has been demonstrated to have tumoricidal effects in cancer patients.

In clinical practice, ultrasound is one of the most widely used therapeutic modalities in addition to superficial heat and cold and electrical stimulating currents.[2] It has been used for therapeutic purposes as a valuable tool in the rehabilitation of many different injuries primarily for the purpose of stimulating the repair of soft-tissue injuries and for relief of pain,[3] although some studies have questioned its efficiency as a treatment modality.[4]

As discussed in Chapter 1, ultrasound is a form of acoustic rather than electromagnetic energy. Ultrasound is defined as inaudible acoustic vibrations of high frequency that may produce either thermal or nonthermal physiologic effects.[5] The use of ultrasound as a therapeutic agent may be extremely effective if the clinician has an adequate understanding of its effects on biologic tissues and of the physical mechanisms by which these effects are produced.[3]

- **Ultrasound** is one of the most widely used modalities in health care.
- Ultrasound and diathermy = deep heating modalities

ULTRASOUND AS A HEATING MODALITY

Chapter 9 discusses heat as a treatment modality. Warm whirlpools, paraffin baths, and hot packs, to name a few, all produce therapeutic heat. However, the depth of penetration of these modalities is superficial and at best only 1–2 cm.[6] Ultrasound, along with diathermy, has traditionally been classified as a "deep heating modality" and has been used primarily for the purpose of elevating tissue temperatures.

Suppose a patient is lacking dorsiflexion. It is determined through evaluation that a tight soleus is the problem, and as a clinician your desire is to use thermotherapy followed by stretching. Will superficial heat adequately prepare this muscle to be stretched? Since the soleus lies deep under the gastrocnemius muscle, it is beyond the reach of superficial heat.

One of the advantages of using ultrasound over other heating modalities is that it can provide deep heating.[7,156] The heating effects of silicate gel hot packs and warm whirlpools have been compared with ultrasound. At an intramuscular depth of 3 cm, a 10-minute hot pack treatment yields an increase of 0.8°C, whereas at this same depth, 1 MHz ultrasound raises muscle temperature nearly 4°C in 10 minutes.[8,9] At 1 cm below the fat surface, a 4-minute warm whirlpool (40.6°C) raises the temperature 1.1°C; however, at this same depth, 3MHz ultrasound raises the temperature 4°C in 4 minutes.[8,10,11]

TRANSMISSION OF ACOUSTIC ENERGY IN BIOLOGIC TISSUES

Unlike electromagnetic energy, which travels most effectively through a vacuum, acoustic energy relies on molecular collision for transmission. Molecules in a conducting medium will cause vibration and minimal displacement of other surrounding molecules when set into vibration, so that eventually this "wave" of vibration has propagated through the entire medium. Sound waves travel in a manner similar to waves created by a stone thrown into a pool of water. Ultrasound is a mechanical wave in which energy is transmitted by the vibrations of the molecules of the biologic medium through which the wave is traveling.[12]

Transverse Versus Longitudinal Waves

Two types of waves can travel through a solid medium, **longitudinal** and **transverse waves**. In a longitudinal wave, the molecular displacement is along the direction in which the wave travels. Within this longitudinal wave pathway are regions of high-molecular density referred to as **compressions** (in which the molecules are squeezed together) and regions of lower molecular density called **rarefactions** (in which the molecules spread out) (Figure 10–1). This is much like the squeezing and spreading action when using a child's "slinky" toy. In a transverse wave, the molecules are displaced in a direction perpendicular to the direction in which the wave is moving. Although longitudinal waves travel both in solids and liquids, transverse waves can travel only in solids. Because soft tissues are more like liquids, ultrasound travels primarily as a longitudinal wave; however, when it contacts bone a transverse wave results.[12]

Frequency of Wave Transmission

The *frequency* of audible sound ranges between 16 and 20 KHz (kilohertz = 1000 cycles/s). Ultrasound has a frequency above 20 kHz. The frequency range for therapeutic ultrasound is

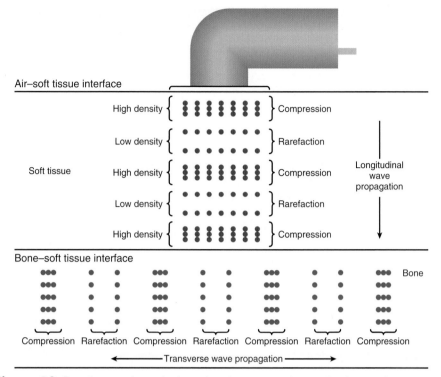

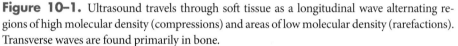

Figure 10–1. Ultrasound travels through soft tissue as a longitudinal regions of high molecular density (compressions) and areas of low molecular density (rarefactions). Transverse waves are found primarily in bone.

between 0.75 and 3 MHz (megahertz = 1,000,000 cycles/s). The higher the frequency of the sound waves emitted from a sound source, the less the sound will diverge and thus a more focused beam of sound will be produced. In biologic tissues, the lower the frequency of the sound waves, the greater the depth of penetration. Higher frequency sound waves are absorbed in the more superficial tissues.

Velocity

The *velocity* at which this vibration or sound wave is propagated through the conducting medium is directly related to the density. Denser and more rigid materials will have a higher velocity of transmission. At a frequency of 1 MHz, sound travels through soft tissue at 1540 m/s and through compact bone at 4000 m/s.[13]

Attenuation

As the ultrasound wave is transmitted through the various tissues, there will be **attenuation** or a decrease in energy intensity. This decrease is owing to either *absorption* of energy by the tissues or *dispersion* and *scattering* of the sound wave that results from reflection or refraction.[12]

Ultrasound penetrates through tissue high in water content and is absorbed in dense tissues high in protein where it will have its greatest heating potential.[14] The capability of acoustic energy to penetrate or be transmitted to deeper tissues is determined by the frequency of the ultrasound as well as the characteristics of the tissues through which ultrasound is traveling. Penetration and absorption are inversely related. Absorption increases as the frequency increases; thus less energy is transmitted to the deeper tissues. Tissues that are high in water content have a low rate of absorption, whereas tissues high in protein have a high absorption rate.[15] Fat has a relatively low-absorption rate, and muscle absorbs considerably more. Peripheral nerve absorbs at a rate twice that of muscle.

Table 10–1 Relationship Between Penetration and Absorption (1 MHz)

MEDIUM	ABSORPTION	PENETRATION
Water	1	1200
Blood plasma	23	52
Whole blood	60	20
Fat	390	4
Skeletal muscle	663	2
Peripheral nerve	1193	1

From Griffin JE. J Am Phys Ther. 1966; 46(1):18–26. Reprinted with permission of the American Physical Therapy Association.

Bone, which is relatively superficial, absorbs more ultrasonic energy than any of the other tissues (Table 10–1).

When a sound wave encounters a boundary or an interface between different tissues, some of the energy will scatter owing to reflection or refraction. The amount of energy reflected, and conversely the amount of energy that will be transmitted to deeper tissues, is determined by the relative magnitude of the **acoustic impedances** of the two materials on either side of the interface. Acoustic impedance may be determined by multiplying the density of the material by the speed at which sound travels inside it. If the acoustic impedance of the two materials forming the interface is the same, all of the sound will be transmitted and none will be reflected. The larger the difference between the two acoustic impedances, the more energy is reflected and the less that can enter a second medium (Table 10–2).[17]

• Penetration and absorption are inversely related.

Sound passing from the transducer to air will be almost completely reflected. Ultrasound is transmitted through fat. It is both reflected and refracted at the muscular interface. At the soft tissue–bone interface virtually all of the sound is reflected. As the ultrasound energy is reflected at tissue interfaces with different acoustic impedances, the intensity of the energy is increased as the reflected energy meets new energy being transmitted, creating what is referred to as a **standing wave** or a **"hot spot."** This increased level of energy has the potential to produce tissue damage. Moving the sound transducer or using pulsed wave ultrasound can help minimize the development of hot spots.[18]

Table 10–2 The Percentage of the Incident Energy Reflected at Tissue Interfaces[16]

INTERFACE	PERCENT REFLECTION
Soft tissue/air	99.9
Water/soft tissue	0.2
Soft tissue/fat	1.0
Soft tissue/bone	15–40

From Ward AR. Electricity Fields and Waves in Therapy. Maricksville, NSW, Australia: Science Press; 1986.

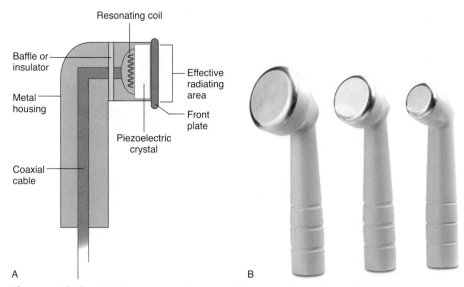

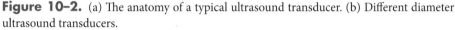

Figure 10–2. (a) The anatomy of a typical ultrasound transducer. (b) Different diameter ultrasound transducers.

BASIC PHYSICS OF THERAPEUTIC ULTRASOUND

Components of a Therapeutic Ultrasound Generator

An ultrasound generator consists of a high-frequency electrical generator connected through an oscillator circuit and a transformer via a coaxial cable to a transducer housed in a type of insulated applicator (Figure 10–2). The oscillator circuit produces a sound beam at a specific frequency that the manufacturer adjusts to the frequency requirements of the transducer. The control panel of an ultrasound unit usually has a timer that can be preset, a power meter, an intensity control, a duty cycle control switch, a selector for continuous or pulsed modes, and possibly output power in response to tissue loading, and automatic shut-off in case of over-heating of the transducer. Recently dual soundheads and dual frequency choices have become standard equipment on ultrasound units (Figure 10–3). Table 10–3 provides a list of the most desirable features in an ultrasound generator.

It must be added that several studies have demonstrated significant differences in the effectiveness of different ultrasound units produced by a variety of manufacturers in raising tissue temperatures.[19,20] It is also critical to make certain that ultrasound units are routinely tested and recalibrated to make certain that selected treatment parameters are actually being produced by the ultrasound unit.[21]

Transducer

The **transducer,** also referred to as an applicator or a soundhead, must be matched to particular units and generally not interchangeable.[22] The transducer consists of some crystal, such as quartz, or synthetic ceramic crystals made of lead zirconate or titanate, barium titanate, or nickel-cobalt ferrite of approximately 2–3 mm in thickness. It is the crystal within the transducer that converts electrical energy to acoustic energy through mechanical deformation of the crystal.

Piezoelectric effect. Crystals that are capable of mechanical distortion (expanding and contracting) are called **piezoelectric crystals**. When a biphasic electrical current generated at the same frequency as the crystal resonance is passed through a piezoelectric crystal, the crystal will expand and contract, creating what is referred to as the **piezoelectric effect**.

There are two forms of this piezoelectric effect (Figure 10–4). An *indirect* or *reverse* piezo-electric effect is created when a biphasic current is passed through the crystal, producing compression or expansion of the crystal. It is this expansion and contraction that causes the crystal

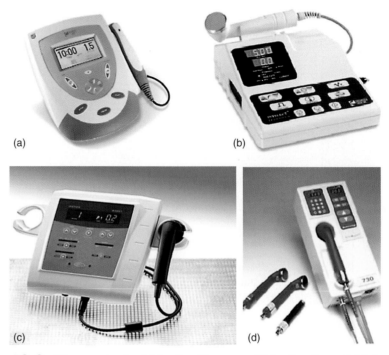

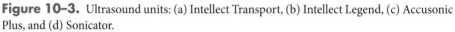

Figure 10–3. Ultrasound units: (a) Intellect Transport, (b) Intellect Legend, (c) Accusonic Plus, and (d) Sonicator.

to vibrate at a specific frequency, producing a sound wave that is transmitted into the tissues. Thus, the reverse piezoelectric effect is used to generate ultrasound at a desired frequency.

A *direct* piezoelectric effect, which has nothing to do with ultrasound, is the generation of an electrical voltage across the crystal when it is compressed or expanded.

Table 10–3   Features of the State-of-the-Art "Ultimate" Ultrasound Machine Offer

Low BNR (4:1)

High ERA (nearly matches the size of the soundhead)

Multiple frequencies (1 and 3 MHz)

Multiple sized soundheads

Sensing device that shuts off the unit when overheating

Well insulated to be used underwater

Output jack for combination therapy

Several pulsed duty cycles

High-quality synthetic crystal

Transducer handle that maintains the operator's wrist in a natural, relaxed position

Durable transducer face that will protect the crystal if dropped

Computer controlled timer that makes adjustments in treatment duration as the intensity is adjusted (much like iontophoresis where the treatment time adjusts according to the dose applied)

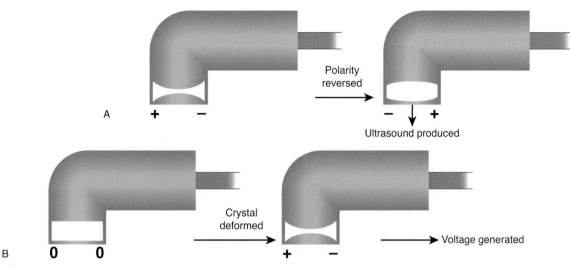

A + −   Polarity reversed   − ↓ +   Ultrasound produced

B **0** **0**   Crystal deformed   **+** **−**   Voltage generated

Figure 10–4. Piezoelectric effect. A. In the reverse piezoelectric effect, as the alternating current reverses polarity, the crystal expands and contracts, producing ultrasound energy. B. In a direct piezoelectric effect, a mechanical deformation of the crystal generates a voltage.

Effective radiating area (ERA). That portion of the surface of the transducer that actually produces the sound wave is referred to as the **effective radiating area (ERA)**. ERA is dependent on the surface area of the crystal and ideally nearly matches the diameter of the transducer faceplate (Figure 10–5).[3] The ERA is determined by scanning the transducer at a distance of 5 mm from the radiating surface and recording all areas in excess of 5% of the maximum power output found at any location on the surface of the transducer. The acoustic energy is contained with a focused cylindrical beam that is roughly the same diameter as the sound-head.[17] The energy output is greater at the center and less at the periphery of the ERA. Likewise the temperature at the center is significantly greater than at the periphery of the ERA.[23]

Because the effective radiating area is always smaller than the transducer surface, the size of the transducer is not indicative of the actual radiating surface. There is significant variability in the effective radiating area and output power of ultrasound transducers.[24] A very common mistake is to assume that because you have a large transducer surface the entire surface radiates ultrasound output. This is generally not true, particularly with larger 10-cm^2 transducers. There is really no point in having a large transducer with a small radiating surface as it only mechanically limits the coupling in smaller areas (see Figure 10–5). The transducer

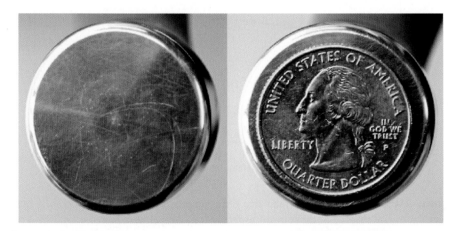

Figure 10–5. (Left) Photo of a quarter-sized crystal mounted to the inside of the transducer faceplate. (Right) A quarter is placed on the transducer face to illustrate that this crystal is smaller than the faceplate. Ideally, they should be closer to the same size.

ERA should match the total size of the transducer as closely as possible for ease of application to various body surfaces, in order to maintain the most effective coupling.

The appropriate size of the area to be treated using ultrasound is two to three times the size of the ERA of the crystal.[25,26] To support this premise, peak temperature in human muscle was measured during 10 minutes of 1 MHz ultrasound delivered at 1.5 W/cm² (Figure 10–6). The treatment size for 10 subjects was 2 ERA, and for the other 10 it was 6 ERA. The 2-ERA group's temperature increased 3.6°C (moderate to vigorous heating), whereas subjects' temperature in the 6-ERA group only increased 1.1°C (mild heating). A similar study showed that 3 MHz ultrasound at an intensity of 1 W/cm² significantly increased patellar tendon temperature at both two times and four times ERA. However, the 2-ERA size provided higher and longer heating than the 4-ERA size.[27] Thus, ultrasound is most effectively used for treating small areas.[28] Hot packs, whirlpools, and -shortwave diathermy have an advantage over ultrasound in that they can be used to heat much larger areas such as heating the entire soulder complex.[160]

Frequency of Therapeutic Ultrasound

Therapeutic ultrasound produced by a piezoelectric transducer has a frequency range between 0.75 and 3.3 MHz. Frequency is the number of wave cycles completed each second. The majority of the older ultrasound generators are set at a frequency of 1 MHz (meaning the crystal is deforming 1 million times per second), whereas some of the newer models also contain the 3 MHz frequency (the crystal is deforming 3 million times per second).[159] Certainly, a generator that can be set between 1 and 3 MHz affords the clinician the greatest treatment flexibility.

A common misconception is that intensity determines the depth of ultrasonic penetration, and therefore high intensities (1.5 or 2 W/cm²) are used for deep heating and low intensities (1 W/cm²) are used for superficial heating. However, depth of tissue penetration is determined by ultrasound frequency and not by intensity.[29] Ultrasound energy generated at 1 MHz

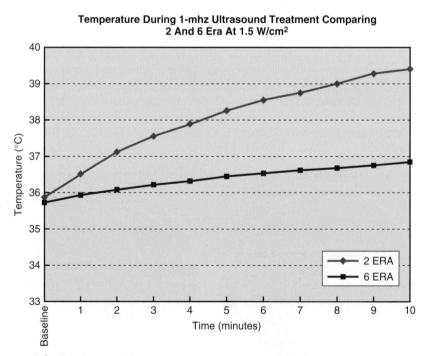

Figure 10–6. This graph illustrates that ultrasound is ineffective in heating areas much larger than twice the size of the transducer face. Mean temperature increase for 2 ERA was 3.4°C, and only 1.1°C for an area six times the effective radiating area (ERA).(From Chudliegh D, Schulthies SS, Draper DO, and Myrer JW: Muscle temperature rise with 1 MHz ultrasound in treatment sizes of 2 and 6 times the effective radiating area of the transducer, *Master's Thesis,* Brigham Young University; July 1997).

is transmitted through the more superficial tissues and absorbed primarily in the deeper tissues at depths of 2–5 cm (Figure 10–7).[8] A 1 MHz frequency is most useful in patients with high-percent body fat cutaneously and whenever desired effects are in the deeper structures, such as the soleus or piriformis muscles.[5] At 3 MHz the energy is absorbed in the more superficial tissues with a depth of penetration between 1 and 2 cm, making it ideal for treating superficial conditions such as plantar fasciitis, patellar tendinitis, and epicondylitis.[13,30]

As previously mentioned, attenuation is the decrease in the energy of ultrasound as the distance it travels through tissue increases. The rate of absorption, and therefore attenuation, increases as the frequency of the ultrasound increases.[31] The 3 MHz frequency is not only absorbed more superficially, it is also absorbed three times faster than 1 MHz ultrasound. This faster rate of absorption results in faster peak heating in tissues. It has been demonstrated that 3 MHz ultrasound heats human muscle three times faster than 1 MHz ultrasound.[8]

Clinical Decision-Making   *Exercise 10–1*

A patient is complaining of pain at the lateral epicondyle of the elbow, which has been diagnosed as tennis elbow. The clinician is trying to decide whether to use 1 or 3 MHz ultrasound. Which would likely be most effective?

The Ultrasound Beam

If the wavelength of the sound is larger than the source that produced it, then the sound will spread in all directions.[17] Such is the case with audible sound, thus explaining why it is possible for a person behind you to hear your voice almost as well as a person in front of you. In the case of therapeutic ultrasound, the sound is less divergent, thus concentrating energy in a limited area (1 MHz at a velocity 1540 m/s in soft tissue and a wavelength of 1.5 mm, emitted from a transducer that is larger than the wavelength at approximately 25 mm in diameter).

The larger the diameter of the transducer, the more focused or **collimated** the beam. Smaller transducers produce a more divergent beam. Also, the beam from ultrasound generated at a frequency of 1 MHz is more divergent than ultrasound generated at 3 MHz (see Figure 10–7).

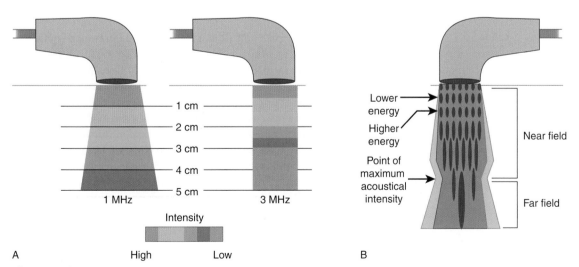

Figure 10–7. (a) The ultrasound energy attenuates as it travels through soft tissue. At 1 MHz, the energy can penetrate to the deeper tissues although the beam diverges slightly. At 3 MHz, the effects are primarily in the superficial tissues and the beam is less divergent. (b) In the near field the distribution of energy is nonuniform. In the far field energy distribution is more uniform but the beam is more divergent.

Near field/far field. Within this cylindrical beam the distribution of sound energy is highly nonuniform, particularly in an area close to the transducer referred to as the **near field** (Figure 10–7b). The near field is a zone of fluctuating ultrasound intensity. The fluctuation occurs because ultrasound is emitted from the transducer in waves. Within each wave there is higher sound energy and between the waves there is less sound energy. Thus within the ultrasound beam close to the transducer in the near field there is variation in ultrasound intensity. As the beam moves away from the transducer, the sound energy becomes more consistent.

$$\text{Length of near field} = \frac{\text{Radius of transducer}^2}{\text{Wavelength of ultrasound}}$$

At the end of the near field, the point of maximum acoustic intensity is where the intensity within the ultrasound beam is at its highest level.[17] The length of the near field from the surface of the transducer and thus the location of the point of maximum acoustic intensity can be determined by the following calculation:[1]

The far field begins just beyond this point of maximum acoustic intensity, where the distribution of energy is much more uniform but the beam becomes more divergent.

Beam nonuniformity ratio. The amount of variability of intensity within the ultrasound beam is indicated by the **beam nonuniformity ratio (BNR).** This ratio is determined by measuring the peak intensity of the ultrasound output over the area of the transducer relative to the average output of ultrasound over the area of the transducer. (Output is measured in Watts per square centimeter.) For example, a BNR of 2 to 1 means the peak output intensity of the beam is 2 W/cm² the average output intensity is 1 W/cm².

The optimal BNR would be 1 to 1; however, because this is not possible, on most ultrasound generators the BNR usually falls between 2:1 and 6:1. Some ultrasound units have BNRs as high as 8:1. Peak intensities of 8 W/cm² have been shown to damage tissue; therefore, the patient runs a risk of tissue damage if intensities greater than 1 W/cm² are used on a machine with an 8:1 BNR. The lower the BNR, the more uniform the output and therefore the lower the chance of developing "hot spots" of concentrated energy. The Food and Drug Administration requires all ultrasound units to list the BNR, and the clinician should be aware of the BNR for that particular unit.[32]

The high-peak intensities associated with high BNRs are responsible for much of the discomfort or periosteal pain often associated with ultrasound treatment.[33] Therefore, the higher the BNR the more important it is to move the transducer faster during treatment to avoid hot spots and areas of tissue damage or cavitation. Figure 10–8 shows the high-beam homogeneity of a low-BNR transducer and the typical beam profile of a high-BNR transducer at 3 MHz output frequency.

Some researchers give little credence to BNR as a factor in good ultrasound equipment and say that it has little effect in treatment quality. Their rationale is that good treatment technique is much more important than the BNR.[34] However, most would agree that a continuous thermal ultrasound treatment is effective only if it is tolerated by the patient, and if it produces uniform heating through the tissues.[20] Some have speculated that a beam flowing from a poor-quality ultrasound crystal might be a reason patients experience pain and might cause uneven heating of tissue. Patient compliance should be better when thermal ultrasound is delivered via an ultrasound device with a low-beam nonuniformity ratio. This will encourage patients to return for needed ultrasound treatments and allow the clinician to increase the intensity to the point where the patient feels local heat. When a heat modality is applied to tissue, it only makes sense that the patient should feel heat. If warmth is not felt, either the clinician is moving the soundhead too fast, or the intensity is too low.

Amplitude, Power, and Intensity

Amplitude is a term that describes the magnitude of the vibration in a wave. Amplitude is used to describe the variation in pressure found along the path of the wave in units of pressure (N/m²).[22] **Power** is the total amount of ultrasound energy in the beam and is expressed in watts. **Intensity** is a measure of the rate at which energy is being delivered per unit area. Because power and intensity are unevenly distributed in the beam, several varying types of intensities must be defined.

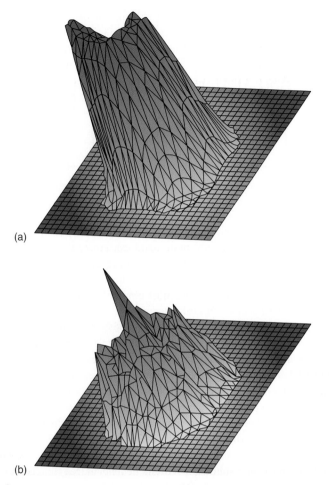

(a)

(b)

Figure 10–8. (a) Graphic representation of a low BNR of 2:1. (b) Graphic representation of a high BNR of 6:1.

- *Spatial-averaged intensity* is the intensity of the ultrasound beam averaged over the entire area of the transducer. It may be calculated by dividing the power output in watts by the total effective radiating area (ERA) of the soundhead in cm² and is indicated in watts per square centimeter (W/cm²). If ultrasound is being produced at a power of 6 W and the ERA of the transducer is 4 cm², the spatial-averaged intensity would be 1.5 W/cm². On many ultrasound units, both the power in watts and the spatial-average intensity in W/cm² may be displayed. If the power output is constant, increasing the size of the transducer will decrease the spatial-averaged intensity.
- *Spatial peak intensity* is the highest value occurring within the beam over time. With therapeutic ultrasound, maximum intensities can range between 0.25 and 3.0 W/cm².
- *Temporal peak intensity*, sometimes also referred to as *pulse-averaged intensity*, is the maximum intensity during the on period with pulsed ultrasound, indicated in W/cm² (see Figure 10–10).
- *Temporal-averaged intensity* is important only with pulsed ultrasound and is calculated by averaging the power during both the on and off periods. For a pulsed sound beam with a duty cycle of 20% with a temporal peak intensity of 2.0 W/cm², temporal-averaged intensity would be 0.4 W/cm². It should be pointed out that on some machines, the intensity setting indicates the temporal peak intensity or on time, whereas on others it shows the temporal-averaged intensity or the mean of the on–off intensity (see Figure 10–10).[6]
- *Spatial-averaged temporal peak (SATP) intensity* is the maximum intensity occurring in time of the spatially averaged intensity. The SATP intensity is simply the spatial average during a single pulse.

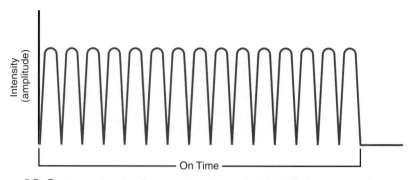

Figure 10–9. In continuous ultrasound, energy is constantly being generated.

No definitive rules govern selection of specific ultrasound intensities during treatment, yet using too much may likely damage tissues and exacerbate the condition.[6] One recommendation is that the lowest intensity of ultrasound energy at the highest frequency that will transmit the energy to a specific tissue should be used to achieve a desired therapeutic effect.[6] Some guidance for selecting intensities has come from published reports from those who have obtained successful, yet subjective, clinical outcomes.[6]

It is important to remember that everyone's tolerance to heat is different, and thus ultrasound intensity should always be adjusted to patient tolerance.[33] At the beginning of the treatment, turn the intensity to the point where the patient feels deep warmth, and then back the intensity down slightly until gentle heating is felt.[28,35] During the treatment, ask the patient for feedback, and make the necessary intensity adjustments. This idea only applies to continuous mode ultrasound because pulsed ultrasound generally does not produce heat. Regardless, the treatment should never produce reports of pain. If the patient reports that the transducer feels hot at the skin surface, it is likely that the coupling medium is inadequate and possible that the piezoelectric crystal has been damaged and the transducer is overheating.

Ultrasound treatments should be temperature dependent, not time dependent. Thermal ultrasound is used in order to bring about certain desired effects, and tissues respond according to the amount of heat they receive.[36,37] Any significant adjustment in the intensity must be countered with an adjustment in the treatment time. Changing the intensity levels during the treatment does not result in optimal heating.[38]

Higher-intensity ultrasound results in greater and faster temperature increase.[39] For this reason, it is likely that the new generation of ultrasound generators will have the capability of automatically decreasing treatment time as the intensity is increased and increasing treatment time as the intensity is decreased (see Figure 10–3).

It should also be added that different ultrasound devices will in all likelihood produce different intensities and different outputs during treatments despite the fact that the selected treatment parameters may be identical. Therefore the therapeutic effects may be different from one therapeutic ultrasound device to the next.[40]

Pulsed versus Continuous Wave Ultrasound

Virtually all therapeutic ultrasound generators can emit either continuous or pulsed ultrasound waves. If **continuous wave ultrasound** is used, the sound intensity remains constant throughout the treatment, and the ultrasound energy is being produced 100% of the time (Figure 10–9).

$$Duty\ cycle = \frac{Duration\ of\ pulse\ (on\ time) \times 100}{pulse\ period\ (on\ time + off\ time)}$$

With **pulsed ultrasound** the intensity is periodically interrupted, with no ultrasound energy being produced during the off period (Figure 10–10). When using pulsed ultrasound, the average intensity of the output over time is reduced. The percentage of time that ultrasound is being generated (pulse duration) over one pulse period is referred to as the *duty cycle.*

Thus, if the pulse duration is 1 millisecond and the total pulse period is 5 milliseconds, the duty cycle would be 20%. Therefore, the total amount of energy being delivered to the

• Depth of tissue penetration is determined by ultrasound frequency and not by intensity.

• 3 MHz = superficial heat
• 1 MHz = deep heat
• Treatment area = 2–3 ERA
• Ultrasound may be continuous or pulsed.

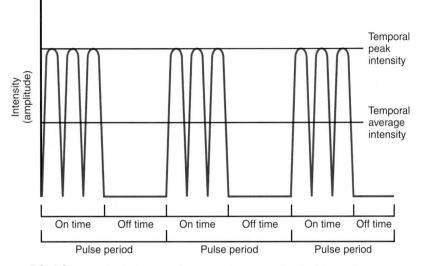

Figure 10–10. In pulsed ultrasound, energy is generated only during the on time. Duty cycle is determined by the ratio of on time to pulse period.

tissues would be only 20% of the energy delivered if a continuous wave was being used. The majority of ultrasound generators have duty cycles that are preset at either 20 or 50%; however, some provide several optional duty cycles. Occasionally the duty cycle is also referred to as the *mark:space* ratio.

Continuous ultrasound is most commonly used when thermal effects are desired. The use of pulsed ultrasound results in a reduced average heating of the tissues. Pulsed ultrasound or continuous ultrasound at a low intensity will produce nonthermal or mechanical effects that may be associated with soft tissue healing.

PHYSIOLOGIC EFFECTS OF ULTRASOUND

Therapeutic ultrasound may induce clinically significant responses in cells, tissues, and organs through both thermal effects and nonthermal biophysical effects.[3,12,13,17,18,29,41–44] Ultrasound will affect both normal and damaged biologic tissues. It has been suggested that damaged tissue may be more responsive to ultrasound than normal tissue.[45] When ultrasound is applied for its thermal effects, nonthermal biophysical effects will also occur that may damage normal tissues.[31] If appropriate, treatment parameters are selected; however, nonthermal effects can occur with minimal thermal effects.

Thermal Effects

The ultrasound wave attenuates as it travels through the tissue. Attenuation is caused primarily by the conversion of ultrasound energy into heat through absorption and to some extent by scattering and beam deflection. Traditionally, ultrasound has been used primarily to produce a tissue temperature increase.[16,46–50] The clinical effects of using ultrasound to heat tissues are similar to other forms of heat that may be applied, including the following:[37]

1. An increase in the extensibility of collagen fibers found in tendons and joint capsules.
2. Decrease in joint stiffness.
3. Reduction of muscle spasm.
4. Modulation of pain.
5. Increased blood flow.
6. Mild inflammatory response that may help in the resolution of chronic inflammation.

It has been suggested that for the majority of these effects to occur the tissues must be raised to a level of 40–45°C for a minimum of 5 minutes.[18] Others are of the opinion that absolute temperatures are not the key, but rather how much the temperature rises above baseline.[36,37,51] They report that tissue temperature increases of 1°C increase metabolism and healing, increases of 2–3°C decrease pain and muscle spasm, and increases of 4°C or greater increase extensibility of collagen and decrease joint stiffness.[25,37,52] It has been shown that temperatures above 45°C may be potentially damaging to tissues, but patients usually experience pain prior to these extreme temperatures.[8]

Ultrasound at 1 MHz with an intensity of 1 W/cm² has been reported to raise soft tissue temperature by as much as 0.86°C/min in tissues with a poor vascular supply.[53] It has been shown that 3 MHz ultrasound at 1 W/cm² raises human patellar tendon temperatures 2°C/min.[27] In muscle, which is quite vascular, 1 and 3 MHz ultrasound at 1 W/cm² increase the temperature 0.2 and 0.6°C/min, respectively.[8] It has also been demonstrated that tissue temperature increases were significantly increased by preheating the treatment area prior to initiating ultrasound treatment.[54]

The primary advantage of ultrasound over other nonacoustic heating modalities is that tissues high in collagen, such as tendons, muscles, ligaments, joint capsules, joint menisci, intermuscular interfaces, nerve roots, periosteum, cortical bone, and other deep tissues, may be selectively heated to the therapeutic range without causing a significant tissue temperature increase in skin or fat.[55] Ultrasound will penetrate skin and fat with little attenuation.[56]

The thermal effects of ultrasound are related to frequency. As indicated earlier, an inverse relationship exists between depth of penetration and frequency. Most of the energy in a sound wave at 3 MHz will be absorbed in the superficial tissues. At 1 MHz, there will be less attenuation, and the energy will penetrate to the deeper tissues, selectively heating them. It has been suggested that 3 MHz ultrasound should be the recommended modality in the heating of tissue structures to a depth level of 2.5 cm. One megahertz treatment will not produce the temperatures (>4°C change or 40°C absolute temperature) needed to heat the structures of the body effectively.[57]

Heating will occur with both continuous and pulsed ultrasound, depending on the intensity of the total current being delivered to the patient.[58] Significant thermal effects will be induced whenever the upper end of the available intensity range is used. Regardless of whether ultrasound is pulsed or continuous, if the spatial-averaged temporal-averaged intensity is in the 0.1–0.2 W/cm² range, the intensity is too low to produce a tissue temperature increase and only nonthermal effects will occur.[18]

Unlike the other heating modalities discussed in this text, whenever ultrasound is used to produce thermal changes, nonthermal changes also simultaneously occur.[42] An understanding of these nonthermal changes, therefore, is essential.

Nonthermal Effects

The nonthermal effects of therapeutic ultrasound include **cavitation** and **acoustic microstreaming** (Figure 10–11). Cavitation is the formation of gas-filled bubbles that expand and compress owing to ultrasonically induced pressure changes in tissue fluids.[12,18] Cavitation may be classified as being either *stable* or *unstable*. In stable cavitation, the bubbles expand and contract in response to regularly repeated pressure changes over many acoustic-cycles. In unstable or transient cavitation, violent large excursions in bubble volume occur before implosion and collapse occur after only a few cycles. Therapeutic benefits are derived only from stable cavitation, whereas the collapse of bubbles is thought to create increased pressure and high temperatures that may cause local tissue damage. Unstable cavitation clearly should be avoided. It is likely that high intensity, low-frequency ultrasound may produce unstable cavitation, particularly if standing waves develop at tissue interfaces.[18]

Cavitation results in an increased flow in the fluid around these vibrating bubbles. Microstreaming is the unidirectional movement of fluids along the boundaries of cell membranes resulting from the mechanical pressure wave in an ultrasonic field.[12,18] Microstreaming

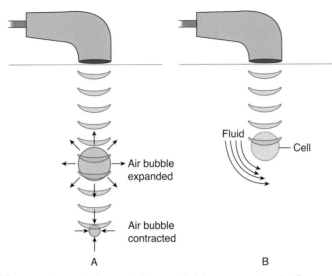

Figure 10–11. Nonthermal effects of ultrasound. (a) Cavitation is the formation of gas-filled bubbles, which expand and compress due to ultrasonically induced pressure changes in tissue fluids. (b) Microstreaming is the unidirectional movement of fluids along the boundaries of cell membranes resulting from the mechanical pressure wave in an ultrasonic field.

produces high-viscous stresses, which can alter cell membrane structure and function due to changes in cell membrane permeability to sodium and calcium ions important in the healing process. As long as the cell membrane is not damaged, microstreaming can be of therapeutic value in accelerating the healing process.[18]

It has been well documented that the nonthermal effects of therapeutic ultrasound in the treatment of injured tissues may be as important as, if not more important than, the thermal effects. Therapeutically significant nonthermal effects have been identified in soft tissue repair via stimulation of fibroblast activity, which produces an increase in protein synthesis, tissue regeneration, blood flow in chronically ischemic tissues, bone healing and repair of nonunion fractures, and phonophoresis.[45,59,60] Treatment with therapeutic levels of ultrasound may alter the course of the immune response. Ultrasound affects a number of biologic processes associated with injury repair.

The literature provides a number of examples in which exposure of cells to therapeutic ultrasound under nonthermal conditions has modified cellular functions. Nonthermal levels of ultrasound are reported to modulate membrane properties, alter cellular proliferation, and produce increases in proteins associated with inflammation and injury repair.[61] Combined, These data suggest that nonthermal effects of therapeutic ultrasound can modify the inflammatory response. The concept of the absorption of ultrasonic energy by enzymatic proteins leading to changes in the enzymes' activity is not novel.[61] However, recent reports demonstrating that ultrasound affects enzyme activity and possibly gene regulation provide sufficient data to present a probable molecular mechanism of ultrasound's nonthermal therapeutic action. The frequency resonance hypothesis describes two possible biologic mechanisms that may alter protein function as a result of the absorption of ultrasonic energy. First, absorption of mechanical energy by a protein may produce a transient conformational shift (modifying the three-dimensional structure) and alter the protein's functional activity. Second, the resonance or shearing properties of the wave (or both) may dissociate a multimolecular complex, thereby disrupting the complex's function.[61]

The nonthermal effects of cavitation and microstreaming can be maximized while minimizing the thermal effects by using a spatial-averaged temporal-averaged intensity of 0.1–0.2 W/cm^2 with continuous ultrasound. This range may also be achieved using a low-temporal-averaged intensity by pulsing a higher temporal-peak intensity of 1.0 W/cm^2 at a duty cycle of 20%, to give a temporal average intensity of 0.2 W/cm^2.

• Ideal BNR = 1:1

Clinical Decision-Making *Exercise 10–2*

A clinician is treating an ankle sprain on day 2 postinjury. To facilitate the healing process, she is using ultrasound for its nonthermal effects. What treatment parameters are required to ensure that there will be no thermal effects during the treatment?

ULTRASOUND TREATMENT TECHNIQUES

The principles and theories of therapeutic ultrasound are well understood and documented. However, specific practical recommendations as to how ultrasound may best be applied to a patient therapeutically are quite controversial and are based primarily on the experience of the clinicians who have used it. Even though there are numerous laboratory and clinically based reports in the literature, treatment procedures and parameters are highly variable, and many contradictory results and conclusions have been presented in the literature.[6]

Frequency of Treatment

It is generally accepted that acute conditions require more frequent treatments over a shorter period of time, whereas more chronic conditions require fewer treatments over a longer period of time.[6] Ultrasound treatments should begin as soon as possible following injury, ideally within hours but definitely within 48 hours to maximize effects on the healing process.[62–64] Acute conditions may be treated using low intensity or pulsed ultrasound once or even twice daily for 6–8 days until acute symptoms such as pain and swelling subside. In chronic conditions, when acute symptoms have subsided, treatment may be done on alternating days.[65] Ultrasound treatment should continue as long as there is improvement. Assuming that appropriate treatment parameters are chosen and the ultrasound generator is functioning properly, if no improvement is noted following three or four treatments, ultrasound should be discontinued, or different parameters (i.e., duty cycle, frequency) employed.

The question is often asked, How many ultrasound treatments can be given? Most of the research regarding treatment longevity has been performed on animals, and it takes quite a leap of logic to assume that the same negative effects would occur in humans. If the correct parameters are followed using a high-quality, recently calibrated ultrasound machine, treatments could occur daily for several weeks. In the past, it has been recommended that ultrasound be limited to 14 treatments in the majority of conditions, although this has not been documented scientifically. More than 14 treatments can reduce both red and white blood cell counts. After these 14 treatments some authors advise avoiding ultrasound use for 2 weeks.[5]

Duration of Treatment

In the past, modality textbooks have been quite vague with respect to treatment time, and generally the suggested duration has been too short.[33,66] Typically recommended treatment times have ranged between 5 and 10 minutes in length; however, these times may be insufficient. The length of the treatment is dependent on several factors: the size of the area to be treated; the intensity in W/cm^2; the frequency; and the desired temperature increase. As stated previously, specific temperature increases are required to achieve beneficial effects in tissue. The clinician must determine what the desired effects of the treatment are before a treatment duration is set (Figure 10–12). There is little research defining the application duration needed to increase tissue temperature to the target range during ultrasound at varying application intensities. Likewise, there are few data describing the effect of ultrasound intensity on the final temperature reached.[67]

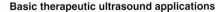

Basic therapeutic ultrasound applications

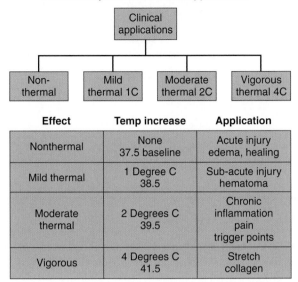

Effect	Temp increase	Application
Nonthermal	None 37.5 baseline	Acute injury edema, healing
Mild thermal	1 Degree C 38.5	Sub-acute injury hematoma
Moderate thermal	2 Degrees C 39.5	Chronic inflammation pain trigger points
Vigorous	4 Degrees C 41.5	Stretch collagen

Figure 10–12. It is important to have a treatment goal, and to adjust the ultrasound treatment time accordingly. (Courtesy of Castel JC: *Sound advice*, PTI, Inc., 1995. Reprinted with permission.).

An accepted recommendation is that ultrasound be administered in an area two times the ERA (roughly twice the size of the soundhead). If thermal effects are desired in an area larger than this, obviously the treatment time needs to be increased.

The higher the intensity applied in W/cm^2, the shorter the treatment time and vice versa. It just does not make clinical sense to treat one patient at 1 W/cm^2 and another at 2 W/cm^2 at identical treatment durations when both patients require vigorous heating. Based on this scenario, it could be hypothesized that patient two will produce tissue temperature increases of twice that of patient one. However, it has been shown that an ultrasound treatment using a 1 MHz frequency and an intensity level of 1.0 W/cm^2 increases intramuscular tissue to higher temperatures than a 2.0 W/cm^2 intensity at a depth of 4 cm.[67]

Ultrasound frequency (MHz) not only determines the depth of penetration but also determines the rate of heating. The energy produced with 3 MHz ultrasound is absorbed three times faster than that produced from 1 MHz ultrasound, the result of which is faster heating. Ultrasound at 3 MHz consistently heats tissues three times faster than 1 MHz, thus reducing the required treatment duration by one-third.[8,68] It has been questioned whether 1 MHz ultrasound is capable of reaching the desired 4-degree increase needed to achieve therapeutic effects.[69]

The desired temperature increase is also a factor in determining the duration of an ultrasound treatment. Table 10–4 displays the rate of muscle temperature increase per minute, per W/cm^2, and at various intensities and frequencies.[8] Based on this information, the clinician can determine the appropriate duration of an ultrasound treatment. For example, a patient has limited range of motion because of scar tissue buildup from a chronic hamstring strain at the musculotendinous junction. An appropriate goal would be to vigorously heat the muscle (an increase of 4°C) and immediately perform passive hamstring stretching. If 1 MHz ultrasound were used at an intensity of 2 W/cm^2, the 4°C increase would take about 10 minutes. At 2 minutes into the treatment, however, the patient complains that the treatment is too hot. Most of us would respond by decreasing the intensity, but we may forget to increase the treatment time. In this case, if we decreased the intensity to 1.5 W/cm^2, we would need to add 2 minutes to the treatment time in order to ensure a 4°C increase in muscle temperature. It is important to note that this chart requires a treatment size of two to three ERA, and these temperatures were reported in muscle. It has also been suggested that tendon heats over three times faster than muscle.[27]

Table 10–4 Ultrasound Rate of Heating per Minute[8]

INTENSITY (W/cm²)	1 MHz (°C)	3 MHz (°C)
0.5	0.04	0.3
1.0	0.2	0.6
1.5	0.3	0.9
2.0	0.4	1.4

Clinical Decision-Making *Exercise 10–3*

A patient is being treated with ultrasound for muscle guarding in the upper trapezius. The clinician wishes to achieve a mild heating effect by increasing the temperature by 30°C. If 1 MHz ultrasound at an intensity of 1.5 W/cm² is being used, how long must the treatment be to achieve this temperature increase?

Coupling Methods

- Water soluble gels = best coupling medium

The greatest amount of reflection of ultrasonic energy occurs at the air–tissue interface. To ensure that maximal energy will be transmitted to the patient, the face of the transducer should be parallel with the surface of the skin so that the ultrasound will strike the surface at a 90 degrees angle. If the angle between the transducer face and the skin is greater than 15 degrees, a large percentage of the energy will be reflected and the treatment effects will be minimal.[15]

Reflection at the air–tissue interface can be further reduced by applying the ultrasound via the use of some coupling agent. The purpose of the **coupling medium** is to exclude air from the region between the patient and the transducer so that ultrasound can get to the area to be treated.[17] The acoustical impedance of the coupling medium should match the impedance of the transducer and should be slightly higher than the skin. Also, the medium should have a low coefficient of absorption to minimize attenuation in the coupling medium. It is important that the medium remains free of air bubbles during treatment. The coupling agent should be viscous enough to act as a lubricant as the transducer is moved over the surface of the skin.[6]

The coupling medium should be applied to the skin surface and the ultrasound transducer should be in contact with the coupling medium before the power is turned on. If the transducer is not in contact with the skin via the coupling medium, or if for some reason the transducer is lifted away from the treatment area, the piezoelectric crystal may be damaged and the transducer can overheat.

A number of studies have looked at the efficacy of different coupling media in transmitting ultrasound.[18,26,56,70] Water, light oils, topical analgesics,[41,71] gel packs,[72,73] gel pads,[74] and various brands of ultrasonic gel have been recommended as coupling agents. The recommendations of these studies have proven to be somewhat contradictory. Essentially it appears that all of these agents have very similar acoustic properties and are effective as coupling agents.[75]

When using ultrasound in the treatment of patients with partial and full-thickness wounds, treatments are performed over a hydrogel sheet (i.e., Nu-Gel, ClearSite, etc.) or semipermeable film dressing (i.e., J&J Bioclusive, Tegaderm). Transmissivity of wound care products used to deliver acoustic energy during ultrasound treatment of wounds varies greatly among dressing products.[72]

Water is an effective coupling medium, but its low viscosity reduces its suitability in surface application. To reach the temperature increase obtained with gel, higher intensities need to be used with water.[76] Light oils, such as mineral oil and glycerol, have relatively higher

Table 10–5 Technique for Checking the Relative Transmission Capability of a Medium

Encircle the transducer with tape while leaving about 2 cm of tape exposed (making a tape tube).

Fill the tape tube with 1 cm thickness of ultrasound gel medium.

Fill the tube to the top with water.

Adjust the intensity and watch the water bubble.

Repeat the procedure but substitute the gel with the medium you are testing.

If the water has little or no bubbles, your desired medium is not a good couplant after all.

absorption coefficients and are somewhat difficult to clean up following treatment. Water-soluble gels seem to have the most desirable properties necessary for a good coupling medium.[56,75] Perhaps the only disadvantage is that the salts in the gel may damage the metal face of the transducer with improper cleaning. For convenience, some clinicians have used massage lotion instead of ultrasound gel; however, experience has revealed that massage lotion is not an adequate ultrasound conducting medium. Table 10–5 describes a technique that can be used to check the relative transmission capability of a medium.

Clinical Decision-Making *Exercise 10–4*

The clinician is using ultrasound to treat an inversion ankle sprain. Unfortunately, the ultrasound generator only has a 10 cm² transducer, and the clinician is worried about maintaining good direct contact over the treatment area. What alternative couple techniques could potentially be used?

Exposure Techniques

Direct Contact

Direct application of ultrasound involves actual contact between the applicator and the skin, with a sufficient amount of couplant between. A layer of gel should be applied to the treatment area in sufficient amounts to maintain good contact and lubrication between the transducer and the skin, but not so much that air pockets may form from movement of the transducer. A thin film of gel should also be applied directly to the transducer face before transmission begins (Figure 10–13).[6] A direct technique of exposure may be used as long as the surface being treated is larger than the diameter of the transducer. If a smaller surface area is to be treated, a smaller transducer should be used so that direct application can still be performed.

Heating the ultrasound gel prior to treatment has been recommended to improve the thermal effects of ultrasound in deeper tissues; however, this is not actually the case. Because ultrasound heats only through conversion of mechanical vibration to heat and not through conduction, heating the gel will have no effect in the deeper tissues.[77] The only rationale for heating cold ultrasound gel is strictly for patient comfort and compliance.

Recently several manufacturers of analgesic creams have been promoting their use as ultrasound couplants (i.e., Biofreeze, T-prep).[71,78–80,161] Patients are treated with ultrasound via a conducting medium of gel mixed with their product.[81,80] One company recommended a mixture of two parts gel to one part analgesic cream (this has recently been changed to 80% gel

• Ultrasound accelerates the inflammatory process.

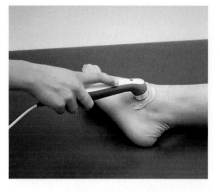

Figure 10–13. Ultrasound may be applied directly through some gel-like coupling medium.

to 20% cream), whereas another recommended a 50/50 ratio of ultrasound gel and their analgesic cream. Small mixtures of analgesic creams with 80% or 90% gel may produce significant heating, but as yet have not been tested. Some of these products have been shown to actually impede the transmission of ultrasound. Many of these over-the-counter medications presently used are only minimally effective as ultrasound couplants.[82] If a patient wants the added benefits of heat and analgesia, first massage the balm into the area; then apply 100% ultrasound gel followed by ultrasound. Perceptions of heat by the patient may not indicate actual temperature increases within the muscle when using analgesic creams.[80] Until further research is performed in this area, it is suggested that the practice of using analgesic creams mixed with ultrasound gel be discontinued when vigorous heating is desired. Figure 10–14 displays the results of research involving two such products and their effect on muscle temperature increase via ultrasound.

Treatment Protocols: Ultrasound
(Direct Coupling)

1. Apply indicated technique: Select continuous or pulsed output and verify output intensity is at 0 before turning unit power on.
2. Apply layer of coupling gel to treatment surface.
3. Establish treatment duration dependent on size of area to be treated (i.e., 5 minutes for each 16-square-inch area).
4. Maintain contact between soundhead and treatment surface, moving soundhead in circular or linear overlapping strokes at a rate of 2–4 inch/s; observe for air bubble formation.
5. Adjust treatment intensity: 0.5–1.0 W/cm² for superficial tissues and 1.0–2.0 W/cm² for deeper tissues.

FLEX-ALL V/S BIOFREEZE

Depth	50/50 flex-all; gel	50/50 biofreeze; gel	100% gel
3cm	2.8°C	1.8°C	3.4°C
5cm	1.8°C	1.3°C	2.5°C

Muscle temperature increase from continuous 1-MHz ultrasound at 1.5 W/cm² for 10 minutes.

Figure 10–14. Two popular analgesic creams were mixed with ultrasound gel and used as coupling media. Only the treatments that used 100% ultrasound gel as the couplant yielded temperatures consistent with vigorous heating. We conclude that these creams, although they might decrease pain perception, actually impede ultrasound transmission. *Note*: These manufacturers are now recommending mixtures of 80% ultrasound gel with 20% of their product.

Immersion

Although direct application with gel has been shown to be the most effective application technique, water immersion is warranted in some instances. The immersion technique is recommended if the area to be treated is smaller than the diameter of the available transducer or if the treatment area is irregular with bony prominences (Figure 10–15). A plastic, ceramic, or rubber basin should be used because a metal basin or whirlpool will reflect some of the ultrasound, increasing the intensity near the basin walls. Tap water seems to be just as effective as degassed water as a coupling medium for the immersion technique and less likely to produce surface heating than mineral oil or glycerin.[26,62] The transducer should be moved parallel to the surface being treated at a distance of 0.5–1 cm.[13] If air bubbles accumulate on the transducer or over the treatment area, they may be wiped away quickly during the treatment. In order to ensure adequate heating, the intensity should be increased, possibly as much as 50%.[83]

Treatment Protocols: Ultrasound
(Underwater Coupling)

1. Fill a plastic or ceramic nonconductive basin with tepid degassed water of sufficient depth to cover treatment surface.

2. Immerse the body part into the basin.

3. Establish treatment duration dependent on size of area to be treated (i.e., 5 minutes for each 16-square-inch area).

4. Maintain soundhead parallel to treatment surface at a distance of 0.5–3 cm, moving soundhead in circular or linear overlapping strokes at a rate of 2–4 inch/sec; observe for air bubble formation on soundhead and wipe away.

5. Adjust treatment intensity: 0.5–1.0 W/cm² for superficial tissues and 1.0–2.0 W/cm² for deeper tissues; intensity may need to be increased.

6. Monitor patient response during treatment; if patient reports warmth or ache, reduce intensity by 10% and continue treatment.

7. Fill a plastic or ceramic nonconductive basin with tepid degassed water of sufficient depth to cover treatment surface.

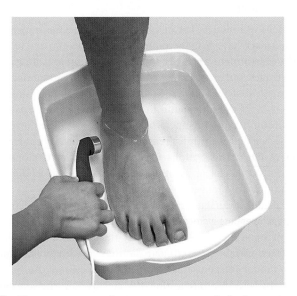

Figure 10–15. The immersion technique is recommended when using ultrasound over irregular surfaces.

Bladder Technique

If for some reason the treatment area cannot be immersed in water, a bladder technique can be used in which a balloon, surgical glove, or even a condom can be filled with water, and the ultrasound energy is transmitted from the transducer to the treatment surface through this bladder (Figure 10–16). Generally the use of the bladder technique is not recommended. Nevertheless it is occasionally used. Both sides of the balloon should be coated with gel to assure better contact. Recently, commercial gel packs have gained popularity and several studies have demonstrated their efficacy as a coupling medium.[72,73,84] Treatments using a bladder filled with either gel or silicone have also been used at higher ultrasound intensities.[70] When ultrasound is applied over bony prominences, a gel pad should be covered with ultrasound gel on both sides to ensure optimal heating[85] (Figure 10–16b).

Treatment Protocols: Ultrasound
(Bladder Coupling)

1. Fill a balloon with tepid, degassed water or use an Aquaflex Gel Pad.
2. Apply layer of coupling gel to bladder.
3. Apply layer of coupling gel to treatment surface.
4. Place bladder over treatment surface.
5. Establish treatment duration dependent on size of area to be treated (i.e., 5 minutes for each 16-square-inch area).
6. Maintain contact between soundhead and treatment surface, moving soundhead in circular or linear overlapping strokes at a rate of 2–4 inch/s; observe for air bubble formation.
7. Adjust treatment intensity: 0.5–1.0 W/cm² for superficial tissues and 1.0–2.0 W/cm² for deeper tissues; intensity may need to be increased.
8. Monitor patient response during treatment; if patient reports warmth or ache, reduce intensity by 10% and continue treatment.

Moving the Transducer

In the past, treatment techniques that involve both moving the transducer and holding the transducer stationary have been recommended. The stationary technique was most often used when the treatment area was small or when pulsed ultrasound was used at a low-temporal-averaged intensity. However, because of the nonuniformity of the ultrasound beam, the energy distribution in the tissue is uneven, thus creating potential tissue-damaging "hot spots."[13] If the ultrasound beam is stationary, the spatial-peak intensity determines the point of maximal temperature increase. With the moving technique, the spatial-averaged intensity gives the most reasonable measure of the average rate of heating within the treatment area.[12] This stationary technique has been demonstrated to produce disruption of blood flow, platelet aggregation, and damage to the venous system; therefore the stationary technique is no longer recommended.[86]

Moving the transducer during treatment leads to a more even distribution of energy within the treatment area, especially if the unit has a low BNR.[52] This can reduce the damaging effects of standing waves, particularly those that are most likely to occur at bone–tissue interfaces. Overlapping circular motions or a longitudinal stroking pattern can be used. Very similar intramuscular temperature increases can be observed among ultrasound treatments with transducer velocities of 2–3, 4–5, and 7–8 cm/s.[87] In general, it has been recommended that the transducer should be moved slowly at approximately 4 cm/s, covering a treatment area that is two to three times larger than the ERA of the

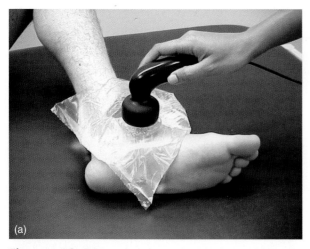

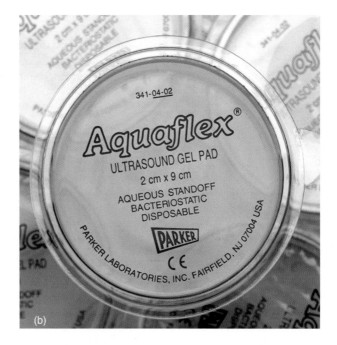

Figure 10–16. (a) Although not recommended, the bladder technique can be used over uneven surfaces. (b) A commercially available Aquaflex gel pad can be used for the same purposes as a bladder (Part b courtesy of Parker Laboratories Inc.).

transducer.[7,88] Movement speed of the transducer is BNR-dependent, and the higher the BNR the more important it is to move the transducer faster during treatment to avoid periosteal irritation and transient cavitation.[33,66] However, moving the transducer too rapidly decreases the total amount of energy absorbed per unit area. Rapid movement of the transducer causes the clinician to slip into treating a larger area; thus, the desired temperatures may not be attained.

Equipment with a low BNR usually allows for a slower stroking movement of the ultrasound transducer. Slow strokes are more controlled and can easily be contained to a small area (2 ERA). Slow movement of the transducer results in evenly distributed sound waves throughout the area, whereas a fast moving transducer will not allow for adequate absorption of the sound waves, and sufficient heating will not occur. If the patient complains of pain, decrease the output intensity, while making the appropriate adjustments in treatment duration. The transducer should be kept in maximum contact with the skin via some coupling agent.

During the administration of ultrasound, it is possible that the amount of pressure at the transducer may affect the physiologic response to and the outcome of the treatment.[89] It has been demonstrated that applying an excessive amount of pressure could decrease the acoustic transmissivity, damage the crystal in the transducer, or make the patient uncomfortable. It is recommended that the clinician apply firm, consistent pressure during treatment.[89]

An ultrasound unit currently on the market has an applicator with multiple piezoelectric crystals that are microprocessor controlled to move the ultrasound output, mimicking human movement, at the prescribed rate of 4 cm/s automatically without having to manually move the transducer (Figure 10–17).

Recording Ultrasound Treatments

It is recommended that the clinician report or record the specific parameters used in an ultrasound treatment when completing treatment records or progress notes so that the treatment may be reproduced or altered. The parameters that should be recorded include frequency, spatial-averaged temporal peak intensity, whether the beam is pulsed or continuous, the duty factor (if pulsed), effective radiating surface area of the transducer, duration of the treatment, and the number of treatments per week.[6] A typical treatment might be recorded as 3 MHz, at 1.0 W/cm², pulsed at 20% (0.2) duty factor, 5-cm transducer head, 5 minutes, four times per week.

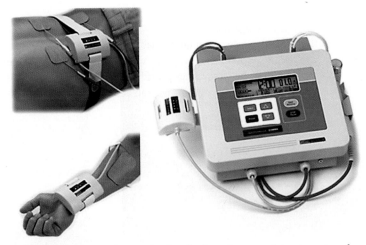

Figure 10–17. Autosound provides hands-free ultrasound treatment and combination ultrasound and electrical stimulation.

CLINICAL APPLICATIONS FOR THERAPEUTIC ULTRASOUND

Ultrasound is generally recognized clinically as one of the most widely used modalities in the treatment of many soft-tissue and bony lesions. Considering the extensive use of ultrasound in treating soft-tissue injuries, until the past decade there has been relatively little documented evidence from the medical community concerning the efficacy of this modality (however, research in this area is increasing). Many of the decisions as to how ultrasound should be used are empirically based on personal opinion and experience. This section summarizes the various clinical applications of therapeutic ultrasound used in a clinical setting.

Clinical Decision-Making *Exercise 10–5*

How may the clinician best use ultrasound to treat patellar tendinitis?

Soft-Tissue Healing and Repair

Soft-tissue healing and repair may be accelerated by both thermal and nonthermal ultrasound.[3,90–92] Repair of soft tissues involves three phases of healing: inflammation, proliferation, and remodeling. Ultrasound does not seem to have any anti-inflammatory effects; rather, it is thought to accelerate the inflammatory phase of healing. It also appears the ultrasound has little if any effect in treating delayed onset muscle soreness.[155]

It has been shown that a single treatment with ultrasound can stimulate the release of histamine from mast cells.[93] The mechanism for this may be attributed primarily to nonthermal effects involving cavitation and streaming that increase the transport of calcium ions across the cell membrane, thus stimulating release of histamine by the mast cells.[18] Histamine attracts polymorphonuclear leukocytes that "clean up" debris from the injured area, along with monocytes whose primary function is to release chemotactic agents and growth factors that stimulate fibroblasts and endothelial cells to form a collagen-rich, well-vascularized tissue used for the development of new connective tissue that is essential for rapid repair. Thus, ultrasound can be effective in facilitating the process of inflammation, and therefore healing, if applied after bleeding has stopped but still within the first few hours after injury during the early stages of inflammation.[18,157] It has been suggested that this response occurs using pulsed ultrasound at 0.5 W/cm^2 with a duty cycle of 20% for 5 minutes or continuous ultrasound at 0.1 W/cm^2.[42]

These treatments have been described as being "proinflammatory" and are of value in accelerating repair in short-term or acute inflammation.[94] However, in chronic inflammatory conditions, the proinflammatory effects are of questionable value.[93] If an inflammatory stimulus such as overuse remains, the response to therapeutic ultrasound is of questionable value.[84]

Pitting edema is a condition that sometimes provides a challenge for clinicians. Pitting edema may be treated with continuous 3 MHz ultrasound at intensities of 1–1.5 W/cm². The heat seems to liquefy the "gel-like" cellular debris. The limb is then elevated, or massaged, or EMS is used to pump the fluid and promote lymphatic drainage.

During the proliferative phase of healing, a connective tissue matrix is produced into which new blood vessels will grow. Fibroblasts are mainly responsible for producing this connective tissue. Fibroblasts exposed to therapeutic ultrasound are stimulated to produce more collagen that gives connective tissue most of its strength.[95] Again, cavitation and streaming alter cell membrane permeability to calcium ions that facilitate increases in collagen synthesis and in tensile strength. The intensity levels of therapeutic ultrasound that produce these changes during the proliferative phase are too low to be entirely thermal. It has been demonstrated that heating with continuous ultrasound may be more effective than stretching alone for increasing the extensibility of dense connective tissue.[96]

Ultrasound does not appear to be effective in enhancing postexercise muscle strength recovery or in diminishing delayed-onset muscle soreness.[97,98,155] Although treatment with pulsed ultrasound can promote the satellite cell proliferation phase of the myoregeneration, it does not seem to have significant effects on the overall morphologic manifestations of muscle regeneration.[99]

Scar Tissue and Joint Contracture

During remodeling, collagen fibers are realigned along lines of tensile stresses and strains, forming scar tissue. This process may continue for months or even years. In scar tissue, collagen never attains the same pattern and remains weaker and less elastic than normal tissue prior to injury. Scar tissue in tendons, ligaments, and capsules surrounding joints can produce joint contractures that limit range of motion. Increased tissue temperatures increase the elasticity and decrease the viscosity of collagen fibers. Because the deeper tissues surrounding joints that most often restrict range are rich in collagen, ultrasound is the treatment modality of choice.[13,100]

A number of studies have investigated the effects of ultrasound treatment on scar tissue and joint contracture. Ultrasound has been demonstrated to increase mobility in mature scars.[101] A greater residual increase in tissue length with less potential damage is produced through preheating with ultrasound prior to stretching, or by putting the joint on stretch while insonating.[10,102,103] Tissue extensibility increases when continuous ultrasound is applied at higher intensities causing vigorous heating of tissues.[104] Thigh, periarticular structures, and scar tissues become significantly more extensible following treatment with ultrasound involving thermal effects at intensities of 1.2–2.0 W/cm².[102] Scar tissue can be softened if treated with ultrasound at an early stage.[64] Dupuytren's contracture shows a beneficial effect on long-standing contracted bands of scar and a decrease in pain when treated early on with ultrasound.[105]

The majority of the earlier studies attributed the effectiveness of ultrasound to thermal effects and used continuous moderate intensities between 0.5 and 2.0 W/cm².

Stretching of Connective Tissue

Collagenous tissue when stressed is fairly rigid, yet when heated it becomes much more yielding.[102,104] However, the combination of heat and stretching theoretically produces a residual lengthening of connective tissue, which increases according to the force applied.[106]

Prevent heating and stretching to improve range of motion are commonly recommended before exercise in an attempt to prevent musculotendinous injury. Active exercise appears to be more effective than ultrasound for increasing intramuscular temperature; however, the temperature increases do not appear to influence range of motion.[107]

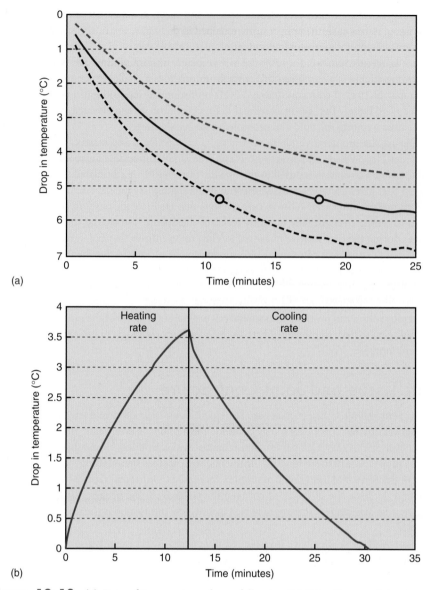

Figure 10–18. (a) Rate of temperature decay following 3 MHz ultrasound treatments. Solid line = mean temperature decay. Hatched line = 1 standard deviation above and below the mean. Oval = time to pre-ultrasound baseline. (b) Rate of temperature increase during 1 MHz ultrasound applied at 1.5W/cm², followed by the rate of temperature decay at termination of insonation. The thermistor was 4 cm deep in the triceps surae muscle.[109,110]

The time period of vigorous heating when tissues will undergo the greatest extensibility and elongation is referred to as the ***stretching window.***[10,103] The existence of this stretching window is theoretical and has not been conclusively demonstrated to exist.[108] An analogy to a plastic spoon helps explain this concept.[52] When a plastic spoon is dipped in hot water it softens, and by pulling on the ends, we are able to stretch it. As the plastic cools, however, it hardens and is no longer able to be stretched. Likewise, if we vigorously heat tissue it becomes more pliable and less resistant to stretch, yet as the tissue cools it resists stretching and can actually be damaged if too great a force is applied.

The rate of tissue cooling following continuous ultrasound at both 1 and 3 MHz frequencies has been determined (Figure 10–18).[10,103] Thermistor probes were inserted 1.2 cm below the skin's surface and ultrasound was applied. The treatment raised the tissue temperature 5.3°C for the 3-MHz frequency. The average time it took for the temperature to drop each degree as expressed in minutes and seconds was: 1°C = 1:20; 2°C = 3:22; 3°C = 5:50; 4°C = 9:13; 5°C = 14:55. In this case, the temperature remained in the vigorous heating phase for only 3.3 minutes following an ultrasound treatment.

The same methods were used to determine the stretching window at 1 MHz. The temperature was recorded 4 cm deep in the muscle. It took 2 minutes for the temperature to drop 1°C, and a total of 5.5 minutes to drop 2°C. The deeper muscle cools at a slower rate than superficial muscle because the added tissue serves as a barrier to escaping heat. Regardless, tissue heated by ultrasound loses its heat at a fairly rapid rate; therefore, stretching, friction massage, or joint mobilization should be performed immediately postultrasound. To increase the duration of the stretching window, it is recommended that stretching be done during and immediately after ultrasound application.

It appears that ultrasound and stretching increase range of motion more than stretching alone immediately following treatment. However, there is no significant difference between the two techniques over the long term.[111]

Chronic Inflammation

Few clinical or experimental studies discuss the effects of therapeutic ultrasound on the chronic inflammations (tendinitis, bursitis, epicondylitis). Treatment of bicipital tendinitis with ultrasound decreases pain and tenderness and increases range of motion.[112] Although earlier studies have shown ultrasound to be effective in treating pain and increasing range of motion in subacromial bursitis, a more recent study shows no improvement in the general condition of the shoulder when using continuous ultrasound at 1.0–2.0 W/cm^2.[109] Ultrasound applied at an intensity of 1.0–2.0 W/cm^2 at a 20% duty cycle significantly enhanced recovery in patients with epicondylitis.[84]

In these chronic inflammatory conditions, ultrasound seems to be effective in increasing blood flow for healing and for pain reduction through heating.[13]

In acute ligament injury, pulsed ultrasound therapy may stimulate inflammation.[113]

Bone Healing

Since bone is a type of connective tissue, damaged bone progresses through the same stages of healing as other soft tissues, the major difference being the deposition of bone salts.[114] Several researchers have observed acceleration of fracture repair following treatment with ultrasound.[60,115–117] It has been shown that the application of ultrasound within the first 2 weeks postfibular fracture during the inflammatory and proliferative stages increases the rate of healing. Treatment parameters were 0.5 W/cm^2 at a duty cycle of 20% for 5 minutes, four times per week.[118] Ultrasound was effectively used to stimulate bone repair following osteotomy and fixation of the tibia in rabbits.[119]

Treatment given during the first 2 weeks after injury is sufficient to accelerate bony union. However, ultrasound given to an unstable fracture during the phase of cartilage formation may cause proliferation of cartilage and consequent delayed bony union.[3] It appears that nonthermal mechanisms are most responsible for the accelerated bone healing.[6]

Several researchers have looked at the use of ultrasound over growing epiphyses.[2,120,121] Although results have been somewhat inconsistent, some form of damage was observed in each study, including premature closure of the epiphysis, epiphyseal displacement, widening of the epiphyseal, fractures, condyle erosion, and shortening of the bones. The degree of destruction appears to be unpredictable; therefore, it is not recommended that ultrasound be applied to growing bone.[5]

Ultrasonic Bone Growth Stimulators

Two types of bone growth stimulators currently exist: electrical and ultrasonic. An electrical bone growth stimulator (EBS) uses electric current to promote bone healing. The current may generate a direct, direct pulsating, or pulsating electromagnetic field (PEMF). An ultrasonic bone growth stimulator uses ultrasound for accelerated fracture healing.[115] It is a pulsed, low-intensity, ultrasound device that provides nonthermal, specifically programmed

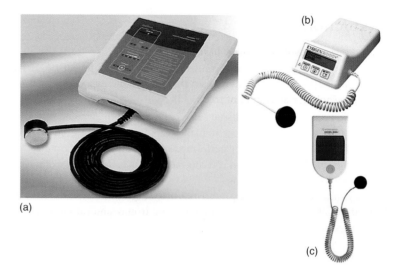

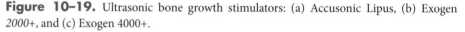

Figure 10–19. Ultrasonic bone growth stimulators: (a) Accusonic Lipus, (b) Exogen *2000+*, and (c) Exogen 4000+.

ultrasonic stimulation to accelerate bone repair. The device is characterized by a main operating unit with an external power supply connected to a treatment head module affixed to a mounting fixture centered over the fracture site (Figure 10–19). This nonthermal device is specifically programmed to promote accelerated fracture healing, but does not increase the temperature of the tissue and therefore can be administered by the patient at home in one daily 20-minute treatment. Healing times of fresh fractures appear to be significantly decreased among those receiving low-intensity ultrasound stimulation.[115]

Absorption of Calcium Deposits

No documented evidence exists that ultrasound treatment can cause reabsorption of calcium deposits. However, it has been suggested that ultrasound may help reduce inflammation surrounding a calcium deposit, thus reducing pain and improving function.[13]

Myositis ossificans is calcification within the muscle following acute or repeated trauma. This condition may be exacerbated by applying heat or massaging the area. Thus ultrasound is contraindicated in acute hematomas, and it is a large leap of logic to assume it capable of reducing the size of the mature calcification.

Ultrasound in Assessing Stress Fractures

The use of ultrasound as a reliable technique for identifying stress fractures has been recommended.[69] Using a continuous beam at 1 MHz with a small transducer and a water-based coupling medium, the clinician moves the transducer slowly over the injured area while gradually increasing the intensity from 0 to 2.0 W/cm^2 until the patient indicates that he or she feels uncomfortable (periosteal irritation), at which point the ultrasound is turned off. If the patient reports a feeling of pressure, bruising, or aching, then a stress fracture may be present. Another technique is to first apply 1 MHz continuous ultrasound in the stationary mode to the contralateral limb. The intensity is slowly increased until the individual reports pain. This is then repeated on the affected area. Typically with a stress fracture, pain will be reported at a lower intensity than on the opposite site. Either a radiograph or a bone scan is then necessary to confirm this diagnosis.

Clinical Decision-Making *Exercise 10–6*

An clinician is treating a patient with a myofascial trigger point. She has been using thermal ultrasound for about 1 week with less than desirable results. How might she alter the treatment to possibly achieve better results?

Pain Reduction

Many of the studies discussed previously have noted that reduction in pain occurs with ultrasound treatment, even though the treatment was given for other purposes. Several mechanisms have been proposed that might explain this pain reduction. Ultrasound is thought to elevate the threshold for activation of free nerve endings through thermal effects.[17] Heat produced by ultrasound in large-diameter myelinated nerve fibers may reduce pain through the gating mechanism.[6,122] Ultrasound may also increase nerve conduction velocity in normal nerves, creating a counterirritant effect through thermal mechanisms.[31] There is no consensus of opinion in the literature as to the exact mechanism of pain reduction.

Pain reduction following application of ultrasound has been reported in patients with lateral epicondylitis,[101] shoulder pain, plantar fasciitis, surgical wounds, bursitis, prolapsed intervertebral disks, ankle sprains, reflex sympathetic dystrophy, and various other soft-tissue injuries.[9,91,101,123–127]

Plantar Warts

Plantar warts are occasionally seen on the weight-bearing areas of the feet owing to either a virus or trauma. These lesions contain thrombosed capillaries in a whitish-colored soft core covered by hyperkeratotic epithelial tissue. Among other more conventional techniques, several studies have recommended ultrasound as being an effective painless method for eliminating plantar warts.[53,128,129] Intensities average 0.6 W/cm^2 for 7–15 minutes.[130]

Placebo Effects

Whereas the physiologic effects of ultrasound have been discussed in detail, it should also be mentioned that ultrasound can have significant therapeutic psychologic effects.[18] A number of studies have demonstrated a placebo effect in patients receiving sham ultrasound.[48,93,131]

CASE STUDY 10–1
ULTRASOUND

Background: An 18-year-old college freshman sustained a fracture of the fifth metacarpal of the left hand during a prank in the dormitory. The fracture required gauntlet cast immobilization for 6 weeks. At the time of cast removal the patient noted significant restriction of motion and weakness in the left wrist. A referral was initiated. Physical examination revealed flexion 0–45 degrees, extension 0–30 degrees with radial and ulnar deviation unaffected. There was point tenderness at the callus site on the shaft of the fifth metacarpal. Finger motion was grossly within normal limits at all constituent joints.

Impression: Wrist capsule motion restriction secondary to immobilization, muscular weakness secondary to immobilization.

Treatment Plan: A course of therapeutic ultrasound was initiated to decrease joint stiffness through increased collagen-connective tissue extensibility. Given the small and irregular surface of the wrist joint, underwater coupling was chosen as the mode of ultrasound delivery. After checking the left wrist and hand for any rashes or open wounds and verifying that sensation and circulation were normal in the distal portion of the extremity the left forearm, wrist, and hand were immersed in a plastic basin filled with warm water. An ultrasound treatment of 1.5 W/cm^2 for 6 minutes was applied to the dorsal aspect of the left wrist. Patient reported a mild sensation of warmth. At the conclusion of the treatment the patient was instructed in active and active-assistive wrist mobilization exercises.

Response: Following initial ultrasound treatment and exercise patient experienced a 10-degree improvement in both flexion and extension range of motion. At the completion of the sixth treatment wrist range of motion was within normal limits, and the patient was aggressively pursuing a wrist curl strengthening regimen. Ultrasound treatments were discontinued at that time with efforts focused on strengthening and functional use of the left upper extremity.

The rehabilitation professional employs therapeutic agent modalities to create an optimum environment for tissue healing

---

CASE STUDY 10–1 *(continued)*
ULTRASOUND

while minimizing the symptoms associated with the trauma or condition.

Discussion Questions

- What tissues were injured or affected?
- What symptoms were present?
- What phase of the injury healing continuum did the patient present for care in?
- What are the therapeutic agent modality's biophysical effects (direct, indirect, depth, and tissue affinity)?

- What are the therapeutic agent modality's indications and contraindications?
- What are the parameters of the therapeutic agent modality's application, dosage, duration, and frequency in this case study?
- What are the parameters of the therapeutic agent modality's application, dosage, duration, and frequency in this case study? What other therapeutic agent modalities could be utilized to treat this injury or condition? Why? How?

CASE STUDY 10-2
ULTRASOUND

Background: A 12-year-old junior high school student sustained a deep bruise of the left quadriceps muscle in a fall from his skateboard. The parents were advised by their pediatrician to apply cold initially and then moist heat until the problem resolved. At this time, 1 month postinjury, there remains significant restriction of left knee motion. A referral was initiated to physical therapy at the parent's request. Physical examination revealed active knee motion of only 10–65 degrees. There was point tenderness and a well-demarcated hematoma palpable in the middle third of the vastus lateralis.

Impression: Knee motion restriction secondary to soft-tissue contusion and hematoma formation.

Treatment Plan: A course of pulsed therapeutic ultrasound was initiated to decrease the hematoma formation through increased collagen-connective tissue extensibility and reabsorption of the extracellular debris from the original contusion. The patient reported a mild sensation of warmth. At the conclusion of the treatment, the patient was instructed in active and active-assistive knee range-of-motion exercises.

Response: Following initial US treatment and exercise, patient experienced a 10-degree improvement in knee flexion and extension range of motion. At the completion of the tenth treatment session, knee range of motion was within normal limits, and the patient was aggressively pursuing a quadriceps-strengthening regimen. Ultrasound treatments were discontinued at that time with efforts focused on strengthening and functional use of the left lower extremity.

The rehabilitation professional employs physical agent modalities to create an optimum environment for tissue healing while minimizing the symptoms associated with the trauma or condition.

Discussion Questions

- What tissues were injured/affected?
- What symptoms were present?
- What phase of the injury-healing continuum did the patient present for care in?
- What are the physical agent modality's biophysical effects (direct/indirect/depth/tissue affinity)?
- What are the physical agent modality's indications/contraindications?
- What are the parameters of the physical agent modality's application/dosage/duration/frequency in this case study?
- What other physical agent modalities could be utilized to treat this injury or condition? Why? How?

Further Discussion Questions

- Which ultrasound frequency would be optimal for this patient's condition?
- Could you utilize continuous ultrasound output? Why? Why not?
- What would be your response to the patient's complaint of a "dull ache" during the treatment?
- Given the patient's age, are there any additional precautions you should take in utilizing ultrasound?

PHONOPHORESIS

Phonophoresis is a technique in which ultrasound is used to enhance delivery of a selected medication into the tissues.[108,154] Perhaps the greatest advantage of phonophoresis is that medication can be delivered via a safe, painless, noninvasive technique as is the case with iontophoresis (discussed in Chapter 6) that uses electrical energy to deliver a medication. It is thought that active transport occurs as a result of both thermal and nonthermal mechanisms that together increase permeability of the stratum corneum, although using thermal parameters seems to be most beneficial.[15] This allows a medication to diffuse across the skin because of differences in concentration from the outside to the inside. Although the medication tends to follow the path of the beam, it must be stressed that once the medication penetrates the stratum corneum, the vascular circulation will cause diffusion from the highly concentrated delivery site, spreading it throughout the body.[108]

Unlike iontophoresis, phonophoresis transports whole molecules into the tissues as opposed to ions.[78] Consequently phonophoresis is not as likely to damage or burn skin. Also, the potential depth of penetration with phonophoresis is substantially greater than with iontophoresis.

Medications commonly applied through phonophoresis most often are either anti-inflammatories such as hydrocortisone, cortisol, salicylates, or dexamethasone or analgesics such as lidocaine. When applying phonophoresis, it is important to select the appropriate drug for the pathology. Because phonophoresis may increase drug penetration, it may also increase the clinical benefits as well as the risks of topical drug application.[132] The clinician should remember that most of the medications used in phonophoresis must be prescribed by a physician.

The most widespread use of the phonophoresis technique has been to deliver hydrocortisone, which has anti-inflammatory effects. Typically, either 1 or 10% hydrocortisone cream is used in treatments along with thermal ultrasound.[133] The 10% hydrocortisone preparation appears to be superior to the 1% preparation.[134] Several studies have looked at the efficacy of this technique.[135,136] Using phonophoresis with hydrocortisone was shown to be superior to ultrasound alone in alleviating pain and reducing inflammation in patients with arthritic disorders.[120] It has been used in treating patients with various inflammatory disorders including bursitis, tendinitis, and neuritis.[134,153] It has also been used to treat temporomandibular joint dysfunction.[137,138] Griffin,[99] Kleinkort,[134] and coworkers have demonstrated the effective penetration of corticosteroids into tissue with ultrasound. However, Benson and McElnay[139] have shown that many phonophoresis treatments are ineffective.

It appears that many clinicians are now using dexamethasone sodium phosphate (Decadron) as an alternative to hydrocortisone.[140] Dexamethasone is best used with thermal ultrasound for 2–3 days.[50,60] Ketoprofen has also been used with phonophoresis.[141]

Salicylates are compounds that evoke a number of pharmocologic effects including analgesia and decreased inflammation due to a reduction in prostaglandins. There are few reports that suggest that phonophoresis using salicylates enhances analgesic or anti-inflammatory effects. However, it has been reported that salicylate phonophoresis may be used to decrease delayed-onset muscle soreness without promoting cellular changes that mimic an inflammatory response.[142]

Lidocaine is a commonly used local anesthetic drug. The use of phonophoresis with lidocaine was found to be effective in treating a series of trigger points.[143]

The efficacy of various coupling media has been discussed previously. The addition of an active ingredient into the coupling medium is common practice. However, topical pharmacologic products are usually not formulated to optimize their efficiency as ultrasound coupling media.[139,158] For example, 1 or 10% hydrocortisone usually comes in a thick, white cream base that has been demonstrated to be a poor conductor of ultrasound. Clinicians have tried mixing this preparation with ultrasound gel (which is known to be a good transmitter) without improvement in transmission capabilities. The use of topical preparations with poor transmission capabilities may negate the effectiveness of ultrasound therapy. Unfortunately few suitable products are available, and there is clearly a need for appropriate active ingredients in gel

Table 10–6 Ultrasound Transmission by Phonophoresis Media[132]	
PRODUCT	TRANSMISSION RELATIVE TO WATER (%)
MEDIA THAT TRANSMIT ULTRASOUND WELL	
Lidex gel, fluocinonid 0.05%[*]	97
Thera-Gesic cream, methyl salicylate 15%[†]	97
Mineral oil[‡]	97
US gel[§]	96
US lotion[‖]	90
Betamethasone 0.05% in US gel[§]	88
MEDIA THAT TRANSMIT ULTRASOUND POORLY	
Diprolene ointment, betamethasone 0.05%[#]	36
Hydrocortisone (HC) powder 1%[b] in US gel[§]	29
HC powder 10%[†] in US gel[§]	7
Cortril ointment, HC 1%[††]	0
Eucerin cream[‡‡]	0
HC cream 1%[§§]	0
HC cream 10%[§§]	0
HC cream 10%[§§] mixed with equal weight US gel[§]	0
Myoflex cream, trolamine salicylate 10%[‡‡]	0
Triamcinolone acetonide cream 0.1%[§§]	0
Velva HC cream 10%[†]	0
Velva HC cream 10%[†] with equal weight US gel[§]	0
White petrolatum[¶¶]	0
OTHER	
Chempad-L[##]	68
Polyethylene wrap[***]	98

[*]Syntex Laboratories Inc, 3401 Hillview Ave., PO Box 10850, Palo Alto, CA 94303.
[†]Missions Pharmacal Co, 1325 E. Durango, San Antonio, TX 78210.
[‡]Pennex Corp, Eastern Ave. at Pennex Dr., Verona, PA 15147.
[§]Ultraphonic, Pharmaceutical Innovations Inc., 897 Frelinghuysen Dr., Newark, NJ 07114.
[‖]Polysonic, Parker Laboratories Inc, 307 Washington St., Orange, NJ 07050.
[#]Schering Corp., Galloping Hill Rd., Kenilworth, NJ 07033.
[††]Pfizer Labs Division, Pfizer Inc., 253 E 42nd St., New York, NY 10017.
[‡‡]Beiersdorf Inc., PO Box 5529, Norwalk, CT 06856-5529.
[§§]E Fougera & Co., 60 Baylis Rd., Melville, NY 11747.
[¶¶]Universal Cooperatives Inc., 7801 Metro Pkwy., Minneapolis, MN 55420.
[##]Henley International, 104 Industrial Blvd., Sugar Land, TX 77478.
[***]*Saran* Wrap, Dow Brands Inc., 9550 Zionsville Rd., Indianapolis, IN 46268.
From Cameron M, Monroe L. Relative transmission of ultrasound by media customarily used for phonophoresis. *Phys Ther.* 1992;72(2):142–148.
Reprinted with permission from the American Physical Therapy Association.

form. Table 10–6 provides a list of transmission capabilities of various commercially available phonophoresis media.[132]

Because research has shown some of these medications to impede the ultrasound,[50,82] one suggestion is to apply the medication and gel separately. This is accomplished by rubbing the medication directly onto the surface of the treatment area and then applying gel couplant followed by the application of ultrasound. With the direct technique transmission gel should be applied, and with immersion the treatment area with the preparation applied is simply treated underwater.

Both pulsed and continuous ultrasound have been used in phonophoresis. Continuous ultrasound at an intensity great enough to produce thermal effects may induce a proinflammatory response.[42] If the goal is to decrease inflammation, pulsed ultrasound with low spatial-averaged temporal peak intensity may be the best choice.[5] If the treatment goal is to reduce pain, it has been demonstrated that regardless of whether pulsed phonophoresis was used or not, stretching, strengthening, and cryotherapy were significantly more effective in decreasing levels of perceived pain.[144]

Treatment Protocols: Phonophoresis

1. Cleanse treatment surface with alcohol or soap and water.
2. Apply medication in glycerol cream, oil, or other vehicle in lieu of coupling gel.
3. Establish treatment duration dependent upon size of area to be treated (i.e., 5 minutes for each 16-square-inch area).
4. Maintain contact between soundhead and treatment surface, moving soundhead in circular or linear overlapping strokes at a rate of 2–4 inch/s; observe for air bubble formation.
5. Adjust treatment intensity: 0.5–1.0 W/cm^2 for superficial tissues and 1.0–2.0 W/cm^2 for deeper tissues. Intensity may need to be decreased.
6. Monitor patient response during treatment; if patient reports warmth or ache, reduce intensity by 10% and continue treatment.
7. Cleanse treatment surface with alcohol or soap and water.

Clinical Decision-Making *Exercise 10–7*

A clinician is treating a patient who has painful muscle spasms of the entire low back on both sides. How can the clinician use ultrasound to treat this problem?

USING ULTRASOUND IN COMBINATION WITH OTHER MODALITIES

In a clinical setting, it is not uncommon to combine modalities to accomplish a specific treatment goal. Ultrasound is frequently used with other modalities including hot packs, cold packs, and electrical stimulating currents. Unfortunately, there is very little documented evidence in the literature to substantiate the effectiveness of ultrasound and electrical-currents; however, recent studies of cooling or heating the area prior to ultrasound application have produced interesting results.[22,97,145] In fact it is possible that combining treatment modalities may actually interfere with the effectiveness of a treatment.[146]

Ultrasound and Hot Packs

Hot packs, like continuous or high-intensity ultrasound, are used primarily for their thermal effects. Heat is effective in reducing muscle spasm and muscle guarding and is useful in pain reduction. For these reasons heat and ultrasound used in combination can be effective for accomplishing these treatment goals.[147] A couple of studies have shown that a 15-minute hot pack application prior to ultrasound had an additive heating effect.[54,148] It was suggested that the ultrasound treatment duration can be decreased 3–5 minutes when tissues are preheated with hot packs.[28] However, it should be pointed out that because hot packs produce an increase in blood flow particularly to the superficial tissues, creating a less dense medium for transmission of ultrasound, attenuation may be increased and the depth of penetration of ultrasound reduced.

Ultrasound and Cold Packs

Some authors have provided a rationale for ultrasound use immediately after ice.[162] According to this premise, the application of a cold pack to human tissues initiates physiologic responses such as vasoconstriction and decreased blood flow. Thus cooling the area not only results in decreased local temperature, but it may assist in temporarily increasing the density of the tissue to be heated. This occurs by decreasing superficial attenuation and facilitating transmission to deeper tissues and consequently improving the thermal effects of ultrasound.[37,97,145] Although this theory sounds good, two recent studies appear to refute such claims.[97,145] Whether an ice pack was applied for 5 or 15 minutes, significant cooling took place in the muscle, reducing the rate and intensity of muscle temperature rise via ultrasound (Figure 10–20). It just does not make sense to cool something that you immediately want to heat.

When treating acute and postacute injuries, however, the combination of cold to reduce blood flow (i.e., swelling) and produce analgesia and low-intensity ultrasound for its nonthermal effects that promote soft-tissue healing may be the treatment of choice. Cold packs are most often used for analgesia and to decrease blood flow acutely following injury. Because cold is such an effective analgesic, caution must be exercised when using ultrasound at higher intensities that produce thermal effects since the patient's perception of temperature and pain

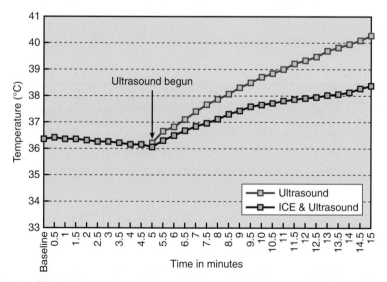

Figure 10–20. When an ice pack was applied for 5 minutes, it impeded the heat produced from ultrasound. The increase in muscle temperature was greater and faster during the ultrasound treatment (increase of 4°C) than during the ice/ultrasound treatment (increase of 1.8°C).(From Draper DO, Schulthies S, Sorvisto P, Hautala A. Temperature changes in deep muscles of humans during ice and ultrasound therapies: an in-vivo study. *J Orthop & Sports Phys Therapy.* 1995;21:153–157).

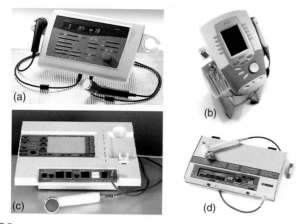

Figure 10–21. Combination ultrasound and electrical stimulating units: (a) Vectorsonic Combi, (b) Intellect Legend XT Combination System, (c) MedCon VC, and (d) Theramini 3C.

are diminished. Pulsed ultrasound, however, could be used after ice application if the goal is pain reduction and healing in the acute stage.[25,52]

Ultrasound and Electrical Stimulation

Ultrasound and electrical stimulating currents are frequently used in combination[163] (Figure 10–21). Using these two modalities in combination is thought to have positive clinical benefits.[149] Electrical stimulating currents are used for analgesia or producing muscle contraction. Ultrasound and electrical stimulating currents in combination have been recommended in the treatment of myofascial trigger points.[150,151] Both modalities provide analgesic effects, and both have been shown to be effective in reducing the pain–spasm–pain cycle, although the specific mechanisms responsible are not clearly understood.

Electrical stimulating currents were discussed in Chapter 5. When using ultrasound and electrical stimulating currents together, the ultrasound transducer serves as one electrode and thus delivers both acoustic energy and electrical energy. (Figure 10–22) The electrical energy

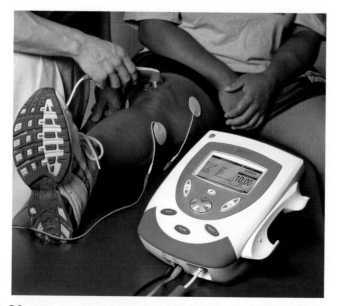

Figure 10–22. When using ultrasound and electrical stimulating currents together, the ultrasound transducer serves as one electrode and thus delivers both acoustic energy and electrical energy.

should be sufficient to cause a muscle contraction when the transducer passes over the trigger point, while the ultrasound should cause at least a moderate increase in tissue temperature. Because trigger points are found within the muscle, it is likely that 3 MHz ultrasound will be more effective in reaching the deeper tissue. The transducer should be moved slowly (4 cm/s) in a small circular pattern over the trigger point. Stretching the muscle during the application of ultrasound and an electrical stimulating current can also be helpful in treating a myofascial trigger point.

TREATMENT PRECAUTIONS

Table 10–7 provides a summary of indications and contraindications for using therapeutic ultrasound. In addition, there are a number of treatment precautions to the use of therapeutic ultrasound.

1. The use of continuous ultrasound with a high spatial-averaged temporal peak intensity should be avoided in acute and postacute conditions because of the associated thermal effects.
2. Caution should be used when treating areas of decreased sensation, particularly when there is a problem in perceiving pain and temperature.
3. In areas of decreased circulation, caution must be exercised owing to excessive heat build-up that can potentially damage tissues.
4. Individuals with vascular problems involving thrombophlebitis should not receive ultrasound because of the possibility of dislodging a clot and creating an embolus.
5. Ultrasound should not be applied around the eye because heat is not dissipated well, and both the lens and the retina may be damaged.
6. Ultrasound should not be applied over reproductive organs, especially the testes because temporary sterility may result. Caution should be used in treating the abdominal region of the female during the reproductive years or immediately following menses.
7. The use of ultrasound is contraindicated during pregnancy because of potential damage to the fetus.
8. Some precaution should be used when treating areas around the heart due to potential changes in ECG activity. Ultrasound can certainly interfere with normal function of a pacemaker.
9. Ultrasound should not be used over a malignant tumor. It appears that using ultrasound may increase the size of the tumor and perhaps cause metastases. There is also danger in using ultrasound even in patients who have a history of malignant tumors, because it is always possible that small tumors may remain without their knowledge. Thus it is best for the clinician to check with the patient's physician or oncologist before using ultrasound in cancer patients.
10. As previously mentioned, ultrasound should never be used over epiphyseal areas in young children.
11. Ultrasound may be used safely over metal implants because it has been shown that there is no increase in temperature of tissue adjacent to the implant because metal has high-thermal conductivity and thus heat is removed from the area faster than it can be absorbed. However, in cases of total joint replacement, the cement used (methyl methacrylate) absorbs heat rapidly and may be overheated, damaging surrounding soft tissues.

GUIDELINES FOR THE SAFE USE OF ULTRASOUND EQUIPMENT

Currently, ultrasound units are the only therapeutic modality for which Federal Performance Standards exist.[152] Ultrasound units produced since 1979 are required to indicate the magnitudes of ultrasound power and intensity with an accuracy of ±20% and accurately control

Table 10–7 Summary of Indications and Contraindications for Using Ultrasound

INDICATIONS

Acute and postacute conditions (ultrasound with nonthermal effects)

Soft tissue healing and repair

Scar tissue

Joint contracture

Chronic inflammation

Increase extensibility of collagen

Reduction of muscle spasm

Pain modulation

Increase blood flow

Soft tissue repair

Increase in protein synthesis

Tissue regeneration

Bone healing

Repair of nonunion fractures

Inflammation associated with myositis ossificans

Plantar warts

Myofascial trigger points

CONTRAINDICATIONS

Acute and postacute conditions (ultrasound with thermal effects)

Areas of decreased temperature sensation

Areas of decreased circulation

Vascular insufficiency

Thrombophlebitis

Eyes

Reproductive organs

Pelvis immediately following menses

Pregnancy

Pacemaker

Malignancy

Epiphyseal areas in young children

Total joint replacements

Infection

treatment time. It is recommended that intensity output, pulse regime accuracy, and timer accuracy be checked at regular intervals by qualified personnel who have access to the appropriate testing equipment. The effective radiating area and the beam nonuniformity ratio of the transducer should be accurately provided by the manufacturer. The following treatment protocol will help to ensure patient safety:

Treatment Protocol: Ultrasound

1. Question patient (contraindications/previous treatments).
2. Position patient (comfort, modesty).
3. Inspect part to be treated (check for rashes, infections, or open wounds).
4. Obtain appropriate soundhead size.
5. Determine ultrasound frequency (1 MHz for deep, 3 MHz for superficial).
6. Set duty cycle (choose either continuous or pulsed setting).
7. Apply couplant to area.
8. Set treatment duration (vigorous heat = 10–12 min at 1 MHz and 3–4 min at 3 MHz).
9. Maintain contact between the skin and the applicator (move at a rate of 4 cm/s, for 2 ERA).
10. Adjust intensity to perception of heat. (If this gets too hot, turn down the intensity or move applicator slightly faster.)
11. If goal is increased joint ROM, put part on stretch (for the last 2–3 minutes of insonation, and maintain stretch or friction massage 2–5 minutes after termination of treatment).
12. Terminate treatment. (Turn all dials to zero; clean gel from unit.)
13. Assess treatment efficacy. (Inspect area, feedback from client.)
14. Record treatment parameters.

Note: Ultrasound units should be recalibrated every 6–12 months, depending on the frequency of use.

SUMMARY

1. Ultrasound is defined as inaudible, acoustic vibrations of high frequency that may produce either thermal or nonthermal physiologic effects.
2. Ultrasound travels through soft tissue as a longitudinal wave at a therapeutic frequency of either 1 or 3 MHz.
3. As the ultrasound wave is transmitted through the various tissues, energy intensity attenuates or decreases owing to either absorption of energy by the tissues or dispersion and scattering of the sound wave.
4. Ultrasound is produced by a piezoelectric crystal within the transducer that converts electrical energy to acoustic energy through mechanical deformation via the piezoelectric effect.
5. Ultrasound energy travels within the tissues as a highly focused collimated beam with a nonuniform intensity distribution.

6. Although continuous ultrasound is most commonly used when the desired effect is to produce thermal effects, pulsed ultrasound or continuous ultrasound at a low intensity will produce nonthermal or mechanical effects.

7. Therapeutic ultrasound when applied to biologic tissue may induce clinically significant responses in cells, tissues, and organs through both thermal effects, which produce a tissue temperature increase, and nonthermal effects, which include cavitation and microstreaming.

8. Recent research has provided answers to many of the contradictory results and conclusions of numerous previous laboratory and clinically based reports in the literature.

9. Therapeutic ultrasound is most effective when an appropriate coupling medium and technique using either direct contact, immersion, or a bladder is combined with a moving transducer.

10. Even though there is relatively little documented evidence from the clinical community concerning the efficacy of ultrasound, it is most often used for soft-tissue healing and repair, with scar tissue and joint contracture, for chronic inflammation, for bone healing, with plantar warts, and for placebo effects.

11. Phonophoresis is a technique in which ultrasound is used to drive molecules of a topically applied medication, usually either anti-inflammatories or analgesics, into the tissues.

12. In a clinical setting, ultrasound is frequently used in combination with other modalities, including hot packs, cold packs, and electrical stimulating currents, to produce specific treatment effects.

13. Although ultrasound is a relatively safe modality if used appropriately, the clinician must be aware of the various contraindications and precautions.

14. For ultrasound to be effective, the clinician must pay particular attention to correct parameters such as intensity, frequency, duration, and treatment size.

REVIEW QUESTIONS

1. What is therapeutic ultrasound, and what are its two primary physiologic effects?
2. How does an ultrasound wave travel through biologic tissues, and what happens to the acoustic energy within those tissues?
3. How does the transducer convert electrical energy into acoustic energy?
4. How does the frequency affect the ultrasound beam within the tissues?
5. What are the differences between continuous and pulsed ultrasound?
6. What are the potential thermal effects of ultrasound?
7. How can the nonthermal effects of ultrasound facilitate the healing process?
8. What is the relationship between treatment intensity and treatment duration in effecting a temperature increase in the tissues?
9. What are the various coupling agents and exposure techniques that may be used when treating a patient with ultrasound?
10. What are the various clinical applications for using ultrasound in treating injuries?
11. What is the purpose of using a phonophoresis treatment?
12. How should ultrasound be used in combination with other therapeutic modalities?

SELF-TEST QUESTIONS

True or False

1. Penetration and absorption are inversely related.
2. Three MHZ frequency ultrasound is absorbed deeper and faster than 1 MHz.
3. A low beam nonuniformity ratio (BNR) results in uneven heating.

Multiple Choice

4. The decrease in energy intensity of the ultrasound wave as it is scattered and dispersed while traveling through various tissues is known as which of the following?

   a. Acoustic impedance
   b. Attenuation
   c. Rarefaction
   d. Compression

5. A(n) may develop when standing waves form at tissue interfaces and reflected energy meets transmitted energy increasing the intensity.

   a. Hot spot
   b. Impedance
   c. Rarefaction
   d. Collimated beam

6. Which of the following is NOT a nonthermal effect of ultrasound?

   a. Acoustic microstreaming
   b. Cavitation
   c. Increased collagen extensibility
   d. Increased fibroblast activity

7. Which of the following is the LEAST effective ultrasound coupling method?

   a. Massage lotion
   b. Ultrasonic gel
   c. Water immersion
   d. Bladder technique

8. Ultrasound may be used to treat which of the following?

   a. Bone fracture
   b. Pain
   c. Plantar warts
   d. All of the above

9. uses ultrasound to drive molecules of medication into the skin.

   a. "Combo therapy"
   b. Iontophoresis
   c. Phonophoresis
   d. None of the above

10. In order to increase tissue temperature 2°C, how long must the ultrasound treatment time be at a setting of 1 MHz and 1.0 W/cm²?

    a. 5 minutes
    b. 10 minutes
    c. 7.5 minutes
    d. 15 minutes

SOLUTIONS TO CLINICAL DECISION-MAKING EXERCISES

10–1

The lower the frequency, the less the energy is absorbed in the superficial tissues, and thus the deeper it penetrates. The majority of the sound waves generated from the 3 MHz treatment would be absorbed in the muscle or tendon. Also, when treating subcutaneous structure, 3 MHz heats more rapidly and is more comfortable than 1 MHz.

10–2

The nonthermal effects of cavitation and microstreaming can be maximized while minimizing the thermal effects by using a spatial-averaged, temporal-averaged intensity of 0.1–0.2 W/cm² with continuous ultrasound. This range may also be achieved using a low-temporal-averaged intensity by pulsing a higher temporal peak intensity of 1.0 W/cm^2 at a duty cycle of 20% to give a temporal-averaged intensity of 0.2 W/cm^2.

10–3

Since temperature increase is frequency dependent, at 1 MHz with an intensity of 1.5 W/cm^2, temperature will elevate at a rate of 0.30°C/min. Therefore, a 10-minute treatment will be necessary.

10–4

When using a large soundhead to treat over boney prominences, the immersion technique using a plastic or rubber tub can be effective. Also the bladder technique could be used to make certain that contact between the soundhead and the coupling medium is consistent.

10–5

Phonophoresis would likely be a reasonable choice. The physician could prescribe a topical anti-inflammatory medication that could be administered to the patient topically. In phonophoresis, ultrasound is used to enhance delivery of a medication into the tissues.

10–6

Since the patient does not seem to be getting better, the clinician might try combining ultrasound with an electrical stimulating current. Stretching during treatment is also recommended.

10–7

In this case, the best treatment choice is not to use ultrasound at all. A better decision would be to use either hydrocollator packs or diathermy, both of which are more useful in treating larger areas. If depth of penetration is a concern, then shortwave diathermy would be the treatment modality of choice.

REFERENCES

1. Kremkau F. Diagnostic Ultrasound: Principles and Instruments. Philadelphia: W.B. Saunders; 2002.
2. Delacerda FG. Ultrasonic techniques for treatment of plantar warts in patients. *J Orthop Sports Phys Ther*. 1979;1:100
3. Dyson M. The use of ultrasound in sports physiotherapy. In: Grisogono V, ed. *Sports Injuries (International Perspectives in Physiotherapy)*, Edinburgh: Churchill Livingstone; 1989.
4. Baker KG, Robertson VJ, Duck FA. A review of therapeutic ultrasound: biophysical effects. *Phys Ther*. 2001;81:1351–1358.
5. Gann N. Ultrasound: current concepts. *Clin Manage*. 1991;11(4):64–69.
6. McDiarmid T, Burns PN. Clinical applications of therapeutic ultrasound. *Physiotherapy*. 1987;73:155.
7. Michlovitz S. *Thermal agents in rehabilitation*. Philadelphia, PA: FA Davis; 1996.
8. Draper DO, Castel JC, Castel D. Rate of temperature increase in human muscle during 1 MHz and 3 MHz continuous ultrasound. *J Orthop Sports Phys Ther*. 1995;22:142–150.
9. Middlemast S, Chatterjee DS. Comparison of ultrasound and thermotherapy for soft tissue injuries. *Physiotherapy*. 1978;64:331.
10. Draper DO, Ricard MD. Rate of temperature decay in human muscle following 3 MHz ultrasound: the stretching window revealed. *J Athl Train*. 1995;30:304–307.
11. Myrer JW, Draper DO, Durrant E. Contrast therapy and intramuscular temperature in the human leg. *J Athl Train*. 1994;29:318–322.
12. Ter Haar C. Basic physics of therapeutic ultrasound, *Physiotherapy*. 1987;73(3):110–113.
13. Ziskin M, McDiarmid T, Michlovitz S. Therapeutic ultrasound. In: Michlovitz S, ed. *Thermal Agents in Rehabilitation*. Philadelphia, PA: FA Davis; 1996.
14. Griffin JE, Karsalis TC. *Physical Agents for Physical Therapists*. Springfield, IL: Charles C Thomas; 1987.
15. Summer W, Patrick MK. *Ultrasonic Therapy*. New York: American Elsevier; 1964.
16. Ward AR. *Electricity Fields and Waves in Therapy*. Marrickville, NSW, Australia: Science Press; 1986.
17. Williams R. Production and transmission of ultrasound. *Physiotherapy*. 1987;73(3):113–116.
18. Dyson M. Mechanisms involved in therapeutic ultrasound. *Physiotherapy*. 1987;73(3):116–120.
19. Holcomb W, Joyce C. A comparison of temperature increases produced by 2 commonly used ultrasound units. *J Athl Train*. 2003;38(1):24–27.
20. Holcomb W, Joyce C. A comparison of the effectiveness of two commonly used ultrasound units. *J Athl Train* (Suppl.). 2001;36(2S):S-89.

21. Artho PA, Thyne JG, Warring BP, et al. A calibration study of therapeutic ultrasound units. *Phys Ther.* 2002;82:257–263.

22. Docker MF. A review of instrumentation available for therapeutic ultrasound. *Physiotherapy.* 1987;73(4):154.

23. Miller M, Longoria J, Cheatham C. A comparison of the tissue temperature difference between the midpoint and peripheral effective radiating area during 1 and 3 MHz ultrasound treatments (abstract). *J Athl Train.* 2007;42(2):S-40.

24. Johns L, Straub S, Howard S. Variability in effective radiating area and output power of new ultrasound transducers at 3 MHz. *J Athl Train.* 2007;42(1):22.

25. Castel JC. Therapeutic ultrasound. *Rehab and Therapy Products Review.* 1993;Jan/Feb:22–32.

26. Reid DC, Cummings GE. Factors in selecting the dosage of ultrasound with particular reference to the use of various coupling agents. *Physiother Can.* 1973;63:255.

27. Chan AK, Myrer JW, Measom G, Draper D. Temperature changes in human patellar tendon in response to therapeutic ultrasound. *J Athl Train.* 1998;33(2):130–135.

28. Draper DO. The latest research on therapeutic ultrasound: clinical habits may need to be changed. Presented at the 46th Annual Meeting and Clinical Symposium of the National Athletic Trainers' Association, Indianapolis, IN, June 16; 1995.

29. Fyfe MC, Bullock M. Therapeutic ultrasound: some historical background and development in knowledge of its effects on healing. *Aust J Physiother.* 1985;31(6):220–224.

30. Hayes B, Merrick M, Sandrey M. Three-MHz ultrasound heats deeper into the tissues than originally theorized. *J Athl Train.* 2004;39(3):230–234.

31. Kitchen S, Partridge C. A review of therapeutic ultrasound: part 2, the efficacy of ultrasound. *Physiotherapy.* 1990;76(10):595–599.

32. Ferguson BA. *A practitioner's guide to ultrasonic therapy equipment standard.* U.S. Dept. of Health and Human Services, Public Health Service, Food and Drug Administration, Rockville, MD; 1985.

33. Hecox B, Mehreteab TA, Weisbergm J. *Physical Agents: A Comprehensive Text for Physical Therapists.* Norwalk, CT: Appleton & Lange; 1994.

34. Gatto J, Kimura IF, Gulick D. Effect of beam nonuniformity ratio of three ultrasound machines on tissue phantom temperature. *J Athl Train.* 1999;34(2):S-69.

35. Draper DO. Ten mistakes commonly made with ultrasound use: current research sheds light on myths. *Athl Train Sports Health Care Perspect.* 1996;2:95–107.

36. Lehmann JF, de Lateur BJ, Silverman DR. Selective heating effects of ultrasound in human beings. *Arch Phys Med Rehab.* 1966;46:331.

37. Lehmann JF, de Lateur BJ. Therapeutic heat. In Lehmann JF, ed. *Therapeutic Heat and Cold.* 4th ed. Baltimore, MD: Williams & Wilkins.

38. Burr P, Demchak T, Cordova M. Effects of altering intensity during 1-MHz ultrasound treatment on increasing triceps surae temperature. *J Sport Rehab.* 2004;13(4):275–286.

39. Morrisette D, Brown D, Saladin M. Temperature change in lumbar periarticular tissue with continuous ultrasound. *J Orthop Sports Phys Ther.* 2004;34(12):754–760.

40. Merrick MA, Bernard KD, Devor ST. Identical 3-MHz ultrasound treatments with different devices produce different intramuscular temperatures. *J Orthop Sports Phys Ther.* 2003;33(7):379–385.

41. Boone L, Ingersol CD, Cordova ML. Passive hip flexion does not increase during or following ultrasound treatment of the hamstring musculature. *J Athl Train.* 1999;34(2):S-70.

42. Dyson M. Therapeutic application of ultrasound. In: Nyborg WL, Ziskin MC, eds. *Biological Effects of Ultrasound*, Edinburgh: Churchill-Livingstone; 1985.

43. Kitchen S, Partridge C. A review of therapeutic ultrasound: part 1, background and physiological effects. *Physiotherapy.* 1990;76(10):593–595.

44. Partridge CJ. Evaluation of the efficacy of ultrasound. *Physiotherapy.* 1987;73(4):166–168.

45. Dyson M, Luke DA. Induction of mast cell degranulation in skin by ultrasound. *IEEE Trans Ultrasonics Ferroelectrics Freq Control.* 1986; UFFC-33:194.

46. Black K, Halverson JL, Maierus K, Soderbere GL. Alterations in ankle dorsiflexion torque as a result of continuous ultrasound to the anterior tibial compartment. *Phys Ther.* 1984;64(6):910–913.

47. Frizell LA, Dunn F. Biophysics of ultrasound; bioeffects of ultrasound. In: Lehmann JF, ed. *Therapeutic Heat and Cold.* 3rd ed. Baltimore, MD, Williams & Wilkins; 1982.

48. Lowden A. Application of ultrasound to assess stress fractures. *Physiotherapy.* 1986;72(3):160–161.

49. MacDonald BL, Shipster SB. Temperature changes induced by continuous ultrasound. *S Afr J Physiother.* 1981;37(1):13–15.

50. Saliba S, Mistry D, Perrin D. Phonophoresis and the absorption of dexamethsone in the presence of an occlusive dressing. *J Athl Train.* 2007;42(3):349–354.

51. Lehman JF, de Lateur BJ, Stonebridge JB, Warren G. Therapeutic temperature distribution produced by ultra-sound as modified by dosage and volume of tissue exposed. *Arch Phys Med Rehab.* 1967;48:662–666.

52. Castel JC. Electrotherapy application in clinical for neuromuscular stimulation and tissue repair. Presented at the 46th Annual Clinical Symposium of the National Athletic Trainer's Association, June 16, 1995, Indianapolis.

53. Quade AG, Radzyminski SF. Ultrasound in verruca plantaris. *J Am Podiatric Assoc.* 1966;56:503.

54. Holcomb WR, Blank C, Davis C. The effect of superficial pre-heating on the magnitude and duration of temperature elevation with 1 MHz ultrasound. *J Athl Train.* 2000;35(2):S-48.

55. Ter Haar G, Hopewell JW. Ultrasonic heating of mammalian tissue in vivo. *Br J Cancer.* 1982;45 (Suppl. V):65–67.

56. Draper DO, Sunderland S. Examination of the law of Grotthus-Draper: does ultrasound penetrate subcutaneous fat in humans? *J Athl Train*. 1993;28:246–250.

57. Hayes B, Sandrey M, Merrick M. The differences between 1 MHz and 3 MHz ultrasound in the heating of sub-cutaneous tissue. *J Athl Train* (Suppl.). 2001;36(2S):S-92.

58. Gallo J, Draper D, Brody L. A comparison of human muscle temperature increases during 3-mhz continuous and pulsed ultrasound with equivalent temporal average intensities. *J Orthop Sports Phys Ther*. 2004;34(7):395–401.

59. Hogan RD, Burke KM, Franklin TD. The effect of ultrasound on microvascular hemodynamics in skeletal muscle: effects during ischemia. *Microvasc Res*. 1982;23:370.

60. Pilla AA, Figueiredo M, Nasser P, et al. Non-invasive low intensity pulsed ultrasound: a potent accelerator of bone repair. Proceedings of the 36th Annual Meeting, Orthopaedic Research Society, New Orleans; 1990.

61. Johns L. Nonthermal effects of therapeutic ultrasound. *J Athl Train*. 2002;37(3):293–299.

62. Fyfe MC, Chahl LA. The effect of single or repeated applications of "therapeutic" ultrasound on plasma extravasation during silver nitrate induced inflammation of the rat hindpaw ankle joint. *Ultrasound Med Biol*. 1985;11:273.

63. Oakley EM. Application of continuous beam ultrasound at therapeutic levels. *Physiotherapy*. 1978;64(4):103–104.

64. Patrick MK. Applications of pulsed therapeutic ultrasound. *Physiotherapy*. 1978;64(4):3–104.

65. Strapp E, Guskiewicz K, Hackney A. The cumulative effects of multiple phonophoresis treatments on dexamethasone and cortisol concentrations in the blood. *J Athl Train*. 2000;35(2):S-47.

66. Starkey C. *Therapeutic Modalities for Athletic Trainers*. Philadelphia, PA: F.A. Davis; 2004.

67. Leonard J, Merrick M, Ingersoll C. A comparison of ultrasound intensities on a 10 minute 1.0 MHz ultrasound treatment. *J Athl Train* (Suppl.). 2001;36(2S):S-91.

68. Draper DO. Guidelines to enhance therapeutic ultrasound treatment outcomes. *Athletic Therapy Today*. 1998;3(6):7.

69. Leonard J, Merrick M, Ingersoll C. A comparison of intramuscular temperatures during 10-minute 1.0-MHz ultrasound treatments at different intensities. *J Sport Rehab*. 2004;13(3):244–254.

70. Balmaseda MT, Fatehi MT, Koozekanani SH. Ultrasound therapy: a comparative study of different coupling medium. *Arch Phys Med Rehab*. 1986;67:147.

71. Pesek J, Kane E, Perrin D. T-Prep ultrasound gel and ultrasound does not effect local anesthesia. *J Athl Train* (Suppl.). 2001;36(2S):S-89.

72. Klucinec B, Scheidler M, Denegar C. Transmission of coupling agents used to deliver acoustic energy over irregular surfaces. *J Orthop Sports Phys Ther*. 2000;30(5):263–269.

73. Mihaloyvov MR, Roethmeier JL, Merrick MA. Intramuscular temperature does not differ between direct ultrasound application and application with commercial gel packs. *J Athl Train*. 2000;35(2):S-47.

74. Merrick MA, Mihalyov MR, Roethemeier JL. A comparison of intramuscular temperatures during ultrasound treatments with coupling gel or gel pads. *J Orthop Sports Phys Ther*. 2002;32(5):216–220.

75. Docker MF, Foulkes DJ, Patrick MK. Ultrasound couplants for physiotherapy. *Physiotherapy*. 1982;68(4):124–125.

76. Jennings Y, Biggs M, Ingersoll C. The effect of ultra-sound intensity and coupling medium on gastrocnemius tissue temperature. *J Athl Train* (Suppl.). 2002;37(2S):S-42.

77. Ferguson HN. Ultrasound in the treatment of surgical wounds. *Physiotherapy*. 1981;67:12.

78. Anderson M, Draper D, Schulthies S. A 1:3 mixture of Flex-All and ultrasound gel is as effective a couplant as 100 % ultrasound gel, based upon intramuscular temperature rise (Abstract). *J Athl Train* (Suppl.). 2005; 40(2): S-89–S-90.

79. Draper D, Anderson M. Combining topical analgesics and ultrasound, part 1. *Athletic Therapy Today*. 2005;10(1):26–27.

80. Myrer J, Measom G, Fellingham G. Intramuscular temperature rises with topical analgesics used as coupling agents during therapeutic ultrasound. *J Athl Train*. 2001;36(1):20–26.

81. Anderson M, Eggett D, Draper D: Combining topical analgesics and ultrasound, Part 2. *Athletic Therapy Today*. 2005;10(2):45.

82. Ashton DF, Draper DO, Myrer JW: Temperature rise in human muscle during ultrasound treatments using Flex-All as a coupling agent. *J Athl Train*. 1998;33(2):136–140.

83. Draper DO, Sunderland S, Kirkendall DT, Ricard MD. A comparison of temperature rise in the human calf muscles following applications of underwater and topical gel ultrasound. *J Orthop Sports Phys Ther*. 1993;17:247–251.

84. Bishop S, Draper D, Knight K. Human tissue temperature rise during ultrasound treatments with the Aquaflex Gel Pad. *J Athl Train*. 2004;39(2):126–131.

85. Bishop S, Draper D, Knight K. Human tissue-temperature rise during ultrasound treatments with the Aquaflex Gel Pad. *J Athl Train*. 2004;39(2):126–131.

86. Zarod AP, Williams AR. Platelet aggregation in vivo by therapeutic ultrasound. *Lancet*. 1977;1:1266.

87. Weaver S, Demchak T, Stone M. Effect of transducer velocity on intramuscular temperature during a 1-MHz ultrasound treatment. *J Orthop Sports Phys Ther*. 2006;36(5):320–325.

88. Kramer JF. Ultrasound: evaluation of its mechanical and thermal effects. *Arch Phys Med Rehab*. 1984;65:223.

89. Klucinec B, Denegar C, Mahmood R. The transducer pressure variable: its influence on acoustic energy transmission. *J Sport Rehab*. 1997;6(1):47–53.

90. Dyson M, Pond JB. The effect of pulsed ultrasound on tissue regeneration. *J Physiother*. 1970;105–108.

91. Finucane S, Sparrow K, Owen J. Low-intensity ultrasound enhances MCL healing at 3 and 6 weeks post injury. *J Athl Train* (Suppl.). 2003;38(2S):S-23.

92. Karnes JL, Burton HW. Continuous therapeutic ultrasound accelerates repair of contraction-induced skeletal muscle damage in rats. *Arch Phys Med Rehab*. 2002;83(1):1–4.

93. Hashish I, Harvey W, Harris M. Antiinflammatory effects of ultrasound therapy: evidence for a major placebo effect. *Br J Rheumatol.* 1986;25:77.

94. Snow CJ, Johnson KA. Effect of therapeutic ultrasound on acute inflammation. *Physiother Can.* 1988;40:162.

95. Harvey W, Dyson M, Pond JB. The simulation of protein synthesis in human fibroblasts by therapeutic ultrasound. *Rheumat Rehab.* 1975;14:237.

96. Reed B, Ashikaga T, Flemming BC. Effects of ultra-sound and stretch on knee ligament extensibility. *J Orthop Sports Phys Ther.* 2000;30(6):341–347.

97. Plaskett C, Tiidus PM, Livingston L. Ultrasound treatment does not affect post exercise muscle strength recovery or soreness. *J Sport Rehab.* 1999;8(1):1–9.

98. Tiidus P, Cort J, Woodruf S. Ultrasound treatment and recovery from eccentric-exercise-induced muscle damage. *J Sport Rehab.* 2002;11(4):305–314.

99. Rantanen J, Thorsson O, Wollmer P, et al. Effects of therapeutic ultrasound on the regeneration of skeletal myofibers after experimental muscle injury. *Am J Sports Med.* 1999;27(1):54–59.

100. Lehmann JF. Effect of therapeutic temperatures on tendon extensibility. *Arch Phys Med Rehab.* 1970;51:481.

101. Bierman W. Ultrasound in the treatment of scars. *Arch Phys Med Rehab.* 1954;35:209.

102. Lehmann JF. Clinical evaluation of a new approach in the treatment of contracture associated with hip fracture after internal fixation. *Arch Phys Med Rehab.* 1961;42:95.

103. Rose S, Draper DO, Schulthies SS, Durrant E. The stretching window part two: rate of thermal decay in deep muscle following 1 MHz ultrasound. *J Athl Train.* 1996;31:139–143.

104. Gersten JW: Effect of ultrasound on tendon extensibility. *Am J Phys Med.* 1955;34:662.

105. Markham DE, Wood MR. Ultrasound for Dupytren's contracture. *Physiotherapy.* 1980;66(2):55–58.

106. Merrick MA. Ultrasound and range of motion examined. *Athletic Therapy Today.* 2000;5(3):48–49.

107. Crumley M, Nowak P, Merrick M. Do ultrasound, active warm-up and passive motion differ on their ability to cause temperature and range of motion changes? *J Athl Train (Suppl.).* 2001; 36(2S):S-92.

108. Bly N, McKenzie A, West J, Whitney J. Low dose ultrasound effects on wound healing: a controlled study with Yucatan pigs. *Arch Phys Med Rehab.* 1992;73:656–664.

109. Downing DS, Weinstein A. Ultrasound therapy of subacromial bursitis (abstract). *Phys Ther.* 1986;66:194.

110. Lundeberg T, Abrahamsson P, Haker E. A comparative study of continuous ultrasound, placebo ultrasound and rest in epicondylalgia. *Scand Rehab Med.* 1988;20:99.

111. Draper DO, Anderson C, Schulthies SS. Immediate and residual changes in dorsiflexion range of motion using an ultrasound heat and stretch routine. *J Athl Train.* 1998;33(2):141–144.

112. Echternach JL. Ultrasound: an adjunct treatment for shoulder disability. *Phys Ther.* 1965;45:565.

113. Leung M, Ng G, Yip K. Effect of ultrasound on acute inflammation of transected medial collateral ligaments. *Arch Phys Med Rehab.* 2004;85(6):963–966.

114. Woolf N. *Cell, Tissue and Disease.* 2nd ed. London: Bailliere Tindall; 1986.

115. Conner C: Use of an ultrasonic bone-growth stimulator to promote healing of a Jones fracture. *Athletic Therapy Today.* 2003;8(1):37–39.

116. Stein T. Ultrasound: exploring benefits on bone repair, growth and healing. *Sports Med Update.* 1998;13(1):22–23.

117. Werden SJ, Bennell KK, McMeeken JM. Can conventional therapeutic ultrasound units be used to accelerate fracture repair? *Phys Ther Rev.* 1999;4(2):117–126.

118. Dyson M, Brookes M. Stimulation of bone repair by ultrasound (abstract). *Ultrasound Med Biol (Suppl.).* 1982;8(50):50.

119. Brueton RN, Campbell B. The use of geliperm as a sterile coupling agent for therapeutic ultrasound. *Physiotherapy.* 1987;73:653.

120. Griffin JE, Echternach JL, Price RE. Patients treated with ultrasonic-driven hydrocortisone and ultrasound alone. *Phys Ther.* 1967;47:594–601.

121. Vaughen IL, Bender LF. Effect of ultrasound on growing bone. *Arch Phys Med Rehab.* 1959;40:158.

122. Currier DP, Kramer IF. Sensory nerve conduction: heating effects of ultrasound and infrared. *Physiother Can.* 1982;34:241.

123. Clarke GR, Stenner L. Use of therapeutic ultrasound. *Physiotherapy.* 1976;62(6):85–190.

124. Gorkiewicz R. Ultrasound for subacromial bursitis. *Phys Ther.* 1984;64:46.

125. Makuloluwe RT, Mouzas GL. Ultrasound in the treatment of sprained ankles. *Practitioner.* 1977;218:586–588.

126. Nwuga VCB. Ultrasound in treatment of back pain resulting from prolapsed intervertebral disc. *Arch Phys Med Rehab.* 1983;64:88.

127. Portwood MM, Lieberman SS, Taylor RG. Ultra-sound treatment of reflex sympathetic dystrophy. *Arch Phys Med Rehab.* 1987;68:116.

128. Kent H. Plantar wart treatment with ultrasound. *Arch Phys Med Rehab.* 1959 40:15.

129. Vaughn DT. Direct method versus underwater method in treatment of plantar warts with ultrasound. *Phys Ther.* 1973;53:396.

130. Draper DO. Current research on therapeutic ultrasound and pulsed short-wave diathermy. Presented at Physio Therapy Research Seminars Japan, Sendai, Japan November 17; 1996.

131. El Hag M, Coghlan K, Christmas P. The anti-inflammatory effects of dexamethasone and therapeutic ultrasound in oral surgery. *Br J Oral Maxillofac Surg.* 1985;23:17.

132. Cameron M, Monroe L. Relative transmission of ultrasound by media customarily used for phonophoresis. *Phys Ther*. 1992;72(2):142–148.

133. Fahey S, Smith M, Merrick M. Intramuscular temperature does not differ among hydrocortisone preparations during exercise. *J Athl Train*. 2000;35(2):S–47.

134. Kleinkort IA, Wood F. Phonophoresis with 1 percent versus 10 percent hydrocortisone. *Phys Ther*. 1975;1320;5.

135. Holdsworth LK, Anderson DM. Effectiveness of ultrasound used with hydrocortisone coupling medium or epicondylitis clasp to treat lateral epicondylitis: pilot study. *Physiotherapy*. 1993;79(1):19–25.

136. Kuntz A, Griffiths C, Rankin J. Cortisol concentrations in human skeletal muscle tissue after phonophoresis with 10% hydrocortisone gel. *J Athl Train*. 2006;41(3):32.

137. Kahn J. Iontophoresis and ultrasound for post-surgical temporomandibular trismus and paresthesia. *Phys Ther*. 1980;60(3):307–308.

138. Wing M. Phonophoresis with hydrocortisone in the treatment of temporomandibular joint dysfunction. *Phys Ther*. 1982;62:32–33.

139. Benson HAE, McElnay IC. Transmission of ultrasound energy through topical pharmaceutical products. *Physiotherapy*. 1988;74:587.

140. Darrow H, Schulthies S, Draper D. Serum dexamethasone levels after Decadron phonophoresis. *J Athl Train*. 1999;34(4):338–341.

141. Cagnie B, Vinck E, Rimbaut S, Vanderstraeten G. Phonophoresis versus topical application of ketoprofen: comparison between tissue and plasma levels. *Phys Ther*. 2003;83:707–712.

142. Ciccone C, Leggin B, Callamaro J. Effects of ultrasound and trolamine salicylate phonophoresis on delayed-onset muscle soreness. *Phys Ther*. 1991;71(9):666–675.

143. Moll MJ. A new approach to pain: lidocaine and decadron with ultrasound. *USAF Medical Service Digest*, May–June 8, 1977.

144. Penderghest C, Kimura I, Gulick D. Double blind clinical efficacy study of pulsed phonophoresis on perceived pain associated with symptomatic tendinitis. *J Sport Rehab*. 1998; (7):9–19.

145. Draper DO, Schulthies S, Sorvisto P, Hautala A. Temperature changes in deep muscles of humans during ice and ultrasound therapies: an in-vivo study. *J Orthop Sports Phys Ther*. 1995;21:153–157.

146. Gum SL, Reddy GK, Stehno-Bittel L, Enwemeka CS. Combined ultrasound, electrical stimulation, and laser promote collagen synthesis with moderate changes in tendon biomechanics. *Am J Phys Med Rehab*. 1997;76(4):288–296.

147. Holcomb W, Blank C. The effects of superficial heating before 1-MHz ultrasound on tissue temperature. *J Sport Rehab*. 2003;12(2):95–103.

148. Draper DO, Harris ST, Schulthies S. Hot pack and 1-MHz ultrasound treatments have an additive effect on muscle temperature increase. *J Athl Train*. 1998;33(1):21–24.

149. Palko A, Krause B, Starkey C. The efficacy of combination therapeutic ultrasound and electrical stimulation (abstract). *J Athl Train*. 2007;42(2):S-134.

150. Girardi CQ, Seaborne D, Savard-Goulet F. The analgesic effect of high voltage galvanic stimulation combined with ultrasound in the treatment of low back pain: a one group pretest/posttest study. *Physiother Can*. 1984;36(6):327–333.

151. Lee JC, Lin DT, Hong C. The effectiveness of simultaneous thermotherapy with ultrasound and electrotherapy with combined AC and DC current on the immediate pain relief of myofascial trigger points. *J Musculoskeletal Pain*. 1997;5(1):81–90.

152. DEPARTMENT OF HEALTH AND HUMAN SERVICES. Performance standards for sonic, infrasonic, ultrasonic radiation emitting products:21 CFR 1050:10. *Federal Register*. 1978;43(8):7116.

153. Antich TJ. Phonophoresis: the principles of the ultrasonic driving force and efficacy in treatment of common orthopedic diagnosis. *J Orthop Sports Phys Ther*. 1982;4(2):99–103.

154. Bly N. The use of ultrasound as an enhancer for transcutaneous drug delivery: phonophoresis. *Phys Ther*. 1995;75(6):89–95.

155. Craig JA, Bradley J, Walsh DM, et al. Delayed onset muscle soreness: lack of effect of therapeutic ultrasound in humans. *Arch Phys Med Rehab*. 1999;80(3):318–323.

156. Demchak T, Stone M. Effectiveness of Clinical Ultrasound Parameters on Changing Intramuscular Temperature. *J Sport Rehabil*. 2008;17(3):220.

157. Johns L, Colloton P. Effects of ultrasound on spleenocyte proliferation and lymphokine production. *J Athl Train* (Suppl.). 2002;37(2S):S-42.

158. Klucinec B, Scheidler M, Denegar C, et al. Effectiveness of wound care products in the transmission of acoustic energy. *Phys Ther*. 2000;80:469–476.

159. Merrick MA. Does 1-MHz ultrasound really work? *Athletic Therapy Today*. 2001;6(6):48–54.

160. Munting E. Ultrasonic therapy for painful shoulders. *Physiotherapy*. 1978;64:180.

161. Myrer JW, Measom G, Fellingham GW. Significant intramuscular temperature rise obtained when topical analgesics Nature's Chemist and Biofreeze were used as coupling agents during ultrasound treatment. *J Athl Train*. 2000;35(2):S-48.

162. Rimington S, Draper DO, Durrant E, Fellingham GW. Temperature changes during therapeutic ultrasound in the precooled human gastrocnemius muscle. *J Athl Train*. 1994;29:325–327.

163. Williams AR, McHale I, Bowditchm M. Effects of MHz ultrasound on electrical pain threshold perception in humans. *Ultrasound Med Biol*. 1987;13:249.

SUGGESTED READINGS

Abramson DI. Changes in blood flow, oxygen uptake and tissue temperatures produced by therapeutic physical agents I: effect of ultrasound. *Am J Phys Med.* 1960;39:51.

Aldes IH, Grabin S. Ultrasound in the treatment of intervertebral disc syndrome. *Am J Phys Med.* 1958;37:199.

Allen KGR, Battye CK. Performance of ultrasonic therapy instruments. *Physiotherapy.* 1978;64(6):174–179.

Antich TJ. Physical therapy treatment of knee extensor mechanism disorders: comparison of four treatment modalities. *Journal of Orthopedic and Sports Physical Therapy.* 1986;8(5):255–259.

Aspelin P, Ekberg O, Thorsson O, Wilhelmsson M. Ultra-sound examination of soft tissue injury in the lower limb in patients. *Am J Sports Med.* 1992;20(5):601–603.

Banties A, Klomp R. Transmission of ultrasound energy through coupling agents. *Physiother Sport.* 1979;3:9–13.

Bare A, McAnaw M, Pritchard A. Phonophoretic delivery of 10% hydrocortisone through the epidermis of humans as determined by serum cortisol concentration. *Phys Ther.* 1996;76(7):738–749.

Bearzy HJ. Clinical applications of ultrasonic energy in the treatment of acute and chronic subacromial bursitis. *Arch Phys Med Rehab.* 1953;34:228.

Behrens BJ, Michlovitz SL. *Physical Agents: Theory and Practice for the Physical Therapy Assistant.* Philadelphia, PA: F.A. Davis; 1996.

Benson HA, McElnay JC, Harland RL. Use of ultrasound to enhance percutaneous absorption of benzydamine. *Phys Ther.* 1989;69(2):113–118.

Bickford RH, Duff RS. Influence of ultrasonic irradiation on temperature and blood flow in human skeletal muscle. *Circ Res.* 1953;1:534.

Billings C, Draper D, Schulthies S. Ability of the Omnisound 3000 Delta T to reproduce predictable temperature increases in human muscle. *J Athl Train (Suppl.).* 1996;31:S-47.

Bondolo W. Phenylbutazone with ultrasonics in some cases of anhrosynovitis of the knee. *Arch Orthopaed.* 1960;73: 532–540.

Borrell RM, Parker R, Henley EJ. Comparison of in vitro temperatures produced by hydrotherapy paraffin wax treatment and fluidotherapy. *Phys Ther.* 1984;60:1273–1276.

Brueton RN, Blookes M, Heatley FW. The effect of ultra-sound on the repair of a rabbit's tibial osteotomy held in rigid external fixation. *J Bone Joint Surg.* 1987;69B:494.

Buchan JF. Heat therapy and ultrasonics. *Practitioner.* 1972;208:130–131.

Buchtala V. The present state of ultrasonic therapy. *Br J Phys Med.* 1952;15:3.

Bundt FB. Ultrasound therapy in supraspinatus bursitis. *Phys Ther Rev.* 1958;38:826.

Burns PN, Pitcher EM. Calibration of physiotherapy ultrasound generators. *Clin Phys Physiol Measure.* 1984;5:37 (abstract).

Byl N. The use of ultrasound as an enhancer for transcutaneous drug delivery: phonophoresis. *Phys Ther.* 1995;75(6):539–553.

Callam MJ, Harper DR, Dale JJ, et al. A controlled trial of weekly ultrasound therapy in chronic leg ulceration. *Lancet.* 1987;2(8552):204.

Cerino LE, Ackerman E, Janes JM. Effects of ultrasound on experimental bone tumor. *Surg For.* 1965;16:466.

Chan AK, Siealmann RA, Guy AW. Calculations of therapeutic heat generated by ultrasound in fat-muscle-bone layers. *Inst Electric Electron Eng Trans Biomed Eng BME-2t.* 1973;280–284.

Cherup N, Urben J, Bender LF. The treatment of plantar warts with ultrasound. *Arch Phys Med Rehab.* 1963;44:602.

Cline PD. Radiographic follow-up of ultrasound therapy in calcific bursitis. *Phys Ther.* 1963;43:16.

Coakley WT. Biophysical effects of ultrasound at therapeutic intensities. *Physiotherapy.* 1978;94(6):168–169.

Conger AD, Ziskin MC, Wittels H. Ultrasonic effects on mammalian multicellular tumor spheroids. *Clin Ultrasound.* 1981;9:167.

Conner-Kerr T, Franklin M, Smith S. Efficacy of using phonophoresis for the delivery of dexamethasone to human transdermal tissues. *J Orthop Sports Phys Ther.* 1996;23(1):79.

Costentino AB, Cross DL, Harrington RJ, Sodarberg GL. Ultrasound effects on electroneuromyographic measures in sensory fibres of the median nerve. *Phys Ther.* 1983;63(11):1788–1792.

Creates V. A study of ultrasound treatment to the painful perineum after childbirth. *Physiotherapy.* 1987;73:162.

Currier DF, Greathouse D, Swift T. Sensory nerve conduction: effect of ultrasound. *Arch Phys Med Rehab.* 1978;59:181.

DeDeyne P, Kirsh-Volders M. In vitro effects of therapeutic ultrasound on the nucleus of human fibroblasts. *Phys Ther.* 1995;75(7):629–634.

Demchak T, Meyer L, Stemmans C. Therapeutic benefits of ultrasound can be achieved and maintained with a 20-minute 1MHz, 4-ERA ultrasound treatment (abstract). *J Athl Train.* 2006;41(2):S-42.

Demchak T, Meyer L. Therapeutic benefits of ultrasound can be achieved and maintained with a 20-minute 1MHz 4-ERA ultrasound treatment. *J Athl Train.* 2006;41(Supplement):S42.

Demchak T, Stone M. Effectiveness of clinical ultrasound parameters on changing intramuscular temperature. *J Sport Rehabil.* 2008;17(3):220.

Demchak T, Straub S. Ultrasound heating is curvilinear in nature and varies between transducers from the same manufacturer. *J Sport Rehabil.* 2007;16(2):122.

DiIorio A, Frommelt T, Svendsen L. Therapeutic ultra-sound effect on regional temperature and blood flow. *J Athl Train (Suppl).* 1996; 31:S-14.

Draper D, Oates D. Restoring wrist range of motion using ultrasound and mobilization: a case study. *Athl Ther Today.* 2006;11(1):45.

Draper D, Mahaffey C, Kaiser D. Therapeutic ultrasound softens trigger points in upper trapezius muscles. *J Athl Train.* 2007;42(2):S-40.

Draper D, Mahaffey C. Therapeutic ultrasound softens trigger point in upper trapezius muscles. *J Athl Train.* 2007;42 (Supplement):S40.

Draper D. Will thermal ultrasound and joint mobilizations restore range of motion to post-operative. *J Athl Train.* 2006;41(Supplement):S42.

Draper D. Will thermal ultrasound and joint mobilizations restore range of motion to post operative hypomobile wrists (abstract). *J Athl Train.* 2006;41(2):S-42.

Duarte LR. The stimulation of bone growth by ultrasound. *Arch Orthop Trauma Surg.* 1983;101:153–159.

Dyson M, Pond JB. The effect of pulsed ultrasound on tissue regeneration. *Physiotherapy.* 1970;56(6):134–142.

Dyson M, Suckling J. Stimulation of tissue repair by ultrasound: a survey of mechanisms involved. *Physiotherapy.* 1978;64:105.

Dyson M, ter Haar GR. The response of smooth muscle to ultra-sound (abstract). In: *Proceedings from an International Symposium on Therapeutic Ultrasound*, Winnipeg, Manitoba; September 10, 1981.

Dyson M, Woodward B, Pond JB. Flow of red blood cells stopped by ultrasound. *Nature.* 1971;232:572–573.

Dyson M. The production of blood cell stasis and endothelial damage in the blood vessels of chick embryos treated with ultrasound in a stationary wave field. *Ultrasound Med Biol.* 1974;11:133.

Dyson M. The stimulation of tissue regeneration by means of ultrasound. *Clin Sci.* 1968;35:273.

Eberhardt M, Bova S, Miller M. Effects of ultrasound heating on intramuscular blood flow characteristics in the gastrocnemius. *J Athl Train.* 2009;44(Supplement):S57.

Edvalston C, Draper D, Knight K. The ability of a new thinner gel pad to conduct ultrasound energy and increase tissue temperature of the Achilles tendon. *J Athl Train.* 2009;44(Supplement):S58.

Edwards MI. Congenital defects in guinea pigs: prenatal retardation of brain growth of guinea pigs following hyperthermia during gestation. *Teratology* 2:329; 1969.

Enwemeka CS. The effects of therapeutic ultrasound on tendon healing. *Am J Phys Med Rehab.* 1989;68(6):283–287.

Evaluation of ultrasound therapy devices. *Physiotherapy.* 1986;72:390.

Falconer J, Hayes KW, Ghang RW. Therapeutic ultra-sound in the treatment of musculoskeletal conditions. *Arthritis Care Res.* 1990;3(2):85–91.

Farmer WC. Effect of intensity of ultrasound on conduction of motor axons. *Phys Ther.* 1968;4:1233–1237.

Faul ED, Imig CJ. Temperature and blood flow studies after ultrasonic irradiation. *Am J Phys Med.* 1955;34:370.

Fieldhouse C. Ultrasound for relief of painful episiotomy scars. *Physiotherapy.* 1979;65:217.

Fincher A, Trowbridge C, Ricard M. A comparison of intramuscular temperature increases and uniformity of heating produced by hands free Autosound and manual therapeutic ultrasound techniques (abstract). *J Athl Train.* 2007;42(2):S-41.

Forrest G, Rosen K. Ultrasound: effectiveness of treatments given under water. *Arch Phys Med Rehab.* 1989;70:28.

Fountain FP, Gersten JW, Sengu O. Decrease in muscle spasm produced by ultrasound, hot packs and IR. *Arch Phys Med Rehab.* 1960;41:293.

Franklin M, Smith S, Chenier T. Effect of phonophoresis with dexamethasone on adrenal function. *J Orthop Sports Phys Ther.* 1995;22(3):103–107.

Friedar S. A pilot study: the therapeutic effect of ultrasound following partial rupture of achilles tendons in male rats. *J Orthop Sports Phys Ther.* 1988;10:39.

Fyfe MC, Bullock M. Acoustic output from therapeutic ultrasound units. *Aust J Physiother.* 1986;32(1):13–16.

Fyfe MC, Chahl LA. The effect of ultrasound on experimental oedema in rats. *Ultrasound Med Biol.* 1980;6:107.

Fyfe MC. A study of the effects of different ultrasonic frequencies on experimental oedema. *Aust J Physiother.* 1979;25(5):205–207.

Gallo J, Draper D, Fellingham G. Comparison of temperature increases in human muscle during 3 MHz continuous and pulsed ultrasound with equivalent temporal average intensies (abstract). *J Athl Train (Suppl.).* 2004;39(2):S-25–S-26.

Gantz S. Increased radicular pain due to therapeutic ultrasound applied to the back. *Arch Phys Med Rehab.* 1989;70:493–494.

Garrett AS, Garrett M. Letters: ultrasound for herpes zoster pain. *J Roy College Gen Practice.* 1982; Nov: 709.

Gersten JW. Effect of metallic objects on temperature rises produced in tissues by ultrasound. *Am J Phys Med.* 1958;37:75.

Goddard DH, Revell PA, Cason J. Ultrasound has no anti-inflammatory effect. *Ann Rheum Dis.* 1983;42:582–584.

Gracewski SM, Wagg RC, Schenk EA. High-frequency attenuation measurements using an acoustic microscope. *J Acoustic Soc Am.* 1988;83(6):2405–2409.

Grant A, Sleep J, Mclntosh J, Ashurst H. Ultrasound and pulsed electromagnetic energy treatment for peroneal trauma: a randomized placebo-controlled trial. *Br J Obstet Gynecol.* 1989;96:434–439.

Graves P, Finnegan E, DiMonda R. Effects and duration of treatment of ultrasound and static stretching on external rotation of the glenohumeral joint (abstract). *J Athl Train (Suppl.).* 2005;40(2):S-106.

Grieder A, Vinton P, Cinott W, et al. An evaluation of ultrasonic therapy for temperomandibular joint dysfunction. *Oral Surg.* 1971;31:25.

Griffin JE, Touchstone JC. Low intensity phonophoresis of cortisol in swine, *Phys Ther.* 1968;48(10):1336–1344.

Griffin JE, Touchstone JC. Ultrasonic movement of cortisol into pig tissue, 1: movement into skeletal muscle. *Am J Phys Med.* 1962;42:77–85.

Griffin JE, Touchstone JC, Liu A. Ultrasonic movement of cortisol into pig tissues, II: peripheral nerve, *Am J Phys Med.* 1965;4:20.

Griffin JE. Patients treated with ultrasonic driven cortisone and with ultrasound alone. *Phys Ther.* 1967;47:594.

Griffin JE. Transmissiveness of ultrasound through tap water, glycerin, and mineral oil. *Phys Ther.* 1980;60:1010.

Halle JS, Franklin RJ, Karalfa BL. Comparison of four treatment approaches for lateral epicondylitis of the elbow. *J Orthop Sports Phys Ther.* 1986;8:62.

Halle JS, Scoville CR, Greathouse DG. Ultrasound's effect on the conduction latency of superficial radial nerve in man. *Phys Ther.* 1981 61:345

Hamer J, Kirk JA. Physiotherapy and the frozen shoulder: a comparative trial of ice and ultrasound therapy. *NZ Med.* 1976;83(3):191.

Hansen TI, Kristensen JH. Effects of massage: shortwave and ultrasound upon 133Xe disappearance rate from muscle and subcutaneous tissue in the human calf. *Scand J Rehab Med.* 1973;5:197.

Harris S, Draper D, Schulthies S. The effect of ultrasound on temperature rise in preheated human muscle. *J Athl Train (Suppl.).* 1995; 30:S-42.

Hashish I, Hai HK, Harvey W, et al. Reduction of post-operative pain and swelling by ultrasound treatment: a placebo effect. *Pain.* 1988;33:303–311.

Hill CR, ter Haar G. Ultrasound and non-ionizing radiation protection. In: Suess MJ, ed. *WHO Regional Publication, European Series No. 10.* Copenhagen: World Health Organization; 1981.

Hogan RD, Burke KM, Franklin TD. The effect of ultrasound on microvascular hemodynamics in skeletal muscle: effects during ischemia. *Microvasc Res.* 1982;23:370.

Hone C-Z, Liu HH, Yu J. Ultrasound thermotherapy effect on the recovery of nerve conduction in experimental compression neuropathy. *Arch Phys Med Rehab.* 1988;69:410–414.

Hustler JE, Zarod AP, Williams AR. Ultrasonic modification of experimental bruising in the guinea-pig pinna. *Ultrasound.* 1978;16:223–228.

Imig CJ, Randall BF, Hines HM. Effect of ultra-sonic energy on blood flow. *Am J Phys Med.* 1954;53:100–102.

Inaba MK, Piorkowski M. Ultrasound in treatment of painful shoulder in patients with hemiplegia. *Phys Ther.* 1972;52:737.

Jedrzejczak A, Chipchase L. The availability and usage frequency of real time ultrasound by physiotherapists in South Australia: an observational study. *Physiother Res Int.* 2008;13(4):231.

Johns L, Demchak F, Straub S. Quantative Schlieren assessment of physiotherapy ultrasound fields may aid in describing variations between the tissue heating rates of different transducers (abstract). *J Athl Train.* 2007;42(2):S-42.

Johns L, Demchak T. Quantitative Schlieren assessment of physiotherapy ultrasound fields may aid in describing variations between the tissue heating rates of different transducers. *J Athl Train.* 2007;42(Supplement):S41.

Johns L, Howard S, Straub S. Comparison of lateral beam profiles between ultrasound manufacturers (abstract). *J Athl Train* (Suppl.). 2005;40(2):S-50.

Johns L, Straub S, LeDet E. Ultrasound beam profiling: comparative analysis of 4 new ultrasound heads at both 1 and 3.3 Mhz shows variability within a manufacturer (abstract). *J Athl Train* (Suppl.). 2004;39(2):S-26.

Jones RI. Treatment of acute herpes zoster using ultrasonic therapy. *Physiotherapy.* 1984;70:94.

Klemp P, Staberg B, Korsgard J, et al. Reduced blood flow in fibromyotic muscles during ultrasound therapy. *Scand J Rehab Med.* 1982;15:21–23.

Konin J. Ultrasound Prep. *Athl Ther Today.* 2006;11(4):11.

Kramer JF. Effect of ultrasound intensity on sensory nerve conduction velocity. *Physiother Can.* 1985;37:5–10.

Kramer JF. Effects of therapeutic ultrasound intensity on subcutaneous tissue temperature and ulnar nerve conduction velocity. *Am J Phys Med.* 1985;64:9.

Kramer JF. Sensory and motor nerve conduction velocities following therapeutic ultrasound. *Aust J Physiother.* 1987;33(4):235–243.

Kuitert JH, Harr ET. Introduction to clinical application of ultrasound. *Phys Ther Rev.* 1955;35:19.

Kuitert JH. Ultrasonic energy as an adjunct in the management of radiculitis and similar referred pain. *Am J Phys Med.* 1954;33:61.

Kuntz A, Multer C, McLoughlin T. Effect of phonophoresis vs. ultrasound on tissue cortisol levels (abstract). *J Athl Training* (Suppl.). 2005;40(2):S-49.

LaBan MM. Collagen tissue: implications of its response to stress in vitro. *Arch Phys Med Rehab.* 1962;43:461.

Lehmann JF, Biegler R. Changes of potentials and temperature gradients in membranes caused by ultrasound. *Arch Phys Med Rehab.* 1954;35:287.

Lehmann JF, Brunner GD, Stow RW. Pain threshold measurements after therapeutic application of ultrasound. microwaves and infrared. *Arch Phys Med Rehab.* 1958;39:560.

Lehmann JF, Erickson DJ, Martin GM. Comparative study of the efficiency of shortwave, microwave and ultrasonic diathermy in heating the hip joint. *Arch Phys Med Rehab.* 1959;40:510.

Lehmann JF, Stonebridge JB, de Lateur BJ, et al. Temperatures in human thighs after hot pack treatment followed by ultrasound. *Arch Phys Med Rehab.* 1978;59:472–475.

Lehmann JF, Warren CC, Scham SM. Therapeutic heat and cold. *Clin Orthop.* 1974;99:207–245.

Lehmann JF. Heating of joint structures by ultrasound. *Arch Phys Med Rehab* 49:28; 1968.

Lehmann JF. Heating produced by ultrasound in bone and soft tissue. *Arch Phys Med Rehab*. 1967;48:397.

Lehmann JF. Therapeutic temperature distribution produced by ultrasound as modified by dosage and volume of tissue exposed. *Arch Phys Med Rehab*. 1967;48:662.

Lehmann JF. Ultrasound effects as demonstrated in live pigs with surgical metallic implants. *Arch Phys Med Rehab*. 1959;40:483.

Lehmann JR, Henrick JF. Biologic reactions to cavitation: a consideration for ultrasonic therapy. *Arch Phys Med Rehab*. 1953;34:86.

Leonard J, Tom J, Ingersoll C. Intramuscular tissue temperature after a 10-minute 1 Mhz ultrasound treatment tested with thermocouples and thermistors (abstract). *J Athl Train* (Suppl.). 2004;39(2):S-24.

Levenson JL, Weissberg MP. Ultrasound abuse: a case report. *Arch Phys Med Rehab*. 1983;64:90–91.

Lloyd JJ, Evans JA. A calibration survey of physiotherapy equipment in North Wales. *Physiotherapy*. 1988;74(2):56–61.

Lota MI, Darling RC. Change in permeability of the red blood cell membrane in a homogeneous ultrasonic field. *Arch Phys Med Rehab*. 1955;36:282.

Lyons ME, Parker KJ. Absorption and attenuation in soft tissues II: experimental results. *Inst Electric Electron Eng Trans Ultrason Ferroelect Freq Contr*. 1988;35:4.

Madsen PW, Gersten JW. Effect of ultrasound on conduction velocity of peripheral nerves *Arch Phys Med Rehab*. 1963;42:645–649.

Massoth A, Draper D, Kirkendall D. A measure of superficial tissue temperature during 1 MHz ultrasound treatments delivered at three different intensity settings. *J Athl Train*. 1993;28(2):166.

Maxwell L. Therapeutic ultrasound and the metastasis of a solid tumor. *J Sport Rehab*. 1995;4(4):273–281.

Maxwell L. Therapeutic ultrasound: its effects on the cellular and molecular mechanisms of inflammation and repair. *Physiotherapy*. 1992;78(6):421–425.

McBrier N, Lekan J. Therapeutic ultrasound decreases mechano-growth factor messenger ribonucleic acid expression after muscle contusion injury. *Arch Phys Med Rehabil*. 2007;88(7):936-940.

McBrier N, Merrick M, Devor S. The effects of ultrasound delivery method and energy transfer on skeletal muscle regeneration (abstract). *J Athl Train* (Suppl.). 2005;40(2):S-50.

McCutchan E, Demchak T, Brucker J. A comparison of the heating efficacy of the Autosound TM with traditional ultrasound methods (abstract). *J Athl Train*. 2007;42(2):S-41.

McDiarmid T, Burns PN, Lewith GT. Ultrasound and the treatment of pressure sores. *Physiotherapy*. 1985;71:661.

McLaren J. Randomized controlled trial of ultrasound therapy for the damaged perineum (abstract). *Clin Phys Physiol Measure*. 1984;5:40.

Meakins A, Watson T. Longwave ultrasound and conductive heating increase functional ankle mobility in asymptomatic subjects. *Phys Ther Sport*. 2006;7(2):74-80.

Michlovitz SL, Lynch PR, Tuma RF. Therapeutic ultrasound: its effects on vascular permeability (abstract). *Fed Proc*. 1761;4;1982.

Mickey D, Bernier J, Perrin D. Ice and ice with nonthermal ultrasound effects on delayed onset muscle soreness. *J Athl Train* (Suppl.). 1996;31:S-19.

Miller DL. A review of the ultrasonic bioeffects of microsonation, gas body activation and related cavitation-like phenomena. *Ultrasound Med Biol*. 1987;13(8):443–470.

Miller M, Longoria J. A comparison of tissue temperature differences between the midpoint and peripheral effective radiating area during 1 and 3 MHz ultrasound treatments. *J Athl Train*. 2007;42(Supplement):S40.

Mortimer AJ, Dyson M. The effect of therapeutic ultrasound on calcium uptake in fibroblasts. *Ultrasound Med Biol*. 1988;14:499–508.

Mummery CL. The effect of ultrasound on fibroblasts in vitro. *PhD Thesis*, London University; 1978.

National Council on Radiation Protection and Measurements (NCRP) Report No 74 (BioloSica): Effects of ultrasound, mechanisms and clinical applications, NCRP, Bethesda MD, p. 197; 1983.

Newman MK, Kill M, Frampton G. Effects of ultrasound alone and combined with hydrocortisone injections by needle or hydrospray. *Am J Phys Med*. 1958;37:206.

Novak EJ. Experimental transmission of lidocaine through intact skin by ultrasound. *Arch Phys Med Rehab*. 1964;45:231.

Oakley EM. Evidence for effectiveness of ultrasound treatment in physical medicine. *Br J Cancer* (Suppl.). 1982;45(V):233–237.

Olson S, Bowman J, Condrey K. Transdermal delivery of hydrocortisone, lidocaine, and menthol in subjects with delayed onset muscle soreness. *J Orthop Sports Phys Ther*. 1994;19(1):69.

Paaske WP, Hovind H, Seyerson P. Influence of therapeutic ultrasonic irradiation on blood flow in human cutaneous, sub-cutaneous and muscular tissues. *Scand J Clin Lab Invest*. 1973;31:389.

Palko A, Krause B. The efficacy of combination therapeutic ultrasound and electrical stimulation. *Journal of Athletic Training*. 2007;42(Supplement):S134.

Paul B. Use of ultrasound in the treatment of pressure sores in patients with spinal cord injury. *Arch Phys Med Rehab*. 1960;41:438.

Payne C. Ultrasound for post-herpetic neuralgia. *Physiotherapy*. 1984;70:96.

Penderghest C, Kimura I, Sitler M. Double blind clinical efficacy study of dexamethasone-lidocaine pulsed phonophoresis on perceived pain associated with symptomatic tendinitis. *J Athl Train (Suppl.).* 1996; 31:S-47.

Pineau J, Filliard J, Bocquet M. Ultrasound techniques applied to body fat measurement in male and female athletes. *J Athl Train.* 2009;44(2)142.

Popspisilova L, Rottova A. Ultrasonic effect on collagen synthesis and deposition in differently localised experimental granulomas. *Acta Chirurgica Plastica.* 1977;19:148–157.

Reid DC. Possible contraindications and precautions associated with ultrasound therapy. In: Mortimer A, Lee N, eds. *Proceedings of the International Symposium on Therapeutic Ultrasound.* Winnipeg: Canadian Physiotherapy Association; 1981.

Reynolds NL. Reliable ultrasound transmission (letter). *Phys Ther.* 1992;72(8):611.

Roberts M, Rutherford JH, Harris D. The effect of ultrasound on flexor tendon repairs in the rabbit. *Hand.* 1982;14:17.

Robinson S, Buono M. Effect of continuous-wave ultrasound on blood flow in skeletal muscle. *Phys Ther.* 1995;75(2):145–150.

Roche C, West J. A controlled trial investigating the effects of ultrasound on venous ulcers referred from general practitioners. *Physiotherapy.* 1984;70(12):475–477.

Rowe RJ, Gray IM. Ultrasound treatment of plantar warts. *Arch Phys Med Rehab.* 1965;46:273.

Rubley M, Touton T. Thermal ultrasound: it's more than power and time. *Athl Ther Today.* 2009;14(1):5.

Shambereer RC, Talbot TL, Tipton HW, et al. The effect of ultrasonic and thermal treatment of wounds. *Plast Reconstruct Surg.* 1981;68(6):880–870.

Sicard-Rosenbaum L, Lord D, Danoff J. Effects of continuous therapeutic ultrasound on growth and metastasis of subcutaneous murine tumors. *Phys Ther.* 1995;75(1):3–12.

Smith W, Winn F, Farette R. Comparative study using four modalities in shinsplint treatments. *J Orthop Sports Phys Ther.* 1986;8:77.

Sokoliu A. Destructive effect of ultrasound on ocular tissues. In: Reid JM, Sikov MR, eds. *Interaction of Ultrasound and Biological Tissues.* Washington, DC, DHEW Pub (FDA) 73–8008; 1972.

Soren A. Evaluation of ultrasound treatment in musculoskeletal disorders, *Physiotherapy.* 1965;61:214–217.

Soren A. Nature and biophysical effects of ultrasound. *J Occup Med.* 1965;7:375.

Stevenson JH. Functional, mechanical, and biochemical assessment of ultrasound therapy on tendon healing in chicken toe. *Plast Reconstruct Surg.* 1986;77:965.

Stewart HF, Abzug JL, Harris GF. Considerations in ultrasound therapy and equipment performance. *Phys Ther.* 1980;80(4):424–428.

Stewart HF. Survey of use and performance of ultrasonic therapy equipment in Pinelles County. *Phys Ther.* 1974;54:707.

Stoller DW, Markholf KL, Zager SA, Shoemaker SC. The effects of exercise ice and ultrasonography on torsional laxity of the knee joint. *Clin Orthop Rel Res.* 1983;174:172–150.

Stratford PW, Cevy DR, Gauldie S, et al. The evaluation of phonophoresis and friction massage as treatments for extensor carpi radialis tendinitis: a randomized controlled trial. *Physiother Can.* 1989;41:93.

Stratton SA, Heckmann. R, Francis RS. Therapeutic ultra-sound: its effect on the integrity of a nonpenetrating wound. *J Orthop Sports Phys Ther.* 1984;5:278.

Straub, S Johns L. ERA measurements of 1 cm² ultrasound transducers operating at 3.3 MHz. *J Athl Train.* 2007;42(Supplement):S41.

Straub S, Johns L, Howard S. ERA measurements of 1 cm² ultrasound transducers operating at 3.3 MHz (abstract), *J Athl Train.* 2007;42(2):S-42.

Talaat AM, El-Dibany MM, El-Garf A. Physical therapy in the management of myofascial pain dysfunction syndrome. *Am Otol Rhinol Laryngol.* 1986;95:225.

Tashiro T, Sander T, Zinder S. Site of ultrasound application over the hamstrings during stretching does not enhance knee extension range of motion (abstract). *J Athl Train(Suppl.).* 2004;39(2):S-25.

Taylor E, Humphry R. Survey of therapeutic agent modality use. *Am J Occup Ther.* 1991;46(10):924–931.

Ter Haar C, Dyson M, Oakley EM. The use of ultrasound by physiotherapists in Britain, 1985. *Ultrasound Med Biol.* 1987;13:659.

Ter Haar G, Wyard SJ. Blood cell banding in ultrasonic standing waves: a physical analysis. *Ultrasound Med Biol.* 1978;4:111–123.

Ter Haar G. Basic physics of therapeutic ultrasound. *Physiotherapy.* 1978;64(4):100–103.

Tom J, Leonard J, Ingersoll C. Cutaneous vesiculations on anterior shin in 3 research subjects after a 1 Mhz, 1.5 W/cm2, continuous ultrasound treatment (abstract). *J Athl Train (Suppl.).* 2004;39(2):S-24–S-25.

Van Levieveld DW. Evaluation of ultrasonics and electrical stimulation in the treatment of sprained ankles: a controlled study. *Ugesrk-Laeger.* 1979;141(16):1077–1080.

Walker N, Denegar C, Preische J. Low-intensity pulsed ultrasound and pulsed electromagnetic field in the treatment of tibial fractures: a systematic review. *J Athl Train.* 2007;42(4):530.

Ward A, Robertson V. Comparison of heating of nonliving soft tissue produced by 45 KHz and 1 MHz frequency ultrasound machines. *J Orthop Sports Phys Ther.* 1996;23(4):258–266.

Warden S, Avin K, Beck E. Low-intensity pulsed ultrasound accelerates and a nonsteroidal anti-inflammatory drug delays knee ligament healing (abstract). *J Orthop Sports Phys Ther.* 2006;36(1):A6.

Warden S, Fuchs R, Kessler C. Ultrasound produced by a conventional therapeutic ultrasound unit accelerates fracture repair. *Phys Ther.* 2006;86(8):1118.

Warren CG, Koblanski IN, Sigelmann RA. Ultrasound coupling media: their relative transmissivity. *Arch Phys Med Rehab.* 1976;57:218.

Warren CG, Lehmann JF, Koblanski N. Heat and stretch procedures: an evaluation using rat tail tendon. *Arch Phys Med Rehab.* 1976;57:122.

Wells PE, Frampton V, Bowsher D, eds. *Pain: Management and Control in Physiotherapy.* London: Heinemann; 1988.

Wells PN. *Biomedical Ultrasonics.* London: Academic Press; 1977.

Williams AR, McHale I, Bowditch M. Effects of MHz ultrasound on electrical pain threshold perception in humans. *Ultrasound Med Biol.* 1987;13:249.

Williamson JB, George TK, Simpson DC, et al. Ultrasound in the treatment of ankle sprains. *Injury.* 1986;17:76–178.

Wilson AG, Jamieson S, Saunders R. The physical behaviour of ultrasound. *NZ J Physiotherapy.* 1984;12(1):30–31.

Wong R, Schumann B. A Survey of Therapeutic ultrasound use by physical therapists who are orthopaedic certified specialists. *Phys Ther.* 2007;87(8):986.

Wood RW, Loomis AL. The physical and biological effects of high frequency waves of great intensity. *Philosoph Mag.* 1927;4:417.

Wright ET, Haase KH. Keloid and ultrasound. *Arch Phys Med Rehab.* 1971;52:280.

Wyper DJ, McNiven DR, Donnelly TJ. Therapeutic ultra-sound and muscle blood flow. *Physiotherapy.* 1978;64:321.

Zaino A, Straub S, Johns L. Independent analysis of ERA at 1 and 3MHz across five manufacturers (abstract). *J Athl Train (Suppl.).* 2005;40(2): S-51.

Zankei HT. Effects of physical agents on motor conduction velocity of the ulnar nerve. *Arch Phys Med Rehab.* 1966;47:787–792.

GLOSSARY

acoustic microstreaming The unidirectional movement of fluids along the boundaries of cell membranes resulting from the mechanical pressure wave in an ultrasonic field.

amplitude The variation in pressure found along the path of the wave in units of pressure (N/m²).

attenuation A decrease in energy intensity as the ultrasound wave is transmitted through various tissues owing to scattering and dispersion.

cavitation The formation of gas-filled bubbles that expand and compress because of ultrasonically induced pressure changes in tissue fluids.

collimated beam A focused, less divergent beam of ultrasound energy produced by a large-diameter transducer.

continuous wave ultrasound The sound intensity remains constant throughout the treatment and the ultrasound energy is being produced 100% of the time.

coupling medium A substance used to decrease the acoustical impedance at the air–skin interface and thus facilitate the passage of ultrasound energy.

intensity A measure of the rate at which energy is being delivered per unit area.

longitudinal wave The primary waveform in which ultrasound energy travels in soft tissue with the molecular displacement along the direction in which the wave travels.

phonophoresis A technique in which ultrasound is used to enhance delivery of a selected medication into the tissues.

power The total amount of ultrasound energy in the beam, expressed in watts.

pulsed ultrasound The intensity is periodically interrupted with no ultrasound energy being produced during the off period. When using pulsed ultrasound, the average intensity of the output over time is reduced.

rarefactions Regions of lower molecular density (i.e., a small amount of ultrasound energy) within a longitudinal wave.

transverse wave Occurring only in bone, the molecules are displaced in a direction perpendicular to the direction in which the ultrasound wave is moving.

LAB ACTIVITY

Ultrasound

DESCRIPTION

Therapeutic ultrasound is a physical agent modality utilized in sports medicine for the purpose of elevating tissue temperature, stimulating the repair of musculoskeletal soft tissues, modulating pain, and in the case of phonophoresis, driving medicinal molecules into a local tissue. Ultrasound is a high frequency, inaudible acoustic sound wave that may produce either thermal or nonthermal physiologic effects within the body. When applied to biologic tissues ultrasound may induce significant responses in cells, tissues, and organs. Ultrasound is one of the most widely utilized physical agent modalities in addition to the thermotherapies and electrotherapies.

Physiologic Effects

Thermal effects
Elevated tissue temperature
Increased blood flow
Increased tissue extensibility
Increased local metabolism
Altered nerve conduction velocity

Nonthermal effects
Cavitation
Fluid movement
Increased cellular membrane permeability
Acoustic microstreaming
Stimulation of fibroblast activity

Therapeutic Effects

Increased collagen tissue extensibility
Decreased joint stiffness
Reduction of muscle spasm
Modulation of pain
Increased blood flow

Mild inflammatory response
Stimulation of tissue regeneration

Indications

The primary indication for the use of therapeutic ultrasound by the therapist is in the acute and chronic treatment of soft tissue dysfunction, that is, strains, sprains, contusions with associated symptoms of pain, and muscular spasm. Ultrasound has also been successfully employed to enhance soft tissue and bone healing. Ultra-sound can also be employed to percutaneously deliver selected medications to areas of inflammation.

Contraindications

- Areas of impaired pain or temperature sensation
- Areas of impaired circulation
- Epiphyseal areas in children
- Not over reproductive organs
- Not over eyes, heart, spinal cord, or cervical/stellate ganglia
- Not over cemented joint prostheses
- Not over malignancies

ULTRASOUND

PROCEDURE	EVALUATION		
	1	2	3
1. Check supplies and equipment.			
a. Obtain appropriate ultrasound unit (1 or 3 MHz), towels, and coupling gel.			
2. Question patient.			
a. Verify identity of patient.			
b. Verify the absence of contraindications.			
c. Ask about previous ultrasound treatments and check previous treatment notes.			
3. Position patient.			
a. Place patient in a well-supported, comfortable position.			
b. Expose body part to be treated.			
c. Drape patient to preserve patient's modesty, protect clothing, but allow access to body part.			
4. Inspect body part to be treated.			
a. Check sensation.			
b. Check circulatory status.			

c. Verify that there are no rashes or open wounds.			
d. Assess function of body part (e.g., ROM, strength, irritability).			
5. Apply indicated technique: select continuous or pulsed output and verify output intensity is at 0 before turning unit power on.			
a. Direct coupling.			
i. Apply layer of coupling gel to treatment surface.			
ii. Establish treatment duration dependent on size of area to be treated (i.e., 5 minutes for each 16-square-inch area).			
iii. Maintain contact between soundhead and treatment surface, moving soundhead in circular or linear overlapping strokes at a rate of 2–4 inch/s; observe for air bubble formation.			
iv. Adjust treatment intensity: 0.5–1.0 W/cm^2 for superficial tissues and 1.0–2.0 W/cm^2 for deeper tissues.			
v. Monitor patient response during treatment; if patient reports warmth or ache, reduce intensity by 10% and continue treatment.			
b. Bladder coupling.			
i. Fill a balloon or condom with tepid, degassed water.			
ii. Apply layer of coupling gel to bladder.			
iii. Apply layer of coupling gel to treatment surface.			
iv. Place bladder over treatment surface.			
v. Establish treatment duration dependent on size of area to be treated (i.e., 5 minutes for each 16-square-inch area).			
vi. Maintain contact between soundhead and treatment surface, moving soundhead in circular or linear overlapping strokes at a rate of 2–4 inch/s; observe for air bubble formation.			
vii. Adjust treatment intensity: 0.5–1.0 W/cm^2 for superficial tissues and 1.0–2.0 W/cm^2 for deeper tissues, intensity may need to be increased.			
viii. Monitor patient response during treatment; if patient reports warmth or ache, reduce intensity by 10% and continue treatment.			
c. Underwater coupling.			
i. Fill a plastic or ceramic nonconductive basin with tepid degassed water of sufficient depth to cover treatment surface.			
ii. Immerse the body part into the basin.			
iii. Establish treatment duration dependent on size of area to be treated (i.e., 5 minutes for each 16-square-inch area).			
iv. Maintain soundhead parallel to treatment surface at a distance of 0.5–3 cm, moving soundhead in circular or linear overlapping strokes at a rate of 2–4 inch/s; observe for air bubble formation on soundhead and wipe away.			

v. Adjust treatment intensity: 0.5–1.0 W/cm² for superficial tissues and 1.0–2.0 W/cm² for deeper tissues, intensity may need to be increased.			
vi. Monitor patient response during treatment; if patient reports warmth or ache, reduce intensity by 10% and continue treatment.			
d. Phonophoresis.			
i. Cleanse treatment surface with alcohol or soap and water.			
ii. Apply medication in glycerol cream, oil, or other vehicle in lieu of coupling gel.			
iii. Establish treatment duration dependent upon size of area to be treated (i.e., 5 minutes for each 16-square-inch area).			
iv. Maintain contact between soundhead and treatment surface, moving soundhead in circular or linear overlapping strokes at a rate of 2–4 inch/s; observe for air bubble formation.			
v. Adjust treatment intensity: 0.5–1.0 W/cm² for superficial tissues and 1.0–2.0 W/cm² for deeper tissues. Intensity may need to be decreased.			
vi. Monitor patient response during treatment; if patient reports warmth or ache, reduce intensity by 10% and continue treatment.			
6. Terminate treatment.			
a. Zero out ultrasound unit control before removing soundhead.			
b. Clean soundhead of excess gel or medication in vehicle.			
c. Clean treatment surface of excess gel or medication in vehicle.			
d. Visually inspect the treated area.			
e. Remove draping material and have patient dress.			
7. Assess treatment efficacy.			
a. Ask the patient how the treated area feels.			
b. Record treatment parameters.			
8. Instruct the patient in any indicated exercise.			
9. Return equipment to storage after cleaning.			

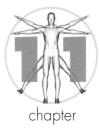

Extracorporeal Shockwave Therapy

Charles Thigpen

OBJECTIVES

Following completion of this chapter, the student will be able to:

➤ Describe the mechanical characteristics of extracorporeal shockwaves.

➤ Identify musculoskeletal pathologies that may benefit from extracorporeal shockwave therapy.

➤ Discuss the cellular effects of extracorporeal shockwave therapy on bone and tendons.

➤ Discuss why these effects may be beneficial to these tissues.

HISTORY OF EXTRACORPOREAL SHOCKWAVE THERAPY (ESWT)

Therapeutic shock waves were first introduced into medicine over 20 years ago for the treatment of kidney stones. Shock waves have since become the primary treatment choice for urinary, biliary, and salivary calculi. More recently, extracorporeal shock wave therapy has been utilized to treat musculoskeletal conditions such as lateral epicondylitis and plantar fasciitis in the United States[33] (Figure 11–1).

This is especially important in the treatment of patients with chronic tendinopathies that are difficult to treat. It is becoming clear that "chronic inflammation" is not present and regeneration of tendocytes is needed to facilitate healing.[1] The biologic effects of ESWT have shown to be effective in stimulating growth of these collagen building cells.[2,3] Furthermore, other musculoskeletal disorders have been treated in Europe including; pseudoarthrosis, nonunion fractures, and during total joint revisions. There have been a number of prospective trials examining the effects of ESWT in the last 10 years with mixed results. The disparity in results suggest there is a need define more accurate indications to optimize therapeutic outcomes.[4] This chapter will clarify the terminology and principles of shock wave therapy, discuss the potential biologic effects of shock waves, and review the current use of ESWT in the treatment of musculoskeletal conditions. Finally, evidence-based clinical guidelines for use of ESWT will be presented.

ESWT will continue to be used more especially in the treatment what has traditionally been referred to as chronic tendonitis. It is important to discuss this topic briefly before we begin. Traditionally, physical therapists, athletic trainers, and physicians have concluded that longstanding symptoms of tendonitis were the result of the healing process being "stuck" in the inflammatory phase. However it is becoming clear that this is not the mechanism underlying

417

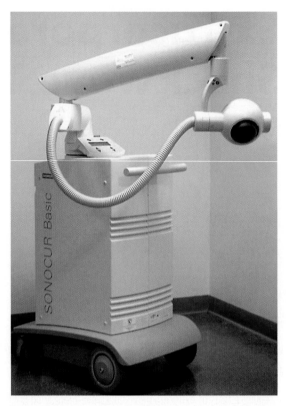

Figure 11-1. The Sonocur is an example of an extracorporeal shockwave therapy unit.

this chronic condition. Current recommendations include a period of rest, followed by aggressive eccentric exercise to stimulate tendon regeneration.[1-3,5-9] ESWT's demonstrated biologic effects of decreasing pain and promoting tissue regeneration make it an ideal adjunct to the rehabilitation process. We explore ESWT and its potential benefits in musculoskeletal rehabilitation.

PHYSICAL CHARACTERISTICS OF EXTRACORPOREAL SHOCK WAVE

To understand the potential biologic effects of the mechanical energy of shock waves, it is helpful to understand their physical properties. A shock wave is a sonic pulse that is characterized by the following physical parameters: a high peak pressure (sometimes as high as 100 MPa but usually around 50–80 MPa), a fast initial rise in pressure (less than 10 ns), a low-tensile amplitude, a short of life cycle (usually less than 10 μs), and a broad frequency spectrum (16–20 Hz)[10,11] (Figure 11–2).

These characteristics are in contrast to ultrasound waves whose peak pressure is much lower with frequencies in the range of 1–3 MHz. Additionally, velocity of an ultrasound wave is in the 1400–1600 m/sec where shockwave velocities are greater than 350 m/sec but less than 1000 m/sec. The high peak pressure of a shock wave is result of the combination of the velocity and frequency of the shockwave. The very high velocities of these wavelets when passed through a medium generate what is essentially a controlled explosion due to the pressure differential from the wavelets. This energy is then dissipated and reflected at tissue interfaces according to the mechanical properties of the tissues through which it passes.[10,11]

The shock wave's pressure disturbance is propagated three dimensionally due to the sudden rise in ambient pressure of the cell relative to the maximum pressure of the wave. This sudden rise in cell pressure causes an expansion and contraction within the medium causing tensile, compression, and shear stresses within the cell membrane. These stresses are usually in the

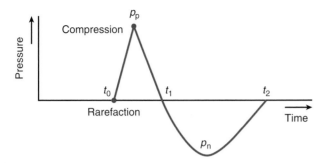

Figure 11–2. Two dimensional graph of positive and negative pressures generated within biologic tissues by shockwaves. p_p, maximum positive pressure (MPa); p_n, maximum negative pressure (MPa); t_0, beginning of shockwave; t_1, rarefaction begins causing negative pressure initiating cavitation; t_2, end of 1 shockwave cycle.

direction of wave propagation but the impedance and dampening at tissue boundaries reflect and refract within tissues causing steepening and attenuation of the wave. The drastic changes in pressure within the cell cause cavitation within the cells. The resulting collapsing of the cavitating bubbles yields water jets, which are proposed to cause cellular-level tissue damage.[12]

The impedance and dampening of the acoustic energy is similar to ultrasound waves. The attenuation of shock waves in air is 1000 times more than through water since the attenuation is dependent on the velocity of the wave and density of the tissue. Shock waves are generated within a water medium and applied through water-based coupling gel on the basis of the assumption that the human body's makeup is similar to water (Figure 11–3).

Therefore, the amount of attenuation and steepening that occurs at the tissue boundaries accounts for most of the loss of energy. It has been suggested that the increased efficiency relative to ultrasound allows for more focused and well controlled energy to be applied to the biologic tissues. Even with this control, biologic tissues respond differently to the same energy on the basis of differences in structural makeup. Keeping in mind these differences in tissue structure are important when applying therapeutic shock waves.[10,13,14]

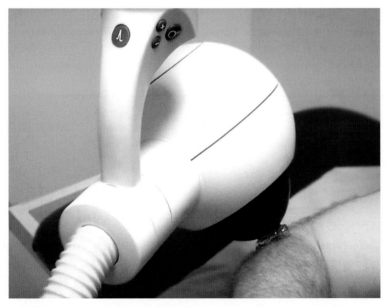

Figure 11–3. Patient is positioned adequate coupling gel in an appropriate position Attenuation of the shockwave is minimized by ensuring contact of the transmitting source with the coupling gel similar to ultrasound application. This position is used for treating lateral epicondylitis.

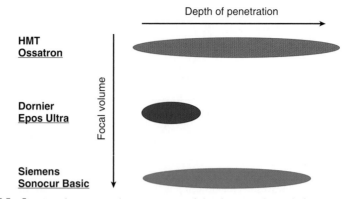

Figure 11–4. Two dimensional comparison of shock waves from different sources.

SHOCK WAVE GENERATION

There are three methods of shock wave generation currently in use in the United States: electrohydraulic, electromagnetic, and piezoelectric. Each of these techniques converts electrical energy into a mechanical shock wave. Currently, electrohydraulic and electromagnetic techniques are both being studied by the FDA. Each method generates shock waves with different volumes and amounts of energy penetrating to variable tissue depths[13] (Figure 11–4).

Electrohydraulic shock wave devices create a spark that discharges rapidly into the water and vaporizes the surrounding water creating a gas bubble filled with the water vapor. The gas bubble produces a sonic pulse and the subsequent implosion and a reverse pulse that causes another shock wave. The expanding shock waves are reflected by the surface of the ellipsoid and refocused into the focal point. Electrohydraulic shock wave devices are usually characterized by high-energy waves in focal volumes with fairly large axial diameters.[13]

Electromagnetic devices use a metal membrane and an opposing electromagnetic coil. An electric current is passed through a coil producing a strong magnetic field. The resulting variable magnetic field forces the metal membrane away compressing the surrounding fluid medium and creating a shock wave. The wave is passed through a lens to focus it at the desired target tissue. Electromagnetic shock wave devices tend to be used to create low-energy waves.[10,11]

Piezoelectric shock wave devices pass electrical current through large numbers of piezocrystals mounted on the inside of a sphere. The resulting expansion and contraction of the piezocrystals creates a shock wave. The piezocrystals are arranged in the sphere so that the resulting shock wave is very focused allowing for a high-energy density within a defined focal volume.[13]

Clinical Decision-Making *Exercise 11–1*

How can the clinician make adjustments in the sound wave to target deeper tissues?

PHYSICAL PARAMETERS OF SHOCK WAVES

Physical parameters used to describe shock waves are **focal volume, pressure field, total acoustical energy, energy flux, and energy flux density.** It is not clear which of these parameters are most important for therapeutic effectiveness. It has been suggested, however, that pressure field distribution, energy density, and total acoustical energy are the most important.[13] The focal volume is manipulated to ensure that the target tissue is treated. This is similar to choosing the frequency of ultrasound before treatment to achieve the desired depth of penetration. This is most commonly controlled by feedback from the patient, termed "**clinical focusing**" while several studies have used ultrasound and fluoroscopic imaging to locate the treatment site.[10] The

Table 11-1 Comparison of Physical Parameters for Shockwave Devices			
	HMT	DORNIER	SIEMENS
PARAMETER	OSSATRON	EPOS ULTRA	SONOCUR BASIC
Positive Peak Pressure in MPa	40.6–71.9	7.3–80.4	5.5–25.6
Focal Area in mm (Maximum dimensions from lowest to highest energy level settings)	6.6 × 6.8 × 67.6	7.7 × 7.7 × 20.0	6.0 × 6.0 × 58
Positive Energy Flux Density in mJ/mm²	0.09–0.34	0.03–0.98	0.016–0.22
Total Energy Flux Density in mJ/mm²	0.12–0.40	0.13–1.70	0.04–0.56

pressure field is measured in peak pulse engery (MPa) as a function of time. The pressure field varies across the focal volume and is greatest at the focal center (Table 11–1).

It is reflective of the maximum amount of acoustical energy that is within the field. The focal region is defined about three axes to describe the focal volume. The amount of acoustical energy within the focal volume is referred to as energy flux density and is calculated as the area below the squared pressure versus time curve. It is a measure of energy per square area for each sonic pulse and expressed in mJ/mm². Energy flux density is considered when calculating the threshold values for biologic tissues.[10,13] The most effective energy flux density is not known, however, Rompe et al.[2] have suggested a classification of energy flux density defined as: low <0.08 mJ/mm², medium 0.08–0.28 mJ/mm², and high >0.28 mJ/mm². This classification system is based on the response of tendons to shockwave treatment and seems to be an excellent guideline for treatment of bone and tendons. The MPa is determined from a pressure profile and is important when considering the maximum amount of pressure generated by a shock wave within a tissue. The pressure field distribution is the energy flux concentrated within the focal area. When ultrasound wave physics are considered, the focal area may be expanded to a larger wave volume where the peak pressure is half its original value. The biologic effects of the energy within the wave volume should be considered when treating each specific tissue. The total acoustical energy is the energy summed for the entire beam and describes the energy per shock wave. It has been suggested that total acoustical energy is the most important of the physical parameters when treating biological tissues. Consideration of the potential biologic effects of shock waves will enable the most appropriate acoustical energy to be applied.[10,11,14]

BIOLOGIC EFFECTS

The direct and indirect stresses of shock waves on biologic tissues should be considered. Tensile and shear stresses are created in the direction of shock wave propagation in biologic tissues. The tensile forces are greater than the tensile strength of water and generate bubbles (cavitation). Oscillation of the bubble diameters increase and decrease the volume of the bubble. Bubbles will fail dependent on the viscosity of the fluid and the pressure of the wave. The more viscous the fluid is the less the oscillation and therefore the less the pressure. The collapse of the bubbles creates microscopic high-energy water jets. This indirect effect can cause an increase in tissue temperature and damage cells.[2,3,13] The impact of cavitation and the water jets has been reported to depend strongly on the water content of the tissue and time between shock wave applications; however, no recommendations on appropriate hydration or time intervals have been made.[15] The micro-jets from the reflected shock waves occurring at tissue boundary areas and are where the most biologic effects are expected.[13]

Bone

The effect of shock waves on bony tissue is thought to occur primarily at the interface between cortical and cancellous bone. It is thought that acoustic streaming causes cavitation and

Table 11–2 Dose Related Effects of Shockwaves[2]

AMOUNT OF ENERGY	EFFECT ON TENDON	PROPOSED CLASSIFICATION
0.08 J/mm^2	No effect seen	Low
0.28 J/mm^2	Transiet swelling	Medium
0.60 J/mm^2	Paratendious inflammation and increase in diameter of tendon	High*

*Levels above 0.28 J/mm^2 are not recommended in the treatment of tendons.

increases cell permeability allowing increased vascularity and bony regeneration. More specifically, an increase in stromal cells seems to allow osteogenesis.[3] Additionally, the increase in osteoprogenitor cells coupled with local increases in growth factor, neovascularization, and protein synthesis suggest that shockwaves can improve the tissue environment for healing to occur.[3,6–9] However, results from both Rompe et al.[2] and Wang et al.[3] suggest that it is possible for too much damage to occur and the resulting cellular activity is unable overcome the damage. This is in contrast to inducing an amount of damage that allows for increases in vascularity and osteogenesis in bone that is not appropriately healed. To prevent cell damage from the short-time effect of high-energy shock wave dosages it has been suggested that less than 2000 pulses are needed to safely stimulate bone remodeling.[6] The use of high-energy devices have been reported in the literature in the treatment of nonunions and pseudoarthrosis.[10] It has been suggested that osteocyte damage and growth plate dysplasia resulting from the use of high-energy shock wave devices (>0.28 mJ/mm^2) may delay fracture healing and mechanical instability.[2] Durst et al.[16] is the only documented case identified in the literature, which reported these suggested adverse effects of ESWT. Humeral head osteonecrosis was confirmed by MRI and X-ray 3 years after treatment for calcific tendonitis. The dosage was 1600–1700 pulses at 12–13 kV for three treatments over a month. Given the nonstandard values reported it is unclear whether the energy density was high, medium, or low. Additionally, most other studies utilized shock wave devices designed specifically for orthopedic use and not a lithotripser. Insufficient detail was given about the device used to compare between studies. However, osteonecrosis may be a complication based on reports in the literature seen in urological cases.[10,11]

Tendon

The suggested mechanisms for biological effects of shock waves on tendons are the same as bone. Direct mechanical stresses cause tensile and shear failure within the cellular matrix of the tendon. The resulting cavitation and indirect microjets cause the most damage at the interface of the tendon and bone.[13] Rompe et al.[2] is the only study identified in the literature comparing the effects of shock waves on tendons. On the basis of their results they have suggested that doses over 0.28 mJ/mm2 are harmful to the musculotendinous complex and may place the complex at risk for rupture (Table 11–2). No complications have been published in the literature in the treatment of musculotendinous complexes.

CLINICAL APPLICATIONS

Fractures

Clinical success has been reported by several authors in the treatment of nonunion,[17–19] pseudarthorses,[20,21] acute fractures of the tibia,[22,23] femoral head necrosis,[24] and total hip revisions.[25] Through the aforementioned biologic mechanisms extracorporeal shock waves

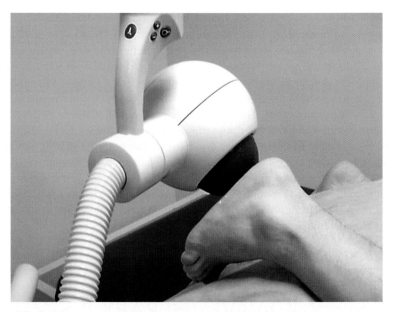

Figure 11–5. Patient positioning for treatment of plantar fasciitis.

are applied at high-energy doses to stimulate bone remodeling. Success rates range from 62–83% for nonunions and pseudarthroses.[11] Limited results are reported in the literature on the effectiveness for acute fractures, femoral head necrosis, and total hip revisions. Each of these conditions have been reported to be successfully treated when traditional treatments failed but it is unclear at this time if shock wave therapy should be considered as an initial treatment. Kuderna and Schaden[17] have suggested that the cost per injury to be 4–5 times less and recovery on average 2 months faster for tibial nonunion fractures treated acutely with high-energy extracorporeal shock waves when compared with traditional surgical intervention.

Plantar Fasciitis

The most studied use of extracorporeal shock wave therapy has been for the treatment of plantar fasciitis (Figure 11–5).

Use of low-energy shock waves have been approved by the FDA for use in the United States.[6] Success rates range from 56% to 75% dependent on the number of pulses applied, exact tissue treated, and previous treatment received by the patient.[10] There did not seem to be a pattern with any of these variables that would predict successful outcomes in these studies.[10,26–28] In a similar manner a recent prospective cohort was unable to identify any factors that predicted positive outcomes. However, they did find that patients with increasing age, diabetes mellitus, and psychological issues negatively influenced outcomes.[29] These factors may be important for clinicians to consider.

Several randomized controlled trials have reported positive results suggesting that shock wave therapy may be a viable option in the treatment of plantar fasciitis.[26–28,30] Boddeker et al.[31] concluded after a biometrical review of the literature that effectiveness of shock wave therapy could be neither confirmed nor denied due to the 21 studies reviewed not meeting all of the guidelines for a biometrical review. The results by Buchbinder et al.[26] from a randomized control trial also did not support the use of shock wave therapy when compared to a placebo ultrasound treatment for pain, function, and quality of life at 6 and 12 weeks post treatment. The conclusions of these authors are in contrast to others who have supported the use of shock wave therapy in the treatment of plantar fasciitis.[2,27,30] Differences in authors' conclusions are likely due to several factors including: method of patient selection, focusing of the shockwave, and definition of plantar fasciitis. Studies who have randomly assigned patients to a treatment groups with only a diagnosis of plantar fasciitis do not reflect actual clinical application of this device. Selection of patients with a well defined area of heel pain seems to respond better than those who are diagnosed with "plantar fasciitis." Differing methods of choosing the area to be treated likely have influenced these outcomes. Studies using "clinical focusing" where the most painful area is treated versus using a radiological guide to apply the shockwave appear to achieve different results. Reviewed literature seems to support "clinical focusing" suggesting that reduction of pain is primary benefit of shock wave therapy. The definition of plantar fasciitis was either not stated or differed between studies ultimately meaning that the comparisons between the studies are limited.

Success rates were based on pain at the initial treatment time and 6–12 months after treatment. Several other clinical trials suggest improved outcomes for patients who had plantar fasciitis for more than 6 months.[30,32–35] Good to excellent outcomes were reported by 70.7% at 3 months and 77.2% at 12 months.[29] This suggests that all plantar fasciitis patients do not appear to be appropriate for ESWT treatment. As the evidence for improvement seems to be with more chronic, troublesome cases.

CASE STUDY 11–1
EXTRACORPOREAL SHOCK WAVE THERAPY (ESWT)

Background: A 22-year-old male presented with a 6-month history of bilateral heel pain (R > L). He noted that his symptoms started approximately 2 weeks after beginning his new job working at a machine shop where he stands 8 or more hours per day on a concrete floor in stiff-soled safety shoes. The patient relates a history of the gradual onset of dull pain in his feet at the end of the work day that he initially attempted to treat with self-administered over-the-counter anti-inflammatories and some shoe inserts he purchased at a local store. He then noticed sharp, stabbing pains through his heels and feet when first standing in the morning and sought the care of his family physician. Currently the patient is taking prescription-strength NSAID and has been referred for further conservative care. On examination the patient was noted to exhibit a pes cavus foot, restricted passive dorsiflexion of the ankle (0°) secondary to tight gastrocsoleus-achilles complex, and point tenderness bilaterally just proximal to the calcaneal insertion of the plantar fascia.

Impression: Bilateral plantar fasciitis (R > L), chronic.

Treatment Plan: The patient was advised to continue his medication regimen. He was fitted with gel heel cushions for continuous wear while ambulatory and assigned light duty at work that reduced his standing time to 4 h/day. He underwent a 1× /week ESWT treatment of his right foot with a medium intensity (0.28 J/mm2) series of shock waves. This was followed by low-intensity prolonged static stretching exercise of the gastrocsoleus–achilles complex and completed with static icing to control transient, localized soft-tissue swelling that accompanies the treatment.

Response: The patient's symptoms diminished (pain decreased from 7/10 to 2/10 on VAS) in the right foot over the course of 6 weeks. Following successful intervention with the right foot, a course of treatment was undertaken for the left foot with similar outcomes. The patient was able to return to full duty without restrictions following a regimen of graduated standing time.

Discussion Questions

- What tissues were injured or affected? What symptoms were present?
- What phase of the injury-healing continuum did the patient present for care in?
- What are the physical agent modality's biophysical effects (direct, indirect, depth, and tissue affinity)?
- What are the physical agent modality's indications and contraindications?
- What are the parameters of the physical agent modality's application, dosage, duration, and frequency in this case study?
- What other physical agent modalities could be used to treat this injury or condition? Why? How?
- What is the significance of a positive Tinel sign? Would compression over the tarsal tunnel reproduce the symptoms?
- Why does the patient experience sharp, piercing pain with his first steps of the day and dull pain after prolonged standing?
- Is there another potential source of the patient's symptoms?

The rehabilitation professional employs physical agent modalities to create an optimum environment for tissue healing while minimizing the symptoms associated with the trauma or condition.

Clinical Decision–Making *Exercise 11–2*

A clinician is using ESWT for a patient with plantar fasciitis 50-year-old marathon runner. What things would suggest that this patient was appropriate for ESWT? What factors would suggest ESWT is not appropriate for treatment?

Medial–Lateral Epicondylitis

Use of the low-energy extracorporeal shock waves in the treatment of lateral epicondylitis has been approved by the FDA (see Figure 11–3). Success rates for shock wave therapy of tendinitis of the elbow are good for lateral epicondylitis ranging from 47% to 81%, but poor for a small sample of patients with medial epicondylitis.[10] Relief of pain and assessment of function have been used as outcome measures with all studies reviewed reporting significant improvement in the groups treated with extracorporeal shock wave therapy when compared to conventional treatments.[36–40] However, a systematic review and meta-analysis of ESWT studies for treatment of plantar fasciitis determined that ESWT provides little or no benefit in terms of pain and function in lateral elbow pain. It is important to note that the difference in conclusions likely lies within the selection of studies. Similar to plantar fasciitis, it appears that more chronic lateral elbow pain, which has not responded to other conservative treatments are most appropriate for ESWT treatment.[41–44] Even so it seems that low-energy extracorporeal shock wave therapy is a viable modality in the treatment of lateral epicondylitis. More studies should be done before any conclusions can be drawn about the treatment of medial epicondylitis or the treatment of tendinopathies in general.

Clinical Decision–Making *Exercise 11–3*

A clinician is determining if ESWT is the best course of treatment for a industrial line worker who has a 9-month history of lateral elbow pain and the MRI indicates a clear area of tendinopathy at the insertion of ECRB. Which type of ESWT should the clinician select and under what dosage parameters?

Calcific Tendinitis of the Shoulder

Treatment of calcific tendinitis of the shoulder with extracorporeal shock waves has been widely used in Europe and Canada with positive outcomes reported in the literature.[45–50] Success rates range from 60% to 85% using pain, function, and size of calcific deposits as outcome measures. When ultrasound or fluoroscopy has been used to focus the shock waves on the calcification outcomes have been improved over 80%.[45] Rompe et al.[49] treated noncalcific rotator cuff tendonitis with extracorporeal shock waves, and while there was an improvement, it was not more than the placebo effect. Haake et al.[48] have reported similar outcomes when comparing surgical intervention and ESWT for analogous shoulder tendinopathies. However, reported total cost was 93% less for those patients treated with ESWT. The majority (65%) of this difference in total cost was accounted for attributable to the productivity losses in the workplace. Recent studies have shown effectiveness for treatment of calcific tendinitis but noted about half the patients failing to achieve a satisfactory outcome and required surgical excision. Additionally, many patients found the procedure painful.[51–53] Similar to the differences in outcomes in the treatment of plantar fasciitis, these studies vary according to patient selection criteria, application of ESWT, and randomization. On the whole, the literature suggests that use of shock wave therapy for treatment of calcific tendonitis is useful and is improved when focused by an imaging technique and provides an reasonable opportunity to avoid surgery for excision of the calcific lesion.

Clinical Decision-Making   *Exercise 11–4*

A clinician is considering using ESWT for a patient with chronic shoulder pain. What are the risks and benefits the clinician should counsel the patient concerning ESWT treatment when considering ESWT? What measures should be taken to increase the likelihood of positive outcomes?

EVALUATION OF ESWT LITERATURE FOR EVIDENCED-BASED PRACTICE

It is important to understand several concepts regarding ESWT in an evaluation of the literature regarding ESWT. The parameters and criteria are outlined below:

1. *The difference in tendonitis/fasciitis and tendinosis/ fasciosis in regards to pathophysiology and the implications in patient selection.*[54–56]

   a. This frames the rationale in choosing treatments that are likely to be effective on a scientific basis. It is likely no accident that the patients who seem to respond to ESWT clearly have chronic tendinosis or fasciosis on a clinical basis (i.e., duration of at least six months and failure of other conservative measures, especially NSAIDS and/or steroid injection). Observations that those who respond best have failed steroid injection and other conservative therapies likely indicate a better selection of those patients who have no inflammatory component to their condition.

2. *The success of ESWT treatment appears to be dependent upon delivery of sufficient shock wave energy within a specific time frame.*[2,3,12]

   a. The amount of delivered energy in both intensity and total volume must be great enough to effect the structural and physiological changes that result in relief of symptoms (pain) and healing (heralded by neovascularity). This appears to require both a direct shock wave effect and cavitation events.

   b. Shock wave energy must be delivered within a relatively short time frame to be effective.

3. *The success or failure of shock wave therapy should be assessed at a point in time after completion of the last ESWT application, which allows for the effects of the shock waves to become clinically manifest with regards to symptoms.* At least 12 weeks is suggested by animal studies.[3]

4. *The success of ESWT appears to be dependent on accurate focusing of the shock wave energy to the precise area of tendinosis/fasciosis pathology.* Studies that have used imaging to select the treatment area have been less effective than those that use pain guided "clinical focusing."[10,26,38,40,49]

   a. Only clinical focusing using patient feedback can consistently accomplish accurate targeting.

   b. X-ray, fluoroscopy, and ultrasound are of minimal value since one cannot "see" pain with these devices.

SUMMARY

1. Studies seem to suggest moderate to good success, lack of consistency in the number of pulses, number of treatments, amount of energy, and application technique limits the ability to compare these studies.

2. ESWT appears to impact biological tissues in a way that is beneficial for chronic, poorly healing musculoskeletal conditions.

3. As with any treatment patient selection is paramount. It appears long standing soft-tissue disorders that have not responded to other treatment are most appropriate for ESWT treatment. Development of evidence-based criteria to guide treatment is needed.

4. Current evidence suggests location of pain, poor treatment progression longer than 3 months, and significant pain reduction upon initial treatment can be used to guide treatment at this time.

5. The non-invasive nature, lack of adverse side effects, possible decrease in cost, and treatment effectiveness reported support the use of ESWT in the treatment of chronic tendinopathies and nonunion fractures.

REVIEW QUESTIONS

1. List and define the five major mechanical characteristics of extracorporeal shockwaves.
2. How do shockwaves stimulate tissue healing?
3. Describe the characteristics of pathologies that may benefit from ESWT.
4. List three criteria when selecting patients for ESWT use.
5. What are the suggested dose parameters for treatment of tendonopathies?
6. Describe the four criteria when evaluating and applying ESWT evidence.

SELF TEST QUESTIONS

True or False

1. The most important parameter to know when assessing therapeutic effectiveness is energy flux density of the ESWT unit.
2. ESWT is thought to be effective in promoting tendon healing primarily by breaking down cell membranes through direct tensile and shear forces
3. ESWT has been shown to be an effective in the treatment of rotator cuff tendinopathy.

Multiple Choice

4. When considering the effect of ESWT on biologic tissues one should first know the
   a. Focal volume
   b. Pressure field
   c. Total acoustical energy
   d. Energy flux density

5. When choosing the appropriate dosage of ESWT for tendons, dosage should not exceed
   a. .04 J/mm^2
   b. .28 J/mm^2
   c. .60 J/mm^2
   d. 1.2 J/mm^2

6. The mechanisms outlined by which bone healing is thought to be promoted include changes in all except
   a. Neovascularization,
   b. Cell permeability
   c. Stromal cells
   d. Inflammation

7. _____ energy ESWT at no more than _____ pulses are suggested to stimulate bone growth without overwhelming the potential for healing.
   a. High, 1000
   b. Low, 2000
   c. High, 2000
   d. Low, 1000

8. Which of the following patients is most likely to respond to ESWT after failing conservative treatment for the 9 months prior to seeing you?
   a. 50-year-old male after falling and straining his rotator cuff
   b. 50-year-old female after developing lateral elbow pain

c. 24-year-old male after nonunion femoral neck fracture

d. 24-year-old female after developing plantar fasciitis

9. All of the following clinical benefits are true for ESWT treatment except

a. Decreased cost of care

b. Ideal adjunct for steroid injections

c. Decreased pain

d. Improved tissue healing

10. A 45-year-old male is treated for his lateral elbow pain with good pain relief over the first 6 visits. He completes his course of treatment at 9 visits in 8 weeks and complains that his pain has returned. You should counsel him that

a. Research suggests it takes 12 weeks or more for the tendon to start healing so he shouldn't worry.

b. Since his pain is not better he should seek a surgical consult next week.

c. The increase in pain is a sign of inflammation and the tendon is healing.

d. Research suggests it takes 20 weeks or more for the tendon to start healing so he shouldn't worry.

SOLUTIONS TO CLINICAL DECISION-MAKING EXERCISES

11–1

The depth of the sound wave is determined by the frequency of the sound wave. The application device should be adjusted to decrease the frequency to target deeper tissues.

11–2

Evidence suggests low-intensity ESWT is effective in treating lateral elbow tendinopathies 70% or more of patients responded in 4–6 wks.

11–3

First and foremost a clear diagnosis of plantar fasciitis confirmed by imaging. Additionally, symptoms for longer than 6 months and having failed other conservative management. If the patient reported a history of diabetes or psychological issues.

11–4

There are few risks except for the potential for pain during and after treatment. The possible benefits demonstrated by literature include: 60% likelihood of success, decreased size of the lesion, decreased cost when compared with surgery. Imagings such as fluoroscopy and ultrasound have been shown to improve outcomes for ESWT of calcific tendinitis.

REFERENCES

1. Almekinders LC. and Temple JD. Etiology, diagnosis, and treatment of tendonitis: an analysis of the literature. *Med Sci Sports Exercise* 1998;30:1183–1190.

2. Rompe JD, Kirkpatrick CJ, Kullmer K, Schwitalle M, and Krischek O. Dose-related effects of shock waves on rabbit tendo Achillis. *J Bone Joint Surg (Br)* 1998;80:546–552.

3. Wang FS, Yang RF, Chen RF, Wang CJ, and Sheen-Chen SM. Extracorporeal shock wave promotes growth and differentiation of bone-marrow stromal cells towards osteoprogenitors associated with induciton of TGF-B1. *J Bone Joint Surg (Br)* 2002;84:457–461.

4. Seil R, Wilmes P, and Nuhrenborger C. Extracorporeal shock wave therapy for tendinopathies. *Expert Rev Med Devices* 2006;3:463–470.

5. Hsu RW-W, Hsu W-H, Tai C-L, and Lee K-F. Effect of shock-wave therapy on patellar tendinopathy in a rabbit model. *J Orthopaed Res* 2004;22:221–227.

6. Kusnierczak D, Brocai DRC, Vettel U, and Loew M. The influence of extracorporeal shock-wave application on the biological behaviour of bone cells in vitro. 2000 *3rd International Congress of the ESMST*. Naples, Italy.

7. Wang C-J, Wang FS, Yang KD, et al. Shock wave therapy induces neovascularization at the tendon-bone junction: A study in rabbits. *J Orthop Res* 2003;21:984–989.

8. Wang FS, Wang C-J, Huang H-J, Chung H, Chen RF, and Yang KD. Physical shock wave mediates membrane hyperpolarization and ras activation for osteogenesis in human bone marrow stromal cells. *Biochem Biophys Res Comm* 2001;287:648–655.

9. Wang FS, Yang KD, Wang C-J, et al. Shockwave stimulates oxygen radical-mediated osteogenesis of the mesenchymal cells from human umbilical cord blood. *J Bone Mineral Res* 2004;19:973–982.

10. Chung B and Wiley P. Extracorporeal shockwave therapy: A review. *Sports Med* 2002;34:851–865.

11. Ogden JA, Alvarez RG, Levitt R, and Marlow M. Shock wave therapy (orthotripsy) in musculoskeletal disorders. *Clin Orth Rel Res* 2001;387:22–40.

12. Russo S, Galasso O, Marlinghaus E, Hagelauer U, and Mayer J. The in-vivo cavatation measurement. 1999 *2nd International Congress of the ESMST*. London.

13. Ogden JA, Kischkat AT, and Schultheiss R. Principles of shock wave therapy. *Clin Orth Rel Res* 2001;387:8–17.

14. Thiel M. Application of shock waves in medicine. *Clin Orth Rel Res* 2001;387:18–21.

15. Vara F. Treatment of the troncanteric bursitis with local application of extracorporeal shock wave. 1999 *2nd International Congress of the ESMST*. London.

16. Durst HB, Blatter G, and Kuster MS. Osteonecrosis of the humeral head after extracorporeal shock-wave lithotripsy. *J Bone Joint Surg (Br)* 2002;84:744–746.

17. Kuderna H and Schaden W. Comparison of 30 tibial nonunions: Costs of surgical treatment vs costs of ESWT. 2000 *3rd International Congress of the ESWT*. Naples, Italy.

18. Rompe J-D, Rosendahl T, Schollner C, and Theis C. High-energy extracorporeal shock wave treatment of nonunions. *Clin Orth Rel Res* 2001;387:102–111.

19. Schaden W, Fischer A, and Sailler A. Extracoporeal shock wave therapy of nonunion or delayed osseous union. *Clin Ortho Relat Res* 2001;387:90–94.

20. Haupt G. Use of extracoporeal shock waves in the treatment of pseudoarthorsis, tendinopathy, and other orthopedic diseases. *J Urol* 1997;158:4–11.

21. Kuner EH, Berwarth H, and Lucke SV. Aseptic pseudoarthrosis: Principles of treatment. *Orthopade* 1996;25:394–404.

22. Wang C-J, Chen H-S, Chen C-E, and Yang KD. Treatment of nonunions of long bone fractures with shock waves. *Clin Orth Rel Res* 2001;387:95–101.

23. Wang CJ, Huang H-Y, Chen H-H, Pai C-H, and Yang KD. Effect of shock wave therapy on acute fractures of the tibia. *Clin Orth Rel Res* 2001;387:112–118.

24. Ludwig J, Lauber S, Lauber H-J, Dreisilker U, Raedel R, and Hotzinger H. High-energy shock wave treatment of femoral head necrosis in adults. *Clin Orth Rel Res* 2001;387:119–126.

25. Karpman RR, Magee FP, Gruen TWS, and Mobley T. The lithotriptor and its potential use in the revision of total hip arthroplatsty. *Clin Orth Rel Res* 2001;387:4–7.

26. Buchbinder R, Ptasznik R, Gordon J, Buchanan J, Prabaharan V, and Forbes A. Ultrasound-guided extracorporeal shock wave therapy for plantar fasciitis. *JAMA* 2002;288:1364–1372.

27. Ogden JA, Alvarez R, Levitt R, Cross GL, and Marlow M. Shock wave therapy for chronic proximal plantar fasciitis. *Clin Orth Rel Res* 2001;387:47–59.

28. Rompe J-D, Schoellner C, and Nafe B. Evaluation of low-energy extracorporeal shock-wave application for treatment of chronic plantar fasciitis. *JBJS* 2002;84:335–341.

29. Chuckpaiwong B, Berkson EM, and Theodore GH. Extracorporeal shock wave for chronic proximal plantar fasciitis: 225 patients with results and outcome predictors. *J Foot Ankle Surg* 2009;48:148–155.

30. Chen H-S, Chen L-M, and Huang T-W. Treatment of painful heel syndrome with shock waves. *Clin Orth Rel Res* 2001;387:41–46.

31. Boddeker IR, Schafer H, and Haake M. Extracorporeal shockwave therapy in the treatment of plantar fasciitis-a biometrical review. *Clin Rheumatol* 2001;20:324–330.

32. Buchbinder R, Green SE, Youd JM, Assendelft WJ, Barnsley L, and N. Smidt. Systematic review of the efficacy and safety of shock wave therapy for lateral elbow pain. *J Rheumatol* 2006;33:1351–1363.

33. Gerdesmeyer L, Frey C, Vester J, et al. Radial extracorporeal shock wave therapy is safe and effective in the treatment of chronic recalcitrant plantar fasciitis: Results of a confirmatory randomized placebo-controlled multicenter study. *Am J Sports Med* 2008;36:2100–2109.

34. Gollwitzer H, Diehl P, von Korff A, Rahlfs VW, and Gerdesmeyer L. Extracorporeal shock wave therapy for chronic painful heel syndrome: A prospective, double blind, randomized trial assessing the efficacy of a new electromagnetic shock wave device. *J Foot Ankle Surg* 2007;46:348–357.

35. Kudo P, Dainty K, Clarfield M, Coughlin L, Lavoie P, and Lebrun C. Randomized, placebo-controlled, double-blind clinical trial evaluating the treatment of plantar fasciitis with an extracoporeal shockwave therapy (ESWT) device: A North American confirmatory study. *J Orthop Res* 2006;24:115–123.

36. Ko J-Y, Chen H-S, and Chen L-M. Treatment of lateral epicondylitis of the elbow with shock waves. *Clin Orth Rel Res* 2001;387:60–67.

37. Krischek O, Hopf C, Nafe B, and Rompe J-D. Shock-wave therapy for tennis and golfer's elbow-1 year follow-up. *Arch Orthop Trauma Surg* 1999;119:62–66.

38. Maier M, Steinborn M, Schmitz C, Stabler A, Kohler S, Veihelmann A, Pfahler M, and Refior HJ. Extracorporeal shock-wave therapy for chronic lateral tennis elbow-prediction of outcome by imaging. *Arch Orthop Trauma Surg* 2001;121:379–384.

39. Rompe J-D, Hopf C, Kullmer K, Heine J, and Burger R. Analgesic effect of extracorporeal shock-wave therapy on chronic tennis elbow. *J Bone Joint Surg (Br)* 1996;78:233–237.

40. Rompe J-D, Hopf C, Kullmer K, Heine J, Burger R, and Nafe B. Low-Energy extracorpal shock wave therapy for persistent tennis elbow. *Intr Orth* 1996;20:23–27.

41. Bisset L, Paungmali A, Vicenzino B, and Beller E. A systematic review and meta-analysis of clinical trials on physical interventions for lateral epicondylalgia. *Br J Sports Med* 2005;39:411–422; discussion 411–422.

42. Buchbinder R, Green SE, Youd JM, Assendelft WJ, Barnsley L, and Smidt N. Shock wave therapy for lateral elbow pain. *Cochrane Database Syst Rev* 2005;CD003524.

43. Radwan YA, ElSobhi G, Badawy WS, Reda A, and Khalid S. Resistant tennis elbow: Shock-wave therapy versus percutaneous tenotomy. *Int Orthop* 2008;32:671–677.

44. Staples MP, Forbes A, Ptasznik R, Gordon J, and Buchbinder R. A randomized controlled trial of extracorporeal shock wave therapy for lateral epicondylitis (tennis elbow). *J Rheumatol* 2008;35:2038–2046.

45. Charrin JE and Noel ER. Shockwave therapy under ultrasonographic guidance in rotator cuff calcific tendinitis. *Joint Bone Spine* 2001;68:241–244.

46. Grob MW, Sattler A, Haake M, Schmitt J, Hildebrandt R, Muller H-H, and Engenhart-Cabillic R. The value of radiotherapy in comparsion with extracorporeal shockwave therapy for supraspinatus tendinitis. *Strahlentherapie und Onkologie* 2002;178:314–320.

47. Haake M, Deike B, Thon A, and Schmitt J. Exact focusing of extracorporeal shock wave therapy for calcifying tendinopathy. *Clin Orth Rel Res* 2002;397:323–331.

48. Haake M, Rautmann M, and Wirth T. Extracorporeal shock wave therapy vs surgical treatment in calcifying tendinitis and non calcifying tendinitis of the supraspinatus muscle. *Eur J Orthop Surg Traumatol* 2001;11:21–24.

49. Rompe JD, Rumler F, Hopf C, Nafe B, and Heine J. Extracorporal shock wave therapy for calcifying tendinitis of the shoulder. *Clin Orth Rel Res* 1995;321:196–201.

50. Speed CA, Richards C, Nichols D, et al. Extracoporeal shock-wave therapy for tendonitis of the rotator cuff. *JBJS* 2001;84:509–512.

51. Hearnden A, Desai A, Karmegam A, and Flannery M. Extracorporeal shock wave therapy in chronic calcific tendonitis of the shoulder: is it effective? *Acta Orthop Belg* 2009;75:25–31.

52. Sabeti M, Dorotka R, Goll A, Gruber M, and Schatz KD. A comparison of two different treatments with navigated extracorporeal shock-wave therapy for calcifying tendinitis: A randomized controlled trial. *Wien Klin Wochenschr* 2007;119:124–128.

53. Schofer MD, Hinrichs F, Peterlein CD, Arendt M, and Schmitt J. High- versus low-energy extracorporeal shock wave therapy of rotator cuff tendinopathy: A prospective, randomised, controlled study. *Acta Orthop Belg* 2009;75:452–458.

54. Kahn K, Cook J, Taunton J, and Bonar F. Overuse tendinosis, not tendonitis: Part I: A new paradigm for a difficult clinical problem. *Phys Sportsmed* 2000;28.

55. Kraushaar B, and Nirschl R. Tendinosis of the elbow (tennis elbow).Clinical features and findings of histological, immunochemical and electron microscopy studies. *J Bone Joint Surg (Am)* 1999;81:259–278.

56. Lemont H, Ammirati B, and Usen N. Plantar fascitis: A degenerative process (fasciosis) without inflammation. *J Am Pod Soc* 2003;93:234–237.

GLOSSARY

clinical focusing   Applying the shockwave over the area that causes the most pain as opposed to the area of tissue disruption.

energy flux   A measure of the peak pulse energy within a focal volume.

energy flux density   A measure of the energy flux per square area (usually mm²).

focal volume   The amount of space the shock wave will have a therapeutic effect over.

pressure field   A function of time and space and is a reflection of the effect of energy over the focal volume.

total acoustical energy   The amount of acoustical energy delivered in one shock wave pulse

PART **FIVE**

Electromagnetic Energy Modalities

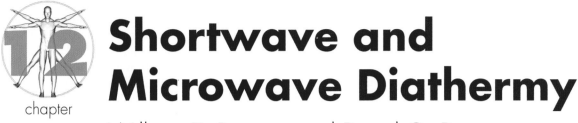

12 chapter

Shortwave and Microwave Diathermy

William E. Prentice and David O. Draper

OBJECTIVES

Following completion of this chapter, the student will be able to:

➤ Evaluate how the diathermies may best be used in a clinical setting.

➤ Explain the physiologic effects of diathermy.

➤ Differentiate between capacitance and inductance shortwave diathermy techniques and identify the associated electrodes.

➤ Compare treatment techniques for continuous shortwave and pulsed shortwave diathermy.

➤ Demonstrate the equipment setup and treatment technique for microwave diathermy.

➤ Discuss the various clinical applications and indications for using continuous short-wave, pulsed shortwave, and microwave diathermy.

➤ Identify the treatment precautions for using the diathermies.

➤ Analyze the rate of heating and how long muscle retains the heat generated from a shortwave diathermy treatment.

➤ Compare and contrast diathermy and ultrasound as deep-heating agents.

Diathermy is the application of high-frequency electromagnetic energy that is primarily used to generate heat in body tissues. Heat is produced by resistance of the tissue to the passage of the energy. Diathermy may also be used to produce nonthermal effects.

Diathermy as a therapeutic agent may be classified as two distinct modalities, shortwave and microwave diathermy. Shortwave diathermy may be either continuous or pulsed. Continuous shortwave diathermy has been used in the treatment of a variety of conditions for some time. For the past 15–20 years, clinicians have not widely used diathermy. It is likely that many young clinicians have never even seen a diathermy unit. However, over the last 5 years there seems to be renewed interest in this treatment modality due in large part to some newly published, evidence-based information that has begun to appear in the professional literature.[1,2,3] In addition, there appears to be renewed effort by equipment manufacturers who are

• Diathermy can have both thermal and nonthermal effects.

433

once again beginning to market pulsed shortwave diathermy units.[4] Shortwave diathermy is a relatively safe modality that can be very effectively incorporated into clinical use. Clinically, shortwave diathermy is much more commonly used than is microwave diathermy.

The effectiveness of a shortwave or microwave diathermy treatment depends on the clinician's ability to tailor the treatment to the patient's needs. This requires that the clinician have an accurate evaluation or diagnosis of the patient's condition and knowledge of the heating patterns produced by various diathermy electrodes or applicators. Many clinicians mistakenly feel that neither shortwave nor microwave diathermy produces heating at the depths desired for the treatment of musculoskeletal injuries. In fact, the depth of penetration is greater than with any of the infrared modalities, and further it has been shown that pulsed shortwave diathermy produces the same magnitude and depth of muscle heating as 1 MHz ultrasound.[4,5]

PHYSIOLOGIC RESPONSES TO DIATHERMY
Thermal Effects

The diathermies are not capable of producing depolarization and contraction of skeletal muscle because the wavelengths are much too short in duration.[6,7,38] Thus, the physiologic effects of continuous shortwave and microwave diathermy are primarily thermal, resulting from high-frequency vibration of molecules.

The primary benefits of diathermy are those of heat in general, such as tissue temperature rise, increased blood flow, dilation of the blood vessels, increased filtration and diffusion through the different membranes, increased tissue metabolic rate, changes in some enzyme reactions, alterations in the physical properties of fibrous tissues (such as those found in tendons, joints, and scars), decreased joint stiffness, a certain degree of muscle relaxation, a heightened pain threshold, and enhanced recovery from injury.[8-16]

Diathermy treatment doses are not precisely controlled, and the amount of heating the patient receives cannot be accurately prescribed or directly measured. Heating occurs in proportion to the square of the current density and in direct proportion to the resistance of the tissue.

$$\text{Heating} = \text{current density}^2 \times \text{resistance}$$

Lehmann stated that temperature increases of 1°C can reduce mild inflammation and increase metabolism, and that moderate heating, an increase of 2–3°C, will decrease pain and muscle spasm. Increasing tissue temperatures more than 3–4°C above baseline will increase tissue extensibility, thus enabling the clinician to treat chronic connective tissue problems.[17]

Opinions differ regarding the desired temperature increases needed to enhance extensibility of collagen. Some believe that optimal heating occurs when the tissue temperature rises above 38–40°C, whereas others believe that a tissue temperature increase of 3–4°C above baseline temperature is optimal.[8,17-19] Presently, no research can validate one opinion over another, but it is clear that the more vigorous the heating with diathermy, the greater chance there is for collagen elongation to occur.

Why certain pathologic conditions respond better to diathermy than other forms of deep heat is not well understood or documented. It probably is more directly related either to the skill of the clinician applying the modality or to some placebo effects associated with tissue temperature increase than it is to the specific effects of diathermy itself.

Subcutaneous adipose tissue thickness may affect the ability of shortwave diathermy to penetrate to deeper tissues.[20]

• Pulsed shortwave diathermy = nonthermal effects

Nonthermal Effects

Pulsed shortwave diathermy (PSWD) has also been used for its nonthermal effects in the treatment of soft-tissue injuries and wounds.[19] The mechanism of its effectiveness has been theorized to occur at the cellular level, relating specifically to cell membrane potential.[21]

Damaged cells undergo depolarization, resulting in cell dsyfunction that might include loss of cell division and proliferation and loss of regenerative capabilities. Pulsed shortwave diathermy has been said to repolarize damaged cells, thus correcting cell dysfunction.[22]

It has also been suggested that sodium tends to accumulate in the cell because of a decrease in activity of the sodium pump during the inflammatory process, thus creating a negatively charged environment. When a magnetic field is induced, the sodium pump is reactivated, thus allowing the cell to regain normal ionic balance.[23]

SHORTWAVE DIATHERMY EQUIPMENT

A shortwave diathermy unit is basically a radio transmitter. **The Federal Communications Commission (FCC)** assigns three frequencies to shortwave diathermy units: 27.12 MHz with a wavelength of 11 m, which is the most widely used; 13.56 MHz with a wavelength of 22 m; and 40.68 MHz with a wavelength of 7.5 m, which is rarely used (see Table 1–2).

The shortwave diathermy unit consists of a power supply that provides power to a radio frequency oscillator (Figure 12–1). This radio frequency oscillator provides stable, drift-free oscillations at the required frequency. The output resonant tank tunes in the patient as part of the circuit and allows maximum power to be transferred to the patient. The power amplifier generates the power required to drive the different types of electrodes.

Control panels on shortwave diathermy units vary considerably from one unit to another. Most modern shortwave diathermy units automatically adjust the output circuit for maximum energy transfer from the output resonant tank, which is similar to tuning in a station on a radio. Some older units have an *output tuning control* that must be manually adjusted. The *output intensity control* adjusts the percentage of maximum power transferred to the patient. This is similar to the volume control on a radio. The *output intensity indicator* monitors only the current that is drawn from the power supply and not the energy being delivered to the patient. Thus, it is only an indirect measure of the energy reaching the patient.

The most critical factor that determines whether a shortwave diathermy unit will increase tissue temperature is the amount of energy absorbed by the tissue. The power output of a shortwave diathermy unit should produce sufficient energy to raise the tissue temperature into a therapeutic range. The **specific absorption rate (SAR)** represents the rate of energy absorbed per unit area of tissue mass. Most shortwave units have a power output of between 80 W and 120 W. Some units are not capable of this level of output, making them safe but ineffective. It is important to remember that the tissue temperature rise with diathermy units can be offset dramatically by an increase in blood flow, which has a cooling effect in the tissue being energized. Therefore, units should be able to generate enough power to provide for an excess of the SAR.

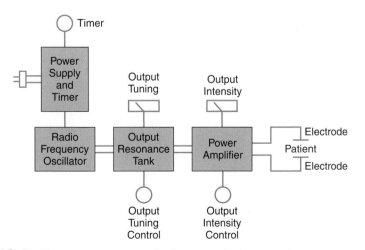

Figure 12–1. The component parts of a shortwave diathermy unit.

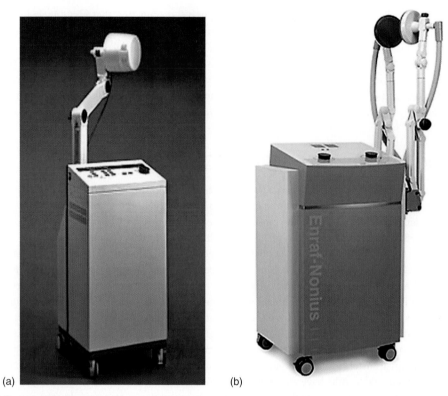

(a)   (b)

Figure 12–2. Shortwave diathermy units. (a) Autotherm. (b) Radarmed 650.

Patient sensation provides the basis for recommendations of continuous shortwave diathermy dosage and thus varies considerably with different patients.[23,24] The following dosage guidelines have been recommended:

Dose I (lowest): No sensation of heat
Dose II (low): Mild heating sensation
Dose III (medium): Moderate (pleasant) heating sensation
Dose IV (heavy): Vigorous heating that is tolerable below the pain threshold

A shortwave diathermy unit that generates a high-frequency electrical current will produce both an **electrical field** and a **magnetic field** in the tissues (Figure 12–2).[25] The ratio of the electrical field to the magnetic field depends on the characteristics of the different units as well as on the characteristics of electrodes or applicators. Shortwave units with a frequency of 13.56 MHz tend to produce a stronger magnetic field than do units with the frequency of 27.12 MHz, which produces a stronger electric field. The majority of the new pulsed shortwave diathermy units use a drum electrode and produce a stronger magnetic field.

Shortwave Diathermy Electrodes

Shortwave diathermy may be delivered to the patient via either **capacitance** or **induction techniques**. Each of these techniques can affect different biologic tissues, and selection of the appropriate electrodes is essential for effective treatment. Shortwave diathermy uses several types of applicators or electrodes, including air space plates, pad electrodes, cable electrodes, or drum electrodes. Table 12–1 summarizes the two shortwave diathermy delivery techniques.

Capacitor Electrodes

The *capacitance* technique, using **capacitor electrodes,** creates a stronger electrical field than a magnetic field. As discussed in Chapter 5, within the body there are many free ions that are

Table 12-1 Summary of Shortwave Diathermy Techniques				
METHOD	FIELD	ELECTRODES	CIRCUIT	TISSUES HEATED
Capacitance	Electric	Capacitor Air space plates Pads	Series-patient part of circuit	Those high in electrolytes (i.e. muscle, blood)
Inductance	Magnetic	Inductor Drum Cable	Parallel-patient not part of circuit	Subcutaneous fat

positively or negatively charged. A positively charged electrode or plate will repel positively charged ions and attract negatively charged ions. Conversely, the negative electrode will repel negative ions and attract positive ions (Figure 12–3).

An electrical field is essentially the lines of force exerted on these charged ions by the electrodes that cause charged particles to move from one pole to the other (Figure 12–4). The intensity of the electrical field is determined by the spacing of the electrodes and is greatest when they are close together. The center of this electrical field has a higher current density than regions at the periphery. When using capacitance electrodes, the patient is placed between two electrodes or plates and becomes part of the circuit. Thus, the tissue between the two electrodes is in a series circuit arrangement (see Chapter 5).

As the electrical field is created in the biologic tissues, the tissue that offers the greatest resistance to current flow tends to develop the most heat. Tissues that have a high fat content tend to insulate and resist the passage of an electrical field. These tissues, particularly subcutaneous fat, tend to overheat when an electrical field is used, which is characteristic of a capacitance type of electrode application.

Air Space Plates. **Air space plates** are an example of a capacitance (strong electrical field) technique or a capacitor electrode (Figure 12–5). This type of electrode consists of two metal plates with a diameter of 7.5–17.5 cm surrounded by a glass or plastic plate guard. The metal plates may be adjusted approximately 3 cm within the plate guard, thus changing the distance from the skin.[26] Air space plates produce high-frequency oscillating current that is passed through each plate millions of times per second. When one plate is overloaded, it discharges to the other plate of the lower potential, and this is reversed millions of times per second.[27]

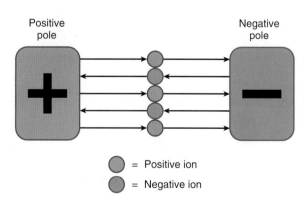

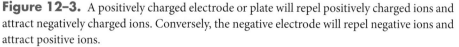

Figure 12–3. A positively charged electrode or plate will repel positively charged ions and attract negatively charged ions. Conversely, the negative electrode will repel negative ions and attract positive ions.

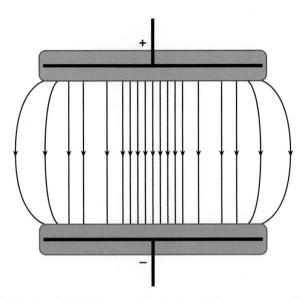

Figure 12–4. An electrical field is essentially the lines of force exerted on these charged ions by the electrodes, which causes charged particles to move from one pole to the other. (Modified from Michlovitz S. *Thermal Agents in Rehabilitation.* Philadelphia: FA Davis, 1990.)

When air space plates are used, the area to be treated is placed between the electrodes and becomes part of the external circuit (Figure 12–6). The sensation of heat tends to be in direct proportion to the distance of the plate from the skin. The closer the plate is to the skin, the better the energy transmission because there is less reflection of the energy. However, it should be remembered that the closer plate will also generate more surface heat in the skin and the subcutaneous fat in that area (Figure 12–7). The greatest surface heat will be under the electrodes. Parts of the body that are low in subcutaneous fat content (e.g., hands, feet, wrists, and ankles) are best treated by this method. Patients who have a very low subcutaneous fat content can be effectively treated in other body areas.[28] This technique is also very effective for treating the spine and the ribs.

Pad Electrodes. **Pad electrodes** are seldom used in the clinical setting; however, they may be available for some units. They are true capacitor electrodes, and they must have

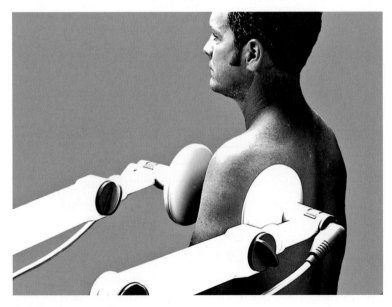

Figure 12–5. Air space plates.

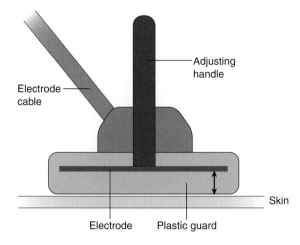

Figure 12–6. Air space plate electrodes consist of a metal plate enclosed in a glass or plastic plate guard. The metal plate may be adjusted approximately 3 cm within the plate guard, thus changing the distance from the skin.

uniform contact pressure on the body part if they are to be effective in producing deep heat, as well as in avoiding skin burns (Figure 12–8). The patient is part of the external circuit. Several layers of toweling are necessary to make sure that there is sufficient space between the skin and the pads. The pads should be separated so they are at least as far apart as the cross-sectional diameter of the pads. In other words, if the pads are 15 cm across, then there should be at least 15 cm between the pads. The closer the spacing of the pads, the higher the current density in the superficial tissues. Increasing the space between the pads will increase the depth of penetration in the tissues (Figure 12–9). The part of the body to be treated should be centered between the pads.[12,25–27]

Clinical Decision-Making   *Exercise 12–1*

An clinician is using pad electrodes to treat a patient who has muscle guarding in the low back. What can be done with these electrodes to increase the depth of penetration without increasing output intensity?

Inductor Electrodes

The inductance technique, using **inductor electrodes,** creates a stronger magnetic field than it does an electrical field. When the induction technique is used in shortwave diathermy, a cable or coil is either wrapped circumferentially around an extremity or it is coiled within an electrode. In either case, when current is passed through a coiled cable, a magnetic field is generated that can affect surrounding tissues by inducing localized secondary currents, called **eddy currents,** within the tissues (Figure 12–10).[21] Eddy currents are small circular electrical fields, and the **intermolecular oscillation (vibration)** of tissue contents causes heat generation.

In the inductance technique, the patient is in a magnetic field and is not part of the circuit. The tissues are in a parallel circuit; thus the greatest current flow is through the tissues

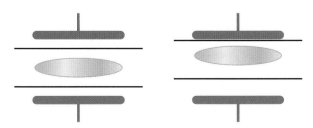

Figure 12–7. As the plate moves closer to the surface of the skin, the electrical field shifts, generating more surface heat in the skin and in the subcutaneous fat.

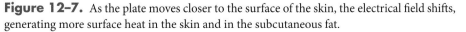

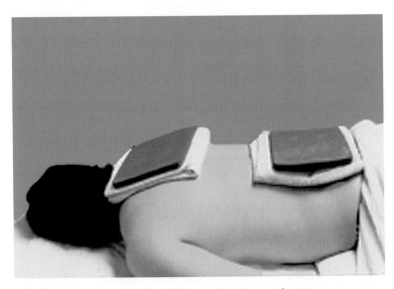

Figure 12–8. Pad electrodes showing correct placement and spacing.

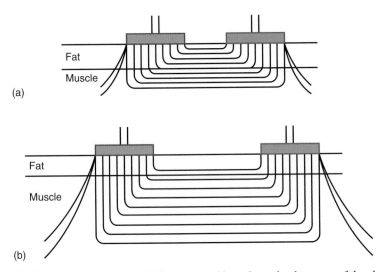

Figure 12–9. Pad electrodes should be separated by at least the diameter of the electrodes. (a) Electrodes placed close together produce more superficial heating. (b) As spacing increases, the current density increases in the deeper tissues.

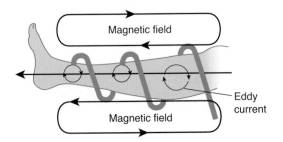

Figure 12–10. When current is passed through a coiled cable, a magnetic field is generated that can affect surrounding tissues by inducing localized secondary currents, called eddy currents, within the tissues. (Modified from Michlovitz S. *Thermal Agents in Rehabilitation.* Philadelphia: FA Davis, 1990.)

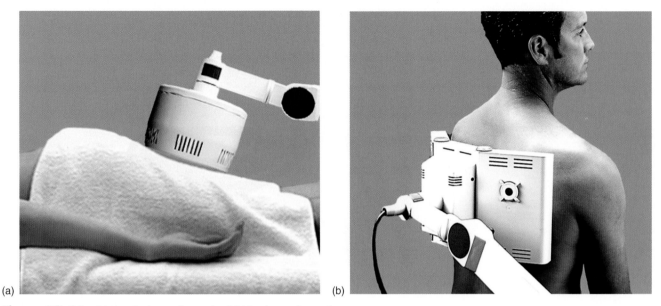

Figure 12–11. (a) Single drum electrode. (b) Tri-drum electrode.

with least resistance (see Chapter 5). When a magnetic field is used with an induction-type setup, the fat does not provide nearly as much resistance to the flow of the energy. Therefore, tissues that are high in electrolytic content (i.e., muscle and blood) respond best to the magnetic field by producing heat. It is important to remember that if the energy is owing primarily to generation of a magnetic field, heating may not be as obvious to the patient because the magnetic field will not provide nearly as much sensation of warmth in the skin as an electrical field.

Drum Electrodes. The **drum electrode** also produces a magnetic field. The drum electrode is made up of one or more monoplanar coils that are rigidly fixed inside some kind of housing (Figure 12–11a). If a small area is to be treated, particularly a small flat area, then a one-drum setup is fine. However, if the area is contoured, then two or more drums, which may be on a hinged apparatus or hinged arm, may be more suitable (Figure 12–11b).

Penetration into the tissues tends to be on the order of 2–3 cm if the skin is no more than 1–2 cm away from the drum.[29] The magnetic field may be significant up to 5 cm away from the drum. A light towel should be kept in contact with the skin and between the drum and the skin. The towel is used to absorb moisture because an accumulation of water droplets would tend to overheat and cause hot spots on the surface. If there is more than 2 cm of fat, tissue temperature under the fat will not increase greatly with a drum setup. The maximum penetration of shortwave diathermy with a drum electrode is 3 cm, provided there is no more than 2 cm of fat beneath the skin. For best absorption of energy, the housing of the drum should be in contact with the towel covering the skin.[28]

Cable Electrodes. The **cable electrode** is an induction electrode, which produces a magnetic field (Figure 12–12). There are two basic types of arrangements: the pancake coil and the wraparound coil. If a pancake coil is used, the size of the smaller circle should be greater than 6 inches in diameter. In either arrangement, there should be at least 1 cm of toweling between the cable and the skin. Stiff spacers should be used to keep the coils or the turns of the pancake or the wraparound coil between 5 and 10 cm between turns of the cable, thus providing spacing consistency. Both the pancake coils and the wraparound coils often provide more even heating because they are better able to follow the contours of the skin than are the drum or the air space plates. It is important that the cables not touch each other because they will short out and cause excessive heat buildup. Diathermy units that operate on a frequency of 13.56 MHz are probably best suited to cable electrode-type applications. This is primarily because the lower frequency is better at producing a magnetic field.[28]

Capacitor Electrodes
- Air space plates
- Pad electrodes

- Pulsed shortwave diathermy uses drum electrodes.

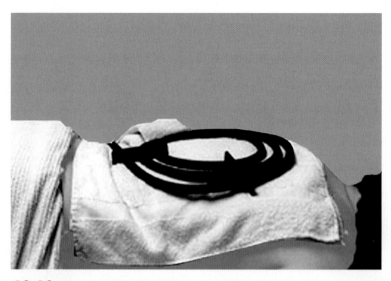

Figure 12–12. Pancake cable electrode.

Pulsed Shortwave Diathermy

Pulsed shortwave diathermy (PSWD), also referred to in the literature as *pulsed electromagnetic energy (PEME), pulsed electromagnetic field (PEMF)*, or *pulsed electromagnetic energy treatment (PEMET)*, is a relatively new form of diathermy.[11] Pulsed diathermy is created by simply interrupting the output of continuous shortwave diathermy at consistent intervals (Figure 12–13). Energy is delivered to the patient in a series of high-frequency bursts or pulse trains. Pulse duration is short, ranging from 20 to 400 sec with an intensity of up to 1000 W per pulse. The interpulse interval or off time depends on the pulse repetition rate, which ranges between 1 and 7000 Hz. The pulse repetition rate may be selected using the pulse-frequency control on the generator control panel.[21] Generally the off time is considerably longer than the on time. Therefore, even though the power output during the on time is sufficient to produce tissue heating, the long off-time interval allows the heat to dissipate. This reduces the likelihood of any significant tissue temperature increase and reduces the patient's perception of heat.

Pulsed diathermy is claimed to have therapeutic value and to produce nonthermal effects with minimal thermal physiologic effects, depending on the intensity of the application. But pulsed shortwave diathermy can also have thermal effects.[30] When pulsed diathermy is used in intensities that create an increase in tissue temperature, its effects are no different from those of continuous shortwave diathermy. Pulsed shortwave diathermy has been shown to increase the temperature of the knee joint capsule.[31] Successful treatments have largely resulted from the application of higher intensities and longer treatment times. Studies that use pulsed shortwave diathermy do not normally compare it with continuous shortwave diathermy but rather with a control group that has received no heat treatment.[13]

With pulsed shortwave diathermy, mean power provides a measure of heat production. Mean power may be calculated by dividing peak pulse power by the pulse repetition frequency to determine the pulse period (on time plus off time).

$$\text{Pulse Period} = \frac{\text{peak pulse power (W)}}{\text{pulse repetition frequency (Hz)}}$$

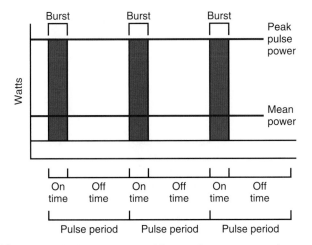

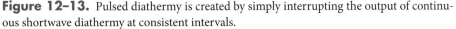

Figure 12–13. Pulsed diathermy is created by simply interrupting the output of continuous shortwave diathermy at consistent intervals.

The percentage on time is calculated by dividing the pulse duration by pulse period.

$$\text{Percentage on time} = \frac{\text{pulse duration (msec)}}{\text{pulse period (msec)}}$$

The mean power is then determined by dividing the peak pulse power by the percentage on time.

$$\text{Mean power} = \frac{\text{peak pulses power (W)}}{\text{percentage on time}}$$

With pulsed shortwave diathermy, the highest mean power output is usually lower than the power delivered with continuous shortwave diathermy.

Generators that deliver pulsed shortwave diathermy typically use a drum type of electrode (Figure 12–14). As with continuous shortwave diathermy, the drum electrode is made of a coil wrapped in a flat circular spiral pattern and housed within a plastic case. The energy is induced in the treatment area via the production of a magnetic field.

Clinical Decision-Making *Exercise 12–3*

A swimmer is complaining of an aching pain and tightness in the shoulder. In this case the clinician decides that heating the joint with pulsed shortwave diathermy rather than ultrasound would be the best treatment choice. What are the potential advantages of using diathermy in this particular situation?

Treatment Time

Treatments lasting only 15 minutes have produced vigorous heating of the triceps surae muscle of humans.[2] A 20- to 30-minute treatment for one body area is probably all that is necessary to reach maximum physiologic effects.[28] The physiologic effects, particularly circulatory, seem to last about 30 minutes.

Treatments in excess of 30 minutes may create a circulatory rebound phenomenon in which the digital temperature may drop after the treatment because of reflex vasoconstriction. If a clinician finds that a diathermy unit has been left on in excess of 30 minutes, it would be wise to check the temperature of the toes or fingers, depending on which extremity has been treated. It has been observed that pulsed shortwave diathermy administered to the triceps surae resulted in peak heating at only 15 minutes into the treatment, and the temperature actually dropped 0.3°C from the 15- to 20-minute mark.[2] Perhaps this can be explained by the increase in blood flow created by the thermal effects of diathermy. The increase in temperature

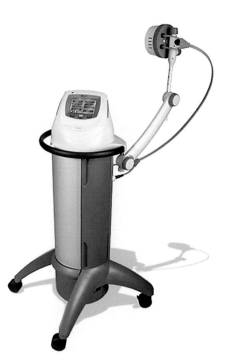

Figure 12–14. Most modern shortwave diathermy units such as the Intellect SWD 100 are capable of delivering pulsed shortwave diathermy (Courtesy Chattanooga Group).

and blood flow engages the body's natural cooling mechanism. Therefore, it may be more difficult to heat muscle tissue than the less vascular tendinous tissue. Perhaps tissue temperatures as high as 45°C, as postulated by other researchers, are too high for the body to tolerate.[2]

It is important to remember that as skin temperature goes up, impedance goes down. Therefore, the unit may need to be returned after 5–10 minutes of treatment.

Treatment Protocols: Shortwave Diathermy

1. Place a single layer of towel on the treatment area.
2. Inductive: Position the drum containing the coil parallel to the body part and in contact with the towel. Capacitive: Position the plates parallel to the body part and about 2.5–7.5 cm away from the body.
3. Turn on the SWD generator; allow to warm up if necessary.
4. Inform the patient that he or she should feel only warmth; if it becomes hot, the patient should inform you immediately.
5. Adjust intensity of SWD to the appropriate level. Set a timer for the appropriate treatment time and give the patient a signaling device. Make sure the patient understands how to use the signaling device.
6. Check the patient's response after the first 5 minutes by asking how it feels.

Clinical Decision-Making   *Exercise 12–4*

In treating a 2-day old rotator cuff strain, what type of diathermy is best used and why?

CASE STUDY 12–1
SHORTWAVE DIATHERMY

Background: A 22-year-old graduate student developed the gradual onset of lumbar paravertebral muscle spasm following a self-made move of his apartment contents. The symptoms were noted the day after the move upon arising and were described as a tightness and restriction of mobility in the low back. He reported no radiation of his symptoms into the buttocks or legs and no difficulty with bowel or bladder function. Physical examination revealed restriction in forward flexion and side rotation of the trunk with tenderness to palpation in the lumbar paravertebral musculature 1 week after the episode of extensive bending and lifting.

Impression: Lumbar paravertebral muscle strain, subacute.

Treatment Plan: The patient was initiated on a course of inductive shortwave diathermy to the lumbar paravertebral musculature, followed by active and active-assisted lumbar region range of motion exercise. Treatment was provided on an every-other-day basis for 2 weeks with increasing emphasis on mobilizing and strengthening the lumbar paravertebral musculature.

Response: The patient experience immediate, but short-duration relief of his low back pain following the initial treatment and enthusiastically pursued his exercise sequence. With each subsequent session, the duration of relief and improved trunk mobility increased. At the 2-week point in the treatment regimen, the patient was independent in the performance of his lumbar exercise regimen and scheduled to attend a back education class prior to discharge.

Discussion Questions

- What tissues were injured/affected?
- What symptoms were present?
- What phase of the injury-healing continuum did the patient present for care in?
- What are the physical agent modality's biophysical effects (direct/indirect/depth/tissue affinity)?
- What are the physical agent modality's indications/contraindications?
- What are the parameters of the physical agent modality's application/dosage/duration/frequency in this case study?
- What other physical agent modalities could be utilized to treat this injury or condition? Why? How?

The rehabilitation professional employs physical agent modalities to create an optimum environment for tissue healing while minimizing the symptoms associated with the trauma or condition.

CASE STUDY 12–2
SHORTWAVE DIATHERMY

Background: A 79-year-old male with a documented history of right knee osteoarthritis, comes to your clinic with a history of increasing pain and swelling over the past 2 months. Gait endurance is beginning to decline. The referral was to initiate quadriceps strengthening, joint protection activities, and gait training as indicated.

Impression: Degenerative joint disease with concurrent muscle inhibition and atrophy.

Treatment Plan: The patient received 15 minutes of capacitive shortwave diathermy prior to initiating quadriceps exercise. He reported short-term relief, which allowed for the performance of his exercise program. Treatment was provided on a twice per week outpatient basis with the patient given specific instructions in the performance of home lower extremity closed-chain exercises two other times per week. At

the tenth visit the patient was discharged as he was adequately self-managing his condition.

Response

Discussion Questions

- What tissues were injured/affected?
- What symptoms were present?
- What phase of the injury-healing continuum did the patient present for care in?
- What are the physical agent modality's biophysical effects (direct/indirect/depth/tissue affinity)?
- What are the physical agent modality's indications/contraindications?
- What are the parameters of the physical agent modality's application/dosage/duration/frequency in this case study?

(continued)

CASE STUDY 12–2 (continued)
SHORTWAVE DIATHERMY

- What other physical agent modalities could be used to treat this injury or condition? Why? How?

Further Discussion Questions

- Was the choice of SWD optimal for this patient's suspected injury?

- What other things would you counsel this patient to be aware of while undergoing diathermy treatment?

The rehabilitation professional employs physical agent modalities to create an optimum environment for tissue healing while minimizing the symptoms associated with the trauma or condition.

MICROWAVE DIATHERMY

Microwave diathermy is seldom used as a clinical treatment modality by clinicians but will be discussed briefly for informational purposes.

Microwave diathermy has two FCC-assigned frequencies in this country, 2456 and 915 MHz. Microwave has a much higher frequency and a shorter wavelength than shortwave diathermy. Microwave diathermy units generate a strong electrical field and relatively little magnetic field. Microwave diathermy cannot penetrate the fat layer as well as shortwave diathermy and thus has less depth of penetration. Heating is caused by the intramolecular vibration of molecules that are high in polarity.[32] If subcutaneous fat is greater than 1 cm, the fat temperature will rise to a level that is too uncomfortable before tissue temperature rises in the deeper tissues.[27] This is less of a problem if the microwave diathermy is of the frequency of 915 MHz. However, very few commercial units operate on that frequency. Almost all the older units have the higher frequency of 2456 MHz. If the subcutaneous fat is 0.5 cm or less, microwave diathermy can penetrate and cause a tissue temperature rise up to 5 cm deep in the tissue. Bone tends to absorb more shortwave and microwave energy than any type of soft tissue.

The microwave electrode beams energy toward the patient, creating the potential for much of the energy to be reflected (Figure 12–15). The electrode should be located so that the maximum amount of energy will be penetrating at a right angle or perpendicular to the skin. Any angle greater or less than perpendicular will create reflection of the energy and significant loss of absorption (cosine law). With appropriate setup of the microwave diathermy unit, less than 10% of the energy is lost from the machine as it is applied to the patient. Contact applicators or electrode are capable of achieving better transmission to the skin.[33]

Microwave diathermy units operating on the frequency 2456 MHz require a specified air space between the electrode and the skin. The manufacturer-suggested distances and power output should be followed closely. In units that have a frequency of 915 MHz, the electrode is placed at a distance of 1 cm from the skin, thus minimizing energy reflection.[12] For this reason 915 MHz is considered to be more effective for therapeutic heating than the more commonly used 2450 MHz diathermy.

Microwave diathermy is best used to treat conditions that exist in areas of the body that are covered with low subcutaneous fat content. The tendons of the foot, hand, and wrist are well treated, as are the acromioclavicular and sternoclavicular joints, the patellar tendon, the distal tendons of the hamstrings, the Achilles tendon, and the costochondral joints and sacroiliac joints in lean individuals.

Clinical Decision-Making   *Exercise 12–5*

A clinician is treating an abdominal strain. Would the better choice be to use shortwave or microwave diathermy? Explain your rationale.

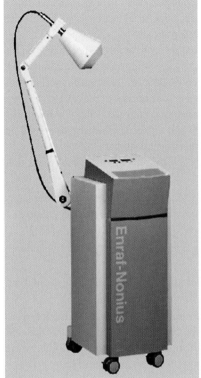

Figure 12–15. Microwave diathermy unit.

Clinical Applications for Diathermy

For the most part, the clinical applications for the diathermies are similar to those of other physical agents that are capable of producing thermal effects resulting in a tissue temperature increase.[34] In addition to the diathermies, thermotherapy discussed in Chapter 9 and ultrasound discussed in Chapter 10 are commonly used as heating modalities. The diathermies have been used in the treatment of a variety of musculoskeletal conditions, including muscle strains, contusions, ligament sprains, tendinitis, tenosynovitis, bursitis, joint contractures, myofascial trigger points, and osteoarthritis.[35]

Continuous shortwave diathermy is used most often for a variety of thermal effects, including inducing local relaxation by decreasing muscle guarding and pain, increasing circulation and improving blood flow to an injured area to facilitate resolution of hemorrhage and edema and removal of the by-products of the inflammatory process, and reducing both subacute and chronic pain.[13,21,36]

Diathermy has been used for selectively heating joint structures for the purpose of improving joint range of motion by decreasing stiffness and increasing the extensibility of the collagen fibers and the resilience of contracted soft tissues.[37] The role of diathermy in increasing range of motion and flexibility has been studied with mixed results.[38,39] One study showed that diathermy and short-duration stretching were no more effective than short-duration stretching alone at increasing hamstring flexibility.[40] A second study indicated that pulsed shortwave diathermy used before prolonged long-duration static stretching appeared to be more effective than stretching alone in increasing flexibility over a 3-week period. After 14 treatments, prolonged long-duration stretching combined with pulsed shortwave diathermy followed by ice application caused greater immediate and net range-of-motion increases than prolonged long-duration stretching alone.[41] It has also been shown that hamstring flexibility can be greatly improved when shortwave diathermy is used in conjunction with prolonged stretching.[42] However the same researcher in a subsequent study found that pulsed shortwave diathermy application prior to stretching does not appear to aid hamstring flexibility.[43] Flexibility gains in normal ankles with 3 weeks of training were retained for at least 3 weeks after training ceased. The application of pulsed, shortwave diathermy during stretching did not appear to influence the chronic retention of flexibility gains in normal subjects.[44]

Deep heating using shortwave diathermy in the absence of stretching increases tissue extensibility more than superficial heating or no heating. Superficial heating is more effective than no heating, but the difference was not statistically significant.[45]

The majority of recent clinical studies relative to diathermy have focused primarily on the efficacy of pulsed shortwave diathermy in facilitating tissue healing, and to date results have been inconclusive at best.[22,46] Various claims have been made as to the specific mechanisms that facilitate healing, including an increase in the number and activity of the cells in the area, reduced swelling and inflammation, resorption of hematoma, increased rate of collagen deposition and organization, and increased nerve growth and repair. These claims are based on a limited number of clinical studies and even fewer experimental studies.[19]

A number of conditions may potentially occur in clinical settings that would make diathermy the treatment of choice.

- If for any reason the skin or some underlying soft tissue is very tender and will not tolerate the loading of a moist heat pack or pressure from an ultrasound transducer, then diathermy should be used.
- Shortwave diathermy is more capable of increasing temperatures to a greater tissue depth than any of the thermotherapy modalities.
- When the treatment goal is to increase tissue temperatures in a large area (i.e., throughout the entire shoulder girdle, in the low back region), diathermy should be used.[47]
- In areas where subcutaneous fat is thick and deep heating is required, the induction technique using either cable or drum electrodes should be used to minimize heating of the subcutaneous fat layer. The capacitance technique with shortwave diathermy and microwave diathermy is more likely to heat selectively more superficial subcutaneous fat.
- The clinician should never underestimate the placebo effects that a treatment with any large machine may be capable of producing.

COMPARING SHORTWAVE DIATHERMY AND ULTRASOUND AS THERMAL MODALITIES

The use of therapeutic ultrasound was discussed in detail in Chapter 10. Ultrasound and pulsed shortwave diathermy are both clinically effective modalities for heating superficial and deep tissues; however, ultrasound is used much more frequently than shortwave diathermy. In surveys of physical therapists in Canada and Australia, only 0.6% and 8% of respondents, respectively, used shortwave diathermy daily, yet 94% and 93%, respectively, used ultrasound daily.[48,49]

Recent research has demonstrated that shortwave diathermy may be more effective as a heating modality than ultrasound in treating certain conditions.[5,50] A study was done to determine the rate of temperature increase during pulsed shortwave diathermy and the rate of temperature decay postapplication. A 23-gauge thermistor was inserted 3 cm below the skin surface of the anesthetized left medial triceps surae muscle belly of 20 subjects. Diathermy was applied to the muscle belly for 20 minutes at 800 Hz, a pulse duration of 400 sec, and an intensity of 150 W. Temperature changes were recorded every 5 minutes during the treatment. The mean baseline temperature was 35.8°C, and the temperature peaked at 39.8°C in 15 minutes, then dropped slightly (0.3°C) during the last 5 minutes of treatment. After the treatment terminated, intramuscular temperature dropped 1°C in 5 minutes and 1.8°C by the tenth minute. Based on these findings, it appears that shortwave diathermy compares favorably with heating rates of 1 MHz ultrasound (1 W/cm² for 12 min creates a 4°C temperature increase at 3 cm intramuscularly) (Figure 12–16).

Shortwave diathermy, however, may be a better modality than ultrasound in some situations, and diathermy appears to have several advantages over ultrasound.

1. Because the surface of the shortwave applicator drum is 25 times larger than a typical ultrasound treatment area, it heats a much larger area. (A standard drum heating area for a diathermy unit is 200 cm², or approximately 25 times that of ultrasound.)

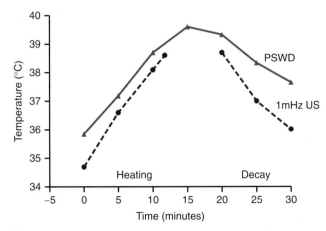

Figure 12–16. Intramuscular temperatures during heating and 10 minutes of decay resulting from 20 minutes of shortwave diathermy (PSWD: triangles) and 12 minutes of 1-MHz ultrasound (US: squares) application. Ultrasound data are from previous studies in our laboratory.[6,13] This illustrates that shortwave diathermy and 1-MHz ultrasound have similar heating rates, yet muscle heated with shortwave diathermy will retain its heat 2–3 times longer.

2. Unlike ultrasound, which causes a fluctuating tissue heating rate as the transducer is moved, diathermy's applicator is stationary so the heat applied to the area is more constant.

3. The rate of temperature decay is slower following diathermy application. Muscle heated with pulsed shortwave diathermy will retain heat over 60% longer than identical muscle depths heated with 1 MHz ultrasound.[5,51] This is important because it provides the clinician more time for stretching, friction massage, and joint mobilization before the temperature drops to an ineffective level.

4. Application of diathermy does not require constant monitoring by the clinician, whereas ultrasound application requires constant monitoring. Thus, a clinician can work with another patient while one is receiving diathermy treatment. This enables the clinician to be more efficient.

DIATHERMY TREATMENT PRECAUTIONS, INDICATIONS, AND CONTRAINDICATIONS

The use of shortwave, and especially microwave, diathermies probably has more treatment precautions and contraindications than any of the other physical agents used in a clinical setting[52,53] (see Table 12–2).

A survey of over 42,000 physical therapists found a modest increase in the risk of miscarriage of pregnant therapists who were regularly exposed to microwave diathermy.[3] Regular exposure to shortwave diathermy during pregnancy, however, did not increase the risk of miscarriage.

Diathermy is known to produce a tissue temperature rise and may be contraindicated in any condition where this increased temperature may produce negative or undesired effects, including traumatic musculoskeletal injuries with acute bleeding; acute inflammatory conditions; areas with reduced blood supply (ischemia); and areas with reduced sensitivity to temperature or pain.[17,21,54] It is important to keep in mind that the power meter on the diathermy units does not indicate the energy entering the tissues. Therefore, the clinician must rely on the sensation of pain for a warning that the patient's tolerance levels have been exceeded.[55]

Because diathermy selectively heats tissues that are high in water content, caution must be exercised when using diathermy over fluid-filled areas or organs. Joint effusion may be exacerbated by heating with diathermy. The increase in temperature may cause an increase in synovitis.[17]

TABLE 12–2 Indications and Contraindications for Shortwave Diathermy

INDICATIONS

Postacute musculoskeletal injuries

Increased blood flow

Vasodilation

Increased metabolism

Changes in some enzyme reactions

Increased collagen extensibility

Decreased joint stiffness

Muscle relaxation

Muscle guarding

Increased pain threshold

Enhanced recovery from injury

Joint contractures

Myofascial trigger points

Improved joint range of motion

Increased extensibility of collagen

Increased circulation

Reduced subacute and chronic pain

Resorption of hematoma

Increased nerve growth and repair

CONTRAINDICATIONS

Acute traumatic musculoskeletal injuries

Acute inflammatory conditions

Areas with ischemia

Areas of reduced sensitivity to temperature or pain

Fluid-filled areas or organs

Joint effusion

Synovitis

Eyes

Contact lenses

Moist wound dressings

Malignancies

Infection

Pelvic area during menstruation

CONTRAINDICATIONS

Testes

Pregnancy

Epiphyseal plates in adolescents

Metal implants

Unshielded cardiac pacemakers

Intrauterine devices

Watches or jewelry

Because of the high fluid content, it should not be used around the eyes for any prolonged periods of time or for repeated treatments, nor should it be used with contact lenses.[56,57]

In most cases, toweling should be used to absorb perspiration.[28] A single layer of toweling should be used with both the drum and air space plates. However, with other types of applicators, such as pads and cables, the toweling should be more dense and thicker, up to 1 cm or more.[9] Toweling is not necessary with microwave diathermy. There should be no overlapping of skin surfaces. If the buttocks area is to be treated, a towel should be placed in the cleavage between the buttocks. If the shoulder area is to be treated, a towel should be placed between the skin folds in the axilla.

If clothing is permitted in the exposed area, the treatment should be closely monitored. In most cases, however, pulsed shortwave diathermy can be applied over some clothing such as a cotton T-shirt. Be aware that many of the synthetic fabrics worn today allow for no evaporation of moisture, serving as a vapor barrier allowing moisture to accumulate. Similarly, moisture can accumulate in patients taped with adhesive tape or wearing compressive wraps or supportive braces. This moisture can create extreme hot spots with diathermy treatments.[58] Diathermy should not be used over moist wound dressings, again because of potential for rapid heating of moisture.[21]

Diathermy should not be applied to the pelvic area of the female who is menstruating, since this can increase blood flow.[17]

Exposure of the gonads to diathermy also should be avoided.[34,58,59] The testes are more superficial and thus are more susceptible to injury from microwave treatment than the ovaries. Minimal evidence exists that diathermy may potentially cause damage to the human fetus, and because research in this area is impossible, it is recommended that caution be used in treating the pregnant female.[39]

Caution should be used when using diathermy over bony prominences to avoid burning the overlying soft tissue.[34] The epiphysis in children should not be vigorously heated.[17]

The patient should not come in contact with any of the cables connecting the generator with the air space plates, pad, cable, or drum electrodes. There should be no crossover of the lead cables with any electrode setup. At no time should the antenna within the microwave applicator ever come in contact with skin, because this would cause a buildup of energy sufficient to cause severe burns.

It is very important to use diathermy units at a safe distance from other types of medical electrical devices or equipment that is transistorized. Transcutaneous electrical nerve stimulation units and other low-frequency current units often have transistor-type circuits, and these can be damaged by the reflected or stray radiation that shortwave and microwave diathermy units produce.[46] Unshielded cardiac pacemakers may also be damaged by diathermy.[60]

Metal chairs or metal tables should not be used to support the patient during treatment. The area being treated should also be free of metal implants. Women wearing intrauterine devices should not be treated in the low back or lower abdomen. There should be no watches or jewelry in the area because the electromagnetic energy will tend to magnetize the watch, and the electromagnetic energy may heat up the jewelry.[17]

The patient must remain in a reasonably comfortable position for the duration of the treatment so that the field does not change because of movement during treatment.

The skin should be inspected before and after a diathermy treatment. It is recommended that the part being treated either be horizontal or elevated during treatment.

Clinicians who are knowledgeable in the physics and biophysics of diathermy, as well as its applications to a variety of cases, tend to achieve good results. Clinicians who work with shortwave and microwave diathermy units must spend considerable time experimenting with equipment setup and the application of different types of electrodes on a variety of uninjured parts of the body if they are to develop the skills necessary to use diathermy safely and effectively on injured tissue.[58]

SUMMARY

1. Diathermy is the application of high-frequency electromagnetic energy that is primarily used to generate heat in body tissues. Diathermy as a therapeutic agent may be classified as two distinct modalities, shortwave diathermy and microwave diathermy. Shortwave diathermy may be continuous or pulsed.

2. The physiologic effects of continuous shortwave and microwave diathermies are primarily thermal, resulting from high-frequency vibration of molecules. Pulsed shortwave diathermy has been used for its nonthermal effects in the treatment of soft-tissue injuries and wounds.

3. A shortwave diathermy unit that generates a high-frequency electrical current will produce both an electrical field and a magnetic field in the tissues. The ratio of the electrical field to the magnetic field depends on the characteristics of the different units as well as on the characteristics of electrodes or applicators.

4. The capacitance technique, using capacitor electrodes (air space plates and pad electrodes), creates a strong electrical field that is essentially the lines of force exerted on charged ions by the electrodes that cause charged particles to move from one pole to the other.

5. The inductance technique, using inductor electrodes (cable electrodes and drum electrodes), creates a strong magnetic field when current is passed through a coiled cable. It may affect surrounding tissues by inducing localized secondary currents, called eddy currents, within the tissues.

6. Pulsed diathermy is created by simply interrupting the output of continuous shortwave diathermy at consistent intervals. Generators that deliver pulsed shortwave diathermy typically use a drum type of electrode to induce energy in the treatment area via the production of a magnetic field.

7. Microwave diathermy units generate a strong electrical field and relatively little magnetic field through either circular or rectangular-shaped applicators that beam energy to the treatment area.

8. The diathermies have been used in the treatment of a variety of musculoskeletal conditions, including muscle strains, contusions, ligament sprains, tendinitis, tenosynovitis, bursitis, joint contractures, and myofascial trigger points.

9. Microwave diathermy probably has more treatment precautions and contraindications than any of the other physical agents used in a clinical setting.

10. Effective treatments using the diathermies require practice in application and adjustment of techniques to the individual patient.

11. Four advantages for the use of diathermy over ultrasound are larger heating area, more uniform heating, longer stretching window, and more clinician freedom.

REVIEW QUESTIONS

1. What is diathermy and what are the different types of diathermy?
2. What are the potential physiologic effects of using continuous shortwave, pulsed shortwave, or microwave diathermies?

3. What determines the ratio of the electrical field to the magnetic field in shortwave diathermy?

4. What are the differences between shortwave diathermy techniques that use capacitance or induction?

5. How is pulsed shortwave diathermy used, and what type of electrode is most typically used?

6. How should microwave diathermy be set up to achieve the most effective results?

7. What are the various clinical applications and indications for using continuous shortwave, pulsed shortwave, and microwave diathermies?

8. What are the most important treatment precautions for using the diathermies?

9. What are the major differences between microwave and shortwave diathermies?

10. What are the advantages and disadvantages of using diathermy or ultrasound as deep-heating modalities?

SELF-TEST QUESTIONS

True or False

1. Diathermy can create both thermal and nonthermal effects.

2. Microwave diathermy is more suited for use in areas with little subcutaneous fat.

3. Shortwave diathermy penetrates more superficially than microwave diathermy.

Multiple Choice

4. Shortwave capacitor electrodes are called which of the following?

   a. air space plates
   b. pad electrodes
   c. both a and b
   d. neither a nor b

5. The drum electrode is an example of a(n) _____.

   a. capacitor electrode
   b. induction electrode
   c. cable electrode
   d. none of the above

6. Microwave diathermy units produce a strong _____ and a weak _____.

   a. electrical field, magnetic field
   b. magnetic field, electrical field
   c. magnetic field, eddy current
   d. eddy current, electrical field

7. What type of diathermy should be used to heat a large area on a patient with thick subcutaneous fat?

   a. capacitance technique
   b. pulsed shortwave diathermy
   c. pad electrodes
   d. induction technique

8. Which of the following is a contraindication for diathermy?

   a. watches or jewelry
   b. improving range of motion
   c. muscle guarding
   d. increased blood flow

9. What conditions may be treated with diathermy?

    a. postacute muscle strain

    b. tendinitis

    c. joint contractures

    d. all of the above

10. Toweling must be used with thermal diathermy primarily to

    a. avoid contact with machine

    b. avoid moisture accumulation

    c. maintain patient modesty

    d. ensure even heating

SOLUTIONS TO CLINICAL DECISION-MAKING EXERCISES

12–1

The depth of penetration can be increased by simply moving the pad electrodes further apart. As the spacing is increased, the current density will be increased in the deeper issues.

12–2

In areas where subcutaneous fat is minimal, the capacitance technique using either airspace or pad electrodes should be used. The capacitance technique with shortwave diathermy is more likely to selectively heat more superficial tissues that are not covered by fat.

12–3

Pulsed shortwave diathermy is capable of heating a much larger area than ultrasound; the applicator is stationary so the heat applied to the area is more constant; the rate of temperature decay is slower following diathermy application, allowing more time for stretching; using diathermy doesn't require constant monitoring.

12–4

Pulsed shortwave diathermy would likely be better then either continuous shortwave or microwave diathermy since the nonthermal effects of pulsed shortwave would assist in the healing process of the injured cell without causing any significant increase in temperature. Heating in this phase of the healing process would be contraindicated.

12–5

Since there is likely to be a significant amount of subcutaneous fat in the abdominal area, shortwave diathermy, which heats using a magnetic field, would likely be more effective in penetrating the fat layer than would microwave diathermy, which produces electrical field heating.

REFERENCES

1. Castel JC, Draper DO, Knight K, Fujiwara T, and Garrett C. Rate of temperature decay in human muscle after treatments of pulsed shortwave diathermy. *J Athl Training* 1997;32: S–34.

2. Draper DO, Castel JC, Knight K, et al. Temperature rise in human muscle during pulsed short wave diathermy: does this modality parallel ultrasound? *J Athl Training* 1997;32:S–35.

3. Hellstrom RO and Stewart WF. Miscarriages among female physical therapists who report using radio- and microwave-frequency electromagnetic radiation. *Am J Epidemiol* 1993;138(10):775–785.

4. Merrick MA. Do you diathermy? *Athlet Ther Today* 2001;6(1):55–56.

5. Draper DO, Castel JC, and Castel D. Rate of temperature increase in human muscle during 1 MHz and 3 MHz continuous ultrasound. *J Orthop Sports Phys Ther* 1995;22: 142–150.

6. Delpizzo V, and Joyner KH. On the safe use of microwave and shortwave diathermy units. *Aust J Physiother* 1987;33(3):152–162.

7. Low J and Reed A. *Electrotherapy Explained: Principles and Practice*, London, : Butterworth-Heinemann, 1990.

8. Behrens BJ and Michlovitz SL. *Physical Agents: Theory and Practice for the Physical Clinician Assistant*, Philadelphia, PA: FA Davis, 2005.

9. Brown M and Baker RD. Effect of pulsed shortwave diathermy on skeletal muscle injury in rabbits. *Phys Ther* 1987;67(2):208–213.

10. Fenn JE. Effect of pulsed electromagnetic energy (Diapulse) on experimental haematomas. *Can Med Assoc J* 1969;100:251.

11. Hansen TI and Kristensen JH. Effect of massage, shortwave diathermy and ultrasound upon Xe disappearance rate from muscle and subcutaneous tissue in the human calf. *Scand J Rehab Med* 1973;5:179–182.

12. Lehmann JF. Diathermy. In Krusen FH (ed). *Handbook of Physical Medicine and Rehabilitation.* Philadelphia, PA: WB Saunders, 1990.

13. Lehmann JF. *Therapeutic Heat and Cold*, 4th ed, Baltimore, MD: Williams & Wilkins, 1990.

14. Millard JB. Effect of high frequency currents and infra-red rays on the circulation of the lower limb in man. *Ann Phys Med* 1961;6:45.

15. Wilson DH. Treatment of soft tissue injuries by pulsed electrical energy. *Br Med J* 1972;2:269.

16. Wright GG. Treatment of soft tissue and ligamentous injuries in professional footballers. *Physiotherapy* 1973;59(12).

17. Lehmann JF. Comparison of relative heating patterns produced in tissues by exposure to microwave energy with exposures at 2450 and 900 megacycles. *Arch Phys Med Rehab* 1965;46:307.

18. Abramson DI, Burnett C, Bell Y, and Tuck S. Changes in blood flow, oxygen uptake and tissue temperatures produced by therapeutic physical agents. *Am J Phys Med* 1960;47:51–62.

19. Kitchen S and Partridge C. Review of shortwave diathermy continuous and pulsed patterns. *Physiotherapy* 1992;78(4):243–252.

20. Crowder C, Trowbridge C, and Ricard M. The effect of subcutaneous adipose on intramuscular temperature during and after pulsed shortwave diathermy (abstract). *J Athl Training* (suppl.) 2007;42(2):S-103.

21. Kloth L and Ziskin M. Diathermy and pulsed electromagnetic fields. In Michlovitz SL (ed). *Thermal Agents in Rehabilitation*, 2nd ed, Philadelphia, PA: FA Davis, 1990.

22. Low J. Dosage of some pulsed shortwave clinical trials. *Physiotherapy* 1995;81(10):611–616.

23. Sanseverino EG. Membrane phenomena and cellular processes under the action of pulsating magnetic fields. Presented at the Second International Congress for Magneto Medicine, Rome, 1980.

24. Lehmann JF and deLateur BJ. Diathermy and superficial heat and cold. In Krusen FH (ed). *Krusen's Handbook of Physical Medicine and Rehabilitation*, 3rd ed, Philadelphia, PA: W.B. Saunders, 1990.

25. Griffin JE. Update on selected physical modalities. Paper presented in Chicago, December, 1981.

26. Health devices shortwave diathermy units, Proceedings of the Emergency Care Research Institute, Meeting in Plymouth, PA, June 1979, pp. 175–193.

27. Griffin JE, Santiesleban AJ, and Kloth L. Electrotherapy for instructors. Paper presented in Lacrosse, WI, August 1982.

28. Griffin JE and Karselis TC. The diathermies. In *Physical Agents for Physical Therapists*, 2nd ed., Springfield, IL: Charles C Thomas, 1987.

29. DeLateur BJ, Lehmann JF, Stonebridge JB, et al. Muscle heating in human subjects with 915 MHz microwave contact applicator. *Arch Phys Med* 1970;51:147–151.

30. Murray CC and Kitchen, S. Effect of pulse repetition rate on the perception of thermal sensation with pulsed shortwave diathermy. *Physiother Res Int* 2000;5(2):73–84.

31. Draper D, Anderson M, and Hopkins T. An exploration of knee joint intracapsular temperature rise following pulsed shortwave diathermy, in vivo (abstract). *J Athl Training* (suppl.) 2005;40(2):S-88.

32. Kitchen S and Partridge C. A review of microwave diathermy. *Physiotherapy* 1991;77(9):647–652.

33. Guy AW and Lehmann JF. On the determination of an optimum microwave diathermy frequency for a direct contact applicator. *Inst Electric Electron Eng Trans Biomed Eng* 1966;13:76–87.

34. Schliephake E. Carrying out treatment. In Thom H (ed). *Introduction to Shortwave and Microwave Diathermy,* 3rd ed, Springfield, IL: Charles C Thomas, 1966.

35. Marks R, Ghassemi M, Duarte R, and Van Nguyen JP. A review of the literature on shortwave diathermy as applied to osteo-arthritis of the knee. *Physiotherapy* 1999;85(6):304–316.

36. Low J. The nature and effects of pulsed electromagnetic radiations. *NZ Physiother* 1978;6:18.

37. Smith DW, Clarren SK, and Harvey MA. Hyperthermia as a possible teratogenic agent. *J Pediatr* 1978;92:878.

38. Brantley S, Crawford C, and Joslyn E. The acute effects of diathermy and stretch versus stretch alone of the hamstring muscle (poster session). *J Orthop Sports Phys Ther* 2003;33(2):A–29.

39. Trowbridge C, Ricard M, and Schoor M. Short term effects of pulsed shortwave diathermy and passive stretch on the torque-angle relationship of the tricep surae muscles (abstract). *J Ath Train* (suppl.) 2007;42(2):S-132.

40. Draper D, Miner L, and Knight K. The carry-over effects of diathermy and stretching in developing hamstring flexibility. *J Athl Training* 2002;37(1):37–42.

41. Peres S, Draper D, and Knight K. Pulsed shortwave diathermy and long-duration stretching increase dorsiflexion range of motion more than identical stretching without diathermy. *J Athl Training* 2002;37(1):43–50.

42. Draper D, Castro J, Feland B. Shortwave diathermy and prolonged stretching increase hamstring flexibility more

than prolonged stretching alone. *J Orthop Sports Phys Ther* 2004;34(1):13–20.

43. Miner L, Draper D, and Knight KL. Pulsed shortwave diathermy application prior to stretching does not appear to aid hamstring flexibility. *J Athl Training* 2000;35(2):S–48.

44. Brucker J, Knight K, and Rubley M. An 18-day stretching regimen, with or without pulsed, shortwave diathermy, and ankle dorsiflexion after 3 weeks. *J Athl Training* 2005;40(4):276.

45. Robertson V, Ward A, and Jung P. The effect of heat on tissue extensibility: A comparison of deep and superficial heating. *Arch Phys Med and Rehab* 2005;86(4):819–825.

46. Hill J. Pulsed short-wave diathermy effects on human fibroblast proliferation. *Arch Phys Med Rehab* 2002;83(6) 832–836.

47. Draper D, Knight KL, and Fujiwara T. Temperature change in human muscle during and after pulsed shortwave diathermy. *J Orthop Sports Phys Ther* 1999;29(1):13–18.

48. Lindsay DM, Dearness J, and McGinley CC. Electrotherapy usage trends in private physiotherapy practice in Alberta. *Physiother Can* 1995;47(1):30–34.

49. Lindsay DM, Dearness J, Richardson C, et al. A survey of electromodality usage in private physiotherapy practices. *Aust J Physiother* 1990;36(4):249–256.

50. Draper DO. Current research on therapeutic ultrasound and pulsed short-wave diathermy, presented at Physio Therapy Research Seminars Japan, Nov. 17, Sendai, Japan, 1996.

51. Rose S, Draper DO, Schulthies SS, and Durrant E. The stretching window part two: Rate of thermal decay in deep muscle following 1 MHz ultrasound. *J Athl Training* 1996;31:139–143.

52. Shields N. Contra-indications to shortwave diathermy: Survey of Irish physiotherapists *Physiotherapy* 2004;90(1): 42–53.

53. Shields N. Short-wave diathermy: Current clinical and safety practices. *Physiother Res Int* 2002;7(4):191–202.

54. Fischer C and Solomon S. Physiologic responses to heat and cold. In Licht S (ed). *Therapeutic Heat and Cold*, New Haven, CT: Elizabeth Licht, 1972.

55. Lehmann JF, Warren CG, and Scham SM. Therapeutic heat and cold. *Clin Orthop* 1974;99:207.

56. Konarska I and Michneiwicz L. Shortwave diathermy of diseases of the anterior portion of the eye. *Klin Oczna* 1955;25:185.

57. Seiger C and Draper D. Use of pulsed shortwave diathermy and joint mobilization to increase ankle range of motion in the presence of surgical implanted metal: A case series. *J Orth Sports Phys Ther* 2006;36(9):669–677.

58. American Physical Therapy Association. *Progress Report*. Virginia: American Physical Therapy Association, June, 1980.

59. Van Demark NL and Free MJ. Temperature effects. In Johnson AD (ed). *The Testis.*, Vol. 3, New York: Academic Press, 1973.

60. Smyth H. The pacemaker patient and the electromagnetic environment. *JAMA* 1974;227:1412 .

SUGGESTED READINGS

Abramson DI, Bell Y, Rejal H, et al. Changes in blood flow, oxygen uptake and tissue temperatures produced by therapeutic physical agents. *Am J Phys Med* 1960;39:87–95.

Abramson DI, Chu LSW, Tuck S, et al. Effect of tissue temperature and blood flow on motor nerve conduction velocity. *JAMA* 1966;198:1082–1088.

Abramson DI. Physiologic basis for the use of physical agents in peripheral vascular disorders, *Arch Phys Med Rehab* 1965;46:216.

Adey WR. Electromagnetic field effects on tissue. *Physiol Rev* 1981;61(3):436–514.

Adey WR. Physiological signaling across cell membranes and co-operative influences of extremely low frequency electromagnetic fields. In Frohlich H (ed). *Biological Coherence and Response to External Stimuli*, Heidelberg: Springer Verlag, 1988.

Allberry J. Shortwave diathermy for herpes zoster. *Physiotherapy* 1974;60:386.

Aronofsky D. Reduction of dental post-surgical symptoms using non-thermal pulsed high-peak-power electromagnetic energy. *Oral Surg* 1971;32(5)688–696.

Babbs CF and Dewitt DP. Physical principles of local heat therapy for cancer. *Med Instrument USA* 1981;15:367–373.

Balogun J and Okonofua F. Management of chronic pelvic inflammatory disease with shortwave diathermy: a case report. *Phys Ther* 1988;68(10):1541–1545.

Bansal PS, Sobti VK, and Roy KS. Histomorphochemical effects of shortwave diathermy on healing of experimental muscle injury in dogs. *Ind J Exp Biol* 1990;28:766–770.

Barclay V, Collier RJ, and Jones A. Treatment of various hand injuries by pulsed electromagnetic energy. *Physiotherapy* 1983;69(6):186–188.

Barker AT, Barlow PS, Porter J, et al. A double-blind clinical trial of low power pulsed shortwave therapy in the treatment of a soft tissue injury. *Physiotherapy* 1985;71(12):500–504.

Barnett M. SWD for herpes zoster. *Physiotherapy* 1975;61:217.

Bassett C. The development and application of pulsed electromagnetic fields (PEMFs) for united fractures and arthrodeses. *Orthop Clin North Am* 1984;15(10):61–89.

Benson TB and Copp EP. The effect of therapeutic forms of heat and ice on the pain threshold of the normal shoulder. *Rheumatol Rehab* 1974;13:101–104.

Bentall RH and Eckstein HB. A trial involving the use of pulsed electromagnetic therapy on children undergoing orchidopexy. *Kinderchirugie* 1975;17(4):380–389.

Bernal G. Turning up the heat. *Rehab Management: The Interdisciplinary Journal of Rehabilitation* 2009;22(5):28–31.

Brown M and Baker RD. Effect of pulsed shortwave diathermy on skeletal muscle injury in rabbits. *Phys Ther* 1987;67(2):208–214.

Brown-Woodnan PDC, Hadley JA, Richardson L, et al. Evaluation of reproductive function of female rats exposed to radio frequency fields (27.12 MHz) near a shortwave diathermy device. *Health Phys* 1989;56(4):521–525.

Burr B. Heat as a therapeutic modality against cancer, Report 16, U.S. National Cancer Institute, Bethesda, MD, 1974.

Cameron BM. Experimental acceleration of wound healing. *Am J Orthopaed* 1961;3:336–343.

Cameron MH. Diathermy for wound care. *Adv Dir Rehab* 2003;12(1):71.

Chamberlain MA, Care G, and Gharfield B. Physiotherapy in osteo-arthrosis of the knee, *Ann Rheum Dis* 1982;23:389–391.

Cole A and Eagleston R. The benefits of deep heat: ultrasound and electromagnetic diathermy. *Phys Sportsmed* 1994;22(2):76–78, 81–82, 84.

Constable JD, Scapicchio AP, and Opitz B. Studies of the effects of Diapulse treatment on various aspects of wound healing in experimental animals. *J Surg Res* 1971;11:254–257.

Coppell R. Survey of stray electromagnetic emissions from microwave and shortwave diathermy equipment. *NZ J Physiother* 1988;16(3):9–12, 14.

Currier DP and Nelson RM. Changes in motor conduction velocity induced by exercise and diathermy. *Phys Ther* 1969;49(2):146–152.

Daels J. Microwave heating of the uterine wall during parturition. *J Microwave Power* 1976;11:166.

de la Rosette J, de Wildt M, and Alivizatos G. Transurethral microwave thermotherapy (TUMT) in benign prostatic hyperplasia: placebo versus TUMT. *Urology* 1994;44(1):58–63.

Department of Health and Welfare (Canada). Canada wide survey of non-ionising radiation-emitting medical devices, 80-EHD-52, 1980.

Department of Health and Welfare (Canada). Safety code 25: Shortwave diathermy guidelines for limited radio frequency exposure, 80-EHD-98, 1983.

Department of Health. Evaluation report: Shortwave therapy units. *J Med Eng Technol* 1987;11(6):285–298.

Doyle JR and Smart BW. Stimulation of bone growth by shortwave diathermy. *J Bone Joint Surg* 1963;45A:15.

Draper D, Castel J, and Castel D. Low-watt pulsed shortwave diathermy and metal-plate fixation of the elbow. *Athlet Ther Today* 2004;9(5):28.

Engel JP. The effects of microwaves on bone and bone marrow and adjacent tissues. *Arch Phys Med Rehab* 1950;31:453.

Erdman WJ. Peripheral blood flow measurements during application of pulsed high frequency currents. *Am J Orthopaed* 1960;2:196–197.

Feibel H and Fast H. Deepheating of joints: A reconsideration. *Arch Phys Med Rehab* 1976;57:513.

Fenn JE. Effect of pulsed electromagnetic energy (Diapulse) on experimental haematomas. *Can Med Assoc J* 1969;100:251–253.

Foley-Nolan D, Barry C, Coughlan RJ, et al. Pulsed high frequency (27MHz) electromagnetic therapy for persistent neck pain. *Orthopaedics* 1990;13(4):445–451.

Foley-Nolan D, Moore K, and Codd M. Low energy high frequency pulsed electromagnetic therapy for acute whiplash injuries. A double blind randomized controlled study. *Scand J Rehab Med* 1992;24(1):51–59.

Foster P. Diathermy burns. *Nursing RSA Verpleging* 1987;2(10):4–5, 7–9.

Frankenberger L. Making a comeback: diathermy is an effective therapeutic agent and should be part of every therapist's armamentarium. *Adv Dir Rehab* 2001;10(5):43–46.

Fukuda T and Ovanessian V. Pulsed short wave effect in pain and function in patients with knee osteoarthritis. *J Appl Res,* 2008;8(3):189–198.

Gibson T, Grahame R, Harkness J, et al. Controlled comparison of shortwave diathermy treatment with osteopathic treatment in non-specific low back pain. *Lancet* 1985;1:1258–1261.

Ginsberg AJ. Pulsed shortwave in the treatment of bursitis with calcification. *Int Rec Med* 174(2):71–75.

Goldin JH and Broadbent NRG, Nancarrow JD, and Marshall T. The effect of diapulse on healing of wounds: A double blind randomized controlled trial in man. *Br J Plastic Surg* 1981;34:267–270.

Grant A, Sleep J, McIntosh J, and Ashurst H. Ultrasound and pulsed electromagnetic energy treatment for peroneal trauma: A randomised placebo-controlled trial. *Br J Obstet Gynaecol* 1981;96:434–439.

Guy AW, Lehmann JF, and Stonebridge JB. Therapeutic applications of electromagnetic power. *Proc Inst Electric Electr Eng* 1974;62:55–75.

Guy AW, Lehmann JF, Stonebridge JB, and Sorensen CC. Development of a 915 MHz direct contact applicator for therapeutic heating of tissues. *Inst Electric Electr Eng Microwave Theory Techn* 1978;26:550–556.

Guy AW. Analyses of electromagnetic fields induced in biological tissues by thermographic studies on equivalent phantom models. *IEEE Trans Microwave Theory Tech Vol MTT* 1971;19:205.

Guy AW. Biophysics of high frequency currents and electromagnetic radiation. In Lehmann JF (ed). *Therapeutic Heat and Cold*, 4th ed, Baltimore, MD: Williams & Wilkins, 1990.

Hall EL. Diathermy generators. *Arch Phys Med Rehab* 1952;33:28.

Hansen TI and Kristensen JH. Effect of massage, shortwave diathermy and ultrasound upon 133Xe disappearance rate from muscle and subcutaneous tissue in the human calf. *Scand J Rehabil Med* 1973;5:179–182.

Harris R. Effect of shortwave diathermy on radio-sodium clearance from the knee joint in the normal and in rheumatoid arthritis. *Phys Med Rehab* 1961;42:241.

Hayne R. Pulsed high frequency energy: Its place in physiotherapy. *Physiotherapy* 1984;70(12):459–466.

Herrick JF, Jelatis DG, and Lee GM. Dielectric properties of tissues important in microwave diathermy. *Fed Proc* 1950;9:60.

Herrick JF and Krusen FH. Certain physiologic and pathologic effects of microwaves, *Elect Eng* 1953;72:239.

Hoeberlein T, Katz J, and Balogun J. Does indirect heating using shortwave diathermy over the abdomen and sacrum affect peripheral blood flow in the lower extremities? *Phys Ther* 1996;76(5):S67.

Hollander JL. Joint temperature measurement in evaluation of antiarthritic agents. *J Clin Invest* 1951;30:701.

Hutchinson WJ and Burdeaux BD. The effects of shortwave diathermy on bone repair. *J Bone Joint Surg* 1951;33A:155.

Jan M, Chai H, and Wang C. Effects of repetitive shortwave diathermy for reducing synovitis in patients with knee osteoarthritis: An ultrasonographic study. *Phys Ther* 2006;86(2):236.

Johnson CC and Guy AW. Nonionizing electromagnetic wave effects in biological materials and systems. *Proc Inst Electric Electr Eng* 1972;66:692.

Jones SL. Electromagnetic field interference and cardiac pacemakers. *Phys Ther* 1976;56:1013.

Justice-Stevenson P. Pulsed electromagnetic field therapy: electrotherapy unplugged. *Acute Care Perspectives* 2008;17(2):1, 3–5.

Kantor G and Witters DM. The performance of a new 915 MHz direct contact applicator with reduced leakage—a detailed analysis, HHS Publication (FDA) S3–8199, April 1983.

Kantor G. Evaluation and survey of microwave and radio frequency applicators. *J Microwave Power* 1981;(2)16:135.

Kaplan EG and Weinstock RE. Clinical evaluation of Diapulse as adjunctive therapy following foot surgery. *J Am Ped Assoc* 1968;58:218–221.

Kloth LC, Morrison M, and Ferguson B. Therapeutic microwave and shortwave diathermy: A review of thermal effectiveness, safe use, and state-of-the-art-1984, Center for Devices and Radiological Health, DHHS, FDA 85-8237, Dec. 1984.

Krag C, Taudorf U, Siim E, and Bolund S. The effect of pulsed electromagnetic energy (Diapulse) on the survival of experimental skin flaps. *Scand J Plas Reconstr Surg* 1979;13:377–380.

Landsmann MA. Rehab products: Equipment focus. Defending diathermy: recently fallen out of favor, this modality deserves a second look. *Adv Dir Rehab* 2002;11(11):61–62.

Lehmann JF, DeLateur BJ, and Stonebridge JB. Selective muscle heating by shortwave diathermy with a helical coil. *Arch Phys Med Rehab* 1969;50:117.

Lehmann JF, Guy AW, deLateur BJ, et al. Heating patterns produced by shortwave diathermy using helical induction coil applicators. *Arch Phys Med* 1968;49:193–198.

Lehmann JF, McDougall JA, Guy AW, et al. Heating patterns produced by shortwave diathermy applicators in tissue substitute models. *Arch Phys Med Rehab* 1983;64:575–577.

Lehmann JF Microwave therapy: stray radiation, safety and effectiveness, *Arch Phys Med Rehab* 1979;60:578.

Lehmann JF Review of evidence for indications, techniques of application, contraindications, hazards and clinical effectiveness for shortwave diathermy DHEW/FDA HFA510, Rockville, MD, 1974.

Leung M and Cheing G Effects of deep and superficial heating in the management of frozen shoulder. *J Rehab Med* 2008;40(2):145–150.

Licht S (ed). *Therapeutic Heat and Cold.* 2nd ed., New Haven, CT: Elizabeth Licht,1972.

Marek M, Fincher L, and Trowbridge C. The thermal effects of pulsed shortwave diathermy on muscle force production electromyography and mechanomyography (abstract). *J Athl Training* (suppl.) 2007;42(2):S–132.

Marek S and Fincher A. The thermal effects of pulsed shortwave diathermy on muscle force production, electromyography and mechanomyography. *J Athl Training* 2007;42(suppl.):S132.

Martin C, McCallum H, and Strelley S. Electromagnetic fields from therapeutic diathermy equipment: A review of hazards and precautions. *Physiotherapy* 1991;77(1):3–7.

McDowell AD and Lunt MJ. Electromagnetic field strength measurements on Megapulse units. *Physiotherapy* 1991;77(12):805–809.

McGill SN. The effect of pulsed shortwave therapy on lateral ligament sprain of the ankle. *NZ J Physiother* 1988;10:21–24.

McNiven DR and Wyper DJ. Microwave therapy and muscle blood flow in man. *J Microwave Power* 1976;11:168–170.

Michaelson SM. Effects of high frequency currents and electromagnetic radiation. In Lehmann HF (ed). *Therapeutic Heat and Cold,* 4th ed, Baltimore, MD: Williams & Wilkins, 1990.

Millard JB. Effect of high frequency currents and infrared rays on the circulation of the lower limb in man. *Ann Phys Med* 1961;6(2):45–65.

Morrissey LJ. Effects of pulsed shortwave diathermy upon volume blood flow through the calf of the leg: plethysmography studies. *J Am Phys Ther Assoc* 1966;46:946–952.

Mosely H and Davison M. Exposure of physiotherapists to microwave radiation during microwave diathermy treatment. *Clin Phys Physiol Meas* 1981;3(2):217.

Nadasdi M. Inhibition of experimental arthritis by athermic pulsing shortwave in rats. *Am J Orthopaed* 1960;2:105–107.

Nelson AJM and Holt JAG. Combined microwave therapy. *Med J Aust* 1978;2:88–90.

Nicolle FV and Bentall RM. The use of radiofrequency pulsed energy in the control of post-operative reaction to blepharoplasty. *Anaesth Plast Surg* 1982;6:169–171.

Nielson NC, Hansen R and Larsen T. Heat induction in copper bearing IUDs during shortwave diathermy. *Acta Obstet Gynaecol Scand* (Stockholm) 1972;58:495.

Nwuga GB. A study of the value of shortwave diathermy and isometric exercise in back pain management. Proceedings of the IXth International Congress of the WCPT, Legitimerader Sjukgymnasters Riksforbund, Stockholm, Sweden, 1982.

Oliver D. Pulsed electromagentic energy—what is it? *Physiotherapy* 1984;70(12):458–459.

Osborne SL and Coulter JS. Thermal effects of shortwave diathermy on bone and muscle. *Arch Phys Ther* 1938;38:281–284.

Paliwal BR. Heating patterns produced by 434 MHz erbotherm UHF69. *Radiology* 1980;135:511.

Pasila M, Visuri T, and Sundholm A. Pulsating shortwave diathermy: Value in treatment of recent ankle and foot sprains. *Arch Phys Med Rehab* 1978;59:383–386.

Patzold J. Physical laws regarding distribution of energy for various high frequency methods applied in heat therapy. *Ultrason Biol Med* 1956;2:58.

Quirk AS, Newman RJ, and Newman KJ. An evaluation of interferential therapy, shortwave diathermy and exercise in the treatment of osteo-arthrosis of the knee. *Physiotherapy* 1985;71(2):55–57.

Rae JW, Herrick JF, Wakim KG, and Krusen FH. A comparative study of the temperature produced by MWD and SWD. *Arch Phys Med Rehab* 1949;30:199.

Raji AM. An experimental study of the effects of pulsed electromagnetic field (diapulse) on nerve repair. *J Hand Surg* 1984;9B(2):105–112.

Reed MW, Bickerstaff DR, Hayne CR, et al. Pain relief after inguinal herniorrhaphy: Ineffectiveness of pulsed electromagnetic energy. *Br J Clin Pract* 1987;41(6):782–784.

Religo W and Larson T. Microwave thermotherapy: New wave of treatment for benign prostatic hyperplasia. *J Am Acad Phys Assist* 1994;7(4):259–267.

Richardson AW. The relationship between deep tissue temperature and blood flow during electromagnetic irradiation. *Arch Phys Med Rehab* 1950;31:19.

Rubin A and Erdman W. Microwave exposure of the human female pelvis during early pregnancy and prior to conception. *Am J Phys Med* 1959;38:219.

Ruggera PS. Measurement of emission levels during microwave and shortwave diathermy treatments. Bureau of Radiological Health Report, HHS Publication (FDA), 1980, pp. 80–8119.

Schoor M and Ricard M. The effects of pulsed shortwave diathermy and stretch on the torque-angle relation of the calf (plantarflexor) muscles associated with passive stretch both during and after treatment. *J Athl Training* 2008;43(suppl.):S88.

Schwan HP and Piersol GM. The absorption of electromagnetic energy in body tissues. Part I. *Am J Phys Med* 1954;33:371.

Schwan HP and Piersol GM. The absorption of electromagnetic energy in body tissues. Part II. *Am J Phys Med* 1955;34:425.

Schwan HP. Interaction of microwave and radio frequency radiation with biological systems. In Cleary SF (ed). *Biological Effects and Health Implications of Microwave Radiation*, Washington, DC: U.S. Department of Health, Education and Welfare, 1970.

Seiger C and Draper D. Use of pulsed shortwave diathermy and joint mobilization to increase ankle range of motion in the presence of surgical implanted metal: A case series. *J Ortho Sports Phys Therapy* 2006;36(9):669–677.

Seiger C and Draper D. Will pulsed shortwave diathermy and joint mobilizations restore range of motion in post-operative hypomobile ankles with surgical implanted metal: A case series. *J Athl Training* 2006;41(suppl.):S43.

Shields N. Short-wave diathermy and pregnancy: What is the evidence? *Adv Physiother* 2003;5(1):2–14.

Silberstein N. Diathermy: Comeback, or new technology? An electrically induced therapy modality enjoys a resurgence. *Rehab Manag* 2008;21(1):30–33.

Silverman DR and Pendleton LA. A comparison of the effects of continuous and pulsed shortwave diathermy on peripheral circulation. *Arch Phys Med Rehab* 1968;49:429–436.

Stuchly MA, Repacholi MH, Lecuyer DW, and Mann RD. Exposure to the operator and patient during shortwave diathermy treatments. *Health Phys* 1982;42(3):341–366.

Svarcova J, Trnavsky K, and Zvarova J. The influence of ultrasound, galvanic currents and shortwave diathermy on pain intensity in patients with osteo-arthritis. *Scand J Rheumatol* (suppl.) 1988;67:83–85.

Tamimi M and McCeney M. a case series of pulsed radiofrequency treatment of myofascial trigger points and scar neuromas. *Pain Medicine* 2009;10(60):1140.

Taskinen H, Kyyronen P, and Hemminki K. The effects of ultrasound, shortwaves and physical exertion on pregnancy outcome in physiotherapists. *J Epidemiol Commun Health* 1990;44:96–201.

Thom H. *Introduction to Shortwave and Microwave Therapy*, 3rd ed., Springfield, ILCharles C Thomas, 1966.

Trowbridge C and Ricard M. Short term effects of pulsed shortwave diathermy and passive stretch on the torque-angle relationship of the triceps surae muscles. *J Athl Training* 2007;42(suppl.):S132.

Tzima E and Martin C. An evaluation of safe practices to restrict exposure to electric and magnetic fields from therapeutic and surgical diathermy equipment. *Physiol Measure* 1994;15(2):201–216.

Van Ummersen CA. The effect of 2450 MHz radiation on the development of the chick embryo. In Peyton MF (ed). *Biological Effects of Microwave Radiation*, Vol. 1, New York: Plenum Press, 1961.

Vanharanta H. Effect of shortwave diathermy on mobility and radiological stage of the knee in the development of experimental osteo-arthritis. *Am J Phys Med* 1982;61(2):59–65.

Verrier M, Falconer K, and Crawford JS. A comparison of tissue temperature following two shortwave diathermy techniques. *Physiother Can* 1977;29(1):21–25.

Wagstaff P, Wagstaff S, and Downie M. A pilot study to compare the efficacy of continuous and pulsed magnetic energy (shortwave diathermy) on the relief of low back pain. *Physiotherapy* 1986;72(11):563–566.

Ward AR. Electricity fields and waves in therapy. *Science Press*, AustraliaNSW, 1980.

Wilson DH. Treatment of soft tissue injuries by pulsed electrical energy continuous and pulsed magnetic energy (shortwave diathermy) on the relief of low back pain. *Physiotherapy* 1986;72(11):563–566.

Wilson DH. Comparison of shortwave diathermy and pulsed electromagnetic energy in treatment of soft tissue injuries. *Physiotherapy* 1974;60(10):309–310.

Wilson DH. The effects of pulsed electromagnetic energy on peripheral nerve regeneration. *Ann NY Acad Sci* 1975;238:575.

Wilson DH. Treatment of soft tissue injuries by pulsed electrical energy. *Br Med J* 1972;2:269–270.

Wise CS. The effect of diathermy on blood flow. *Arch Phys Med Rehab* 1948;29:17.

Witters DM and Kantor G. An evaluation of microwave diathermy applicators using free space electric field mapping. *Phys Med Biol* 1981;26:1099.

Worden RE. The heating effects of microwaves with and without ischemia. *Arch Phys Med Rehab* 1948;29:751.

Wyper DJ and McNiven DR. Effects of some physiotherapeutic agents on skeletal muscle blood flow. *Physiotherapy* 1976;63(3):83–85.

GLOSSARY

air space plate   A capacitor type electrode in which the plates are separated from the skin by the space in a glass case. Used with shortwave diathermy.

cable electrodes   An inductance type electrode in which the electrodes are coiled around a body part, creating an electromagnetic field.

capacitance technique   Creates a strong electric field.

capacitor electrodes   Air space plates or pad electrodes that create a stronger electrical field than a magnetic field.

diathermy   The application of high-frequency electrical energy that is used to generate heat in body tissues as a result of the resistance of the tissue to the passage of energy.

drum electrodes   Induction electrodes that produce a strong magnetic field. Primarily used with pulsed shortwave diathermy.

eddy currents   Small circular electrical fields induced when a magnetic field is created that result in intramolecular oscillation (vibration) of tissue contents, causing heat generation.

electrical field   The lines of force exerted on charged ions in the tissues by the electrodes, which cause charged particles to move from one pole to the other.

federal Communications Commission (FCC)   Federal agency charged with assigning frequencies for all radio transmitters, including diathermies.

induction technique   Creates a strong magnetic field.

inductor electrodes   Cable electrodes or drum electrodes that create a stronger magnetic field than electrical field.

intermolecular oscillation (vibration)   Movement between molecules that produces friction and thus heat.

magnetic field   Created when current is passed through a coiled cable affecting surrounding tissues by inducing localized secondary currents, called eddy currents within the tissues.

pad electrodes   Capacitor type electrodes used with shortwave diathermy to create an electrical field.

pulsed shortwave diathermy   Created by simply interrupting the output of continuous shortwave diathermy at consistent intervals, it is used primarily for nonthermal effects.

specific absorption rate (SAR)   Represents the rate of energy absorbed per unit area of tissue mass.

LAB ACTIVITY

SHORTWAVE DIATHERMY

DESCRIPTION

Shortwave diathermy (SWD; *diathermy* means to heat through) uses an alternating current (most commonly 27.12 MHz) passed either through a coiled conductor or to a capacitor plate.

With the coil method, the patient is placed in the magnetic field that is generated when the current passes through the coil; the magnetic field then is absorbed by the molecules in the body, increasing the patient's internal energy. This method is referred to as inductive, because the body acts as a secondary coil, and the current in the body is induced by the current in the primary coil; the body never becomes part of the electrical circuit.

With the second method, there are two capacitor plates that are charged, and the body acts as a lower resistance conductor for the discharge of the capacitive current; thus the term capacitive shortwave diathermy. Again, the molecules of the body absorb the energy and have their internal energy increased. In capacitive SWD, the patient becomes part of the electrical circuit.

Because the motion of a molecule is dependent on its internal energy, when a molecule absorbs any type of energy, its motion increases. Temperature is a reflection of the average kinetic energy of a system, and the kinetic energy is by definition the random molecular motion. Therefore, when the molecular motion increases, the temperature increases. Although there are increased molecular collisions when the thermal energy of a system increases, these collisions do not produce any energy; they merely transfer the energy from one molecule to another. It is a misconception that the "friction" that occurs between the molecules causes the increased temperature.

Although electrical energy is used in SWD, action potentials are not induced in excitable tissue. At such high frequencies, the phase charge of the current is inadequate to alter the membrane voltage enough for the membrane to reach threshold. The amount of heat generated does follow Joule's law

$$Q = I^2Rt$$

where Q is heat, I is current, R is resistance, and t is time. The heat is generated in the tissue that absorbs the energy, and this varies according to the type of SWD used. Inductive SWD is absorbed mostly by tissues that have a high electrical conductivity, such as muscle. Capacitive SWD is absorbed mostly by tissues that have a low electrical conductivity, such as skin and fat. Because of this, capacitive SWD does not penetrate as deeply as inductive SWD, but does produce a more marked sensation of warmth in the patient. The general guideline for the depth of penetration of capacitive SWD is 1 cm, and 3–4 cm for inductive SWD.

PHYSIOLOGIC EFFECTS

Vasodilation
Decreased pain perception
Increased local metabolism
Increased connective tissue plasticity
Decreased isometric strength (transient)

THERAPEUTIC EFFECTS

Decreased pain
Increased soft-tissue extensibility

INDICATIONS

Shortwave diathermy is a heating physical agent; therefore, the indications are the same as for any heating agent. However, the depth of penetration, at least for inductive SWD, is greater than for any of the infrared agents. Ultrasound has a deeper penetration than SWD, but SWD can be used to treat a much larger area.

CONTRAINDICATIONS

- Lack of normal temperature sensibility
- Peripheral vascular disease with compromised circulation
- Over tumors, the testes, open growth plates, acutely inflamed tissue, active hemorrhage, the eyes, or metallic objects
- Pregnancy
- In patients with implanted electrical stimulators (e.g., cardiac pacemakers, phrenic nerve stimulators)

SHORTWAVE DIATHERMY

PROCEDURE	EVALUATION		
	1	2	3
1. Check supplies.			
a. Obtain sheet or towels for draping, timer, signaling device.			
b. Check SWD generator for frayed power cords, integrity cables and drum, shields, and so on.			

c. Verify that the output control is at zero.			
2. Question patient.			
a. Verify identity of patient (if not already verified).			
b. Verify the absence of contraindications.			
c. Ask about previous thermotherapy treatments; check treatment notes.			
3. Position patient.			
a. Place patient in a well-supported, comfortable position. This is particularly crucial, because the patient should not shift positions after the treatment starts.			
b. Expose body part to be treated; have patient remove all jewelry from the area.			
c. Drape patient to preserve modesty, protect clothing, but allow access to body part.			
4. Inspect body part to be treated.			
a. Check light touch perception.			
b. Check circulatory status (pulses, capillary refill).Assess function of body part (e.g., ROM, irritability).			
5. Apply SWD.			
a. Place a single layer of towel on the treatment area.			
b. Inductive: Position the drum containing the coil parallel to the body part and in contact with the towel. Capacitive: Position the plates parallel to the body part and about 2.5–7.5 cm away from the body.			
c. Turn on the SWD generator, allow to warm up if necessary.			
d. Inform the patient that he or she should feel only warmth; if it becomes hot, the patient should inform you immediately.			
e. Adjust intensity of SWD to the appropriate level. Set a timer for the appropriate treatment time and give the patient a signaling device. Make sure the patient understands how to use the signaling device.			
f. Check the patient's response after the first 5 minutes by asking how it feels.			
6. Complete the treatment.			
a. When the treatment time is over, turn the intensity control to zero, and move the generator away from the patient; dry the area with a towel.			
b. Remove material used for draping, assist the patient in dressing as needed.			
c. Have the patient perform appropriate therapeutic exercise as indicated.			
d. Clean the treatment area and equipment according to normal protocol.			
7. Assess treatment efficacy.			
a. Ask the patient how the treated area feels.			
b. Visually inspect the treated area for any adverse reactions.			
c. Perform functional tests as indicated.			

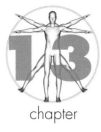

Low-Level Laser Therapy

chapter

Ethan Saliba and Susan Foreman-Saliba

OBJECTIVES

Following completion of this chapter, student will be able to:

➤ Identify the different types of lasers.

➤ Explain the physical principles used to produce laser light.

➤ Contrast the characteristics of the helium neon and gallium arsenide low-power lasers.

➤ Analyze the therapeutic applications of lasers in wound and soft-tissue healing, edema reduction, inflammation, and pain.

➤ Demonstrate the application techniques of low-power lasers.

➤ Describe the classifications of lasers.

➤ Incorporate the safety considerations in the use of lasers.

➤ Be aware of the precautions and contraindications for low-power lasers.

LASER is an acronym that stands for light amplification of stimulated emissions of radiation.

Despite the image presented in science-fiction movies, lasers offer valuable applications in the industrial, military, scientific, and medical environments. Einstein in 1916 was the first to postulate the theorems that conceptualized the development of lasers. The first work with amplified electromagnetic radiation dealt with microwave amplification of stimulated emission of radiation (MASER)s. In 1955, Townes and Schawlow showed that it was possible to produce stimulated emission of microwaves beyond the optical region of the electromagnetic spectrum. This work with stimulated emission soon extended into the optical region of the electromagnetic spectrum, resulting in the development of devices called optical masers. The first working optical maser was constructed in 1960 by Theodore Maiman when he developed the synthetic ruby laser. Other types of lasers were devised shortly afterward. It was not until 1965 that the term laser was substituted for optical masers.[1]

Lasers have been incorporated into numerous everyday applications that range from audio discs and supermarket scanning to communication and medical applications.[2] This chapter deals principally with the application of low-level lasers as they are used in conservative management of medical conditions.

• LASER = Light Amplification for the Stimulated Emission of Radiation

463

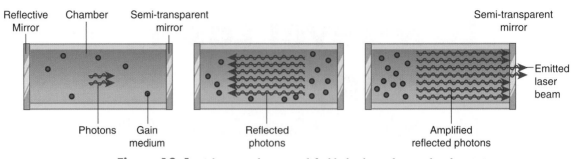

Figure 13-1. A laser produces amplified light through stimulated emissions.

Three Properties of LASER
- Coherence
- Monochromaticity
- Collimation

PHYSICS

A laser is a form of electromagnetic energy that has wavelengths and frequencies that fall within the infrared and visible light portions of the electromagnetic spectrum.[1] Electromagnetic light energy is transmitted through space as waves that contain tiny "energy packets" called **photons**. Each photon contains a definite amount of energy, depending on its wavelength (color).

A laser consists of a **gain medium**, which is a material (gas, liquid, solid) with specific optical properties contained inside an optical chamber (Figure 13–1). When an external power source is applied to the gain medium, photons are released, which are identical in phase, direction, and frequency. To contain them, and to generate more photons, mirrors are placed at both ends of the chamber. One mirror is totally reflective, whereas the other is semitransparent. The photons bounce back and forth reflecting between the mirrors, each time passing through the gain medium, thus amplifying the light and stimulating the emission of other photons. Eventually, so many photons are stimulated that the chamber cannot contain the energy. When a specific level of energy is attained, photons of a particular wavelength are ejected through the semitransparent mirror appearing as a beam of light.[3,4] Thus, amplified light through **stimulated emissions** (LASER) is produced.

The laser light is emitted in an organized manner rather than in a random pattern as from incandescent and fluorescent light sources. Three properties distinguish the laser: **coherence**, **monochromaticity**, and **collimation**.[1]

Coherence means all photons of light emitted from individual gas molecules are of the same wavelength and that the individual light waves are in phase with one another. Normal light, on the other hand, is composed of many wavelengths that superimpose their phases on one another.

Monochromaticity refers to the specificity of light in a single, defined wavelength; if the specificity is in the visible light spectrum, it is of only one color. The laser is one of the few light sources that produces a specific wavelength.

The laser beam is well collimated, that is, there is minimal divergence of the photons.[5] That means the photons move in a parallel fashion, thus concentrating a beam of light (Figure 13–2).

TYPES OF LASERS

There are potentially thousands of different types of lasers, each with specific wavelengths and unique characteristics. Lasers are classified according to the nature of the gain medium placed between two reflecting surfaces. The gain mediums used to create lasers include the following categories: crystal and glass (solid-state), gas, semiconductor, liquid dye, and chemical.

Lasers can be categorized as either high- or low-power, depending on the intensity of energy they deliver. High-power lasers are also known as "hot" lasers because of the thermal responses they generate. These are used in the medical realms in numerous areas, including surgical cutting and coagulation, ophthalmologic, dermatologic, oncologic, and vascular specialties.

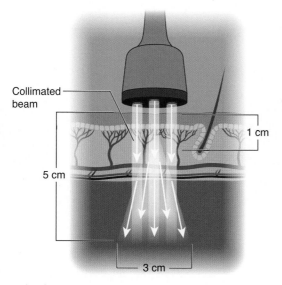

Figure 13–2. Depth of penetration with a GaAs laser. Direct penetration is up to 1 cm with a collimated laser beam. Stimulation causes indirect effects up to 5 cm.

The use of low-power lasers for wound healing and pain management is a relatively new area of application in medicine.[6] These lasers produce a maximal output of less than 1 milliwatt (1 mW = 1/1000 W) in the United States and work by causing photochemical, rather than thermal, effects. No tissue warming occurs. The exact distinction of the power output that delineates a low- versus high-power laser varies. Low-level devices are considered any laser that does not generate an appreciable thermal response. This category can include lasers capable of producing up to 500 W of power.[7]

Clinical Decision-Making *Exercise 13–1*

After watching a show on the use of lasers in surgery, a patient expresses genuine concern to the clinician that using a laser to treat a myofascial trigger point will cause skin burns. What should the clinician explain to the patient to allay his or her fears?

Low-level laser therapy is the dominant term in use today. In the literature low-power laser therapy is also frequently used. Therapeutic laser, low-level laser, low-power laser, or low-energy laser is also used for laser therapy. The term soft laser was originally used to differentiate therapeutic lasers from hard lasers, that is, surgical lasers. Several different designations then emerged, such as MID laser and medical laser. Biostimulating laser is another term, with the disadvantage that one can also give inhibiting doses.[8] The term bioregulating laser has thus been proposed. Other suggested names are low-reactive-level laser, low-intensity-level laser, photobiostimulation laser, and photobiomodulation laser.

Low-level lasers, which have been studied and used in Canada and Europe for the last 30 years, have been investigated in the United States for the last two decades. The two most commonly used low-level lasers are the helium–neon (HeNe) (Figure 13–3a) and the gallium arsenide (GaAs) (Figure 13–3b). HeNe lasers deliver a characteristic red beam with a wavelength of 632.8 nm. The laser is delivered in a continuous wave and has a direct penetration of 2–5 mm and an indirect penetration of 10–15 mm. GaAs lasers are invisible and have a wavelength of 904 nm. They are delivered in a pulse mode and have an average power output of 0.4 mW. This laser has a direct penetration of 1–2 cm and an indirect penetration to 5 cm.

Most commonly used lasers
- Helium neon (HeNe)
- Gallium arsenide (GaAs)

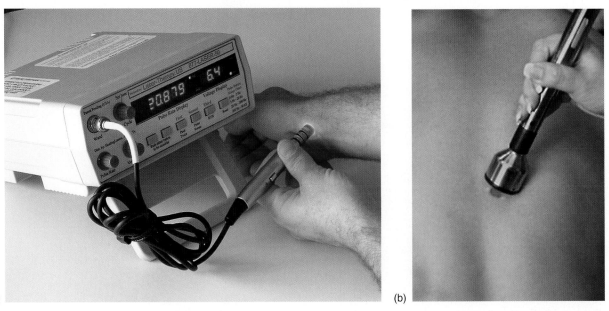

(a)

(b)

Figure 13–3. Low-level lasers. (a) Helium neon laser. (b) Gallium arsenide laser. (Courtesy of ColdLaserEquipment.com.)

The potential applications for low-level lasers include treatment of tendon and ligment injury, arthritis, edema reduction, soft-tissue injury, ulcer and burn care, scar tissue inhibition, and acutherapy.[9]

The laser units available in the United States have the ability to deliver both HeNe and GaAs lasers. The same device can both measure electrical impedance and deliver electrical point stimulation. The impedance detector allows hypersensitive or acupuncture points to be located. The point stimulator can be combined with laser application when treating pain. The electrical stimulation is believed to provide spontaneous pain relief, whereas the laser provides more latent tissue responses.[10]

LASER TREATMENT TECHNIQUES

The method of application of laser therapy is relatively simple, but certain principles should be discussed so the clinician can accurately determine the amount of laser energy delivered to the tissues. For general application, only the treatment time and the pulse rate vary. For research purposes, the investigator should measure the exact energy density emitted from the applicator before the treatments. Dosage is the most important variable in laser therapy.

The laser energy is emitted from a handheld remote applicator. The HeNe lasers contain their components inside the unit and deliver the laser light to the target area via a fiber-optic tube. The fiber-optic assembly is fragile and should not be crimped or twisted excessively. The GaAs laser houses semiconductor elements in the tip of the applicator. The fiber-optics used with the HeNe and the elliptical shape of the semiconductor in the GaAs laser create beam **divergence** with both devices. This divergence causes the beam's energy to spread out over a given area so that as the distance from the source increases, the intensity of the beam lessens.

Lasing Techniques
- Gridding
- Scanning
- Wanding

Lasing Techniques

To administer a laser treatment, the tip should be in light contact with the skin and directed perpendicularly to the target tissue while the laser is engaged for the designated time. Commonly, a treatment area is divided into a grid of square centimeters, with each square centimeter stimulated for the specified time. This gridding technique is the most frequently utilized method of application and should be used whenever possible. Lines and points should not be

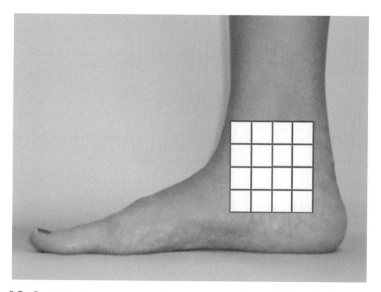

Figure 13–4. Gridding techniques. An imaginary grid can be drawn over the area to be treated and each square centimeter of the injured area should be lasered for the specified time. The laser should be in light contact with the skin.

drawn on the patient's skin because this may absorb some of the light energy (Figure 13–4). If open areas are to be treated, a sterilized clear plastic sheet can be placed over the wound to allow surface contact.

An alternative is a scanning technique in which there is no contact between the laser tip and the skin. With this technique, the applicator tip should be held 5–10 mm from the wound. Because beam divergence occurs, the amount of energy decreases as the distance from the target increases. The amount of energy lost becomes difficult to quantify accurately if the distance from the target is variable. Therefore, it is not recommended to treat at distances greater than 1 cm. When using a laser tip of 1 mm with 30 degrees of divergence, the red laser beam of the HeNe should fill an area the size of 1 cm² (Figure 13–5).

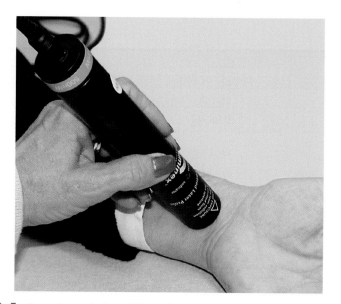

Figure 13–5. Scanning technique. When skin contact cannot be maintained, the applicator should be held in the center of the square centimeter grid at a distance of less than 1 cm and should be at an angle of 30 degrees to the surface being treated.

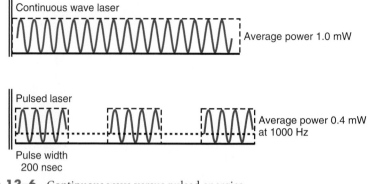

Figure 13–6. Continuous wave versus pulsed energies.

Although the infrared laser is invisible, the same consideration should be given when using the scanning technique. If the laser tip comes into contact with an open wound, the tip should be cleaned thoroughly with a small amount of bleach or other antiseptic agents to prevent cross-contamination.

The scanning technique should be differentiated from the wanding technique, in which a grid area is bathed with the laser in an oscillating fashion for the designated time. As in the scanning technique, the dosimetry is difficult to calculate if a distance of less than 1 cm cannot be maintained. The wanding technique is not recommended because of irregularities in the dosages.

Dosage

The HeNe laser has a 1.0-mW average power output at the fiber tip and is delivered in the continuous wave mode. The GaAs laser has an output of 2 W but has only a 0.4-mW average power when pulsed at its maximum rate of 1000 Hz. The frequency of the GaAs is variable, and the clinician may choose a pulse rate of 1–1000 Hz, each with a pulse width of 200 ns (ns = 10^{-9}) (Figure 13–6). Table 13–1 describes the contrasting specifications of these lasers.

The pulsed modes drastically reduce the amount of energy emitted from the laser. For example, a 2-W laser is pulsed at 100 Hz:

$$\textbf{Average power} = \textbf{pulse rate} \times \textbf{peak power} \times \textbf{pulse width}$$
$$= \textbf{100 Hz} \times \textbf{2 W} \times (\textbf{2} \times \textbf{10}^{-7} \textbf{ s})$$
$$= \textbf{0.04 mW}$$

Table 13-1 Parameters of Low-Output Lasers		
	HELIUM NEON (HeNe)	**GALLIUM ARSENIDE (GaAs)**
Laser type	Gas	Semiconductor
Wavelength (nm)	632.8	904
Pulse rate	Continuous wave	1–1000 Hz
Pulse width	Continuous wave	200 ns
Peak power	3 mW	2 W
Average power (mW)	1.0	0.04–0.4
Beam area (cm)	0.01	0.07
FDA class	Class II laser	Class I laser

Copied with permission from Physio Technology.

This contrasts with the power output of 0.4 mW at the 1000 Hz rate. Therefore, it can be seen that adjustment of the pulse rate alters the average power, which significantly affects the treatment time if a specified amount of energy is required. In the past it was thought that altering the frequency of the laser would increase its benefits. Recent evidence indicates that the total number of joules is more important; therefore, higher pulse rates are recommended to decrease the treatment time required for each stimulation point.[11]

Clinical Decision-Making *Exercise 13-2*

A clinician is treating a postacute inversion ankle sprain with an HeNe laser. How can the clinician ensure that the amount of energy delivered to the injured area is relatively uniform?

The dosage or energy density of laser is reported in the literature as joules per square centimeter (J/cm^2). One joule is equal to 1 W/s. Therefore, dosage is dependent on (1) the output of the laser in mW, (2) the time of exposure in seconds, and (3) the beam surface area of the laser in cm^2.

Dosage should be accurately calculated to standardize treatments and to establish treatment guidelines for specific injuries. The intention is to deliver a specific number of J/cm^2 or mJ/cm^2. After setting the pulse rate, which determines the average power of the laser, only the treatment time per cm^2 needs to be calculated.[11]

$$TA = (E/P_{av}) \times A$$

TA = treatment time for a given area
E = mJ of energy per cm^2
P$_{av}$ = Average laser power in mW
A = beam area in cm^2

For example: To deliver 1 J/cm^2 with a 0.4 mW average-power GaAs laser with a 0.07 cm^2 beam area:

$$TA = (1 \text{ J/cm}^2/0.0004 \text{ W}) \times 0.07 \text{ cm}^2$$
$$= 175 \text{ seconds or 2:55 minutes}$$

To deliver 50 mJ/cm^2 with the same laser, it would only take 8.75 seconds of stimulation. Charts are available to assist the clinician in calculating the treatment times for a variety of pulse rates. The GaAs laser can only pulse up to 1000 Hz, resulting in an average energy of 0.4 mW. Therefore, the treatment times may be exceedingly long to deliver the same energy density with a continuous wave laser (Table 13–2).

Table 13–2 Treatment Times for Low-output Lasers

JOULES PER CENTIMETER SQUARE (J/CM²)

Laser Type	Average Power (mW)	0.05	0.1	0.5	1	2	3	4
HeNe (632.8 nm) continuous wave	1.0		0.5	1.0	5.0	10.0	20.0	30.0	40.0
GaAs (904 nm) pulsed at 1000 Hz	0.4		8.8	17.7	88.4	176.7	353.4	530.1	706.9

Copied with permission from Physio Technology, Topeaka, Kansas.

> ### Clinical Decision-Making *Exercise 13-3*
>
> The clinician is trying to calculate the dosage in J/cm² of a HeNe laser treatment. What factors will need to be taken into account that collectively determine the correct dosage?

Depth of Penetration

Any energy applied to the body can be absorbed, reflected, transmitted, and refracted. Biologic effects result only from the absorption of energy, and as more energy is absorbed, less is available for the deeper and adjacent tissues.

Laser light's depth of penetration depends on the type of laser energy delivered. Absorption of HeNe laser energy occurs rapidly in the superficial structures, especially within the first 2–5 mm of soft tissue. The response that occurs from absorption is termed the **direct effect**. The **indirect effect** is a lessened response that occurs deeper in the tissues. The normal metabolic processes in the deeper tissues are catalyzed from the energy absorption in the superficial structures to produce the indirect effect. HeNe laser has an indirect effect on tissues up to 8–10 mm.[11]

The GaAs, which has a longer wavelength, is directly absorbed in tissues at depths of 1–2 cm and has an indirect effect up to 5 cm (see Figure 13–2). Therefore, this laser has better potential for the treatment of deeper soft-tissue injuries, such as strains, sprains, and contusions.[12] The radius of the energy field expands as the nonabsorbed light is reflected, refracted, and transmitted to adjacent cells as the energy penetrates. The clinician should stimulate each square centimeter of a "grid," although there will be an overlap of areas receiving indirect exposure.

CLINICAL APPLICATIONS FOR LASERS

Because the production of lasers is relatively new, the biologic and physiological effects of this concentrated light energy are still being explored. The effects of low-level lasers are subtle, primarily occurring at a cellular level. Various in vitro and animal studies have attempted to elucidate the interaction of photons with the biologic structures. Although few controlled clinical studies are found in the literature, documented case studies and empirical evidence indicate that lasers are effective in reducing pain and aiding wound healing. The exact mechanisms for action are still uncertain, although proposed physiological effects include an acceleration in collagen synthesis, a decrease in microorganisms, an increase in vascularization, reduction of pain, and an anti-inflammatory action.[11]

Low-level lasers are best recognized for increasing the rate of wound and ulcer healing by enhancing cellular metabolism.[13] Results from animal studies have varied as to the benefits on wound healing, perhaps owing to the fact that the types of lasers, dosages, and protocols used have been inconsistent. In humans, improvement of nonhealing wounds indicates promising possibilities for treatment with lasers.

Wound Healing

The effectiveness of laser in wound healing was discussed in detail in Chapter 3. Early investigations of the effects of low-power laser on biologic tissues were limited to in vitro experimentation. Although it was known that high-power lasers could damage and vaporize tissues, little was known about the effect of small dosages on the viability and stability of cellular structures. It was found that low dosages (<10 J/cm²) of radiation from low-level lasers had a stimulatory action on metabolic processes and cell proliferation compared with incandescent or tungsten light.[14]

Mester conducted numerous in vitro experiments with two lasers in the red portion of the visual spectrum: the ruby laser, wavelength of 694.3 nm, and the HeNe laser, wavelength

632.8 nm. Human tissue cultures showed significant increases in fibroblastic proliferation following stimulation by either laser tested.[15] Fibroblasts are the precursor cells to connective tissue structures such as collagen, epithelial cells, and chondrocytes. When the production of fibroblasts is stimulated, one should expect a subsequent increase in the production of connective tissue. Abergel and associates documented that certain dosages of HeNe and GaAs laser, wavelength 904 nm, caused in vitro human skin fibroblasts to have a threefold increase in procollagen production.[14] This effect was most marked when low-level stimulation (1.94×10^{-7} to 5.84×10^{-6} J/cm^2 of GaAs and dosages of 0.053 to 1.589 J/cm^2 of HeNe) was repeated over 3–4 days versus a single exposure. Samples of tissue showed increases in fibroblast and collagenous structures as well as increases in the intracellular material and swollen mitochondria of cells.[15] Furthermore, cells were undamaged in regard to their morphology and structure after exposure to low-power lasers.[16]

Analysis of the cellular metabolism, with attention to the activity of DNA and RNA, has been made.[14,17,18] Through radioactive markers, it was suggested that laser stimulation enhances the synthesis of nucleic acids and cell division.[19,17] Abergel reported that laser-treated cells had significantly greater amounts of procollagen messenger RNA, further confirming that increased collagen production occurs because of modifications at the transcriptional level.[5]

Low-level lasers were used in animal studies to further delineate both the beneficial applications of laser light and its potential harm. In an early study by Mester and associates, mechanical and burn wounds were made on the backs of mice.[20] Similar wounds on the same animals served as the controls, with the experimental wounds subjected to various doses of ruby laser. Although there were no histologic differences among the wounds, the lased wounds healed significantly faster, especially at a dosage of 1 J/cm^2. It was also demonstrated that repeated laser treatments were more effective than a single exposure.

Other researchers investigated the rate of healing and tensile strength of full-thickness wounds when exposed to laser irradiation.[13,14,15,21,22] There were conflicting reports regarding rates of healing, with some studies showing no change in the rate of wound closure and others showing significantly faster wound healing.[3,13,14,15,21,22,23] Although the experimental results were conflicting, an explanation for the discrepancy may be an indirect systemic effect of laser energy. Mester showed that it was not necessary to irradiate an entire wound to achieve beneficial results because stimulation of remote areas had similar results.[17] Kana and associates described an increase in the rate of healing of both the irradiated and nonirradiated wounds on the same animal compared with nonirradiated animals.[21] This systemic effect was most marked with the argon laser. Several studies that investigated the rate of healing on living animal tissue used a second, nontreated control wound on the same animal. The rate of healing may have been confounded by this systemic effect. Whether this systemic effect involves a humoral component, a circulating element, or immunologic effects has yet to be determined or identified. Bactericidal and lymphocyte stimulation are proposed mechanisms for this phenomenon.[24]

Tensile Strength

The increased tensile strength of lased wounds was confirmed more often.[13,14,15,20,21,23] Wound contraction, collagen synthesis, and increases in tensile strength are fibroblast-mediated functions and were demonstrated most markedly in the early phase of wound healing. Wounds were tested at various stages of healing to determine their breaking point and were compared with a control or nonlased wound. Laser-treated wounds had significantly greater tensile strengths, most commonly in the first 10 to 14 days after injury, although they approached the values of the control after that time.[5,15,23] Hypertrophic scars did not result as tissue responses normalized after a 14-day period. HeNe laser of doses ranging from 1.1 to 2.2 J/cm^2 elicited positive results when lased either twice a day or on alternate days. The increased tensile strength corresponds to higher levels of collagen.

Immunologic Responses

These early studies led to the hypothesis that laser exposure could enhance healing of skin and connective tissue lesions, but the mechanism was still unclear. Biochemical analysis and radioactive tracers were used to delineate the immunologic effects of laser light on human tissue cultures. The laser irradiation caused increased phagocytosis by leukocytes with dosages of 0.05 J/cm^2.[17] This led to the possibility of a bactericidal effect, which was further demonstrated with laser exposures on cell cultures containing Escherichia coli, a common intestinal bacteria in humans. The ruby laser had an increased effect both on cell replication and on the destruction of bacteria via the phagocytosis of leukocytes.[17,20] Mester also concluded that there were immunologic effects with the ruby, HeNe, and argon lasers. Specifically, a direct stimulatory influence on the T- and B-lymphocyte activity occurred, a phenomenon that is specific to laser output and wavelength. HeNe and argon lasers gave the best results, with dosages ranging from 0.5 to 1 J/cm^2.[17] Trelles did similar investigations in vitro and in vivo and reported that laser did not have bactericidal effects alone, but when used in conjunction with antibiotics, it produced significantly higher bactericidal effects compared with controls.[25]

With the confidence that they would cause little or no harm and that they could serve a therapeutic purpose, low-power lasers have been used clinically on human subjects since the 1960s. In Hungary, Mester treated nonhealing ulcers that did not respond to traditional therapy with HeNe and argon lasers with respective wavelengths of 632.8 and 488 nm.[17] The dosages were varied but had a maximum of 4 J/cm^2. By the time of Mester's publication, 1125 patients had been treated, of which 875 healed, 160 improved, and 85 did not respond. The wounds, which were categorized by etiology, took an average of 12–16 weeks to heal. Trelles also showed promising results clinically using the infrared GaAs and HeNe lasers on the healing of ulcers, nonunion fractures, and on herpetic lesions.[25]

Gogia and associates, in the United States, treated nonhealing wounds with GaAs lasers pulsed at a frequency of 1000 Hz for 10 s/cm^2 with a sweeping technique held about 5 mm from the wound surface.[26] This protocol was used in conjunction with daily or twice daily sterile whirlpool treatments and produced satisfactory results, although statistical information was not reported. Empirical evidence by these authors suggested faster healing and cleaner wounds when subjected to GaAs laser treatment three times per week.

Inflammation

Biopsies of experimental wounds were examined for prostaglandin activity to delineate the effect of laser stimulation on the inflammatory process. A decrease in prostaglandin PGE2 is a proposed mechanism for promoting the reduction of edema through laser therapy. During inflammation, prostaglandins cause vasodilation, which contributes to the flow of plasma into the interstitial tissue. By reducing prostaglandins, the driving force behind edema production is reduced.[11] The prostaglandin E and F contents were examined after treatments with HeNe laser at 1 J/cm^2.[17] In 4 days, both types of prostaglandins accumulated more than the controls. However, at 8 days, the PGE2 levels decreased, whereas PGF2 alpha increased. Increased capillarization also occurred during this phase. Data indicate that prostaglandin production is affected by laser stimulation, and these changes possibly reflect an accelerated resolution of the acute inflammatory process.[17]

Scar Tissue

Macroscopic examination of healed wounds was subjectively described after the laser experiments in most studies. In general, the wounds exposed to laser irradiation had less scar tissue and a better cosmetic appearance. Histologic examination showed greater epithelialization and less exudative material.[22]

Studies that utilized burn wounds showed more regular alignment of collagen and smaller scars. Trelles lased third-degree burns on the backs of hairless mice with GaAs and HeNe lasers and showed significantly faster healing in the lased animals.[25] The best results were obtained with the GaAs laser because of its greater penetration. Trelles found increased circulation with the production of new blood vessels in the center of the wounds compared with the controls. Edges of the wounds maintained viability and contributed to the epithelialization and closure of the burn. Because there was less contracture associated with irradiated wounds, laser treatment has been suggested for burns and wounds on the hands and neck, where contractures and scarring can severely limit function.

Clinical Considerations

No ill effects have been reported from laser treatments for wound healing.[27] More controlled clinical data are needed to determine efficacy and to establish dosimetry that elicits reproducible responses. The impressions of low-power lasers are that they have a biostimulative effect on impaired tissues unless higher dosages, in excess of 8–10 J/cm^2, are administered.[5,19] This effect does not influence normal tissue. Beyond these ranges a bioinhibitive effect may occur.

The applications of the low-power laser in a clinical environment are potentially unlimited. Its applications can include wound healing properties on lacerations, abrasions, or infections. Clean procedures should be maintained to prevent cross-contamination of the laser tip. Because the depth of penetration of the infrared laser is about 5 cm, other soft-tissue injuries can be treated effectively by laser irradiation. Sprains, strains, and contusions have been observed by the authors to have faster healing rates with less pain.[28] Acupuncture and superficial nerve sites also can be lased or combined with electrical stimulation to treat painful conditions.

Pain

Lasers have also been effective in reducing pain and have been shown to affect peripheral nerve activity. Rochkind and others produced crush injuries in rats and treated experimental animals with 10 J/cm^2 of HeNe laser energy transcutaneously along the sciatic nerve projection.[29] The amplitude of electrically stimulated action potentials was measured along the injured nerve and compared with controls up till 1 year later. The amplitude of the action potentials was 43% greater after 20 days, which was the duration of laser treatment. By 1 year, all lased nerves demonstrated equal or higher amplitudes than preinjury. The controls followed an expected course of recovery and did not reach normal levels even after 1 year.

Snyder-Mackler and Bork have investigated the effect of HeNe irradiation on peripheral sensory nerve latency in humans.[30] This double-blind study showed that exposure of the superficial radial nerve to low dosages of laser resulted in a significantly decreased sensory nerve conduction velocity, which may provide information about the pain-relieving mechanism of lasers. Other explanations for pain relief may be the result of hastened healing, anti-inflammatory action, autonomic nerve influence, and neurohumoral responses (serotonin, norepinephrine) from descending tract inhibition.[11,10,31,32]

Chronic pain has been treated with GaAs and HeNe lasers, and positive results have been observed empirically and through clinical research. Walker conducted a double-blind study to document analgesia after exposure to HeNe irradiation in chronic pain patients compared with sham treatments.[33] When the superficial sites of the radial, median, and saphenous nerves as well as painful areas were exposed to laser irradiation, there were significant decreases in pain and less reliance on medication for pain control. These preliminary studies suggest positive results, although pain modulation is difficult to measure objectively.

Bone Response

Future uses of laser irradiation include the treatment of other connective tissue structures, such as bone and articular cartilage. Schultz and colleagues studied various intensities of laser on the healing of partial-thickness articular cartilage lesions in guinea pigs.[34] During the surgical procedure, the lesions were irradiated for 5 seconds, with intensities ranging from 25 to 125 J. After 4 weeks, the low-dosage group (25 J) had chondral proliferation, and by 6 weeks the defect had reconstituted to the level of the surface cartilage. Normal basophilia cells were present with staining, indicating normal cellular structures. The higher dosage groups and controls had little or no evidence of restoration of the lesion with cartilage. Bone healing and fracture consolidation have been investigated by Trelles and Mayayo.[18] An adapter was attached to an intramuscular needle so that the laser energy could be directed deeper to the periosteum. Rabbit tibial fractures showed faster consolidation with HeNe treatment of 2.4 J/cm^2 on alternate days. Histologic examination indicated more mature Haversian canals with detached osteocytes in the laser-treated bone. There was also a remodeling of the articular line, which is impossible with traditional therapy.[18,25,35] The use of lasers for the treatment of nonunion fractures has begun in Europe.

> ### Clinical Decision-Making   *Exercise 13–4*
>
> A patient is complaining of pain in the upper back. Following an evaluation, the clinician determines that the pain is radiating from an active trigger point in the upper trapezius. How should this trigger point be treated using a HeNe laser?

SUGGESTED TREATMENT PROTOCOLS

Research suggests some laser densities for treating several clinical models. These average from 0.05 to 0.5 J/cm^2 for acute conditions and range from 0.5 to 3 J/cm^2 for more chronic conditions.[11] The responses of the tissues depend on the dosage delivered, although the type of laser used can also influence the effect. The response obtained with different dosages and with different lasers varies considerably among studies, leaving treatment parameters to be determined largely empirically. In the literature, there seems to be little differentiation when comparing the dosages of HeNe and GaAs lasers, although their depths of penetration differ significantly. The laser units produced in the United States have relatively little average power, so the tendency is to administer dosages in millijoules rather than joules. Three to six treatments may be required before the effectiveness of laser therapy can be determined.

Although higher laser output is recommended to reduce treatment times, overstimulation should be avoided. The Arndt-Schultz principle that states more is not necessarily better is applicable with laser therapy. For this reason, laser should be administered at a maximum of once daily per treatment area. When using large dosages, treatment is recommended on alternate days. If the effects of laser plateau, the frequency of treatments should be reduced or the treatments discontinued for 1 week, time after which the treatment can be reinstated if needed.[25]

Pain

The use of low-power lasers in the treatment of acute and chronic pain can be implemented in various manners.[36] After proper diagnosis of the pain's etiology, the pathology site can be gridded. The entire area of injury should be lased as described previously. Table 13–3 lists some suggested treatment protocols for various clinical conditions. When trigger points are being treated, the probe should be held perpendicular to the skin with light contact. If a specific structure, such as a ligament, is the target tissue, the laser probe should be held in contact with the skin and perpendicular to that structure. When treating a joint, the patient should be positioned so that the joint is open to allow penetration of the energy to the intra-articular areas.

The treatment of acupuncture and trigger points with laser can be augmented with electrical stimulation for pain management. Reference to charts should be made to determine appropriate acupuncture points. The impedance detector in the laser remote enhances the ability to locate these sites. Points should be treated from distal to proximal for best results.

Occasionally patients may experience an increase in pain after a laser treatment. This phenomenon is believed to be the initiation of the body's normal responses to pain that have become dormant.[7] Laser has been found to help resolve the condition by enhancing normal physiological processes needed to resolve the injury. As stated previously, several treatments should be administered before deeming the modality ineffective in pain management.

> ### Treatment Protocols: Low-level Laser
>
> 1. Determine the area to be treated and visualize a grid overlying the treatment area. The grid should be divided into 1-cm squares.
> 2. If the gridding technique is to be used, place the tip of the probe in light contact with the skin and administer the light to each square centimeter of area for the appropriate time to obtain the desired dosage.

Table 13-3 Suggested Treatment Applications

APPLICATION	LASER TYPE	ENERGY DENSITY
Trigger point		
Superficial	HeNe	1–3 J/cm^2
Deep	GaAs	1–2 J/cm^2
Edema reduction		
Acute	GaAs	0.1–0.2 J/cm^2
Subacute	GaAs	0.2–0.5 J/cm^2
Wound healing (superficial tissues)		
Acute	HeNe	0.5–1 J/cm^2
Chronic	HeNe	4 J/cm^2
Wound healing (deep tissues)		
Acute	GaAs	0.05–0.1 J/cm^2
Chronic	GaAs	0.5–1 J/cm^2
Scar tissue	GaAs	0.5–1 J/cm^2

Copied with permission from Physio Technology.

3. If the scanning technique is to be used, hold the tip of the probe within 1 cm of the skin and make sure the aperture of the probe is positioned such that the laser beam will be perpendicular to the skin. Administer the light to each square centimeter of area for the appropriate time to obtain the desired dosage.

4. Ensure that the laser energy will not be directed at the patient's eyes.

5. If the patient reports anything unusual, such as discomfort at the treatment site, nausea, and so on, discontinue the treatment.

6. Continue to monitor the patient during the duration of the treatment.

Wound Healing

Open wounds and ulcerations as well as contusions, abrasions, and lacerations can be treated with laser to hasten healing time and decrease infection.[13,37,38] The wound should be cleaned appropriately and all debris and eschar removed. Heavy exudate that covers the wound will diminish the laser's penetration; therefore, lasing around the periphery of the wound is recommended. The scanning technique should be utilized over open wounds unless a clear plastic sheet is placed over the wound to allow direct contact. Opaque materials can absorb some of the laser energy and are not recommended. Facial lacerations can be treated with laser, although care should be taken not to direct the beam into the patient's eyes. Risk of retinal damage from the low-power lasers used in the United States is low.

Scar Tissue

The laser energy affects only what is metabolically diminished and does not change normal tissue. Hypertrophic scars can be treated with lasers because of the bioinhibitive effects.

Bioinhibition requires prolonged treatment times and may be clinically impractical because of the low power output of the lasers used in the United States. Pain and edema associated with pathologic scars have been effectively treated with low-power lasers. Thick scars have varied vascularity, which makes laser transmission irregular; therefore, it is often recommended to treat the periphery of the scar rather than to use the laser directly over it.

Edema and Inflammation

The primary action of laser application for control of edema and inflammation is through the interruption of the formation of intermediate substrates necessary for the production of inflammatory chemical mediators: kinins, histamines, and prostaglandins. Without these chemical mediators, the disruption of the body's homeostatic state is minimized and the extent of pain and edema is diminished. It is also believed that laser energy can optimize cell membrane permeability, which regulates interstitial osmotic hydrostatic pressures.[39] Therefore, during tissue trauma, the flux of fluid into the intercellular spaces would be reduced. Laser treatment is usually applied by gridding over the involved areas or by treating related acupuncture points if the area of involvement is generalized.

SAFETY

Few safety considerations are necessary with the low-level laser. However, as the variety of lasers evolved and their uses increased in the United States, it became necessary to develop national guidelines not only for safety but also for therapeutic efficacy. The U. S. Food and Drug Administration (FDA)'s Center for Devices and Radiological Health regulates the manufacture and sale of lasers in the United States.

Laser equipment commonly is grouped into four FDA classes, with simplified and well-differentiated safety procedures for each.[22]

- Class I, or "exempt," lasers are considered nonhazardous to the body. All invisible lasers with average power outputs of 1 mW or less are class I devices. These include the GaAs lasers with wavelengths from 820 to 910 nm.[3] The invisible infrared lasers should contain an indicator light to identify when the laser is engaged.
- Class II, or "low-power," lasers are hazardous only if a viewer stares continuously into the source. This class includes visible lasers that emit up to 1 mW average power, such as the HeNe laser.
- Class III, or moderate-risk, lasers can cause retinal injury within the natural reaction time. The operator and patient are required to wear protective eyewear. However, these lasers cannot cause serious skin injury or produce hazardous diffuse reflections from metals or other surfaces under normal use.[34]
- Class IV, or high-power, lasers present a high risk of injury and can cause combustion of flammable materials. Other dangers are diffuse reflections that may harm the eyes and cause serious skin injury from direct exposure. These high-power lasers are seldom used outside research laboratories and restricted industrial environments.[34]

The low-level lasers used in treating most orthopedic injuries are categorized as classes I and II laser devices and class III medical devices. Class III medical devices include new or modified devices not equivalent to any marketed before May 28, 1976.[19] The U. S. FDA has so far had a very strict policy on laser therapy. To use laser therapy on humans, it has been necessary to obtain approval by an Institutional Review Board (IRB), established through a university, a manufacturer, or a hospital. In accordance with a new policy established in 1999, the FDA started to issue so-called Premarket Notifications, labeled 510(k). The FDA does not regulate clinicians in the use of any laser product. They regulate the companies that manufacture and sell the laser products. A company must be approved by the FDA to market a device, and these companies are allowed to promote the medical use of their laser products only for the specifically approved applications. The FDA forbids statements that a treatment can help or cure diseases if scientific studies have not found it to be true. Such an approval means that

---

CASE STUDY 13–1
LOW-LEVEL LASERS

Background: A 44-year-old man who has had Type I diabetes mellitus for 30 years presents for treatment of a non- or slow-healing lesion on his left foot. He has a mild peripheral sensory neuropathy, and developed a blister after going for a long run with new running shoes. The initial injury occurred 3 months ago, and there has been no change in the size of the lesion for the past month. The lesion is on the plantar surface of the foot, under the first metatarsal head. It is a full-thickness lesion, and is approximately 3 cm in diameter. The patient's medical condition is stable, and there are no other complaints.

Impression: Chronic dermal lesion on the left foot.

Treatment Plan: Daily treatment with a helium-neon laser was initiated. After cleansing the wound under aseptic conditions, the entire lesion was exposed to the HeNe light at 632.8 nm wavelength. The scanning technique was used to prevent contamination of the wound and equipment. The entire lesion was treated with an energy density of 4.0 J/cm^2.

Response: Photographs were taken on a weekly basis to document the effects of the treatment. After 3 weeks of daily treatment, the frequency was decreased to three sessions per week. After a total of 21 sessions (5 weeks), the lesion was healed. The patient was taught self-care and techniques to prevent further injuries.

Discussion Questions

- What tissues were injured/affected?
- What symptoms were present?
- What phase of the injury-healing continuum did the patient present for care in?
- What are the physical agent modality's biophysical effects (direct/indirect/depth/tissue affinity)?
- What are the physical agent modality's indications/contraindications?
- What are the parameters of the physical agent modality's application/dosage/duration/frequency in this case study?
- What other physical agent modalities could be utilized to treat this injury or condition? Why? How?
- What is the mechanism of action of the laser energy?
- Why are patients with diabetes mellitus susceptible to cutaneous lesions?
- What precautions must be taken before treating a patient with a low-powered laser?
- What alternative treatment techniques would you consider? What are their advantages and disadvantages as compared to using a laser?

The rehabilitation professional employs physical agent modalities to create an optimum environment for tissue healing while minimizing the symptoms associated with the trauma or condition.

---

the specific laser approved can be sold, but the only claim the manufacturer can make is the indication described in the 510(k). Since 2002, the FDA granted 510(k) approval to several companies to market low-level lasers classified as Class II lasers. Table 13–4 provides a list of low-level lasers that the FDA has approved for study since 2002. To date the low-level laser is indicated for adjunct use in the temporary relief of hand and wrist pain associated with carpal tunnel syndrome.[40] By requiring documentation of the results and side effects of lasers, the FDA regulations serve to generate scientific data to determine safety and efficacy of the device in question.

Clinical Decision-Making *Exercise 13–5*

How can the clinician treat a new abrasion using a laser to facilitate healing time and lessen infection?

Precautions and Contraindications

Table 13–5 lists indications and contraindications for using low-level laser. Lasers deliver non-ionizing radiation; therefore, no mutagenic effects on DNA and no damage to the cells or cell membranes have been found.[11] No deleterious effects have been reported after low-power laser

Table 13–4 List of Low-Level Lasers Approved for Study by the FDA since 2002

- MicroLight 830 (MicroLight Corporation of America, Missouri City, TX) received approval in 2002 for the indication of "adjunctive use in the temporary relief of hand; and wrist pain associated with Carpal Tunnel Syndrome."

- Axiom BioLaser LLL T Series-3 (Axiom Worldwide, Tampa, FL) received approval in 2003 for the indication of "adjunctive use in the temporary relief of hand and wrist pain associated with Carpal Tunnel Syndrome."

- Acculaser Pro4 (PhotoThera, Carlsbad, CA) received approval in 2004 for the indication of "adjunctive use in providing temporary relief of pain associated with iliotibial band syndrome."

- Thor DDII IR Lamp System (Thor International Ltd, Amersham, UK) received approval in 2004 for the indication of "elevating tissue temperature for the temporary relief of minor muscle and joint pain and stiffness, minor arthritis pain, or muscle spasm; the temporary increase in local blood circulation; and/or the temporary relaxation of muscle."

- Thor DDII 830 CL3 Laser System (Thor International Ltd, Amersham, UK) received approval in 2003 for the indication of "adjunctive use in the temporary relief of hand and wrist pain associated with Carpal Tunnel Syndrome."

- Luminex LL Laser System (Medical Laser Systems, Inc, Branford, CT) received approval in 2007 for the indication of "adjunctive use in the temporary relief of hand and wrist pain associated with Carpal Tunnel Syndrome."

exposure, including carcinogenic responses, unless applied to already cancerous cells. Tumorous cells may proliferate when stimulated.[26] The following are some suggestions for laser use.

It is better to underexpose than to overexpose. If clinical results plateau, a reduction in dosage or treatment frequency may facilitate results. Avoid direct exposure into the eyes

Table 13–5 Indications and Contraindications

INDICATIONS
Facilitate wound healing
Pain reduction
Increasing the tensile strength of a scar
Decreasing scar tissue
Decreasing inflammation
Bone healing and fracture consolidation

CONTRAINDICATIONS
Cancerous tumors
Directly over eyes
Pregnancy
Cancerous growths

because of possible retinal burns. If lasing for extended periods, as with wound healing, safety glasses are recommended to avoid exposure from reflection. Although no adverse reactions have been documented, the use of laser during the first trimester of pregnancy is not recommended. A small percentage of patients, especially those with chronic pain, may experience a syncope episode during the laser treatment. Symptoms usually subside within minutes. If symptoms exceed 5 minutes, no further treatments should be given.

CONCLUSION

The use of low-level lasers appears to have nothing but positive effects. This in itself should create a state of professional caution in deeming it a panacea modality. With current power outputs, lasers are recognized as nonsignificant risk devices. However, the FDA has not recognized low-power lasers as a safe or effective modality. Although many empirical and clinical findings show promising results, more controlled studies are essential to determine the types of lasers and dosages that are required to attain reproducible results.

SUMMARY

1. The first working laser was the ruby laser developed in 1960, initially called an optical maser.
2. Light is transmitted through space in waves and comprises photons emitted at distinct energy levels.
3. Stimulated emission occurs when the photon is released from an excited atom and promotes the release of an identical photon to be released from a similarly excited atom.
4. Characteristics of laser light vary from conventional light sources in three manners: laser light is monochromatic (single color or wavelength), coherent (in phase), and collimated (minimal divergence).
5. Laser can be thermal (hot) or nonthermal (low power, soft, or cold). The categories of lasers include solid-state (crystal or glass), gas, semiconductor, dye, or chemical lasers.
6. Helium neon (HeNe; gas) and gallium arsenide (GaAs; semiconductor) lasers are two low-level lasers being investigated by the FDA for application in physical medicine. These low-level lasers are currently being used in the United States and other countries for wound and soft-tissue healing and pain relief.
7. HeNe lasers deliver a characteristic red beam with a wavelength of 632.8 nm. The laser is delivered in a continuous wave and has a direct penetration of 2–5 mm and an indirect penetration of 10–15 mm.
8. GaAs lasers are invisible and have a wavelength of 904 nm. They are delivered in a pulse mode and have an average power output of 0.4 mW. This laser has a direct penetration of 1–2 cm and an indirect penetration of 5 cm.
9. The proposed therapeutic applications of lasers in physical medicine include acceleration of collagen synthesis, decrease in microorganisms, increase in vascularization, and reduction of pain and inflammation.
10. The technique of laser application ideally is done with gentle contact with the skin surface and should be perpendicular to the target surface. Dosage appears to be the critical factor in eliciting the desired response, but exact dosimetry has not been determined. Dosage fluctuates by varying the pulse frequency and the treatment times.
11. The laser is applied by developing an imaginary grid over the target area. The grid comprises 1-cm squares and the laser is applied to each square for a predetermined time. Trigger or acupuncture points are also treated for painful conditions.
12. The FDA considers low-level lasers as low-risk investigational devices. In the United States, they require an IRB approval and informed consent prior to use.
13. Although no deleterious effects have been reported, certain precautions and contraindications exist. Contraindications include lasing over cancerous tissue, directly into the eyes,

and during the first trimester of pregnancy. Occasionally pain may initially increase when laser treatments begin but does not indicate cessation of treatment. A low percentage of patients have experienced a syncope episode during laser treatment, but this is usually self-resolving. If symptoms persist for longer than 5 minutes, future laser treatments are not advised.

REVIEW QUESTIONS

1. What does the acronym LASER stand for?
2. How does the laser use the concept of stimulated emission to produce a laser beam?
3. What are the characteristics of the helium neon and gallium arsenide low-power lasers?
4. What are the various therapeutic applications of lasers in wound and soft-tissue healing, edema reduction, inflammation, and pain reduction?
5. What are the scanning and gridding techniques of application of the laser?
6. What seems to be the most critical treatment parameter in eliciting a desired response?
7. What are the treatment precautions and contraindications for low-power lasers?
8. Where does the low-power laser stand in terms of FDA approval as a therapeutic modality?

SELF-TEST QUESTIONS

True or False

1. An atom containing more energy than normal is considered to be in an excited state.
2. HeNe and AuAg lasers are the most common.
3. Tissue responses occurring from absorption of the laser are direct effects.

Multiple Choice

4. Which of the following is NOT a property of lasers?
   a. monochromaticity
   b. coherence
   c. divergenge
   d. collimation

5. _____ lasers may be used for wound healing and pain management.
   a. High-power
   b. Low-power
   c. Hot
   d. Chemical

6. Wounds treated with low-power lasers were shown to have what?
   a. increased tensile strength
   b. increased collagen synthesis
   c. both a and b
   d. neither a nor b

7. How are lasers thought to influence the inflammatory process?
   a. decrease prostaglandin production
   b. increase lymphocyte activity
   c. realign collagen
   d. increase metabolism

8. What type of laser application technique consists of holding the applicator over each square cm for the appropriate period of time?
   a. dosimetry
   b. wanding

c. scanning

d. gridding

9. Which of the following is a contraindication for low-power lasers?

a. bone fracture

b. cancerous tumors

c. inflammation

d. wounds

10. What energy density range is used in therapeutic applications?

a. 0.05–4 mJ/cm^2

b. 0.05–4 J/cm^2

c. 5–15 mJ/cm^2

d. 5–15 J/cm^2

SOLUTIONS TO CLINICAL DECISION-MAKING EXERCISES

13–1

It should be made clear that the type of laser being used in surgery is different from the one that is going to be used in treating the patient's trigger point. The surgical techniques require a "hot" laser, whereas the clinician will be using a cold laser. The patient will feel nothing during the treatment and there will be no burns or any other residual indication from the laser treatment.

13–2

The clinician should use a gridding technique in which there is contact between the tip of the laser and the skin. Moving the laser at a uniform speed over the predetermined grid area can help to ensure reasonably even coverage.

13–3

Dosage is dependent on the beam surface area of the laser in cm^2, the time of exposure in seconds, and the output of the laser in mW.

13–4

The clinician should use a gridding laser technique with the probe held perpendicular to the skin with light contact. The energy density should be set at 3 J/cm^2. The laser treatment can be combined with electrical stimulation using low-frequency (1–5 Hz), high-intensity current to produce pain modulation via the release of beta-endorphin.

13–5

First the wound should be cleaned appropriately and debrided as necessary. A scanning lasing technique with no direct contact should be done around the periphery of the abrasion. It is recommended that an HeNe laser be used at an energy density of 0.5 to 1 J/cm^2.

REFERENCES

1. Van Pelt W, Stewart H, Peterson R. *Laser fundamentals and experiments*. Rockville, MD: U. S. Dept. HEW; 1970.

2. Hallmark C, Horn D. *Lasers: the light fantastic*. 2nd ed. Blue Ridge Summit, PA: TAB Books; 1987.

3. McComb G. *The laser cookbook: 88 practical projects*. Blue Ridge Summit, PA: TAB Books; 1988.

4. Shaffer B. Scientific basis of laser energy. *Clin Sports Med.* 2002;(4):585–598.

5. Abergel R, Lyons R, Castel J. Biostimulation of wound healing by lasers: experimental approaches in animal models and in fibroblast cultures. *J Dermatol Surg Oncol.* 1987;13:127–133.

6. Gogia P, Hurt B, Zirn T. Wound management with whirlpool and infrared cold laser treatment. *Phys Ther.* 1988;68: 1239–1242.

7. Castel M. Personal communication, Downsview, Ontario. March, 1989, MEDELCO.

8. Fact Sheet. *Laser biostimulation.* Rockville, MD, 1984, Center of Devices and Radiological Health, FDA.

9. McLeod I. Low-level laser therapy in athletic training. *Athletic Therapy Today.* 2004;9(5):17.

10. Cheng R. Combination laser/electrotherapy in pain management, Second Canadian Low Power Laser Conference, Ontario, Canada. March, 1987.

11. Castel M. *A clinical guide to low power laser therapy.* Downsview, Ontario, 1985, PhysioTechnology Ltd.

12. De Bie RA, De Vet HCW, Lenssen TF, et al. Low-level laser therapy in ankle sprains: a randomized clinical trial. *Arch Phys Med Rehab.* 1998;79(11):1415–1420.

13. Hunter J, Leonard L, Wilson R. Effects of low energy laser on wound healing in a porcine model. *Lasers Surg Med.* 1984;3:285–290.

14. Abergel R. Biochemical mechanisms of wound and tissue healing with lasers. *Second Canadian Low Power Medical Laser Conference.* March, 1987.

15. Lyons R, Abergel R, White R. Biostimulation of wound healing in vivo by a helium neon laser. *Ann Plast Surg.* 1987;18:47–77.

16. Bostara M, Jucca A, Olliaro P. In vitro fibroblast and dermis fibroblast activation by laser irradiation at low energy. *Dermatologica.* 1984;168:157–162.

17. Mester E, Mester A, Mester A. Biomedical effects of laser application. *Laser Surg Med.* 1985;5:31–39.

18. Trelles M, Mayayo E. Bone fracture consolidates faster with low power laser. *Lasers Surg Med.* 1987;7:36–45.

19. Enwemeka C. Laser biostimulation of healing wounds: specific effects and mechanisms of action. *J Orthop Sports Phys Ther.* 1988;9:333–338.

20. Mester E, Spiry T, Szende B. Effect of laser rays on wound healing. *Am J Surg.* 1971;122:532–535.

21. Kana J, Hutschenreiter G, Haina D. Effect of low power density laser radiation on healing of open skin wounds in rats. *Arch Surg.* 1981;116:293–296.

22. Longo L, Evangelista S, Tinacci G. Effect of diode-laser silver-arsenide-aluminum (Ag-As-Al) 904 nm on healing of experimental wounds. *Lasers Surg Med.* 1987;7:444–447.

23. Surinchak J, Alago M, Bellamy R. Effects of low-level energy lasers on the healing of full-thickness skin defects. *Lasers Surg Med.* 1983;2:267–274.

24. DeSimone NA, Christiansen C, Dore D. Bactericidal effect of .95 m W helium-neon and indium-gallium-aluminum phosphate laser irradiation at exposure times of 30, 60, and 120 secs

on photosensitized Staphylococcus aureus and Pseudomonas aeruginosa in vitro. *Phys Ther.* 1999;79(9):839–846.

25. Trelles M. Medical applications of laser biostimulation, Second Canadian Low Power Medical Laser Conference. Ontario, Canada. March, 1987.

26. Farnham J. Personal communication. Rockville, MD, March, 1989, Center of Devices and Radiological Health, FDA.

27. Castel J. Laser biophysics, Second Canadian Low Power Medical Laser Conference, Ontario, Canada. March, 1987.

28. Kern C. The use of low-level laser therapy in the treatment of a hamstring strain in an active older male. *J Orthop Sports Phys Ther.* 2006;36(1):45.

29. Rochkind S, Nissan M, Barr-Nea L. Response of peripheral nerve to HeNe laser: experimental studies. *Lasers Surg Med.* 1987;7:441–443.

30. Snyder-Mackler L, Bork C. Effect of helium neon laser irradiation on peripheral nerve sensory latency. *Phys Ther.* 1988;68:223–225.

31. Bartlett W, Quillen W, Creer R. Effect of gallium-aluminum-arsenide triple-diode laser irradiation on evoked motor and sensory action potentials of the median nerve. *J Sport Rehab.* 2002;11(1):12.

32. Bartlett WP, Quillen WS, Gonzalez JL. Effect of gallium aluminum arsenide triple-diode laser on median nerve latency in human subjects. *J Sport Rehab.* 1999;8(2):99–108.

33. Walker J. Relief from chronic pain by low power laser irradiation. *Neurosci Lett.* 1983;43:339–344.

34. Sliney D, Wolkarsht M. *Safety with lasers and other optical sources: a comprehensive hand*book. New York: Plenum Press; 1980.

35. Schultz R, Krishnamurthy S, Thelmo W. Effects of varying intensities of laser energy on articular cartilage: a preliminary study. *Lasers Surg Med.* 1985;5:577–588.

36. Kleinkort J. Low-level laser therapy. new possibilities in pain management and rehab. *Orthopaedic Physical Therapy Practice.* 2005;17(1):48–51.

37. Hopkins J, McLoda T, Seegmiller J. Low-level laser therapy facilitates superficial wound healing in humans: a triple-blind, sham-controlled study. *J Ath Train.* 2004;39(3):223–229.

38. Hopkins J, McCloda T, Seegmiller J. Effects of low-level laser on wound healing. *J Athl Train.* 2003;(Suppl)38(2S):S–33.

39. Maher S. Is low-level laser therapy effective in the management of lateral epicondylitis? *Phy Ther.* 2006;86:1161–1167.

40. Johnson DS. Low-level laser therapy in the treatment of carpal tunnel syndrome. *Athletic Therapy Today.* 2003;8(2):30–31.

SUGGESTED READINGS

Abergel R. Biostimulation of procollagen production by low energy lasers in human skin fibroblast cultures. *J Invest Dermatol.* 1984;82:395.

Armagan O. Long-term efficacy of low level laser therapy in women with fibromyalgia: a placebo-controlled study. *Journal of Back & Musculoskeletal Rehabilitation.* 2006;19(4):135–140.

Bakhtiary A. Ultrasound and laser therapy in the treatment of carpal tunnel syndrome. *Australian Journal of Physiotherapy.* 2004;50(3):147–151.

Bandolier J. Low level laser therapy for painful joints. *Australian Journal of Physiotherapy*. 2004;11 (5):6–7.

Baxter G, Basford J. Low level laser therapy: current status. *Focus on Alternative & Complementary Therapies*. 2008;13 (1):11-3. Baxter G, Bell A, Allen J. Low level laser therapy: current clinical practice in Northern Ireland. *Physiotherapy*. 1991;77: 171–178. Baxter G. *Therapeutic lasers: theory and practice*. New York; Elsevier Health Sciences; 1994.

Beckerman H, de Bie R, Bouter L. The efficacy of laser therapy for musculoskeletal and skin disorders: a criteria-based meta-analysis of randomized clinical trials. *Phy Ther*. 1992;72(7):483–491.

Bjordal J, Lopes-Martins R, Iversen V. A randomised, placebo controlled trial of low level laser therapy for activated Achilles tendinitis with microdialysis measurement of peritendinous prostaglandin E2 concentrations. *Br J Sports Med*. 2006;40(1): 76–80.

Bolton P, Young S, Dyson M. Macrophage response to laser therapy: a dose response study. *Laser Ther*. 1990;2:101–106.

Bolton P, Young S, Dyson M. Macrophage responsiveness to laser therapy with varying power and energy densities. *Laser Ther*. 1991;3:105–112.

Braverman B, McCarthy R, Ivankovich A. Effect on helium neon and infrared laser irradiation on wound healing in rabbits. *Lasers Surg Med*. 1989;9:50–58.

Chow R, Johnson M. Efficacy of low-level laser therapy in the management of neck pain: a systematic review and meta-analysis of randomised placebo or active-treatment controlled trials. *Lancet*. 2009;374 (9705): 1897–908. Chow R. A pilot study of low-power laser therapy in the management of chronic neck pain. *Journal of Musculoskeletal Pain*. 2004;12(2):71–81.

Crous L, Malherbe C. Laser and ultraviolet light irradiation in the treatment of chronic ulcers. *Physiotherapy*. 1988;44: 73–77.

Cummings J. The effect of low energy (HeNe) laser irradiation on healing dermal wounds in an animal model. *Phys Ther*. 1985;65:737.

Djavid G, Mehrdad R. In chronic low back pain, low level laser therapy combined with exercise is more beneficial than exercise alone in the long term: a randomised trial. *Aust J Physiother*. 2007;53(3): 155–160.

Dreyfuss P, Stratton S. The low-energy laser, electro-acuscope, and neuroprobe: treatment options remain controversial. *Phys Sports Med*. 1993;21(8):47–50, 55–57.

Dyson M, Young S. Effects of laser therapy on wound contraction and cellularity in mice. *Laser Surg Med*. 1986;1:125.

Ezzati A, Bayat M. Low-level laser therapy with pulsed infrared laser accelerates third-degree burn healing process in rats. *J Rehabil Res Dev*. 2009;46(4):543–554.

Fisher B. The effects of low power laser therapy on muscle healing following acute blunt trauma. *J Phys Ther Sci*. 2000;12(1):49–55.

Flemming LA, Cullum NA, Nelson EA. A systematic review of laser therapy for venous leg ulcers. *J Wound Care*. 1999;8(3):111–114.

Gogia P, Marquez R. Effects of helium-neon laser on wound healing. *Ostomy Wound Manage*. 1992;38(6):33, 36, 38–41.

Hayashi K, Markel M, Thabit G. The effect of nonablative laser energy on joint capsular properties: an in vitro mechanical study using a rabbit model. *Am J Sports Med*. 1995;23(4):482–487.

Herbert K, Bhusate L, Scott D. Effect of laser light at 820 nm on adenosine nucleotide levels in human lymphocytes. *Lasers Life Sci*. 1989;3:37–45.

Johns L, Zhang X: The effects of low level laser on inflammation. *Journal of Athletic Training*. 2008;43(Suppl):S84.

Karu T, Tiphlova S, Samokhina M. Effects of near infrared laser and superluminous diode irradiation on Escherichia coli division rate. *IEEE J Quant Electron*. 1990;26:2162–2165.

Kazemi-Khoo N. Successful treatment of diabetic foot ulcers with low-level laser therapy. *Foot*. 2006;16(4):184–187.

Kern C. The use of low-level LASER therapy in the treatment of hamstring strain in an active older male. *Journal of Orthopaedic & Sports Physical Therapy*. 2006;36(1):A45.

Kleinkort J. Low-level laser therapy: new possibilities in pain management and rehab. *Orthopaedic Physical Therapy Practice*. 2005;17(1):48–51.

Kopera D. Does the use of low-level laser influence wound healing in chronic venous leg ulcers? *Wound Care*. 2005;14(8):391–394.

Kramer J, Sandrin M. Effect of low-power laser and white light on sensory conduction rate of the superficial radial nerve. *Physiother Can*. 1993;45(3):165–170.

Laakso L, Richardson C, Cramond T. Factors affecting low level laser therapy. *Aust J Physiother*. 1993;39(2):95–99.

Lam T, Abergel R, Meeker C. Biostimulation of human skin fibroblasts: low energy lasers selectively enhance collagen synthesis. *Laser Surg Med*. 1984;3:328.

Lundeberg T, Haker E, Thomas M. Effect of laser versus placebo in tennis elbow. *Scand J Rehab Med*. 1987;19:135–138.

Lyons R, Abergel R, White R. Biostimulation of wound healing in vivo by a helium neon laser. *Ann Plast Surg*. 1987;18: 47–50.

Maher S. Evidence in practice... Is low-level laser therapy effective in the management of lateral epicondylitis? *Physical Therapy*. 2006;86 (8):1161-1167.

Malm M, Lundeberg T. Effect of low power gallium arsenide laser on healing of venous ulcers. Scand *J Reconstruct Hand Surg*. 1991;25:249–251.

Mangus B, Orzechowski K. Low level laser therapy's effect on migration of human skin cells across a standardized wound. *Journal of Athletic Training*. 2007;42(Suppl):S133.

Martin D. An investigation into the effects of low level therapy on arterial blood flow in skeletal muscle. *Physiotherapy*. 1995;81(9):562.

McBrier N, Olczak J. Low Level Laser Therapy for Stimulating Muscle Regeneration Following Injury. *Athletic Therapy Today*. 2009;14(3):20.

McMeeken J, Stillman B. Perceptions of the clinical efficacy of laser therapy. *Aust J Physiother*. 1993;39(2):101–106.

Mester E, Jaszsagi-Nagy E. The effects of laser radiation on wound healing and collagen synthesis. *Studia Biophysica*. 1973;35(3):227.

Nussbaum E, Biemann I, Mustard B. Comparison of ultrasound/ultraviolet-C and laser for treatment of pressure ulcers in patients with spinal cord injury. *Phys Ther* 1994;74(9):812–823.

Palmgren N, Dahlin J, Beck H. Low level laser therapy of infected abdominal wounds after surgery. *Lasers Surg Med*. 1991;(Suppl)3:11.

Penny L. The effectiveness of low-level laser therapy in the treatment of verrucae pedis. *British Journal of Podiatry*. 2005;8(2):45–48.

Rockhind S, Russo M, Nissan M. Systemic effect of low power laser on the peripheral and central nervous system, cutaneous wounds, and burns. *Lasers Surg Med*. 1989;9:174–182.

Saperia D, Glassberg E, Lyons R. Stimulation of collagen synthesis in human fibroblast cultures. *Laser Life Sci*. 1986;1:61–77.

Saunders L. Laser versus ultrasound in the treatment of supraspinatus tendinosis: randomized controlled trial. *Physiotherapy*. 2003;89(6):365–373.

Swenson RS. Therapeutic modalities in the management of nonspecific neck pain. Physical Therapy and Rehabilitation Clinics of North America. 2003.14(3):605–627.

Turner J, Hode L. *Laser therapy: clinical practice and scientific background*. Grängesberg, Sweden: Prima Books; 2002.

Vasseljen O. Low-level laser versus traditional physiotherapy in the treatment of tennis elbow. *Physiotherapy*. 1992;78(5):329–334.

Waylonis G, Wilke S, O'Toole D. Chronic myofascial pain: management by low-output helium-neon laser therapy. *Arch Phys Med Rehab*. 1988;69(12):1017–1020.

Witt JD. Interstitial laser photocoagulation for the treatment of osteoid osteoma. *J Bone Joint Surg*. 2000;82B(8):1125–1128.

Wu S, Maloney R. Low-level laser therapy: a possible new light on wound healing. *Podiatry Management*. 2008;27(6):105–110.

Yeldan I, Cetin E. The effectiveness of low-level laser therapy on shoulder function in subacromial impingement syndrome. *Disabil Rehabil*. 2009;31(11):935–940.

Young S, Dyson M, Bolton P. Effect of light on calcium uptake by macrophages, presented at the Fourth International Biotherapy Association Seminar on Laser Biostimulation, Guy's Hospital, London, 1991.

Young S. Macrophage responsivity to light therapy. *Lasers Surg Med*. 1989;9:497–505.

Yousefi-Nooraie R, Schonstein E. Low level laser therapy for nonspecific low-back pain. *Cochrane Database Syst Rev*. 2008.

GLOSSARY

coherence   Property of identical phase and time relationship. All photons of laser light are the same wavelength.

collimate   To make parallel.

continuous wave   An uninterrupted opposed to pulsed beam of laser light.

direct effect   The tissue response that occurs from energy absorption.

divergence   The bending of light rays away from each other; the spreading of light.

frequency   The number of cycles or pulses per second.

indirect effect   A decreased response that occurs in deeper tissues.

laser   A device that concentrates high energies into a narrow beam of coherent, monochromatic light (Light Amplification by the Stimulated Emission of Radiation).

monochromaticity   The condition that occurs when a light source produces a single color or wavelength.

photon   The basic unit of light; a packet or quanta of light energy.

population inversion   A condition where more atoms exist in a high energy, excited state than atoms that are in a normal ground state. This is required for lasing to occur.

stimulated emission   This occurs when a photon interacts with an atom already in a high energy state and decay of the atomic system occurs, releasing two photons.

wavelength   The distance from peak to the same point on the next peak of an electromagnetic or acoustic wave.

LAB ACTIVITY

LOW-POWER LASER

DESCRIPTION

Low-power lasers produce a coherent, monochromatic, collimated light beam. They are used in the United States principally for pain modulation and wound healing. The two principal wavelengths used are 632.8 nm, produced by the helium neon (HeNe) laser, and 94 nm, produced by the gallium arsenide (GaAs) laser. Low-power (cold) lasers are distinguished from high-power (hot) lasers by the lack of thermal effects by the low-power lasers.

The mechanism of action of low-power laser energy is not clear. Whether the absorbed photons stimulating protein synthesis, thus promoting tissue healing, have a bactericidal effect on the wound or increase angiogenesis has not been established. The potential mechanisms for pain modulation are even less clear.

Although it has been suggested that laser energy may have indirect effects on tissue up to 5 cm deep, there is no convincing evidence of penetration this deep. How light energy absorbed by the superficial cells is conducted to underlying cells when the energy is nonionizing and nonthermal has not been explained.

It must be made crystal clear that the use of low-power lasers for these purposes has not been approved by the U.S. FDA, the regulating body for medical devices. Individuals using low power lasers for these purposes must have an Investigational Device Exemption and should obtain informed consent from each patient before using the laser.

The physiological and therapeutic effects of low-power laser stimulation are not well established. Therefore, the indications, which are derived from the physiological effects, are somewhat speculative.

PHYSIOLOGICAL EFFECTS

Increased collagen synthesis by fibroblasts
Decreased nerve conduction velocity

THERAPEUTIC EFFECTS

Increased rate of wound closure
Increased tensile strength of wounds
Decreased perception of pain

INDICATIONS

Low-power laser stimulation may be helpful to optimize the rate of wound closure, modulate musculoskeletal pain, and remodel established scar tissue.

CONTRAINDICATIONS

There are no established contraindications to low-power laser application, but the light should not be directed at the eyes.

LOW-POWER LASER

PROCEDURE	EVALUATION		
	1	2	3
1. Check supplies.			
a. Obtain towels or sheets for draping.			
b. Check laser equipment for charged battery, broken or frayed cables, and so on.			
2. Question patient.			
a. Verify identity of patient (if not already verified).			
b. Verify the absence of contraindications.			
c. Ask about previous exposure to laser therapy; check treatment notes.			
3. Position patient.			
a. Place patient in a well-supported, comfortable position.			

b. Expose body part to be treated.			
c. Drape patient to preserve patient's modesty, protect clothing, but allow access to body part.			
4. Inspect body part to be treated.			
a. Check light touch perception.			
b. Assess function of body part (e.g., ROM, irritability).			
5. Apply laser stimulation.			
a. Determine the area to be treated and visualize a grid overlying the treatment area. The grid should be divided into 1-cm squares.			
b. If the gridding technique is to be used, place the tip of the probe in light contact with the skin and administer the light to each square centimeter of area for the appropriate time to obtain the desired dosage.			
c. If the scanning technique is to be used, hold the tip of the probe within 1 cm of the skin and make sure the aperture of the probe is positioned such that the laser beam will be perpendicular to the skin. Administer the light to each square centimeter of area for an appropriate time to obtain the desired dosage.			
d. Ensure that the laser energy will not be directed at the patient's eyes.			
e. If the patient reports anything unusual, such as discomfort at the treatment site, nausea, and so on, discontinue treatment.			
f. Continue to monitor the patient during the duration of the treatment.			
6. Complete treatment.			
a. When the treatment time is over, discontinue application of the laser energy.			
b. Remove material used for draping, assist the patient in dressing as needed.			
c. Have the patient perform appropriate therapeutic exercise as indicated.			
d. Clean the treatment area and equipment according to normal protocol.			
7. Assess treatment efficacy.			
a. Ask the patient how the treated area feels.			
b. Visually inspect the treated area for any adverse reactions.			
c. Perform functional tests as indicated.			

PART **SIX**
Mechanical Energy Modalities

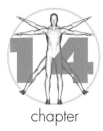

14
chapter

Spinal Traction

Daniel N. Hooker

OBJECTIVES

Following completion of this chapter, the student will be able to:

➤ Analyze the physical effects and therapeutic value of traction on bone, muscle, ligaments, joint structures, nerve, blood vessels, and intervertebral disks.

➤ Evaluate the clinical advantages of using positional lumbar traction and inversion traction.

➤ Describe the clinical applications for using manual lumbar traction techniques including level-specific manual traction and unilateral leg pull manual traction.

➤ Explain the setup procedures and treatment parameter considerations for using mechanical lumbar traction.

➤ Articulate the advantages of using a manual traction technique of the cervical spine.

➤ Demonstrate the setup procedure for mechanical traction techniques for the cervical spine.

Traction has been used since ancient times in the treatment of painful spinal conditions. Traction can be defined as a drawing tension applied to a body segment.[1,2] In the clinical setting, traction may be performed *mechanically*, using a traction machine or ropes and pulleys to apply a traction force, or it may be performed *manually* by a clinician who understands the appropriate positions and intensities of the force being applied to the joints of the spine or the extremities. Some of the concepts of traction discussed in this chapter are generalizable to the treatment of the extremities; however, this discussion has been aimed specifically at cervical and lumbar spinal traction.

THE PHYSICAL EFFECTS OF TRACTION

Effects on Spinal Movement

Traction encourages movement of the spine both overall and between each individual spinal segment.[3] Changes in overall spinal length and the amount of separation or space between each vertebra have been shown in studies of both the lumbar and the cervical spine (Figure 14–1).[4–13]

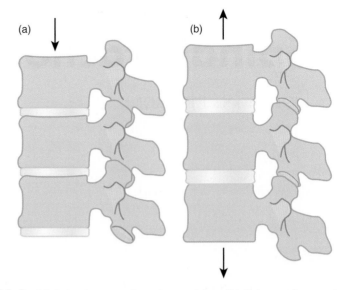

Figure 14–1. (a) Spine in normal resting position. (b) Spine under traction load with overall increase in length and overall increased separation between each vertebra.

The amount of movement varies according to the position of the spine, the amount of force, and the length of time the force is applied. Separations of 1–2 mm per intervertebral space have been reported. This change is very transient, and the spine quickly returns to the previous intervertebral space relationships when traction is released and the erect posture is assumed.[11,14–17] Decreases in pain, paresthesia, or tingling while traction is applied may be caused by the physical separation of the vertebral segments and the resultant decrease in pressure on sensitive structures. If these changes occur while the patient is being treated with traction, the prognosis for the patient is good and traction should be continued as part of the treatment plan.[3,10,18] Any lasting therapeutic changes must be assumed to occur from adjustments or adaptations of the structures around the vertebrae in response to the traction.

Effects on Bone

Bone changes, according to **Wolff's law**, usually occur in response to compressive or distractive loads. Traction places a distractive load on each of the vertebrae affected by the traction load. Although bone tissue adapts relatively quickly, bony changes do not occur fast enough to cause the symptom changes that occur with traction application. An intermittent traction with a rhythmic on and off load cycle not only provides distraction load but also promotes movement. The major effect of traction on the bone may come from the increase in spinal movement that reverses any immobilization-related bone weakness by increasing or maintaining bone density.

Effects on Ligaments

The ligamentous structures of the spinal column are stretched by traction. Structural changes of the ligaments occur relatively slowly in response to mechanical stresses because ligaments have **viscoelastic properties** that allow them to resist shear forces and return to their original form following the removal of a deforming load.[3,10,18]

With rapid loading, the ligaments become stiffer or resistant to changes in length and are able to absorb a high load or force before failure occurs. With this type of loading, overstress could produce a significant injury.[18]

Slow loading rates allow the ligament to lengthen as it absorbs the force of the load. Overstress can still produce injury, but it is not as severe as in the high-loading rates. The amount of **ligament deformation** accompanying a low rate of loading is higher than in rapid loading situations. Loading should be applied slowly and comfortably.[18] The ligament deformation allows the spinal vertebrae to move apart.

In ligaments shortened or contracted by an injury or a long-term postural problem, traction is important in restoring normal length. The traction force provides the stress that encourages the ligament to make adaptive changes in length and strength. The traction force in this instance would have to be heavy enough to stimulate adaptive changes but not heavy enough to overwhelm the ligament. In acute severely sprained ligaments, a traction force may overwhelm the ligament and have a negative effect on the healing process. Traction treatment should be a part of an overall treatment program that includes strengthening and flexibility exercises.[3]

When they are stretched, the ligaments put pressure on or move other structures within the ligamentous structure (**proprioceptive nerves**) and external to the ligament structure (**disk material, synovial fringes**, vascular structures, and nerve roots). This pressure or movement can have a tremendous impact on painful problems if it reduces pressure on a sensitive structure (nerve, vascular). Activation of the proprioceptive system also relieves pain by providing a gating effect similar to a transcutaneous electrical nerve stimulation treatment.[3,19]

Effects on the Disk

The mechanical tension created by the traction has an excellent effect on **disk protrusions and disk-related pain.** Normally, the disk helps to dissipate compressive forces while the spine is in an erect posture (Figure 14–2a). In the normal disk, internal pressure increases but the nucleus pulposus (fluidlike center of the fibrocartilaginous vertebral disk) does not move with changes in the weight-bearing forces as the spine moves from flexion to extension.[11] When an injury occurs to the disk structures and the disk loses its normal fullness, the vertebrae can move closer together. The annular fibers bulge just as an underinflated car tire bulges when compared with a normally inflated one (Figure 14–2b).[11]

If the disk is damaged and movement occurs in a weight-bearing position, the disk nucleus will shift according to fluid-dynamic principles. Pressure on one side squeezes the nucleus in the opposite direction (Figure 14–2c). If tears develop in the annular fibers, the nucleus will tend to take the path of least resistance and move in this direction (Figure 14–2d).

Traction that increases the separation of the vertebral bodies decreases the central pressure in the disk space and encourages the **disk nucleus** to return to a central position. The mechanical tension of the **annulus fibrosus** and ligaments surrounding the disk also tends to force the nuclear material and cartilage fragments toward the center.[3,9,11,16,19,20]

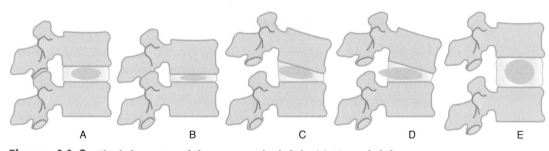

A   B   C   D   E

Figure 14–2. Fluid dynamics of the intervertebral disk. (a) Normal disk in noncompressed position; internal pressure, indicated by arrows, is exerted relatively equally in all directions. The internal annular fibers contain the nuclear materials. (b) Sitting or standing with compression of an injured disk causes the nucleus to become flatter. Pressure in this instance still remains relatively equal in all directions. (c) In an injured disk, movement in the weight-bearing position causes a horizontal shift in the nuclear material. If this was forward bending, the bulge to the left would take place at the posterior annular fibers, whereas the anterior annular fibers would be slackened and narrow. (d) Weakness of the annular wall would allow the nuclear material to create a herniation and possibly put pressure on sensitive structures in the area. (e) When placed under traction, the intervertebral space expands, lowering the disk pressure. The taut annulus creates a centripetally directed force. Both these factors encourage the nuclear material to move and decrease the herniation and its effects.

Movement of these materials relieves pain and symptoms if they are compressing nervous or vascular structures. Decreasing the compressive forces also allows for better fluid interchange within the disk and spinal canal.[3,19] The reduction in **disk herniation** is unstable and the herniation tends to return when compressive forces return (Figure 14–2d and e).[17,20]

The positive effect of traction in this instance may be destroyed by allowing the patient to sit after treatment. Minimizing compressive forces after treatment may be equally as important to the treatment's success as the traction.[3] The sitting posture increases the disk pressure, causing the nucleus to follow the path of least resistance and a return of the disk herniation.

Effects on Articular Facet Joints

The articular joints of the spine (**facet joints**) can be affected by traction, primarily through increased separation of the joint surfaces. **Meniscoid structures**, synovial fringes, or osteochondral fragments (calcified bone chips) impinged between joint surfaces are released and a dramatic reduction in symptoms is noticed when joint surfaces are separated. Increased joint separation decompresses the articular cartilage, allowing the synovial fluid exchange to nourish the cartilage. The separation may also decrease the rate of degenerative changes from osteoarthritis. Increased proprioceptive discharge from the facet joint structures provides some decrease in pain perception.[3,14,18,20]

Effects on the Muscular System

The vertebral muscles can be effectively stretched by traction provided that the positions of the spine during traction are selected to optimize the stretch of particular muscle groups. The initial stretch should come from body positioning, and the addition of traction then provides some additional stretch. Electromyographic recordings of the spinal erector muscles during traction showed some decrease in electromyographic activity in most patients, indicating a muscular relaxation.[21,22] This effect can be enhanced by palpating the erector muscles and focusing the patient's attention on relaxing them. The muscular stretch lengthens tight muscle structures or creates relaxation of contraction, allowing better muscular blood flow, and also activates muscle proprioceptors, providing even more of a gating influence on the pain. All these properties lead to a decrease in muscular irritation.[3,14,23–26]

Ligaments may be progressively stretched with traction.

Effects on the Nerves

The nerve is the structure at which traction's effects are most often directed. Pressure on nerves or roots from bulging disk material, irritated facet joints, bony spurs, or narrowed foramen size causes the neurologic malfunctioning often associated with spinal pain. Tingling is usually the first clinical sign indicating that there is pressure on a nerve structure. If the pressure is not relieved or if damage of the nerve as a result of trauma or anoxia has resulted in an inflammation, the tingling may not respond to traction.[7,10,11,13,14,21,27]

Unrelieved pressure on a nerve causes slowing and eventual loss of impulse conduction. The signs of motor weakness, numbness, and loss of reflex become progressively more apparent and are indicative of nerve degeneration. Pain, tenderness, and muscular spasm are also associated with continued pressure on the nerve.

Anything that decreases the pressure on the nerve increases the blood's circulation to the nerve, decreasing edema and allowing the nerve to return to normal functioning. Some degenerative changes are reversible, depending on the amount of degeneration and the amount of fibrosis that occur during the repair process.[3,13,14,27]

Effects on the Entire Body Part

The previous discussion outlined the effect of traction on the major systems involved in spine-related pain and dysfunction. The complexity and interrelationships among these systems make determining specific causes of pain and dysfunction very difficult. Traction is not specific to one system but has an effect on each system, and collectively the effect can be very satisfactory. Traction can affect the pathologic process in any of the systems, and then all the structures involved can begin to normalize. Traction should not stand alone as a treatment but should be considered as part of an overall treatment plan, and each component of any spine-related dysfunction should be treated with other appropriate modalities.[3,4,10,11,18,19,25,28,29]

TRACTION TREATMENT TECHNIQUES

The literature on traction and its clinical effectiveness is somewhat limited.[5,11,12,19,20,23,30,31] Most of the clinical studies go into great depth about the pathology being treated, but unfortunately they provide only a cursory description of the traction setup, making duplication of the traction method difficult.[30]

The following discussion of specific traction setups is organized according to lumbar and cervical traction. Each of these areas will contain discussions of postural, manual, and machine-assisted traction. The traction setups mentioned in this chapter should be used as starting points in a treatment plan. The parameters of time, position, and traction force should be adapted to the patient, rather than forcing the patient to adapt to a predetermined traction setup.

The treatment plan should include the clinical criteria for judging the success and continued use of traction. Positive changes should occur within 5–8 treatment days if traction is going to be successful, for example, if a patient has a positive straight leg raise sign (i.e., pain in the back with a passive straight leg raise). This is a measurable clinical criterion that can be used to judge the treatment's success. If the straight leg raise test is positive at 20 degrees of hip flexion before and after traction and after successive treatments the straight leg raise test is positive at increasing degrees of hip flexion, then the treatment can be considered successful.[32]

Lumbar Positional Traction

Spinal nerve root impingement, from a variety of causes ranging from disk herniation or prolapse to spondylolisthesis, is the leading diagnosis for which traction is prescribed. Traction has also been used to treat joint hypomobility, arthritic conditions of the facet joints, mechanically produced muscle spasm, and joint pain.[3,10,11,13,21,23,31,33]

Normal spinal mechanics allow movements to occur that narrow or enlarge the intervertebral foramina. If the patient is placed in the supine position with hips and knees flexed, the lumbar spine bends forward and the spinous processes separate. This movement increases the size of the intervertebral foramen bilaterally (Figure 14–3). The flexed postures used to treat low back pain are examples of this positional traction.

The greatest **unilateral foramen opening** occurs by positioning the patient sidelying with a pillow or blanket roll between the iliac crest and the lower border of the rib cage. The side on which increased foramen opening is desired should be superior. The roll should be

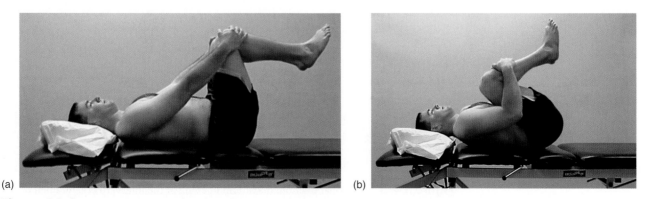

(a) (b)

Figure 14–3. Positional traction: knees to chest posture can be used to increase the size of the lumbar foramen bilaterally. (a) Beginning position. (b) Terminal position.

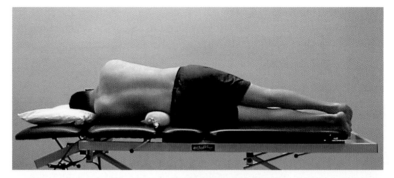

Figure 14–4. Positional traction: patient positioned sidelying with a blanket roll between the iliac crest and the lower border of the rib cage. This increases the intervertebral foramen size of the left side of the lumbar spine.

close to the level of the spine where the traction separation is desired. The spine side bends around the roll (Figure 14–4). The patient's hips and knees are then flexed until the lumbar spine is in a forward-bent position (Figure 14–5a). This accentuates the opening of a foramen. Maximal opening can be achieved by adding trunk rotation toward the side of the superior shoulder (Figure 14–5b).[11–13,27]

Positional traction is normally used when the patient is on a very restricted activity program because of low back pain. The positions are used on a trial-and-error basis to determine maximum comfort and to attempt to relieve pressure on nerve roots. The results of the patient evaluation should be used to determine whether the painful side should be up or down when using the sidelying positional traction technique. Protective scoliosis is the most obvious sign that will help determine patient position. If the patient leans away from the painful side, the painful side should be up (Figure 14–6a). If the patient leans toward the painful side, the painful side should be down (Figure 14–6b). The patient should be evaluated following the first treatment to determine changes in symptoms. Hopefully the patient will describe excellent results, but it is not uncommon to complain of increased pain.

The location of the pressure from the disk herniation was previously believed to cause these signs. Further research suggests that hand dominance may be more of a factor than herniation location in producing this scoliosis. However, the patient may be more compliant with the treatment regimen if simple mechanical explanations such as pushing the herniation back into place are used.[34]

Patients with these symptoms may also be good candidates for unilateral traction.[3,10,11,18,27,29] Facet irritation is capable of causing similar scoliotic curves; in most instances the scoliosis is convex toward the painful side.

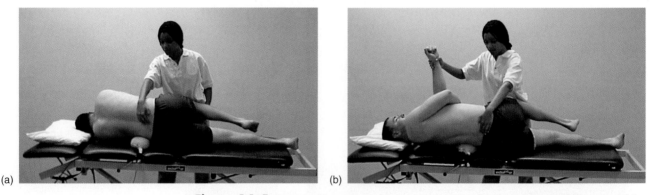

(a)   (b)

Figure 14–5. Positional traction: maximum opening of the intervertebral foramen of the left side of the patient's lumbar spine is achieved by flexing the upper hip and knee and rotating the patient's shoulders so he is looking over the left shoulder (left rotation).

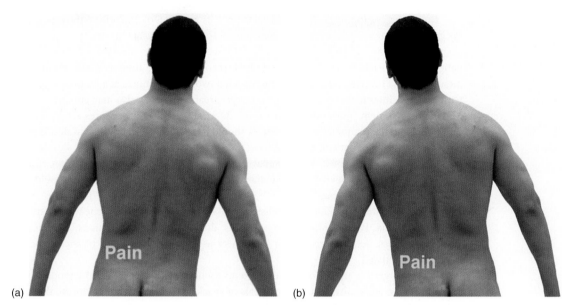

(a)   (b)

Figure 14–6. (a) Patient leaning away from the painful side. The patient's left side should be placed up while sidelying over a blanket roll to open up the upper foramen or the nerve roots away from the lateral herniation or both. (b) Patient leaning toward the painful side. The patient's left side should be placed down while sidelying over a blanket roll to pull the nerve roots away from a medial herniation.

Inversion Traction

Inversion traction, another positional traction, is used for prevention and treatment of back problems.[35-37] Specialized equipment or simply hanging upside down from a chinning bar places a person in the inverted position.[37] The spinal column is lengthened because of the stretch provided by the weight of the trunk. The force of the trunk in this position is usually calculated to be approximately 40% of body weight (Figure 14–7).[38] When the person is comfortable in the inverted position and able to relax, the length of the spinal column increases. These length changes coincide with decreases in spinal muscle activity.[3-5,15,22,39-41]

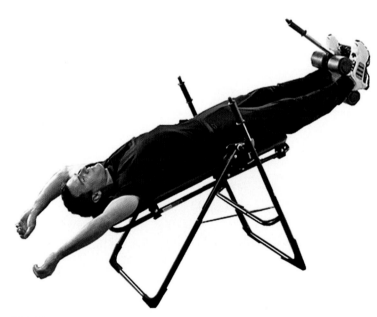

Figure 14–7. Back-A-Traction inversion traction.

No research-supported protocols exist for this method of traction, although a slow progression of time in the inverted position seems to be best. One study suggests the electromyographic activity decreases after 70 seconds in the inverted position. If the patient is comfortable completely inverted, 70 seconds may be used as a minimum treatment time. The inverted position may be repeated two or three times at a treatment session, with a 2- to 3-minute rest between bouts. Longer treatment times also may enhance results. Maximum treatment times range from 10 to –30 minutes. Setup procedures are equipment dependent and the manufacturer's protocols should be followed and modified as necessary to meet the needs of the patient.[3,4,22,35,36,42,43]

Blood pressure should be monitored while the patient is in the inverted position. If a rise of 20 mm of mercury above the resting diastolic pressure is found, the clinician should stop the treatment for that session.[3,22,42]

Contraindications include hypertensive (140/90) individuals and anyone with heart disease or glaucoma. Patients with sinus problems, diabetes, thyroid conditions, asthma, migraine headaches, detached retinas, or hiatal hernias should consult their physicians before treatment is initiated.

Recent surgery or musculoskeletal problems to the lower limb may require modification of the inversion apparatus. In addition, meals or snacks should not be eaten during the hour before treatment to keep the patient comfortable.

One method of testing the patient's tolerance to the inverted position is to have the patient assume the hand–knee position and put his or her head on the floor, holding that position for 60 seconds. Any vertigo, dizziness, or nausea may indicate that this patient is a poor candidate for inversion and that the treatment progression should be very slow (Figure 14–8).[3–5,15,19,22,39–42]

Clinical Decision-Making   *Exercise 14–1*

A patient is complaining of acute low back pain. She is very guarded and is leaning to the right, away from her left side, which she says is most painful. What can the clinician do to make the patient more comfortable immediately?

Manual Lumbar Traction

Manual lumbar traction is used for lumbar spine problems to test the patient's tolerance to traction, to arrive at the most comfortable treatment setup, to make the traction as specific to

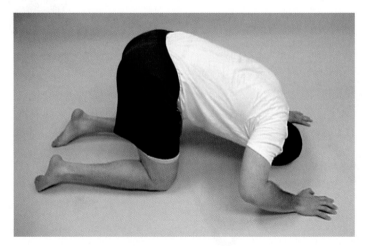

Figure 14–8. Inversion tolerance test position. Any vertigo, dizziness, or nausea may indicate that this patient is a poor candidate for inversion treatment.

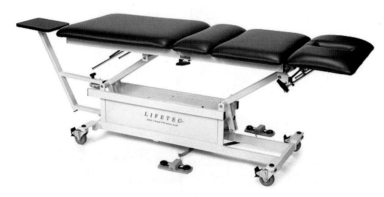

Figure 14–9. Split table with movable section to decrease frictional forces.

one vertebral level as possible, and to provide the specificity needed for a traction mobilization of the spine. If the patient's back pain is diminished by having the clinician flex the patient's hips and knees to 90 degrees each and apply enough pressure under the calves to lift the buttocks off the table, then the patient is a good candidate for spine 90–90-degree traction. The disadvantage is that maintaining the large forces necessary for separation of the lumbar vertebrae for a period is difficult and energy consuming for the athletic trainer.[3,29,44]

Having a split table will eliminate most of the friction between the patient's body segments and the treatment table and is essential for effective delivery of manual lumbar traction (Figure 14–9).[3,13,17,18,27] The clinician's effort does not cause separation of the vertebral segments unless the frictional forces are overcome first.

Level-Specific Manual Traction

To make the traction specific to a vertebral level, the patient is positioned sidelying on the split table. For traction specific to L3–4, L4–5, and L5–S1 levels, the patient's lumbar spine is flexed, using the patient's upper leg as a lever. The clinician palpates the interspinous area between two spinous processes. The upper spinous process is the one at which maximum effect is desired. When the lumbar spine flexes and the clinician feels the motion of the lower spinous process with the palpating hand, the foot is placed against the opposite leg so that further flexion is not allowed (Figure 14–10). The clinician rotates the patient's trunk until the trainer

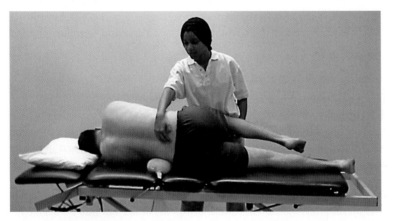

Figure 14–10. Positioning the patient for maximum effect at a specific level. The lumbar spine is flexed, using the patient's upper leg as a lever. The clinician palpates the interspinous area between two spinous processes. The upper spinous process is the one at which maximum effect is desired. When the lumbar spine flexes and the clinician feels the motion of the lower spinous process with the palpating hand, the foot is placed against the opposite leg so that further flexion is not allowed.

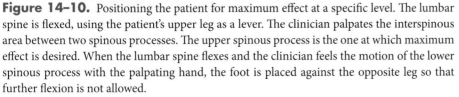

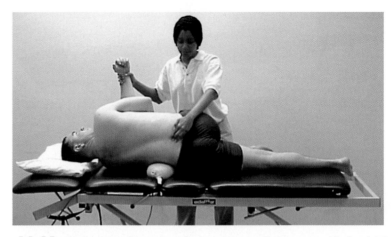

Figure 14–11. Positioning the patient for maximum effect at a specific level. The clinician rotates the patient's trunk until she or he feels motion of the upper spinous process. The clinician should passively produce trunk rotation by positioning the patient's upper arm with hand on the rib cage and pulling on the patient's lower arm, creating trunk rotation toward the upper arm. In this case it is rotation to the left.

feels motion of the upper spinous process. Trunk rotation should be passively produced by the athletic trainer, positioning the patient's upper arm with hand on the rib cage, and pulling on the patient's lower arm, creating trunk rotation toward the upper arm. In this case it is rotation to the left (Figure 14–11).

If lumbar levels T12, L1, L1–2, and L2–3 are to be given specific traction, the patient is again positioned sidelying. These levels require positioning in reverse order from the lower levels. First the trunk is rotated; then the lumbar spine is flexed.[3,18]

In both instances the rotation and flexion tighten and lock joint structures in which these motions have taken place, leaving the desired segment with more movement available than the upper or lower levels. When traction is applied, greater movement of the desired level occurs, whereas movement at other levels is minimized because of the joint locking created by the preliminary positioning.

The split table is then released and the clinician palpates the spinous processes of the selected intervertebral level, places his or her chest against the anterior superior iliac spine of the patient's upper hip, and leans toward the patient's feet. Enough force is used to cause a palpable separation of the spinous processes (Figure 14–12). Intermittent movement is most easily accomplished, whereas sustained traction becomes physically more difficult.[3,18]

Unilateral Leg Pull Manual Traction

Unilateral leg pull traction has been used in the treatment of hip joint problems or difficult lateral shift corrections. A thoracic countertraction harness is used to secure the patient to the table. The clinician grabs the patient's ankle and brings the patient's hip into 30-degree flexion, 30-degree abduction, and full external rotation. A steady pull is applied until a noticeable distraction is felt (Figure 14–13).[18]

In suspected sacroiliac joint problems, a similar setup can be used. A banana strap is placed through the groin on the side to be stretched. This strap will secure the patient in position. The clinician grabs the patient's ankle, brings his or her hip into 30-degree flexion and 15-degree abduction, and then applies a sustained or intermittent pull to create a mobilizing effect on the sacroiliac joint (Figure 14–14).[18]

As a preliminary to mechanical traction, manual traction is helpful in determining what degree of lumbar flexion, extension, or sidebending is most comfortable and will also give an indication of the treatment's success. The most comfortable position is usually the best therapeutic position.[12,18,29]

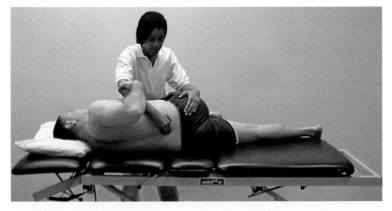

Figure 14–12. Manual lumbar traction with maximum effect at a specific level. The clinician has positioned the patient for maximum effect and is palpating the interspinous area between the two spinous processes where maximum traction effect is desired. The clinician then places his or her chest against the anterior superior iliac spine and the patient's upper hip. The split table is released and the clinician leans toward the patient's feet, using enough force to cause a palpable separation of the spinous processes at the desired level.

Patient comfort may have a bigger impact on the traction's results than the angle of pull, the force used, the mode, or the duration of the treatment. The inability of the patient to relax in any traction setup affects the traction's ability to cause a separation of the vertebrae. The lack of vertebral separation minimizes some of the traction's therapeutic benefits.[12,18,29]

Clinical Decision-Making   *Exercise 14-2*

A patient has been diagnosed with a prolapsed disk at L4, which is impinging the nerve root on the left side. What specific positional traction technique should the clinician recommend to make the patient most comfortable at home?

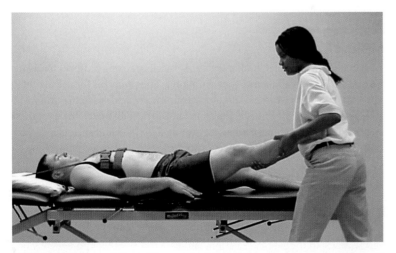

Figure 14–13. Unilateral leg pull traction. With the patient secured to the table with a thoracic countertraction harness, the clinician brings the patient's hip into 30-degree flexion, 30-degree abduction, and maximum external rotation. A steady pull is then applied.

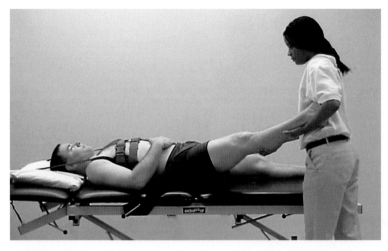

Figure 14–14. Unilateral leg pull traction for sacroiliac joint problems. A strap is placed through the groin and secured to the table. The clinicianbrings the patient's hip into 30-degree flexion and 15-degree abduction, and then applies a traction force to the leg.

Clinical Decision-Making *Exercise 14–3*

A gymnast asks the clinician if it is OK to hang upside down by her knees from the uneven parallel bars because this seems to help her stretch her low back. Should she take any precautions?

Mechanical Lumbar Traction

When using mechanical traction, the clinician will have to select and adjust the following seven parameters of the traction equipment and patient position. Traction will return disk nucleus to a central position.

1. Body position: prone, supine, hip position, bilateral, or unilateral direction of pull
2. Force used
3. Intermittent traction: traction time and rest time
4. Sustained traction
5. Duration of treatment
6. Progressive steps
7. Regressive steps

The research on mechanical lumbar traction gives us a strong protocol for using traction to decrease disk protrusion and nerve root symptoms. The protocols for use in other pathologies are not supported by research, but clinical empiricism and inference from some of the research give a good working protocol. The clinician will need to match the traction treatment to the patient's symptoms and make adjustments based on the clinical results.[9,18,21,29,45]

Traction can relieve pressure on a nerve root.

Patient Setup and Equipment

A split table or other mechanism to eliminate friction between body segments and the table surface is a prerequisite to effective lumbar traction. Otherwise, most of the force applied would be spent overcoming the coefficient of friction (see Figure 14–9).[3,4,13,15,17,18,27,45]

A nonslip traction harness is needed to transfer the traction force comfortably to the patient and to stabilize the trunk while the lumbar spine is placed under traction. A harness lined with a vinyl material is best because it adheres to the patient's skin and does not slip like the cotton-lined harness. Clothing between the harness and the skin will also promote

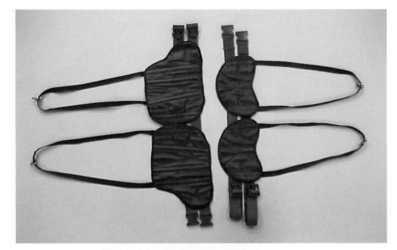

Figure 14–15. Vinyl-backed traction harness.

slipping. The vinyl-sided harness does not have to be as constricting as the cotton-backed harness to prevent slippage, thus increasing the patient's comfort (Figure 14–15).[13,18,27]

The harness can be applied when the patient is standing next to the traction table prior to treatment. The pelvic harness is applied so the contact pads and upper belt are at or just above the level of the iliac crest (Figure 14–16). Shirts should never be tucked under the pelvic harness because some of the tractive force would be dissipated pulling on the shirt material. The contact pads should be adjusted so that the harness loops provide a posteriorly directed pull, encouraging lumbar flexion (Figure 14–17). The harness firmly adheres to the patient's hips.[13,18,27] The rib belt is then applied in a similar manner with the rib pads positioned over the lower rib cage in a comfortable manner. The rib belt is then snugged up and the patient is positioned on the table (Figure 14–18).[13,18,27]

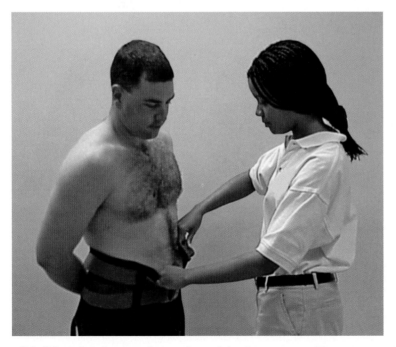

Figure 14–16. Pelvic harness for mechanical lumbar traction. The contact pads are applied so that the upper belt is at or just above the level of the iliac crest.

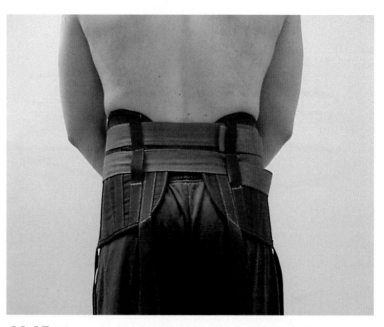

Figure 14–17. The traction straps from the pelvic harness should bracket the patient's buttocks if a lumbar flexion pull is desired. If a straight pull is desired, the pelvic harness should be adjusted so that the straps bracket the patient's lateral hip area.

The standing application of the traction harness is easier and more effective if the patient is to be placed in prone position for treatment (Figure 14–19).[13,18,27] The traction harness can also be applied by laying it out on the traction table and having the patient lie down on top of it. The pads are then adjusted and the belts snugged with the patient lying down.

Body Position

Body position has been reported to have a substantial impact on traction results, but this has been empirically derived rather than research supported. The clinician needs a satisfactory

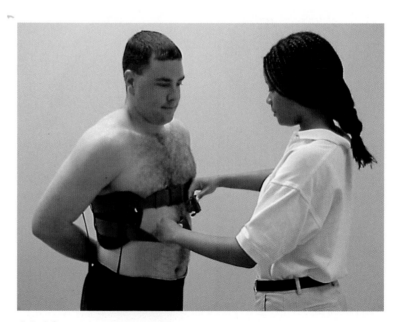

Figure 14–18. Thoracic countertraction harness. Rib pads are positioned over the lower rib cage.

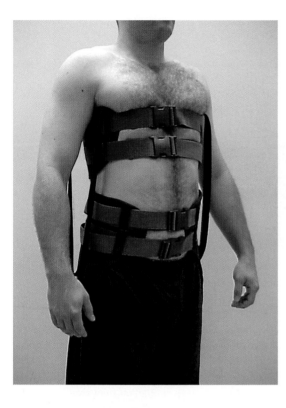

Figure 14–19. Applying the pelvic and thoracic harnesses may be easier if done while the patient is standing.

understanding of the mechanics of the lumbar spine to make decisions about a position that will best affect a patient's symptoms.[3,11,13,18,20,27,45]

Generally, the neutral spinal position allows for the largest intervertebral foramen opening, and it is usually the position of choice whether the patient is prone or supine. Extension beyond neutral lumbar spine causes the bony elements of the foramen to create a narrower opening. Lumbar spinal flexion beyond neutral causes the ligamentum flavum and other soft tissues to constrict the foramen's opening (Figure 14–20).[12,29]

Saunders recommends the prone position with a normal to slightly flattened lumbar lordosis (an abnormal anterior curve) as the position of choice in disk protrusions.[13,27] The amount of lordosis may be controlled by using pillows under the abdomen. The prone position also allows the easy application of other modalities to the pain area and an easier assessment of the amount of spinous process separation (Figure 14–21).[13,18,27]

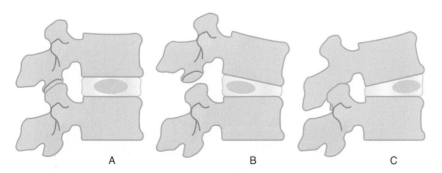

A   B   C

Figure 14–20. (a) Neutral lumbar spine position allows for the largest intervertebral foramen opening before traction is applied. (b) Flexion, while it may tend to increase the posterior opening, puts pressure on the disk nucleus to move posterior. Other soft tissue may also close the foramen opening. (c) Extension beyond neutral tends to close the foramen down as the bony arches come closer together.

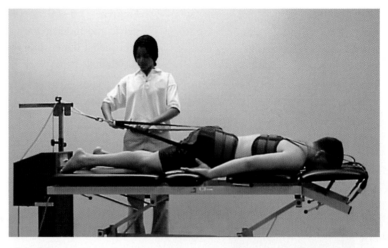

Figure 14–21. Mechanical lumbar traction: patient in the prone position with a pillow under the abdomen to help control lumbar spine extension.

In traction applied to a patient in the supine position, hip position was found to affect vertebral separation. As hip flexion increased from 0 to 90 degrees, traction produced a greater posterior intervertebral space separation (Figure 14–22).[34]

Unilateral pelvic traction also has been recommended when a stronger force is desired on one side of the spine. Patients with protective scoliosis, unilateral joint dysfunction, or unilateral lumbar muscle spasm with scoliosis may do quite well with this approach. Only one side of the pelvic harness is hooked to the traction device to accomplish this technique (Figure 14–23).[13]

In patients with protective scoliosis, when the patient leans away from the painful side, the traction should be applied on the painful side. When the patient leans toward the painful side, the traction should be applied on the nonpainful side (see Figure 14–6).

In patients with scoliosis caused by muscle spasm, the traction force should be applied from the side with the muscle spasm (Figure 14–24). In unilateral facet joint dysfunction, the traction should be applied from the side of most complaint.[12]

Overall, patient positioning for traction should be varied according to a patient's needs and comfort. Experimentation with positioning is encouraged so that the traction's effect on the patient will be maximized. Patient comfort is far more important than relative position in

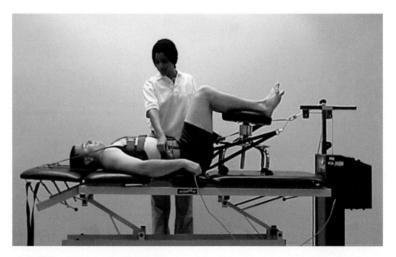

Figure 14–22. Mechanical lumbar traction: patient in the supine position with hips and knees flexed to approximately 90 degrees.

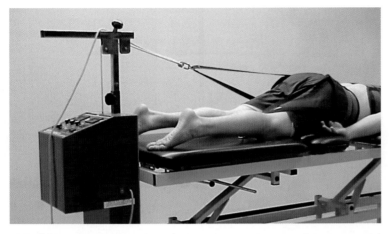

Figure 14–23. Mechanical lumbar traction with a unilateral pull: only one of the pelvic straps is hooked to the traction device.

making patient position decisions. If the patient cannot relax, the traction will not be successful in causing vertebral separation.[13,18,27]

Traction Force

Several researchers have indicated that no lumbar vertebral separation will occur with traction forces less than one quarter of the patient's body weight. The traction force necessary to cause effective vertebral separation will range between 65 and 200 pounds.[3,4,13,17,20,27,32] This force does not have to be used on the first treatment, and progressive steps both during and between treatments are often necessary to comfortably reach these therapeutic loads. A force equal to half the patient's body weight is a good guideline to use in selecting a force high enough to cause vertebral separation. These high weight levels pose no danger, as cadaver research indicates a force of 440 pounds or greater is necessary to cause damage to the lumbar spine components (Figure 14–25).[17,20]

Caution must be used when using traction of the lumbar spine because of a tendency for the nucleus pulposus gel to imbibe fluid from the vertebral body, thus increasing pressure within the disk. This happens in a very short period. When pressure is released and weight is applied to the disk, this excess fluid increases pressure on the annulus and exacerbates the patient's symptoms. Therefore, it is recommended that during an initial treatment with lumbar

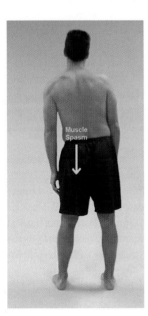

Figure 14–24. In a patient with scoliosis caused by muscle spasm (left), the unilateral traction force should be applied using only the left pelvic strap.

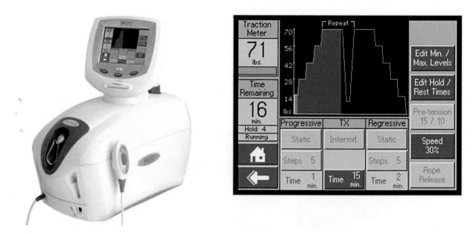

Figure 14–25. Traction device with enlarged screen showing treatment parametor options.

traction, a maximum of 30 pounds be used to determine whether traction will have a negative effect on the symptoms.[14]

The research has been aimed at forces necessary to cause vertebral separation. Traction certainly has effects that are not associated with vertebral separation, and if these effects are desired, less force may be necessary to get them.

Intermittent Versus Sustained Traction

Good results have been reported with both intermittent and sustained traction. In most cases of lumbar disk problems, sustained traction seems to be the treatment of choice. Partial reduction in disk protrusions was observed in 4 minutes of sustained traction.[10,17,20,27,30] Good results also were reported using intermittent traction in the treatment of ruptured intervertebral disk.[23]

Separation of the posterior intervertebral space was noted with a 10-second-hold intermittent traction.[46] Posterior intervertebral separations using 100 pounds of force were similar when intermittent and sustained traction modes were compared.[41] The electromyographic activity of the sacrospinalis musculature showed similar patterns when sustained and intermittent traction were compared.[23]

Traction can stretch paraspinal muscles.

Sustained traction is favored in treating intervertebral disk herniation because sustained traction allows more time with the disk uncompressed to cause the disk nuclear material to move centripetally and reduce the disk herniation's pressure on nerve structures. When used for this purpose, sustained traction may be superior to intermittent traction.[18,27,30]

In deciding on sustained versus intermittent traction, the clinician should follow the guidelines for treating diagnosed disk herniations with sustained traction, whereas most other traction-appropriate diagnoses may be treated with intermittent traction. Intermittent traction, in any case, is usually more comfortable when using higher forces, and increased comfort is one of the primary considerations because there is no conclusive evidence supporting the choice of one method over the other.[3,4,17,18,21,27,30,34]

The timing of the traction and rest phases of intermittent traction has not been researched. Short traction phases (less than 10 seconds) cause only minimal interspace separation but will activate joint and muscle receptors and create facet joint movements.[18,19] Longer traction phases (more than 10 seconds) tend to stretch the ligamentous and muscular tissues long enough to overcome their resistance to movement and create a longer-lasting mechanical separation. When using high-traction forces, the comfort of the patient may dictate the adjustment of the traction time. Also, a longer total treatment time is tolerated with intermittent traction.[14,17–20,27]

Rest phase times should be relatively short but should also be comfort oriented. The rest time should be adjusted to allow the patient to recover and feel relaxed before the next traction cycle. The clinician should monitor the traction patient frequently to adjust traction and rest time adjustments to maintain the patient in a relaxed comfortable state.

Duration of Treatment

The total treatment times of sustained traction and intermittent traction are only partially research based. With sustained traction, Mathews found reduction in disk protrusion after 4 minutes with further reduction at 20 minutes.[40] Complete reduction in protrusions was seen at 38 minutes. Other researchers found no difference in separation of the cervical spine when times of 7, 30, and 60 seconds were compared.[17,19,20]

When dealing with suspected disk protrusions, the total treatment time should be relatively short. As the disk space widens, the pressure inside the disk decreases and the disk nucleus moves centripetally. The projected time for pressure within a disk to equalize is 8–10 minutes. At this point the nuclear material is no longer moving centripetally. With longer time in this position, osmotic forces equalize the pressure within the disk with that of the surrounding tissue. When the pressure equalization occurs, the traction effect on the protrusion is lost. The intradisk pressure may increase when the traction is released if the traction stays on too long. This increased pressure results in increased symptoms. This situation has not been reported when treatment times are kept at 10 minutes or less.[13,27] If this reaction does occur, shorter treatment times or long-hold intermittent traction (60 seconds traction, 10–20 seconds rest) may be necessary to control the symptoms.

Some sources advocate traction times of up to 30 minutes.[17,18,20] The contradiction in philosophy may be because of pathology or the individual anatomy of each patient. However, an adverse reaction to traction (i.e., a dramatic increase in symptoms when the traction is released) is something the clinician should try to avoid.

Total treatment time for sustained traction when treating disk-related symptoms should start at less than 10 minutes. If the treatment is successful in reducing symptoms, the time should be left at 10 minutes or less. If the treatment is partially successful or unsuccessful in relieving symptoms, the clinician may increase the time gradually over several treatments to 30 minutes.

Progressive and Regressive Steps

Some traction equipment is built with progressive and regressive modes. The machine progressively increases the traction force in a preselected number of steps. A gradual increase in pressure lets the patient accommodate slowly to the traction and helps him or her to stay relaxed. A gradual progression of force also allows the clinician to release the split table after the slack in the system has been taken up by several progressions (Figure 14–26).[3,18,28]

Regressive steps do just the opposite and allow the patient to come down gradually from the high loads. Again, patient comfort is the primary consideration because no research supports any protocol (Figure 14–27).[3,18,28]

Some equipment has the capability to be programmed for progressive and regressive steps and also to have minimum traction forces, allowing a sustained force with intermittent peaks (Figure 14–28).[3,18,28] To achieve such traction setups with a machine that is not programmable, manual operation and timing are necessary.

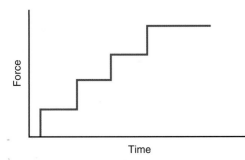

Figure 14–26. Progressive steps for lumbar traction of X pounds. Four steps are used: the first is 1/4 X pounds, the second 2/4 X, and so on. Each lasts for an equal time.

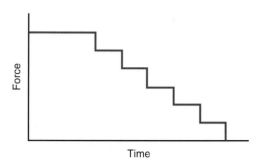

Figure 14–27. Regressive steps for lumbar traction of X pounds. Six equal regressive steps are used: the first drops the traction force from X to 5/6 X, the second to 4/6 X, and so on. Each lasts for an equal time.

Throughout the discussion on lumbar traction, patient comfort comes up again and again in regard to the parameters of the treatment setup. One of the primary keys to successful traction treatment is the relaxation of the patient. The use of appropriate modalities before and during the traction treatment adds to the total effectiveness of the treatment plan. Bracing or appropriate exercise after traction may also enhance the results and prolong the benefits gained. Better technology and more research will help refine the traction art and provide better results from this type of treatment.

CASE STUDY 14–1
MECHANICAL TRACTION

Background: A 49-year-old man developed lower cervical pain 4 days ago after trimming trees in his yard for several hours. He has been referred for symptomatic treatment of his mechanical neck pain; there are no neural deficits, and no signs of a disk lesion. The patient is experiencing pain in the midline of the lower cervical area, and across the upper trapezius area bilaterally. His active range of motion is normal, but is painful at the end of range in all planes, and overpressure increases the symptoms. Extension (back bending) is the most painful motion.

Impression: Soft-tissue injury of the lower cervical spine.

Treatment Plan: To assist in pain relief, a 3-day per week course of intermittent mechanical cervical traction was initiated. The patient was positioned supine on the traction table, and the traction unit was adjusted to produce approximately 20 degrees of cervical flexion during traction. For the initial session, 20 pounds of traction was applied, with four progressive steps up, and four regressive steps down. Each traction cycle consisted of 15 seconds of tension, followed by 20 seconds of rest. Total treatment time was 20 minutes. The target traction force was increased by 10% each session, to a maximum of 40 pounds. In addition to the traction, active exercise was prescribed.

Response: The patient reported a transient increase in symptoms following the first two sessions, then a gradual resolution of the symptoms. There was a marked reduction in symptoms immediately following the third session; the relief persisted for approximately 2 hours. Cervical traction was discontinued after a total of six sessions, and the patient was instructed in a home exercise program. Two weeks later, the patient was asymptomatic.

Discussion Questions

- What tissues were injured/affected?
- What symptoms were present?
- What phase of the injury-healing continuum did the patient present for care in?
- What are the physical agent modality's biophysical effects (direct/indirect/depth/tissue affinity)?
- What are the physical agent modality's indications/contraindications?
- What are the parameters of the physical agent modality's application/dosage/duration/frequency in this case study?
- What other physical agent modalities could be utilized to treat this injury or condition? Why? How?
- What was the mechanism of injury to the cervical spine?
- What were the physiological effects of the cervical traction?
- Why was the supine position used for the treatment?
- What additional physical agents may have been helpful for this patient?
- What are the contraindications to cervical traction?
- Why were the symptoms initially increased?

The rehabilitation professional employs physical agent modalities to create an optimum environment for tissue healing while minimizing the symptoms associated with the trauma or condition.

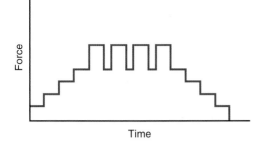

Figure 14–28. Progressive and regressive steps with a minimum sustained traction force.

Manual Cervical Traction

The objectives for using traction in the cervical region do not vary much from the objectives for using traction in the lumbar region.[47] Reasonable objectives for cervical traction include stretch of the muscles and joint structures of the vertebral column, enlargement of the intervertebral spaces and foramina, centripetally directed forces on the disk and soft tissue around the disk, mobilization of vertebral joints, increases and changes in joint proprioception, relief of compressive effects of normal posture, and improvement in arterial venous and lymphatic flow.[14,17,18,29,33,47–52] In the clinical setting, diagnoses and symptoms requiring traction are found infrequently.[10] These diagnoses are more typically found in older populations.

In most cases involving sprains and strains, simple manual traction used to produce a rhythmic longitudinal movement will be very successful in helping decrease pain, muscle spasm, stiffness, and inflammation, and also in reducing joint compressive forces. Manual traction is infinitely more adaptable than mechanical traction, and changes in the direction, force, duration of the traction, and patient position can be made instantaneously as the clinician senses relaxation or resistance.[3,4,18–20,48]

The clinician supports the patient's head and neck. The hand should cradle the neck and provide adequate grip for the effective transfer of the traction force to the mastoid processes. One hand should be placed under the patient's neck with the thenar eminence (base of the thumb) in contact with one mastoid process and the fingers cradling the neck reaching across toward the other mastoid process (Figure 14–29a).[3]

The clinician then provides a gentle (less than 20-pound) pull in a cephalic direction. Intervertebral separation is not desired because of the damage to the ligaments or capsule. A head halter or similar harness may also be used to deliver the force (Figure 14–29b).

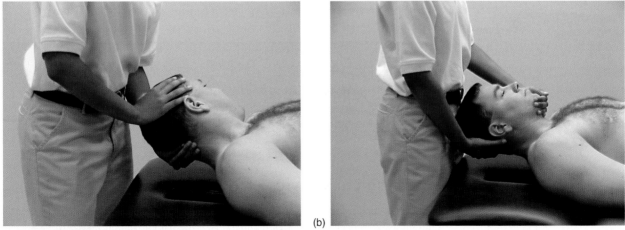

(a)　　　　　　　　　　　　　　　　　　　(b)

Figure 14–29. Manual cervical traction: (a) patient in the supine position with the clinician's fingertips and thenar eminence contacting the mastoid process of the patient's skull. (b) Traction is applied with both hands.

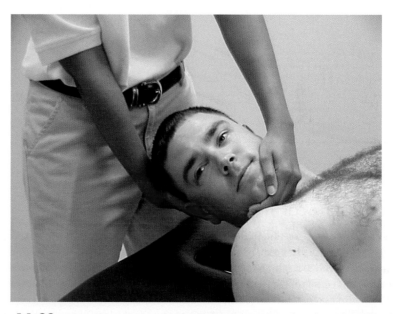

Figure 14–30. Manual cervical traction: patient is positioned with neck in flexion and with some neck rotation to the right. Laterally flexed positions may also be used.

The force should be intermittent, with the traction time between 3 and 10 seconds. The rest time may be very brief, but the traction force should be released almost completely. The total treatment time should be between 3 and 10 minutes.[3,4,18,19]

When pain is limiting or affecting movement, a bout of traction should be followed by a reassessment of the painful motion to determine increases or decreases in pain or motion. Successive bouts of traction can be used as long as the symptoms are improving. When the symptoms stabilize or are worse on the reassessment, the traction should be discontinued.[18]

A variety of head and neck positions can be used in cervical traction. Different head and neck positions will place some vertebral structures under more tension than others. Good knowledge of cervical kinesiology and biomechanics, and good knowledge and skill in joint mobilization, are required before the clinician should experiment with extensive position changes (Figure 14–30).[3,18,19]

At the completion of the traction treatment, in cases of strain or sprain, protection of the neck with a soft collar is often desirable to prevent extremes of motion, minimize compressive forces, and encourage muscle relaxation. Instructions in sleeping positions and regular support postures are also important in caring for patients with cervical problems.[3,18]

Clinical Decision-Making   Exercise 14–4

The clinician has decided to treat a patient with signs and symptoms of a disk protrusion using mechanical traction. What treatment parameters will likely be most effective in treating this problem?

Mechanical Cervical Traction

The literature does provide a relatively clear protocol to use in trying to achieve vertebral separation using a mechanical traction apparatus.[53] The patient should be supine or long-sitting with the neck flexed between 20 and 30 degrees (Figure 14–31). A sitting posture can be used, but this is clinically more cumbersome and is not supported by the research as an optimal position of cervical traction.[13,18,27]

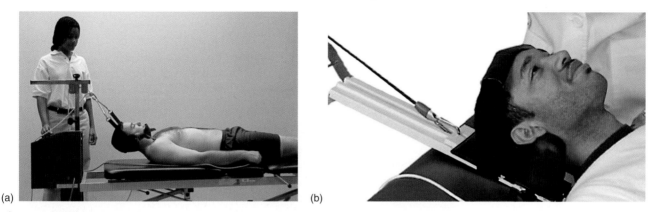

(a)   (b)

Figure 14–31. Mechanical cervical traction: (a) patient in the supine position with traction harness placed so that maximum pull is exerted on the occiput and the athlete is in a position of approximately 20 to 30 degrees of neck flexion. (b) Tru-Trac cervical traction unit.

The traction harness must be arranged comfortably so that the majority of pull is placed on the occiput rather than the chin. Some cervical traction harnesses do not have a chinpiece. These harnesses may have an advantage, provided that the traction force is effectively transferred to the structures of the cervical spine.[14,19]

A traction force above 20 pounds, applied intermittently for a minimum of 7 seconds' traction time and with adequate rest time for recovery is recommended. This traction should be continued over 20 to –25 minutes. Higher forces up to 50 pounds may produce increased separation, but the other parameters should remain the same. The average separation at the posterior vertebral area is 1–1.5 mm per space, whereas the anterior vertebral area separates approximately 0.4 mm per space. Greater separations are expected in the younger population than in the older population. Within 20–25 minutes from the time traction is stopped and normal sitting or standing postures are resumed, the vertebral separation returns to its previous heights. The upper cervical segments do not separate as easily as lower cervical segments.[14,19,20,54] The addition of pain-reducing and heating modalities will add to the benefits gained by the traction.[3,4,14,18,20,55]

Clinical Decision-Making   *Exercise 14–5*

In treating a patient who is complaining of cervical neck pain, the clinician is trying to decide whether to use a manual cervical traction technique or mechanical traction. Which would you recommend?

TREATMENT PROTOCOLS: TRACTION

1. Apply and adjust appropriate halters, harnesses, and belts for indicated traction treatment.
   a. Cervical: Apply head halter beneath the occiput and mandible; attach to spreader bar.
   b. Lumbar: Attach pelvic harness snugly about the waist, beginning just above the iliac crests, thoracic rib belt snugly about the lower rib cage.
2. Attach traction apparatus to unit: Take up and adjust for slack in the line.

3. Position patient for indicated traction treatment.
   a. Cervical: Supine lying with neck flexed 20–30 degrees.
   b. Lumbar: Supine hooklying with hips flexed and legs supported by pillows or stools.
   c. Lumbar: Prone lying in neutral.
4. Apply indicated traction poundage.
   a. Cervical: Adjust traction poundage beginning with 20 pounds or as tolerated by the patient (range 20–50 pounds).
   b. Lumbar: Adjust traction poundage beginning with 65 pounds or as tolerated by the patient (range 65–200 pounds).
5. Adjust traction duty cycle and treatment duration.
   a. Sustained: Less than 10 minutes.
   b. Intermittent: 3–10 seconds, on–off for 20–30 minutes.

CASE STUDY 14–2
SPINAL TRACTION: LUMBAR

Background: A 58-year-old pharmacist has an 11-year history of recurrent low back pain. The onset was insidious, and he has developed episodes of moderately severe low back pain three or four times per year since the initial episode. This episode started 9 days ago after playing 18 holes of golf and is the most severe episode ever. He has constant pain in the right lumbosacral area, with radiation of the pain into the right buttock, and down the posteriolateral aspect of the thigh and leg into the foot, with paresthesia in the lateral foot. He demonstrates weakness in the S1 myotome, a loss of the right ankle jerk, and positive tests for adverse neural tension on the right. He was referred to a neurosurgeon, who obtained an MRI. The MRI revealed a moderately large right posteriolateral bulge of the intervertebral disk at L5S1, with a loss of disk height. The neurosurgeon recommended surgery, but the patient opted for a trial of conservative treatment. The patient was referred for lumbar traction and therapeutic exercise.

Impression: S1 nerve root compression due to L5S1 disk lesion.

Treatment Plan: Motorized static lumbar traction with the patient prone on the traction table was initiated. For the initial treatment session, the traction device was set to apply 14 kilograms (31 pounds) of distractive force, which was equal to one sixth of the patient's body weight. The force was increased in three steps over a 3-minute period, then the force was maintained at 14 kilograms for 4 minutes, then removed in two steps over a 2-minute period. Because this initial session did not exacerbate the patient's symptoms, therapeutic traction was administered on a daily basis starting the next day, with a distraction force of 41 kilograms (90 pounds), or one-half of the patient's body weight. The traction increased to the therapeutic dose in three steps over a 3-minute period, the maximal force was maintained for 10 minutes, then decreased to 0 in two steps over a 2-minute period. The patient then performed therapeutic exercise to maintain a lordosis of the lumbar spine before getting off the table.

Response: Following each treatment session, the patient noted diminished peripheral and central symptoms for approximately 1 hour. There was no sustained improvement after 10 sessions, and the patient elected to return to the neurosurgeon for surgical treatment.

Discussion Questions

- What tissues were injured or affected?
- What symptoms were present?
- What phase of the injury-healing continuum did the patient present for care in?
- What are the physical agent modality's biophysical effects (direct, indirect, depth, and tissue affinity)?
- What are the physical agent modality's indications and contraindications?
- What are the parameters of the physical agent modality's application, dosage, duration, and frequency in this case study?
- What other physical agent modalities could be used to treat this injury or condition? Why? How?

(continued)

CASE STUDY 14–2 (continued)
SPINAL TRACTION: LUMBAR

- Why was the initial treatment applied with such a low force? If the patient had noted an increase in the symptoms following this initial session, how would the therapist have proceeded?
- How much force is needed to achieve distraction of the vertebrae? How much is required to damage the vertebral motion segment?
- Why was the therapeutic distraction force applied for only 10 minutes? What are the advantages and disadvantages of a shorter session? A longer session?

- What is the most likely reason the traction was not successful in this patient? Would the treatment have been more or less likely to be successful if it had been initiated immediately after the onset of the symptoms?

The rehabilitation professional employs physical agent modalities to create an optimum environment for tissue healing while minimizing the symptoms associated with the trauma or condition.

CASE STUDY 14–3
SPINAL TRACTION: CERVICAL

Background: A 47-year-old woman noted an ache in the right midcervical area upon awakening this morning. While driving to work, she turned her head to the right before changing lanes, and noted an audible click with severe pain in the right midcervical area. After arriving at work, she continued to experience localized pain that gradually worsened over the next hour. She presented to the emergency room, where an examination (including radiographic) revealed no neurologic or bony injury. She was referred for treatment of an acute neck sprain. She does not have radiating pain, and the neurologic examination is negative. She holds her head tilted and rotated to the left, and any attempt at side bend or rotation to the right produces severe, localized right midcervical pain. She is very tender over the right articular pillar at C4–5, and passive mobility testing reveals a markedly restricted joint play at C4–5.

Impression: Acute locking of the cervical spine (C4–5).

Treatment Plan: Manual cervical traction. With the patient supine on a treatment table, the therapist placed one hand under the patient's head, with the palm over the occiput, thumb over one mastoid process, and the fingertips over the opposite mastoid process. The therapist's other hand was placed over the patient's forehead to avoid compressive forces on the temporomandibular joint. A gentle distraction force was applied (approximately 5 kilograms), with the line of force parallel to the long axis of the spine. The force was held for 3 seconds, then released for 10 seconds. This was repeated 10 times, with the distraction force gradually increased to a maximum of approximately 15 kilograms.

Response: A reassessment was performed after the 10th force application, and the patient was able to hold her neck in a neutral position. The cycle was repeated four more times, with a gradual improvement in cervical range of motion and a reduction in pain each time. After the fifth cycle, she was able to attain rotation and side bending to the right equal to approximately 80% that of the motion to the left. She was treated the following day with the same approach, and attained full, pain-free range of motion.

Discussion Questions

- What tissues were injured or affected?
- What symptoms were present?
- What phase of the injury-healing continuum did the patient present for care in?
- What are the physical agent modality's biophysical effects (direct, indirect, depth, and tissue affinity)?
- What are the physical agent modality's indications and contraindications?
- What are the parameters of the physical agent modality's application, dosage, duration, and frequency in this case study?
- What other physical agent modalities could be used to treat this injury or condition? Why? How?
- What is the mechanism for acute locking of the cervical spine?
- What are the advantages of manual traction over mechanical (motorized) traction for this patient? Disadvantages?

(continued)

CASE STUDY 14–3 (continued)
SPINAL TRACTION: CERVICAL

- Why was the distraction force applied parallel to the long axis of the spine? What advantages or disadvantages would there be to applying the force along an oblique axis?

The rehabilitation professional employs physical agent modalities to create an optimum environment for tissue healing while minimizing the symptoms associated with the trauma or condition.

Table 14–1 Indications and Contraindications for Spinal Traction
INDICATIONS
Impingement on a nerve root
Disk herniation
Spondylolisthesis
Narrowing within the intervertebral foramen
Osteophyte formation
Degenerative joint diseases
Subacute pain
Joint hypomobility
Discogenic pain
Muscle spasm or guarding
Muscle strain
Spinal ligament or connective tissues contractures
Improvement in arterial, venous, and lymphatic flow
CONTRAINDICATIONS
Acute sprains or strains
Acute inflammation
Fractures
Vertebral joint instability
Any condition in which movement exacerbates the existing problem
Tumors
Bone diseases
Osteoporosis
Infections in bones or joints
Vascular conditions
Pregnancy
Cardiac or pulmonary problems

INDICATIONS AND CONTRAINDICATIONS

As discussed throughout this chapter, spinal traction may be useful for a number of conditions, including cases where there is impingement on a nerve root resulting from disk herniation, spondylolisthesis, narrowing within the intervertebral foramen, or osteophyte formation; degenerative joint diseases; subacute pain; joint hypomobility; discogenic pain; and muscle spasm. Table 14–1 lists indications and contraindications.

Traction, except as a light mobilization, is contraindicated in acute sprains or strains (first 3–5 days), acute inflammation, or any conditions in which movement is either undesirable or exacerbates the existing problem. In cases of vertebral joint instability, traction may perpetuate the instability or cause further strain. Certainly, the serious problems associated with tumors, bone diseases, osteoporosis, and infections in bones or joints are also contraindications. Patients who can potentially experience problems relating to the fitting of a harness, such as those with vascular conditions, pregnant females, or those with cardiac or pulmonary problems, should also avoid traction.

SUMMARY

1. Traction has been used to treat a variety of cervical and lumbar spine problems.
2. The effect of traction on each system involved in the complex anatomic makeup of the spine needs to be considered when selecting traction as a part of a therapeutic treatment plan.
3. The traction protocol should be set up to manage a particular problem rather than applied in the same manner regardless of the patient or pathology.
4. Traction is a flexible modality with an infinite number of variations available. This flexibility allows the clinician to adjust protocols to match the patient's symptoms and diagnosis.
5. Traction is capable of producing a separation of vertebral bodies; a centripetal force on the soft tissues surrounding the vertebrae; a mobilization of vertebral joints; a change in proprioceptive discharge of the spinal complex; a stretch of connective tissue; a stretch of muscle tissue; an improvement in arterial, venous, and lymphatic flow; and a lessening of the compressive effects of posture. Any of these effects can change the symptoms of the patient under treatment and help to normalize the patient's lumbar or cervical spine.
6. Traction techniques in the lumbar region include positional traction; inversion traction; manual traction, which may be done using either level-specific or unilateral leg pull techniques; and mechanical traction.
7. Cervical traction is used less frequently than lumbar traction. Cervical traction techniques include manual traction and mechanical traction.

REVIEW QUESTIONS

1. What is traction and how may it be performed by the clinician?
2. What are the physical effects and therapeutic value of spinal traction on bone, muscle, ligaments, facet joints, nerves, blood vessels, and intervertebral disks?
3. What are the clinical advantages of using positional lumbar traction and inversion traction?
4. What are the clinical applications for using manual lumbar traction techniques, including level-specific manual traction, and unilateral leg pull manual traction?
5. What are the setup procedures and treatment parameter considerations for using mechanical lumbar traction?

6. What are the advantages of using a manual traction technique of the cervical spine?
7. What is the setup procedure for mechanical and wall-mounted traction techniques for the cervical spine?

SELF-TEST QUESTIONS

True or False

1. The goal of traction is to encourage movement of the spine and decrease the patient's symptoms.
2. Ligament deformation due to traction should occur during slow loading.
3. Traction may only be applied with a machine.

Multiple Choice

4. Traction may help reduce disk herniation. In this condition the _____ protrudes.
   a. annulus fibrosus
   b. nucleus pulposus
   c. disk material
   d. synovial fringe
5. Traction has effects on
   a. articular facet joints
   b. paraspinal muscles
   c. nerve roots
   d. all of the above
6. What is the most common problem traction is used to treat?
   a. spondylolisthesis
   b. fibrosis
   c. nerve root impingement
   d. none of the above
7. Which of the following is NOT a contraindication to traction?
   a. muscle strain
   b. acute inflammation
   c. fractures
   d. vertebral joint instability
8. How long should intermittent manual cervical traction be applied?
   a. less than 30 seconds
   b. 1–2 minutes
   c. 3–10 minutes
   d. 10–15 minutes
9. If traction treatments are resulting in no change in symptoms or a worsening of symptoms. The treatments should be
   a. done more often
   b. continued 1 more week
   c. performed in a different position
   d. discontinued
10. What is the appropriate range of force to be used on a patient while performing mechanical lumbar traction?
    a. 0–50 pounds
    b. 65–200 pounds
    c. 200–300 pounds
    d. as great as the athlete can tolerate

SOLUTIONS TO CLINICAL DECISION-MAKING EXERCISES

14–1

The clinician should have the patient lie on the treatment table on her right side with the left side up, supported with a pillow under the right hip. This position and traction technique should help immediately.

14–2

The patient should lie on the right side with a towel rolled up and placed under the right side as near to the appropriate segment as possible creating side bending to the right. The knees should be flexed until the spine is bent forward. Finally, the trunk should rotate to the left.

14–3

The clinician should check to make sure that the gymnast does not have a history of hypertension. Then, an inversion tolerance test should be used to make certain that there is not a significant increase in diastolic blood pressure and that there is no dizziness or vertigo or nausea from being in this position.

14–4

It is recommended that the clinician begin treatments by using sustained traction for a short treatment time of less than 10 minutes at a traction force that would be slightly more than one quarter of that patient's body weight. Treatment time and traction force may be increased as tolerated. If sustained traction exacerbates symptoms, intermittent traction may be used for about 15 minutes initially.

14–5

Manual traction is considerably more adaptable than mechanical traction, and changes in the direction, force, duration of the traction, and patient position can be made instantaneously as the clinician senses relaxation or resistance on the part of the patient.

REFERENCES

1. *Dorland's Illustrated Medical Dictionary.* Philadelphia, PA: WB Saunders; 2007.

2. Paris S. *Course Notes, Basic Course in Spinal Mobilization.* Atlanta, GA; 1977.

3. Burkhardt S. *Course Notes, Cervical and Lumbar Traction Seminar.* Morgantown, WV; 1983.

4. Bridger, R. Effect of lumbar traction on stature. *Spine.* 1990;15:522–524.

5. Gianakopoulos G. Inversion devices: their role in producing lumbar distraction. *Arch Phys Med Rehabil.* 1985;68:100–102.

6. O'Donoghue D. *Treatment of Injuries to Athletes.* Philadelphia, PA: WB Saunders; 1984.

7. Krause M, Refshauge KM, Dessen M, Boland R. Lumbar spine traction: evaluation of effects and recommended application for treatment. *Man Ther.* 2000;5(2):72–81.

8. KeKosz U. Cervical and lumbopelvic traction. *Postgrad Med.* 1986;80(8):187–194.

9. Onel D. Computed tomographic investigation of the effects of traction on lumbar disc herniations. *Spine.* 1989;14: 82–90.

10. Peake N. The effectiveness of cervical traction. *Phys Ther Rev.* 2005;10(4):217–229.

11. Petulla L. Clinical observations with respect to progressive/regressive traction. *J Orthop Sports Phys Ther.* 1986;7: 261–263.

12. Saunders HD. The controversy over traction for neck and low back pain. *Physiotherapy.* 1998;84(6):285–288.

13. Sood N. Prone cervical traction. *Clin Manage Phys Ther.* 1987;7(6):37–42.

14. Harris P. Cervical traction: review of the literature and treatment guidelines. *Phys Ther.* 1977;57:910–914.

15. Kent B. Anatomy of the trunk: part I. *Phys Ther.* 1974;54: 722–744.

16. Kent B. Anatomy of the trunk: part II. *Phys Ther.* 1974;54: 850–859.

17. Mathews J. Dynamic discography: a study of lumbar traction. *Ann Phys Med.* 1968;9:275–279.

18. Erhard R. *Course Notes, Cervical and Lumbar Traction Seminar.* Morgantown, WV; 1983.

19. Grieve G. Neck traction. *Physiotherapy.* 1982;6:260–265.

20. Mathews J. The effects of spinal traction. *Physiotherapy*. 1972;58:64–66.

21. Hood L, Chrisman D. Intermittent pelvic traction in the treatment of the ruptured intervertebral disk. *Phys Ther*. 1968;48:21–30.

22. Oakley P. A history of spine traction. *J Vertebr Subluxation Res*. 2006;2(1):1–12.

23. Hood C. Comparison of EMG activity in normal lumbar sacrospinalis musculature during continuous and intermittent pelvic traction. *J Orthop Sports Phys Ther*. 1981;2:137–141.

24. Jett D. Effect of intermittent, supine cervical traction on the myoelectric activity of the upper trapezius muscle in subjects with neck pain. *Phys Ther*. 1985;65:1173–1176.

25. Letchuman R, Deusinger R. Comparsion of sacrospinalis myoelectric activity and pain levels in patients undergoing static and intermittent lumbar traction. *Spine*. 1993;18:1261–1365.

26. Murphy M. Effects of cervical traction on muscle activity. *Orthop Sports Phys Ther*. 1991;13:220–225.

27. Saunders D. Use of spinal traction in the treatment of neck and back conditions. *Clin Orthop*. 1983;179:31–38.

28. Reilly J. Pelvic femoral position on vertebral separation produced by lumbar traction. *Phys Ther*. 1979;59:282–286.

29. Saunders D. Unilateral lumbar traction. *Phys Ther*. 1981;61:221–225.

30. Stoddard A. Traction for cervical nerve root irritation. *Physiotherapy*. 1954;40:48–49.

31. Fritz J, Lindsay W, Matheson J. Is There a Subgroup of Patients With Low Back Pain Likely to Benefit From Mechanical Traction? Results of a Randomized Clinical Trial and Subgrouping Analysis. *Spine*. 2007;32(26):793–800.

32. Meszaros TF, Olson R, Kulig K. Effect of 10%, 30%, and 60% body weight traction on the straight leg raise test of symptomatic patients with low back pain. *J Orthop Sports Phys Ther*. 2000;30(10):595–601.

33. Strapp EJ. Lumbar traction: suggestions for treatment parameters. *Sports Med Update*. 1998;13(4):9–11.

34. Roaf R. A study of the mechanics of spinal injuries. *J Bone Joint Surg*. 1960;42B:810–819.

35. Draper D. Inversion table traction as a therapeutic modality. Part 2: application. *Athletic Ther Today*. 2005;10(4):40–42.

36. Draper D. Inversion table traction as a therapeutic modality. Part 1: oh my aching back. *Athletic Ther Today*. 2005;10(3):42.

37. Houlding M. Clinical perspective. Inversion traction: a clinical appraisal. *NZ J Physiother*. 1998;26(2):23–24.

38. Klatz R. Effects of gravity inversion on hypertensive subjects. *Phys Sports Med*. 1985;13(3):85–89.

39. Goldman R. The effects of oscillating inversion on systemic blood pressure pulse, intraocular pressure and central retinal arterial pressure. *Phys Sports Med*. 1985;13(3):93–96.

40. LaBan M. Intermittent traction: a progenitor of lumbar radicular pain. *Arch Phys Med Rehabil*. 1992;73:295–296.

41. LeMarr J. Cardiorespiratory responses to inversion. *Phys Sports Med*. 1983;11(11):51–57.

42. Cooperman J, Scheid D. Guidelines for the use of inversion. *Clin Manage*. 1984;4(1):6–10.

43. Gudenhoven R. Gravitational lumbar traction. *Arch Phys Med Rehabil*. 1978;59:510–512.

44. Saunders D. Lumbar traction. *J Orthop Sports Phys Ther*. 1979;1:36–45.

45. Varma S. The role of traction in cervical spondylosis. *Physiotherapy*. 1973;59:248–249.

46. Nosse L. Inverted spinal traction. *Arch Phys Med Rehabil*. 1978;59:367–370.

47. Porter R, Miller C. Back pain and trunk list. *Spine*. 1986;11:596–600.

48. Browder D, Erhard R, Piva, S. Intermittent cervical traction and thoracic manipulation for management of mild cervical compressive myelopathy attributed to cervical herniated disc: a case series. *J Orthop Sports Phys Ther*. 2004;34(11):701–712.

49. Katavich L. Neural mechanisms underlying manual cervical traction. *J Man Manipulative Therapy*. 1999;7(1):20–25.

50. Taskaynatan M. Cervical traction in conservative management of thoracic outlet syndrome. *J Musculoskelet Pain*. 2007;15(1):89–94.

51. Walker G. Goodley polyaxial cervical traction: a new approach to a traditional treatment. *Phys Ther*. 1986;66:1255–1259.

52. Weinert A, Rizzo T. Non-operative management of multilevel lumbar disk herniations in an adolescent patient. *Mayo Clin Proc*. 1992;67:137–141.

53. McGaw S, Fritz J, Bernnan G. Factors related to success with the use of mechanical cervical traction. *J Orthop Sports Phys Ther*. 2006;36(1):A14.

54. Graham N. Mechanical traction for mechanical neck disorders: a systematic review. Cervical Overview Group. *J Rehabil Med*. 2006;38(3):145–152.

55. Moeti P, Marchetti G. Clinical outcome from mechanical intermittent cervical traction for the treatment of cervical radiculopathy: a case series. *J Orthop Sports Phys Ther*. 2001;31(4):207–213.

SUGGESTED READINGS

Alice M, Wong M, Chaupeng I. The traction angle and cervical intervertebral separation. *Spine*. 1992;17(2):136.

Beattie P, Nelson R. Outcomes after a prone lumbar traction protocol for patients with activity-limiting low back pain: a prospective case series study. *Arch Phys Med Rehabil*. 2008;89(2):269.

Beurskens A, de Vet H, Koke A. Efficacy of traction for nonspecific low back pain: a randomised clinical trial. *Lancet*. 1995;346(8990):1596–1600.

Beurskens A, van der Heijden G, de Vet H. The efficacy of traction for lumbar back pain: design of a randomized clinical trial. *J Manipulative Physiol Ther*. 1995;18(3):141–147.

Cevik R, Bilici A. Effect of new traction technique of prone position on distraction of lumbar vertebrae and its relation with different application of heating therapy in low back pain. *J Back Musculoskelet Rehabil.* 2007;20(2/3):71.

Cholewicki J, Lee A. Trunk muscle response to various protocols of lumbar traction. *Man Ther.* 14 (5): 562–566, 2009.

Cleland J, Whitman J, Fritz J. Manual physical therapy, cervical traction and strengthening exercises in patients with cervical radiculopathy: a case series. *J Orthop Sports Phys Ther.* 2005;35(12):802–811.

Constantoyannis C. Intermittent cervical traction for cervical radiculopathy caused by large-volume herniated disks. *J Manipulative Physiol Ther.* 2002;25(3):188–192.

Corkery MJ. The use of lumbar harness traction to treat a patient with lumbar radicular pain: a case report. *J Man Manipulative Ther.* 2001;9(4):191–197.

Creighton D. Positional distraction, a radiological confirmation. *J Man Manipulative Ther.* 1993;1(3):83–86.

Dilulio R. Treating with traction. *Phys Ther Prod.* 2008; 19(9):12.

Donkin RD. Possible effect of chiropractic manipulation and combined manual traction and manipulation on tension-type headache: a pilot study. *J Neuromusc Syst.* 2002;10(3):89–97.

Gilworth G. Cervical traction with active rotation. *Physiotherapy.* 1991;77(11):782–784.

Graham N, Gross A. Mechanical traction for mechanical neck disorders: a systematic review. *J Rehabil Med.* 2006;38(3):145.

Güvenol K. A comparison of inverted spinal traction and conventional traction in the treatment of lumbar disc herniations. *Physiother Theory Pract.* 2000;16(3):151–160.

Hariman D. The efficacy of cervical extension-compression traction combined with diversified manipulation and drop table adjustments in the rehabilitation of cervical lordosis: a pilot study. *J Manipulative Physiol Ther.* 1995;18(5): 323–325.

Harrison D, Jackson B, Troyanovich S. The efficacy of cervical extension-compression traction combined with diversified manipulation and drop table adjustments in the rehabilitation of cervical lordosis: a pilot study. *J Manipulative Physiol Ther.* 1995;18(5):590–596.

Harrison DE. A new 3-point bending traction method for restoring cervical lordosis and cervical manipulation: a nonrandomized clinical controlled trial. *Arch Phys Med Rehabil.* 2002;83(4):447–453.

Harte A. Current use of lumbar traction in the management of low back pain: results of a survey of physiotherapists in the United Kingdom. *Arch Phys Med Rehabil.* 2005;86(6): 1164–1169.

Joghataei M, Arab A, Khaksar H. The effect of cervical traction combined with conventional therapy on grip strength on patients with cervical radiculopathy. *Clin Rehabil.* 2004;18(8):879.

Krause M. Lumbar spine traction: evaluation of effects and recommended application for treatment. *Man Ther.* 2000;5(2):72–81.

Lee RY. Loads in the lumbar spine during traction therapy. *Aust J Physiother.* 2001;47(2):102–108.

Letchuman R, Deusinger R. Comparison of sacrospinalis myoelectric activity and pain levels in patients undergoing static and intermittent lumbar traction. *Spine.* 1993;18(10): 1361–1365.

Ljunggren A, Walker L, Weber H. Manual traction vs. isometric exercise in patients with herniated intervertebral lumbar disks. *Physiother Theory Pract.* 1992;8:207.

Maikowski G, Gill N, Jensen D. Quantification of forces delivered via cervical towel traction. *J Orthop Sports Phys Ther.* 2005;35(1):A64–A65.

McGaw S, Fritz J. Factors related to success with the use of mechanical cervical traction. *J Orthop Sports Phys Ther.* 2006;36(1):A14.

Meszaros TF. Effect of 10%, 30%, and 60% body weight traction on the straight leg raise test of symptomatic patients with low back pain. *J Orthop Sports Phys Ther.* 2000;30(10): 595–601.

Muraki T, Aoki M. Strain on the repaired supraspinatus tendon during manual traction and translational glide mobilization on the glenohumeral joint: a cadaveric biomechanics study. *Man Ther.* 2007;12(3):231.

Nanno M. Effects of intermittent cervical traction on muscle pain: flowmetric and electromyographic studies of the cervical paraspinal muscles. *J Nippon Med School.* 1994;61(2):137–147.

Pal B, Magnion P, Hossian M. A controlled trial of continuous lumbar traction in the treatment of back pain and sciatica. *Br J Rheumatol.* 1989;25:181.

Pellecchia G. Lumbar traction: a review of the literature (review). *J Orthop Sports Phys Med.* 1994;20(5):262–267.

Pio A, Rendina M, Benazzo F. The statics of cervical traction. *J Spinal Disord.* 1994;7(4):337–342.

Taskaynatan M, Balaban B. Cervical traction in conservative management of thoracic outlet syndrome. *J Musculoskelet Pain.* 2007;15(1):89.

Terahata N, Ishihara H, Ohshima H. Effects of axial traction stress on solute transport and proteoglycan synthesis in the porcine intervertebral disc in vitro. *Eur Spine J.* 1994;3(6):325–330.

Tesio L, Merlo A. Autotraction versus passive traction: an open controlled study in lumbar disc herniation. *Arch Phys Med Rehabil.* 1993;74(8):871–876.

Thorpe DL. On "Manual therapy, exercise, and traction for patients with cervical radiculopathy..." Young IA, et al. Phys Ther. 2009;89:632-642. *Phys Ther.* 2009;89(11): 1253.

Trudel G. Autotraction. *Arch Phys Med Rehabil.* 1994;75(2): 234–235.

van der Heijden G, Beurskens A, Koes B. The efficacy of traction for back and neck pain: a systematic, blinded review of randomized clinical trial methods. *Phys Ther.* 1995;75(2):93–104.

Vaughn H. Radiographic analysis of intervertebral separation with a 0 degree and 30 degree rope angle using the Saunders cervical traction device. *Spine.* 2006;31(2):E39–E43.

Vernon H, Humphreys K. Chronic mechanical neck pain in adults treated by manual therapy: a systematic review of change scores in randomized clinical trials. *J Man Physiol Ther.* 2007;30(3):215–227.

Wong A, Leong C, Chen C. The traction angle and cervical intervertebral separation. *Spine.* 1992;17(2):136–138.

Young I, Michener L. Manual therapy, exercise, and traction for patients with cervical radiculopathy: a randomized clinical trial. *Phys Ther.* 2009;89(7):632.

GLOSSARY

annulus fibrosus   The interlacing cross-fibers of fibroelastic tissue that are attached to adjacent vertebral bodies that contain the nucleus pulposus.

disk herniation   The protrusion of the nucleus pulposus through a defect in the annulus fibrosus.

disk material   Cartilaginous material from vertebral body surfaces, disk nucleus, or annulus fibrosus.

disk nucleus   The protein polysaccharide gel that is contained between the cartilaginous endplates of the vertebrae and the annulus fibrosus.

disk protrusion   The abnormal projection of the disk nucleus through some or all of the annular rings.

facet joints   Articular joints of the spine.

ligament deformation   Lengthening distortion of ligament caused by traction loading.

meniscoid structures   A cartilage tip found on the synovial fringes of some facet joints.

proprioceptive nervous system   System of nerves that provide information on joint movement, pressure, and muscle tension.

synovial fringes   Folds of synovial tissue that move in and out of the joint space.

traction   Drawing tension applied to a body segment.

unilateral foramen opening   Enlargement of the foramen on one side of a vertebral segment.

viscoelastic properties   The property of a material to show sensitivity to rate of loading.

Wolff's law   Bone remodels itself and provides increased strength along the lines of the mechanical forces placed on it.

LAB ACTIVITY

MECHANICAL TRACTION

DESCRIPTION

Mechanical traction has been used since ancient times in the treatment of painful spinal conditions. Simply, traction is applying tension to a body segment though a rope attached to various straps, halters, or devices. The therapeutic effect of traction is a function of the position of the spine, amount of traction force, and length of time the force is applied. Mechanical traction results in longitudinal separation of cervical or lumbar spinal segments with associated ligament, discal, neural, and muscular structures.

THERAPEUTIC EFFECTS

Separation of spinal segments
Elongation of muscle, ligament, and capsular tissue
Reduced intradiscal pressure

INDICATIONS

Mechanical traction is indicated to reduce the signs and symptoms of spinal compression. Appropriately applied mechanical traction can stretch facet joint capsules, increase the dimension of the intervertebral foramen thus increasing space for nerve roots, and alter intradiscal pressure. Paraspinal muscle tissues can also be elongated contributing to a reduction in the pain–spasm cycle, which frequently accompanies spinal dysfunction.

CONTRAINDICATIONS

• Spinal infection or malignancy
• Rheumatoid arthritis
• Osteoporosis
• Spinal hypermobility
• Acute stage injury
• Cardiac or respiratory insufficiency
• Pregnancy

MECHANICAL TRACTION

PROCEDURE	EVALUATION		
	1	2	3
1. Check supplies and equipment.			
a. Assemble towels, halters, harnesses, and belts.			
2. Question patient.			
a. Verify identity of patient.			
b. Verify the absence of contraindications.			
c. Ask about previous traction treatments and review treatment record.			
3. Apply and adjust appropriate halters, harnesses, and belts for indicated traction treatment.			
a. Cervical: Apply head halter beneath the occiput and mandible, attach to spreader bar.			
b. Lumbar: Attach pelvic harness snugly about the waist, beginning just above the iliac crests, thoracic rib belt snugly about the lower rib cage.			
c. Attach traction apparatus to unit: Take up and adjust for slack in the line.			
4. Position patient for indicated traction treatment.			
a. Cervical: Supine lying with neck flexed 20–30 degrees.			
b. Lumbar: Supine hooklying with hips flexed and legs supported by pillows or stools.			
c. Lumbar: Prone lying in neutral.			
d. Ensure proper body alignment and pull off traction apparatus.			
4. Apply indicated traction poundage.			
a. Cervical: Adjust traction poundage beginning with 20 pounds or as tolerated by the patient (range 20–50 pounds).			
b. Lumbar: Adjust traction poundage beginning with 65 pounds or as tolerated by the patient (range 65–200 pounds).			
5. Adjust traction duty cycle and treatment duration.			
a. Sustained: Less than 10 minutes.			
b. Intermittent: 3–10 seconds, on–off for 20–30 minutes			
6. Complete the treatment.			
a. Zero out equipment, turn power off.			
b. Slacken traction line.			
c. Remove the traction harness, halter, or belt.			

d. Have patient sit up slowly.			
e. Assess treatment efficacy.			
f. Record treatment parameters.			
7. Instruct the patient in any indicated exercise.			
8. Return equipment to storage after cleaning.			

chapter 15

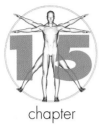

Intermittent Compression Devices

Daniel N. Hooker

OBJECTIVES

Following completion of this chapter, the student will be able to:

- Appraise the effectiveness of external compression on the accumulation and the reabsorption of edema following an athletic injury.
- Outline the setup procedure for intermittent external compression.
- Recognize the effects that changing a parameter might have on edema reduction.
- Review the clinical applications for using intermittent compression devices.

Edema accumulation following trauma is one of the clinical signs at which considerable attention is directed in first aid and therapeutic rehabilitation programs. **Edema** is defined as the presence of abnormal amounts of fluid in the extracellular tissue spaces of the body. Intermittent compression is one of the clinical modalities used to help reduce the accumulation of edema.

Two distinct kinds of tissue swelling are usually associated with injury. **Joint swelling,** marked by the presence of blood and joint fluid accumulated within the joint capsule, is one kind. This type of swelling occurs immediately following injury to a joint. Joint swelling is usually contained by the joint capsule and has the appearance and feel of a water balloon. If pressure is placed on the swelling, the fluid moves but it immediately returns when the pressure is released.

Lymphedema is the other variety of swelling encountered in athletic injuries. This type of swelling in the subcutaneous tissues results from an excessive accumulation of **lymph** and usually occurs over several hours following the injury. Intermittent compression can be used with both varieties, but it is usually more successful with **pitting edema.** The lymphatic system is the primary body system that deals with these injury-induced changes.

THE LYMPHATIC SYSTEM

Purposes of the Lymphatic System

The lymphatic system has four major purposes:

1. The fluid in the interstitial spaces is continuously circulating. As plasma and plasma proteins escape from the small blood vessels, they are picked up by the lymphatic system and returned to the blood circulation.

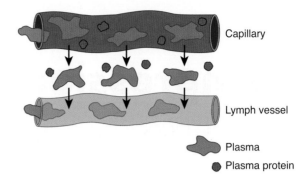

Figure 15–1. Plasma proteins outside the capillaries attract fluid to the intercellular space, leading to an abnormal "wet state" in the intercellular spaces. Plasma is absorbed back into the lymphatic spaces and away from the injured area.

2. The lymphatic system acts as a safety valve for fluid overload and helps keep edema from forming. As the interstitial fluid increases, the interstitial fluid pressure increases, causing an increase in the local lymph flow. The local lymphatic system can be overwhelmed by sudden local increases in the interstitial fluid and pitting edema will be the result.[1]

3. The homeostasis of the extracellular environment is maintained by the lymphatic system. The lymphatic system removes excess protein molecules and waste from the interstitial fluid. The large protein molecules and fluids that cannot reenter the circulatory vessels gain entry back into the blood circulation through the terminal lymphatics.

4. The lymphatic system also cleanses the interstitial fluid and provides a blockade to the spread of infection or malignant cells in the lymph nodes. The lymph nodes' ability is not clearly understood and is highly variable.[2]

Structure of the Lymphatic System

The lymphatic system is a closed vascular system of **endothelial cell–lined** tubes that parallel the arterial and nervous system. The lymphatic capillaries are made of single-layered endothelial cells with **fibrils** radiating from the junctions of the endothelial cells (Figure 15–1). These fibrils support the lymphatic capillaries and anchor them to the surrounding connective tissue. The capillary is surrounded by the interstitial fluid and tissues. These lymphatic capillaries are called the terminal lymphatics, and they provide the entry way into the lymphatic system for the excess interstitial fluid and plasma proteins.

These lymphatic capillaries join in a network of lymphatic vessels that eventually lead to larger collecting vessels in the extremities. The collecting vessels connect with the thoracic duct or the right lymphatic duct, which join the venous system in the left and right cervical area. As the lymph flows centrally up the system, the lymph moves through one or more lymph nodes. These nodes remove the foreign substances and are the primary area of lymphocyte activity.[2]

Peripheral Lymphatic Structure and Function

Deep and superficial lymphatic collecting systems are found in the extremities. The terminal lymphatics in the skin and subcutaneous tissue drain into the superficial branches. Lymph channels in the fascial and bony layers drain into the deep branches.

In the superficial branches, the dermis is packed with two types of lymphatic channels. The channels closer to the surface have no valves, whereas those lying under the dermis and in the subcutaneous tissue do have valves. The valves are located approximately 1 cm apart and are similar in construction to the valves in veins. These structures prevent the back flow of lymph when pressure is applied. As with the blood vessels, the lymph system is concentrated on the medial side of the limbs.[2]

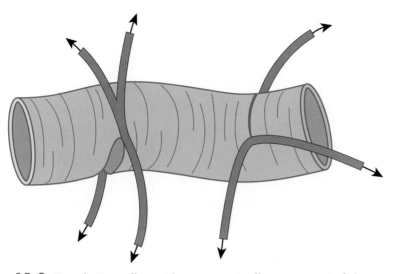

Figure 15–2. Lymphatic capillary with pore open to allow movement of plasma protein out of the intercellular space. As the intercellular fluid accumulates, the fibrils radiating from the seams in the lymphatic capillary pull the seam open to create a pore large enough for plasma proteins to enter.

As the lymphatic system changes from the entry channels to the collecting channels, the lymphatic vessel changes to look similar to venous tissue. These vessels have smooth muscle and appear to have innervation from the sympathetic nervous system.

As the fluid or tissues move in the interstitial spaces, they push or pull on the fibrils supporting the terminal lymphatics (Figure 15–2). This activity forces the endothelial cells to gap apart at their junctions, creating an opening in the terminal lymphatics for the entry of interstitial fluid, cellular waste, large protein molecules, plasma proteins, extracellular particles, and cells into the lymphatic channels. These junctions are constantly being pushed and pulled open and are then allowed to close, depending on the local activity. Once the interstitial fluid and proteins enter these channels, they become lymph. Terminal lymphatics in inflamed areas are dilated and an increased number of gaps in the capillary are present (Figure 15–2).[2,3–6]

If no tissue activity or interstitial volume increase takes place, these endothelial junctions remain closed. The interstitial fluid, however, can still enter the terminal lymphatics by moving across the endothelial cell, or by being transported across in a vesicle or cell organelle. This permeability is similar to the small blood vessels or capillaries (see Figure 15–1).

Muscle activity, active and passive movements, elevated positions, respiration, and blood vessel pulsation all aid in the movement of lymph by compressing the lymphatic vessels and allowing gravity to pull the lymph down the channels. The valves help by maintaining a unidirectional flow of lymph in response to pressure. The collecting lymph channels all have smooth muscle in their walls. These muscles can provide contractible activity that promotes lymph flow. These muscles have a natural firing frequency that simulates a rhythmic pumping action. Studies also indicate increased lymph flow during heating of animal limbs.[5–24]

INJURY EDEMA

Following a closed injury, changes in and around the site of the injury occur that have an impact on the accumulation of extracellular fluid and proteins in the local interstitial spaces. The direct effects of the injury include cell death, bleeding, the release of chemical mediators to initiate and guide the healing process, and changes in local tissue electric currents. The first stage of the healing process is inflammation, which is characterized by local redness, heat, swelling, and pain. In addition, loss of function frequently occurs.

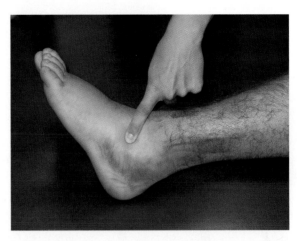

Figure 15–3. Ankle with pitting edema. Finger pressure squeezes fluid out of the intercellular space; an indentation is left when the pressure is removed.

Formation of Pitting Edema

These changes are brought about by changes in the local circulation. Local edema is formed by the plasma, plasma proteins, and cell debris from the damaged cells all moving into the interstitial spaces. This sudden volume change is compounded by the intact local circulatory responses to the chemical mediators of the inflammatory process. The hormones released by the injured cells stimulate the small arterioles, capillaries, and venules to vasodilate, enlarging the size of the vascular pool. This causes the local blood flow to slow down and the pressure within the blood vessels to increase. The endothelial cells in the blood vessel walls then separate or become more loosely bound to their neighboring cell. The permeability of the vessel increases, allowing more plasma, plasma proteins, and leukocytes to escape into the local area. The increase in the plasma proteins in the interstitial spaces causes the osmotic pressure to push more plasma into the area, forming an inflammatory exudate. This exudate forms too quickly for the lymphatic system to maintain the local equilibrium and pitting edema is formed (Figure 15–3). This small increase in the plasma protein in the intercellular spaces causes an increase in the intercellular fluid volume by several hundred percent.[6,7–9,13,23,26]

This fluid in the form of a gel is trapped by both collagen fibers and proteoglycan molecules. The gel prevents the free flow of fluid, as seen in the joint fluid example. Clinically, this state is recognized as pitting edema. After finger pressure on the swollen part is released, a slight pit is left at the finger's previous location. Fluid is squeezed out of the intercellular space and time is needed for the fluid to move slowly back into that space.

Movement of lymph occurs because of:
- Muscle activity
- Active and passive motion
- Elevation
- Respiration
- Contraction of vessels

Formation of Lymphedema

As the intercellular fluid becomes greater, the lymph begins to flow. If the edema causes an overdistention of the lymph capillaries, the entry pores become ineffective and lymphedema results. Constriction of lymph capillaries or larger lymphatic vessels from increased pressure also discourages lymph flow and causes intercellular fluid to increase.[6,7–9,13,23,26]

Using computerized tomography cross-sectional images, Airaksinen reported a 23% increase in the subcutaneous tissue, thickened skin, and muscular atrophy in patients following lower leg fracture and casting. They reported an 8% edema decrease in the subcutaneous compartment after intermittent compression. The mean area of the subfascial compartment remained the same, but the density of the muscle tissue increased after treatment. This study indicates that injury edema follows the path of least resistance and that tissues that have the least natural pressure exerted on them demonstrate the greatest accumulation of extra fluid. The skin and subcutaneous tissue appear to be the major site for pitting edema; the deep muscle and connective tissue have enough pressure to inhibit major accumulations in the deeper tissues.[9]

Clinical measurement of edema is reasonably accurate and correlates extremely well with both CT scan and volumetric measures. The standard clinical circumferential measurement of limb and joint is adequate to determine the treatment effects.[9,11]

Clinical Decision-Making *Exercise 15–1*

A patient comes into the clinic with an extremely swollen knee that she says has been like that for 2 days. How can the clinician determine whether she has joint swelling or pitting lymphedema?

The Negative Effects of Edema Accumulation

Edema compounds the extent of an injury by causing secondary hypoxic cellular death in the tissues surrounding the injured area. The edema increases the distance nutrients and oxygen must travel to nourish the remaining cells. This in turn adds to the injury debris in the damaged area and causes further edema to accumulate, thus perpetuating the cycle.[14]

Other negative effects of edema include the physical separation of torn tissue ends, pain, and restricted joint range of motion. Recovery times become more prolonged. If the edema persists, further problems with extremity function can occur, including infection, muscle atrophy, joint contractures, interstitial fibrosis, and reflex sympathetic dystrophy.[3,13,17]

TREATMENT OF EDEMA

Good first aid can minimize edema (Figure 15–4). The use of ice, compression, electricity, elevation, and early gentle motion retards the accumulation of fluid and keeps the lymphatic system operating at an optimum level. Any treatment that encourages the lymph flow will decrease plasma protein content in the intercellular spaces and therefore decrease edema. The standard methods of treatment in most clinical settings include elevation, compression, and muscular contraction.

Edema is best treated with:

- Elevation
- Compression
- Weight-bearing exercise
- Cryotherapy

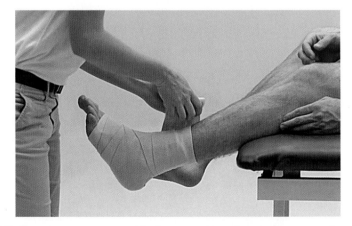

Figure 15–4. Wrapping an injured body part with an elastic wrap to provide compression should be followed by the application of ice, and elevation of the body part to minimize initial swelling.

The force of gravity can be used to augment normal lymph flow. The swollen part can be elevated so that gravity does not resist the flow of lymph but encourages its movement. Elevation of the injured swollen part above heart level is all that is necessary. The higher the elevation, the greater the effect on the lymph flow.[27,28]

In an uninjured population, placing the legs in an elevated position significantly decreased ankle volume after 20 minutes, although the dependent position significantly increased ankle volume. These findings could be expected to be the same in injured subjects, but the dependent position may markedly increase volume, whereas the elevated position may decrease volume less well because of the injury to the tissue. In the majority of studies using postacute ankle sprain edema, elevation alone provided a significant posttreatment reduction in ankle volume,[9,11,27–29] although a more recent study has shown no effect.[30,31]

Rhythmic internal compression provided by muscle contraction also squeezes the lymph through the lymph vessels, improving its flow back to the vascular system. This muscle contraction can be accomplished through isometric or active exercise or through electrically induced muscle contraction. Several authors also advocate the use of noncontractable electric current for edema control and reduction. (See Chapter 5 for a discussion of electrical therapy for edema control.) When elevation is combined with muscle contraction, lymph flow benefits.[10,12,16]

External pressure also can be used to increase lymph flow. Massage, elastic compression, and intermittent pressure devices are the most often used external pressure devices. External compression can be provided by an elastic wrap or by a custom fitted elastic garment such as those made by Jobst (Figure 15–5). This external compression not only moves the lymph along but also may spread the intercellular edema over a larger area, enabling more lymph capillaries to become involved in removing the plasma proteins and water. External pressure from horseshoes and other pads used under elastic wraps are also helpful in minimizing the accumulation or reaccumulation of edema in the injured area.[5,6,14,23]

Gardner has proposed that weight-bearing activities activate a powerful venous pump.[25] The pump consists of the venae comitantes of the lateral plantar artery. It is emptied immediately on weight bearing and flattening of the plantar arch. Because this emptying occurs so rapidly, they believe that this process is mediated by the release of an **endothelial-derived relaxing factor** (EDRF) and is not related to muscular activity of the limb. The EDRF is liberated by sudden pressure changes, and it diffuses locally. Its major action is to relax the smooth muscle and stimulate blood flow rates in the veins.[32]

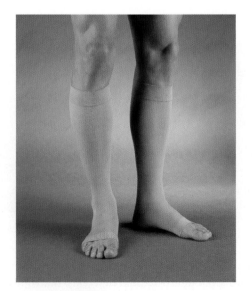

Figure 15–5. Jobst compression garment.

This phenomenon may explain the rapid decrease in edema that occurs when patients switch from a non-weight-bearing gait to a weight-bearing gait. Using this venous pump on lower leg edema is a reason to include early weight bearing in a variety of injury treatment protocols.

Using an intermittent compression device to decrease postacute injury edema has recently been shown to have a good effect. The addition of cryotherapy to the intermittent compression has shown the best results in the reduction of postacute injury edema.[4,7–9,11,18,19,24,29,33,34]

INTERMITTENT COMPRESSION TREATMENT TECHNIQUES

Three parameters are available for adjustment when using most intermittent pressure devices: (i) inflation pressure; (ii) on–off time sequence; and (iii) total treatment time (Figure 15–6). There are also intermittent pressure devices with multiple compartments that inflate distal-to-proximal with gradual reduced pressure in each compartment. These devices try to mimic the massage strokes used in edema removal.[4,18,21,29] Reduction in postacute injury edema does not require this graded sequential action, nor is postinjury edema reduction -significantly enhanced by these devices.[21,29] All intermittent compression devices seem to have similar influences on edema. The treatment parameters include the following:

- Inflation pressure
- On–off times
- Total treatment time

Little research has been done comparing adjustments of these parameters with volumetric results. Empiricism and clinical trials have been used to design the established protocols.

Inflation Pressures

Pressure settings have been loosely correlated with blood pressure and patient comfort to arrive at the therapeutic pressure. A pressure approximating the patient's diastolic blood pressure has been used in most treatment protocols. The arterial capillary pressures are approximately

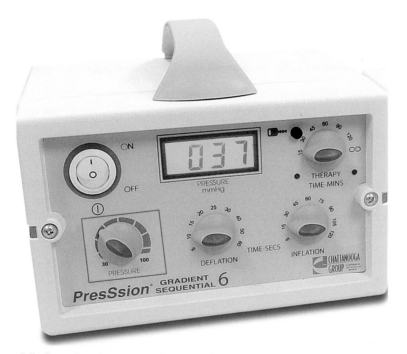

Figure 15–6. A digital pressure indicator and a pressure control knob on the control panel allow the clinician to adjust easily compression pressure.

30 mmHg, and any pressure that exceeds this should encourage reabsorption of the edema and movement of the lymph. Maximum pressure should correspond to the systolic blood pressure. Higher pressure would shut off arterial blood flow and create a potentially uncomfortable tissue response as a result of low blood flow.[3,7–9,17,26,35]

More may not necessarily be better. Enough pressure is needed to squeeze the lymphatic vessels and force the lymph to move. This should be accomplished with relatively low pressures, for example, 30–40 mmHg. The other mechanism in operation is the force of the hydrostatic pressure and pressure in the range of 40–50 mmHg should suffice to raise the interstitial fluid pressure higher than the blood vessel pressures.[17,26,35] Recommended inflation pressures for intermittent compression are 30–60 mm for the upper extremity and 40–80 mm for the lower extremity.

It has also been suggested that the pressures indicated on the control panel may be substantially less than actual pressures in the cuff. Thus it is recommended that cuff target pressures be set at much lower levels than indicated above.[1]

Clinical Decision-Making   *Exercise 15–2*

A patient has swelling in the knee joint from a sprain of the anterior cruciate ligament. What treatment techniques should the clinician use on day 2 postinjury to help eliminate swelling?

Treatment Protocols: Intermittent Compression

1. Attach sleeve to compression pump via tubing.
2. Turn pump on and inflate to <60 mm for the lower extremity, <50 mm for the upper extremity. **Warning: Do not exceed diastolic bp.**
3. Adjust the compression pump to cycle in a 3:1 ratio of on and off time.
4. Set duration of treatment from 30 minutes to 1 hour.
5. Encourage the patient to wiggle his or her fingers or toes during the off cycle.
6. Remove the sleeve at least once during the course of treatment to inspect skin and allow joint motion.

On–Off Sequence

On and off time sequences are even more variable, with some protocols calling for a sequence of 30 seconds on, 30 seconds off; 1 minute on, 2 minutes off; whereas others reverse this to 2 minutes on, 1 minute off. Some others use a 4 minutes on to 1 minute off ratio. One study has recommended using continuous compression for treating delayed onset muscle soreness.[36] If lymphatic massage is the primary vehicle used in this therapy, shorter on–off time sequences may have an advantage. The hydrostatic pressure vehicles require the longer on times. These time periods are not research based, and the clinician is left to his or her own empirical judgment as to the optimum time sequence for each patient. Patient comfort should be the primary deciding factor here. On–off times can be easily adjusted on the control panel of most intermittent compression units (Figure 15–7).

Total Treatment Time

Total treatment times have some basis in research, but again this is convenience or empirically based in many instances. Most of the protocols for primary lymphedema call for 3- to 4-hour treatments. This time frame has been effective for many patients.[4,5,7–9,11,16–19,21,24,27–29,33,35–40]

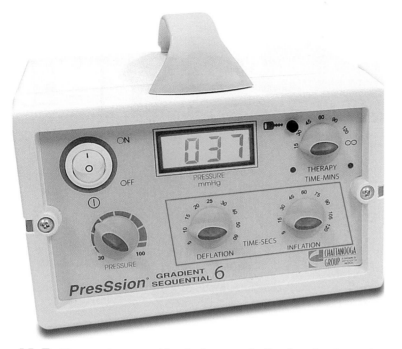

Figure 15–7. Time setting control knobs for on and off cycles of an intermittent compression unit. This illustrates the setting at the beginning of the treatment when the appliance is uninflated. The off-time knob is increased when the proper inflation pressure is reached.

Researchers have shown a marked increase in lymph flow on initiation of massage; this flow decreases over a 10-minute period and stops when the massage is discontinued.[41] Clinical studies show significant gains in limb volume reduction after 30 minutes of compression.[5,7-9,11,16,19,23,28,29,33,34,37,38] In most situations, a 10- to 30-minute treatment seems adequate unless the edema is overwhelming in volume or is resistant to treatment. More treatment times per day may also be an advantage in controlling and reducing edema from various musculoskeletal injuries.

Clinical Decision-Making *Exercise 15–3*

A patient comes into the clinic 3 days postinversion ankle sprain. He now shows signs of pitting lymphedema, and the clinician decides to use an intermittent compression device to help reduce the edema. What would be the appropriate treatment parameters?

Sequential Compression Pumps

Many intermittent compression pumps have incorporated sequentially inflated multiple compartment designs for some time[2,33,42] (Figure 15–8). Recently, these designs have also included a programmable gradient design. This was designed to incorporate the massage effect of a distal-to-proximal pressure with a gradual decrease in the pressure gradient.[4]

The highest pressure is in the distal sleeve and, according to the manufacturer's recommendation, is determined by the mean value of systolic to diastolic pressure at the outset of a specifically determined 48-hour protocol whose purpose is to determine the effectiveness of the device in individual cases.[4] The middle cell is set 20 mm lower than the distal cell, and the proximal cell pressure is reduced an additional 20 mm. There are some sequential units that have as many as six sequential compartments.

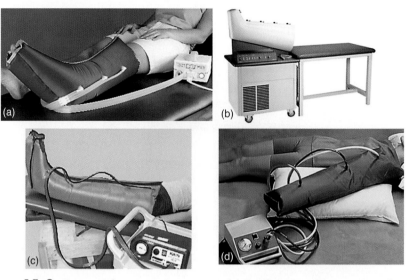

Figure 15–8. Sequential compression pumps. (a) PresSsion gradient sequential pump. (b) CryoPress. (c) BioCryo. (d) KCI Sequential Pump.

The length of each pressure cycle is 120 seconds. The distal cell is pressurized initially and continues pressurization for 90 seconds. Twenty seconds later the middle cell is inflated, and after another 20 seconds the proximal cell inflates. A final 30-second period allows pressure in all three cells to return to 0, after which the cycle repeats itself.

Only a few studies have shown the efficacy of using decreasing pressure in a distal to proximal direction relative to previously existing compression sleeves.[2,15] In a study comparing sequential compression and cold and compression, Lemly found both effective in reducing edema but no significant difference between the devices.[29]

Intermittent compression may also be used in conjunction with a low-frequency pulsed or surging electrical-stimulating current setup to produce muscle-pumping contractions. The combination of these two modalities should facilitate resorption of injury by-products by the lymphatic system.[16]

Patient Setup and Instructions

Patient setup using an intermittent compression device is relatively simple. The patient should have the appropriate-sized compression appliance fitted on the extremity in an elevated position (Figure 15–9). The compression sleeves come as foot and ankle, half-leg, full-leg,

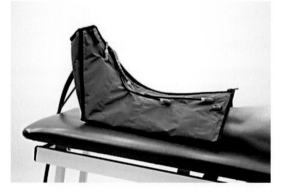

Figure 15–9. Uninflated compression appliance applied to a patient's leg in an elevated position.

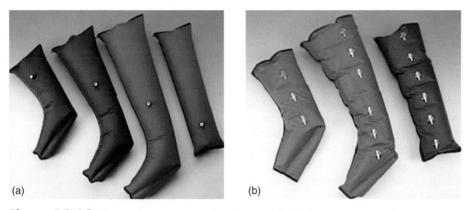

Figure 15–10. Intermittent compression sleeves. (a) Single compartment sleeves. (b) Sequential compartment sleeves.

full-arm, or half-arm. They may be single compartment sleeves or sequential compartment sleeves (Figure 15–10). The deflated compression sleeve is connected to the compression unit via a flexible hose and connecting valve.

Once the machine has been turned on, three parameters may be adjusted: on–off time, inflation pressure, and treatment time. The on time should be adjusted between 30 and 120 seconds. The off time is left at 0 until the sleeve is inflated and the treatment pressure is reached and then may be adjusted between 0 and 120 seconds. When the unit cycles off, the patient should be instructed to move the extremity. A 30-seconds-on, 30-seconds-off setting seems to be both effective and comfortable for the patient. Some compression devices slowly reach the target pressure, whereas others respond more rapidly. It is important that the on and off times take the machine characteristics into account.

When using electrical stimulation in combination with compression, always adjust the current intensity with the sleeve fully pressurized, as this may affect electrode contact and current density (Figure 15–11).

The treatment should last between 20 and 30 minutes. Patients do not seem to tolerate comfortably treatments lasting longer than 30 minutes. On completion of the treatment, the extremity should be measured to see if the desired results have been achieved. The part should be wrapped with elastic compression wraps to help maintain the reduction. If the edema is not reduced, another treatment may be needed after a short recovery time. If not contraindicated, weight bearing should be encouraged to stimulate the venous pump.

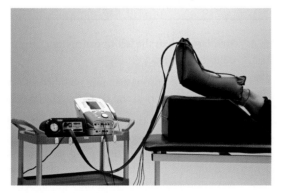

Figure 15–11. Intermittent compression used in combination with electrical-stimulating currents to reduce edema.

CASE STUDY 15–1
INTERMITTENT COMPRESSION

Background: A 48-year-old male developed pain and edema in his right foot and ankle subsequent to stepping in a hole in his yard while mowing his lawn. He was treated at his local hospital's emergency room. He failed to comply with their instructions to elevate and ice the injured extremity and reported to his family physician 48 hours later with a moderately swollen and ecchymotic right ankle. The patient reported the obvious swelling, localized tenderness over the lateral aspect of the ankle, and difficulty with weight-bearing during ambulation. Physical examination revealed point tenderness at the ATF (anterior talofibular ligament), 2 + effusion—figure 8 girth increased by three-fourth inch versus uninvolved side, and reduced ROM of dorsiflexion to 0°/plantarflexion to 35°. The ankle was stable to anterior drawer and talar tilt tests.

Impression: Subacute grade I inversion sprain right ankle.

Treatment Plan: In addition to reinstruction in home care principles; a course of intermittent compression was initiated to the right foot/ankle to mobilize the residual effusion/edema. The right lower extremity was elevated, pretreatment circumferential measurements taken, and stockingnette placed over the extremity. Treatment consisted of 60 mmHg pressure applied intermittently for 30-seconds-on/10-seconds-off cycles for 30 minutes duration. Posttreatment circumferential measures were taken and the patient was encouraged to attempt active and active-assisted ankle pumping exercise. Patient was fitted with a compression stocking and thermoplastic ankle stirrup for ambulation weight-bearing as tolerated.

Response: Postinitial treatment, patient's circumferential measures were reduced by 1/4 inch. Dorsiflexion range of motion increased by 5°. Over the course of five treatment sessions, effusion was resolved and active range of motion approached normal limits. Strengthening exercises were implemented and the patient continued to ambulate with the aid of the ankle stirrup. At the time of discharge, the patient was essentially symptom free, independent in performing his strengthening regimen, and had returned to his yard work.

The rehabilitation professional employs therapeutic agent modalities to create an optimum environment for tissue healing while minimizing the symptoms associated with the trauma or condition.

Discussion Questions

- What tissues were injured or affected?
- What symptoms were present?
- What phase of the injury-healing continuum did the patient present for care in?
- What are the therapeutic agent modality's biophysical effects (direct, indirect, depth, and tissue affinity)?
- What are the therapeutic agent modality's indications and contraindications?
- What are the parameters of the therapeutic agent modality's application, dosage, duration, and frequency in this case study?
- What other therapeutic agent modalities could be utilized to treat this injury or condition? Why? How?

CASE STUDY 15–2
INTERMITTENT COMPRESSION

Background: A 57-year-old woman underwent a modified radical mastectomy on the right 1 year ago, followed by radiation treatment for breast cancer. Over the past 6 months, she has developed progressively increasing swelling in the right upper member, from the hand to the axilla. The swelling is beginning to interfere with her ability to work on the assembly line at an automobile manufacturing plant and her daily activity. She has been referred for assistance in management of the edema. Circumferential measurements of her upper members reveals that the right upper member is

20% larger than the left upper member from the wrist to the deltoid tubercle.

Impression: Postmastectomy lymphedema syndrome due to lymph node removal and damage.

Treatment Plan: Intermittent compression using a full-length upper member sleeve. The inflation pressure was initially set at 40 mmHg, with an on time of 45 seconds, and off time of 60 seconds, and a total treatment time of 30 minutes. The patient was positioned supine, with the right upper member elevated

(continued)

CASE STUDY 15–2 *(continued)*
INTERMITTENT COMPRESSION

on pillows, and she was asked to make and release a fist during the time the sleeve was deflated. Treatment was conducted three days per week for 15 sessions.

Response: There was a light decrease in right upper member circumference following the initial treatment, but the reduction was not maintained. Over the next three sessions, the maximum inflation pressure was gradually increased to 60 mmHg, and the on time was increased to 120 seconds, with an off time of 30 seconds. There was a steady decrease in limb circumference until the eleventh session, after which there were no further gains noted. She was then fitted with a custom elastic garment to assist in maintaining the reduced limb volume. Upon discharge, her right upper member had a circumference that was 8% greater than the left upper member.

Discussion Questions

- What tissues were injured or affected?
- What symptoms were present?
- What phase of the injury-healing continuum did the patient present for care in?
- What are the physical agent modality's biophysical effects (direct, indirect, depth, and tissue affinity)?
- What are the physical agent modality's indications and contraindications?
- What are the parameters of the physical agent modality's application, dosage, duration, and frequency in this case study?

- What other physical agent modalities could be used to treat this injury or condition? Why? How?
- What is the difference in the pathophysiology of postmastectomy lymphedema and the edema noted with musculoskeletal injuries? Is there a difference in treatment techniques? Duration of treatment? Probability of recurrence?
- Would this patient have been more or less likely to develop lymphedema if she had undergone a simple mastectomy? A radical mastectomy?
- What effect did the radiation therapy have on the development of lymphedema? Would a course of chemotherapy have had the same effect? Why or why not?
- Could the development of postmastectomy lymphedema have been prevented in this patient? Why or why not? What measures could have been used in an attempt to prevent the lymphedema?
- What was the rationale for having the limb elevated during the intermittent compression? For the making and releasing a fist? For intermittent as opposed to static compression? For the inflation pressure?
- Would an inflation pressure of 120 mmHg have been more effective at reducing the edema?

The rehabilitation professional employs physical agent modalities to create an optimum environment for tissue healing while minimizing the symptoms associated with the trauma or condition.

COLD AND COMPRESSION COMBINATION

Some manufacturers have coupled intermittent pressure with a coolant (usually water).[43] These devices have the advantage of cooling the injured part as well as compressing it. The Jobst Cryo-Temp is a controlled cold-compression unit that has a temperature adjustment ranging between 10°C and 25°C. Cooling is accomplished by circulating cold water through the sleeve.

The combination of cold and compression has been shown to be clinically effective in treating some edema conditions.[11,16,19,26,29,33,34,44,45] A study comparing a technique using an intermittent compression unit, cold, and elevation with one using an elastic wrap, cold, and elevation showed that the use of the cold-compression device was more effective in edema reduction.[11]

The *Cryo-Cuff*, discussed previously in Chapter 4, the *Game Ready System, the Vital Wrap System Polar Care Cub* are all portable units that make use of both compression and cold (Figure 15–12). These units are inexpensive and are also relatively easy to use. Currently their most common use is in management of postsurgical swelling. The BioCryo unit in Figure 15–8 is an example of a stationary cold-compression unit.

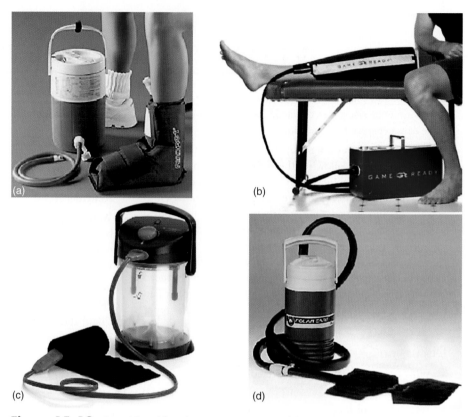

Figure 15–12. Portable cold and compression units. (a) Cryo-Cuff. (b) Game Ready System. (c) Vital Wrap. (d) Polar Cub.

Clinical Decision-Making *Exercise 15–4*

The clinician is treating a swollen ankle with intermittent compression and wants to know whether using electrical-stimulating current or cold or a combination of the two will be more effective in treating lymphedema.

INDICATIONS AND CONTRAINDICATIONS FOR USE

Table 15–1 summarizes indications and contraindications for using intermittent compression. Intermittent compression has been recommended for treating lymphedema; traumatic edema that occurs following injury to soft tissue; chronic edema that occurs in patients with certain types of neurologic diseases owing to an inability to move a limb; stasis ulcers that develop with the presence of fluid in the interstitial spaces for long periods of time; swelling that occurs with limb amputation; patients on dialysis owing to renal insufficiency that tend to develop edema in the extremities and hypothesion; patients with arterial insufficiency, such as in cases of intermittent claudications to increase venous return; edema and contractures in the hand that result from stroke or surgery; and stimulating proteoglycan synthesis in human cartilage.[37,39–42] It has also been used postoperatively to reduce the possibility of developing a deep vein thrombosis resulting from inactivity and coagulation; and to facilitate wound healing following surgery by reducing swelling.[38,46,47]

The clinician should avoid using intermittent compression in patients with known deep vein thrombosis, local superficial infection, congestive heart failure, acute pulmonary edema, and displaced fractures.[48]

Table 15–1 Indications and Contraindications for Intermittent Compression

INDICATIONS
Lymphedema
Traumatic edema
Chronic edema
Stasis ulcers
Intermittent claudications
Wound healing following surgery
CONTRAINDICATIONS
Deep vein thrombosis
Local superficial infection
Congestive heart failure
Acute pulmonary edema
Displaced fractures

Clinical Decision-Making *Exercise 15–5*

In providing initial first aid care to a patient who has suffered and acute contusion to the left gastrocnemius muscle, is it more effective to use an intermittent compression unit or an elastic wrap to control swelling?

SUMMARY

1. Edema following injury or surgery can be effectively managed using a compression pump program.

2. Lymphedema is swelling in the subcutaneous tissues that results from an excessive accumulation of lymph and usually occurs over several hours following the injury.

3. Muscle activity, active and passive movements, elevated positions, respiration, and blood vessel pulsation all aid in the movement of lymph by compressing the lymphatic vessels and allowing gravity to pull the lymph down the channels.

4. The use of ice, compression, electricity, elevation, and early gentle motion retards the accumulation of fluid and keeps the lymphatic system operating at an optimum level.

5. Three parameters may be adjusted when using most intermittent pressure devices: inflation pressure, on–off time sequence, and total treatment time. Adjustments in these parameters should be made using patient comfort as the primary guide.

6. The combination of cold and compression has been shown to be clinically effective in treating some edema conditions.

7. Sequential compression pumps were designed to incorporate the massage effect of a distal-to-proximal pressure with a gradual decrease in the pressure gradient.

REVIEW QUESTIONS

1. What are the various types of edema that can accumulate following trauma?
2. Explain the purpose, structure, and function of the lymphatic system.
3. What is lymphedema?
4. What can be done to facilitate the reabsorption of lymphedema into the lymphatic system?
5. What are the effects of external compression on the accumulation and the reabsorption of edema following an injury?
6. What are the three treatment parameters that should be considered when using intermittent compression?
7. How can intermittent compression be used effectively in combination with other modalities?
8. Are there any clinical advantages to using sequential compression pumps?
9. What are the clinical applications for using intermittent compression devices?

SELF-TEST QUESTIONS

True or False

1. One of the roles of the lymphatic system is to remove excess proteins from interstitial fluid.
2. The lymphatic system runs parallel to the arterial system.
3. None of the lymphatic vessels has muscular linings.

Multiple Choice

4. Excessive accumulation of lymph fluid in subcutaneous tissues is called
   a. edema
   b. lymphedema
   c. joint swelling
   d. pitting edema
5. Lymph is composed of
   a. endothelial cells and fibrils
   b. a transparent, slightly yellow liquid found in lymphatic vessels
   c. the fluid in extracellular space
   d. blood and joint fluid in the joint
6. Which of the following are responsible for lymph movement?
   a. muscle activities
   b. active and passive movements
   c. elevated positions
   d. all of the above
7. At what minimum setting should the pressure be when using intermittent compression devices?
   a. greater than or equal to 30 mmHg
   b. greater than or equal to 100 mmHg
   c. approximately systolic pressure
   d. approximately diastolic pressure
8. How long should most intermittent compression treatments last, bearing in mind patient comfort?
   a. 5–10 minutes
   b. 10–20 minutes
   c. 20–30 minutes
   d. over an hour
9. What may be combined with compression treatment?
   a. cold, via a cold-compression unit
   b. electrical-stimulating current
   c. neither *a* nor *b*
   d. both *a* and *b*

10. Which of the following is *not* a contraindication to intermittent compression?
    a. intermittent claudication
    b. deep vein thrombosis
    c. displaced fracture
    d. local superficial infection

SOLUTIONS TO CLINICAL DECISION-MAKING EXERCISES

15–1

Joint swelling is usually contained in the joint capsule and feels very much like a water balloon. The fluid is easily moved around by simply applying pressure on one side of the joint. Lymphedema occurs in the subcutaneous tissues and has more of a gel-like feeling to it and leaves an indentation after finger pressure is removed.

15–2

The clinician should include cold, elevation, compression, using an -intermittent compression unit, and some weight-bearing exercise to facilitate venous and lymphatic drainage.

15–3

The compression boot should be applied with the inflation pressure set at about 60 mmHg, the on–off time at 30 seconds on 30 seconds off, and a total treatment time of 20 minutes initially. The on–off times and total treatment time can be increased over the next several days as can be tolerated.

15–4

Using electrical-stimulating currents to induce muscle pumping contractions should facilitate removal of edema. Also, it is well documented that using cold in conjunction with compression is clinically effective in treating cases of lymphedema.

15–5

It will be OK to use the intermittent compression unit as long as it also provides cold and the part can still be elevated. It is perhaps a better choice to use an elastic compression wrap if the intermittent compression unit cannot keep the injured part cold during initial management.

REFERENCES

1. Segers P, Belgrado JP, Leduc A, et al. Excessive pressure in multichambered cuffs used for sequential compression therapy. *Phys Ther* 2002;82:1000–1008.
2. Gnepp D. Lymphatics. In Staub N and Taylor A (eds). *Edema*, New York:Raven, 1984, pp. 263–298.
3. Evans P. The healing process at the cellular level: a review, *Physiotherapy* 1980;66:256–259.
4. Klein M, Alexander M, and Wright J. Treatment of lower extremity lymphedema with the Wright Linear Pump: A statistical analysis of a clinical trial. *Arch Phys Med Rehab* 1988;69:202–206.
5. Wilkerson J. Treatment of ankle sprains with external compression and early mobilization *Phys Sports Med* 1985;13(6):83–90.
6. Wilkerson J. External compression for controlling traumatic edema. *Phys Sports Med* 1985;13(6):97–106.
7. Airaksinen O. Changes in post-traumatic ankle joint mobility, pain and edema following intermittent pneumatic compression therapy. *Arch Phys Med Rehab* 1989;70:341–344.
8. Airaksinen O. Treatment of post-traumatic edema in lower legs using intermittent pneumatic compression. *Scand J Rehab Med* 1988;20:25–28.
9. Airaksinen O. Intermittent pneumatic compression therapy in post-traumatic lower limb edema: computed tomography and clinical measurements. *Arch Phys Med Rehab* 1991;72:667–670.
10. Angus J, Prentice W, and Hooker D. A comparison of two intermittent external compression devices and their effect on post acute ankle edema. *J Athl Training* 1994;29(2):179.
11. Brewer K, Prentice W, and Hooker D. The effects of intermittent compression and cold on reducing edema in post-acute ankle sprains. Unpublished master's thesis, University of North Carolina, Chapel Hill, NC, 1990.
12. Brown S. Ankle edema and galvanic muscle stimulation. *Phys Sports Med* 1981;9:137.

13. Capps S and Mayberry B. Cryotherapy and intermittent pneumatic compression for soft tissue trauma. *Athlet Ther Today* 2009;14(1):2.

14. Duffley H and Knight K. Ankle compression variability using elastic wrap, elastic wrap with a horseshoe, edema II boot and air stirrup brace. *J Athl Training* 1989;24:320–323.

15. Elkins E, Herrick J, and Grindley J. Effect of various procedures on the flow of lymph. *Arch Phys Med Rehab* 1953;34:31–39.

16. Flicker M. An analysis of cold intermittent compression with simultaneous treatment of electrical stimulation in the reduction of post acute ankle lymphaedema. Unpublished master's thesis, University of North Carolina, Chapel Hill, NC, May, 1993.

17. Foldi E, Foldi M, and Weissleder H. Conservative treatment of lymphoedema of the limbs. *Angiology* 1985;36:171–180.

18. Kim-Sing C and Basco V. Postmastectomy lymphedema treated with the Wright Linear Pump. *Can J Surg* 1987;30(5):368–370.

19. Starkey J. Treatment of ankle sprains by simultaneous use of intermittent compression and ice packs. *Am J Sports Med* 1976;4:142–144.

20. Tsang K, Hertel J, and Denegar C. Volume decreases after elevation and intermittent compression of postacute ankle sprains are negated by gravity-dependent positioning. *J Athl Training* 2003;38(4):320–324.

21. Wakim K. Influence of centripetal rhythmic compression on localized edema of an extremity. *Arch Phys Med Rehab* 1955;36:98–103.

22. Wilkerson J. Contrast baths and pressure treatment for ankle sprains. *Phys Sports Med* 1979;7:143.

23. Wilkerson J. Treatment of the inversion ankle sprain through synchronous application of focal compression and cold. *J Athl Training* 1991;26:220–237.

24. Winsor T, and Selle W. The effect of venous compression on the circulation of the extremities. *Arch Phys Med Rehab* 1953;34:559–565.

25. Gardner A. Reduction of post-traumatic swelling and compartment pressure by impulse compression of the foot. *J one Joint Surg* 1990;72-B:810–815.

26. Kobl P and Denegar C. Traumatic edema and the lymphatic system. *J Athl Training* 1983;18:339–341.

27. Rucinski T, Hooker D, and Prentice W. The effects of intermittent compression on edema in post-acute ankle sprains, *J Orthop Sports Phys Ther* 1991;14(2):65–69.

28. Sims D. Effects of positioning on ankle edema. *J Orthop Sports Phys Ther* 1986;8:30–33.

29. Lemley T, Prentice W, and Hooker D. A comparison of two intermittent compression devices on pitting ankle edema. *J Athl Training* 1993;28(2):156–157.

30. Tsang K, Hertel J, and Denegar C. The effects of elevation and intermittent compression on the volume of injured ankles. *J Athl Training* (suppl.) 2001;36(2S):S-50.

31. van Veen S, Hagen J, and van Ginkel F. Intermittent compression stimulates cartilage mineralization. *Bone* 1995;17(5):461–465.

32. Hurley J. Inflammation. In Staub N and Taylor A (eds). *Edema,* New York:Raven, 1984, pp. 463–488.

33. Quillen W, and Rouiller L. Initial management of acute ankle sprains with rapid pulsed pneumatic compression and cold. *J Orthop Sports Phys Ther* 1982;4:39–43.

34. Sloan J, Giddings P, and Hain R. Effects of cold and compression on edema. *Phys Sports Med* 1988;16(8):116–120.

35. Kruse R, Kruse A, and Britton R. Physical therapy for the patient with peripheral edema: Procedures for management. *Phys Ther Rev* 1960;80:29–33.

36. Kraemer W, Bush J, and Wickham R. Continuous compression as an effective therapeutic intervention in treating eccentric-exercise-induced muscle soreness. *J Sport Rehab* 2001;10(1):11.

37. Lafeber F. Intermittent hydrostatic compressive force stimulates exclusively the proteoglycan synthesis of osteo-arthritic human cartilage. *Br J Rheumatol* 1992;31(7):437–442.

38. Pflug J. Intermittent compression: A new principle in the treatment of wounds. *Lancet* 1974;2(3):15.

39. Redford J. Experiences in the use of a pneumatic stump shrinker. *Int Clin Inform Bull Prosth Orthot* 1973;12:1.

40. Sanderson R, and Fletcher W. Conservative management of primary lymphedema. *Northwest Med* 1965;64:584–588.

41. Henry J and Windos T. Compensation of arterial insufficiency by augmenting the circulation with intermittent compression of the limbs. *Am Heart J* 1965;70(1):77–88.

42. McCulloch J. Intermittent compression for the treatment of a chronic stasis ulceration: a case report. *Phys Ther* 1981;61:1452–1453.

43. Womochel K, Trowbridge C, and Keller D. Effect of continuous circulating water and cyclical compression on intramuscular temperature and cardiovascular strain. *J Athl Training* 2009;44(suppl):S87.

44. Liu N, and Olszewski W. The influence of local hyperthermia on lymphedema and lymphedematous skin of the human leg. *Lymphology* 1993;26:28–37.

45. Seamon C, and Merrick M. Comparison of intramuscular temperature of the thigh during treatments with the Grimm Cryopress and the game ready accelerated recovery system (abstract). *J Athl Training* 2005;40(2 suppl.)S-99.

46. Carriere B. Edema—its development and treatment using lymph drainage massage. *Clin Manage Phys Ther* 1988;8(5):19–21.

47. Matzdorff A and Green D. Deep vein thrombosis and pulmonary embolism: prevention, diagnosis, and treatment, *Geriatrics* 1992;47(8):48–52, 55–57, 62–63.

48. Fond D and Hecox B. Intermittent pneumatic compression. In Hecox, B, Mehreteab, T, and Weisberg J (eds). *Physical Agents: A Comprehensive Text for Physical Therapists.* Norwalk, CT: Appleton & Lange, 1994.

SUGGESTED READINGS

Aydog S and Özçakar L. A handball player with a tennis leg: Incentive for muscle sonography and intermittent pneumatic compression during the follow up. *J Back Musculoskeletal Rehab* 2007;20(4):181.

Capper C. Product focus. External pneumatic compression therapy for DVT prophylaxis, *Br J Nur* 1998;7(14):851.

Challis M and Jull, G. Cyclic pneumatic soft-tissue compression enhances recovery following fracture of the distal radius: A randomised controlled trial. *Aust J Physiotherapy* 2007;53(4):247.

Chleboun GS, Howell JN, Baker HL, et al. Intermittent pneumatic compression effect on eccentric exercise-induced swelling, stiffness, and strength loss. *Arch Phys Med Rehab* 1995;76(8):744–799.

Christen Y and Reymond M. Hemodynamic effects of intermittent pneumatic compression of the lower limbs during laparoscopic cholecystectomy. *Am J Surg* 1995;170(4):395–398.

Coogan C. Venous leg ulcers and intermittent pneumatic compression therapy: Care of venous leg ulcers. *Ostomy Wound Manage* 1999;45(11):5.

DePrete A, Cogliano T, and Agostinucci J. The effect of circumferential pressure on upper motoneuron reflex excitability in healthy subjects. *Phys Ther* (suppl.) 1994;74(5):S70.

Duffield R and Cannon J. The effects of compression garments on recovery of muscle performance following high-intensity sprint and plyometric exercise. *J Sci Med Sport* 2010;13(1):136.

Eisele R and Kinzl L. Rapid-inflation intermittent pneumatic compression for prevention of deep venous thrombosis. *J Bone Joint Surg* 2007;89(5):1050.

Elliot CG, Dudney TM, Egger M, et al. Calf-thigh sequential pneumatic compression compared with plantar venous pneumatic compression to prevent deep-vein thrombosis after non-lower extremity trauma. *J Trauma Inj Infect Crit Care* 1999;47(1):25–32.

French D and Thompson K. The effects of contrast bathing and compression therapy on muscular performance. *Med Sci in Sports Exer* 2008;40(7):1297.

Gilbart MK, Ogilvie-Harris DJ, Broadhurst C, and Clarfield M. Anterior tibial compartment pressures during intermittent sequential pneumatic compression therapy. *Am J Sports Med* 1995;23(6):769–772.

Hamzeh M, Lonsdale R, and Pratt D. A new device producing ambulatory intermittent pneumatic compression suitable for the treatment of lower limb edema: a preliminary report. *J Med Eng Technol* 1993;17(3):110–113.

Hofman D. Intermittent compression treatment for venous leg ulcers. *J Wound Care* 1995;4(4):163–165.

Iwama H, Suzuki M, Hojo M, et al. Intermittent pneumatic compression on the calf improves peripheral circulation of the leg. *J Crit Care* 2000;15(1):18–21.

Jacobs M. Leg volume changes with EPIC and posturing in dependent pregnancy edema: external pneumatic intermittent compression. *Nurs Res* 1986;35(2):86–89.

Knobloch K and Kraemer R. Microcirculation of the Ankle after Cryo/Cuff Application in Healthy Volunteers. *Int J Sports Med* 2006;27(3):250–255.

Knobloch K. Changes of Achilles midportion tendon microcirculation after repetitive simultaneous cryotherapy and compression using a cryo/cuff (includes abstract). *Am J Sports Med* 2006;34 (12):1953–1959.

Kozanoglu E and Basaran S. Efficacy of pneumatic compression and low-level laser therapy in the treatment of postmastectomy lymphoedema: A randomized controlled trial. *Clin Rehab* 2009;23(2):117.

Lachmann E, Rook J, and Tunkel R. Complications associated with intermittent pneumatic compression. *Arch Phys Med Rehab* 1992;73(5):482–485.

Majkowski R, and Atkins R. Treatment of fixed flexion deformities of the knee in rheumatoid arthritis using the Flowtron intermittent compression stocking. *Br J Rheumatol* 1992;31(1):41–43.

McCulloch J. Physical modalities in wound management: ultrasound, vasopneumatic devices and hydrotherapy. *Ostomy Wound Manage* 1995;41(5):30–32, 34, 36–37.

Murphy K. The combination of ice and intermittent compression system in the treatment of soft tissue injuries. *Physiotherapy* 1988;74(1):41.

Seki K. Lymph flow in human leg. *Lymphology* 1979;12:2–3.

Smith P. The use of intermittent compression in treatment of fixed flexion deformities of the knee. *Physiotherapy* 1989;75(8):494.

Stillwell G. Further studies on the treatment of lymphedema. *Arch Phys Med Rehab* 1957;38:435–441.

Tan X and Qi, W. Intermittent pneumatic compression regulates expression of nitric oxide synthases in skeletal muscles. *Biomechanics* 2006;39(13):2430.

Waller T and Caine M. Intermittent pneumatic compression technology for sports recovery. *Sports Engineering.* 2006;9(4):247.

Wicker P. Clinical feature supplement. Intermittent pneumatic compression therapy for deep vein thrombosis prophylaxis. *Br J Theatre Nurs* 1999;9(3):108.

Yates P, Cornwell J, and Scott, G. Treatment of haemophilic flexion deformities using the Flowtron intermittent compression system. *Br J Haematol* 1992;82(2):384–387.

GLOSSARY

edema The presence of abnormal amounts of fluid in the extracellular tissue spaces of the body.

endothelial cell Cells that line the cavities of vessels.

endothelial-derived relaxing factor Relaxes smooth muscle and stimulates blood flow rates in veins.

fibrils Connective tissue fibers supporting the lymphatic capillaries.

joint swelling Accumulation of blood and joint fluid within the joint capsule.

lymph A transparent slightly yellow liquid found in the lymphatic vessels.

lymphedema Swelling of subcutaneous tissues as a result of accumulation of excessive lymph fluid.

pitting edema A type of swelling that leaves a pitlike depression when the skin is compressed.

LAB ACTIVITY

INTERMITTENT COMPRESSION

DESCRIPTION

Intermittent compression pumps are mechanical units that inflate double-layered fabric sleeves shaped to fit the extremities in order to apply external pressure to facilitate the body's reabsorption of edema resulting from injury or trauma. Units allow the regulation of inflation pressure, on–off time sequence, and total treatment time.

PHYSIOLOGIC EFFECTS

Movement of interstitial fluid to venous and lymphatic drainage sites.

Temporary decrease in peripheral blood flow.

THERAPEUTIC EFFECTS

Reduction of soft-tissue edema.
Decreased pain.
Increased range of motion.

INDICATIONS

The therapist will most frequently employ intermittent compression pumps in the treatment of soft-tissue edema that accompanies musculoskeletal trauma. It may also be utilized in cases of venous insufficiency and lymphedema.

CONTRAINDICATIONS

- Infections
- Arterial insufficiency
- Possibility of blood clots
- Cardiac or kidney dysfunction
- Obstructed lymphatic channels

INTERMITTENT COMPRESSION

PROCEDURE	EVALUATION		
	1	2	3
1. Check supplies.			
a. Obtain compression pump, pneumatic sleeve, and cotton stockingette.			
2. Question patient.			
a. Verify identity of patient.			
b. Verify the absence of contraindications.			
c. Take the patient's blood pressure.			
d. Ask about previous treatments and review treatment notes.			

3. Position patient.			
a. Place patient in a well-supported, comfortable position.			
b. Elevate the extremity to be treated.			
4. Inspect the patient's skin and extremity sensation.			
a. Perform circumferential measures of part to be treated.			
b. Cover extremity with stockingette, insure there are no wrinkles.			
5. Apply compression sleeve over the stockingette covered extremity.			
6. Explain the procedure to the patient.			
7. Begin the indicated procedure.			
a. Attach sleeve to compression pump via tubing.			
b. Turn pump "on" and inflate to: <60 mm for the lower extremity <50 mm for the upper extremity **Warning: Do not exceed diastolic bp.**			
c. Adjust the compression pump to cycle in a 3:1 ratio of on and off time.			
d. Set duration of treatment from 30 minutes to 1 hour.			
e. Encourage the patient to wiggle his or her fingers or toes during the off cycle.			
f. Remove the sleeve at least once during the course of treatment to inspect skin and allow joint motion.			
8. Complete the treatment.			
a. Remove the sleeve and stockingette.			
b. Inspect the skin and check peripheral circulation.			
c. Perform circumferential measures.			
d. Record results of treatment.			
e. Assess treatment efficacy.			
9. Wrap extremity to retain edema reduction and perform any indicated exercise.			
10. Return equipment to storage after cleaning.			

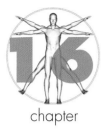

16 Therapeutic Massage

chapter   William E. Prentice

OBJECTIVES

Following completion of this chapter, the student will be able to:

➤ Discuss the physiologic effects of massage differentiating between reflexive and mechanical effects.

➤ Apply specific treatment guidelines and considerations when administering massage.

➤ Demonstrate the various strokes involved with Classic Hoffa massage.

➤ Describe connective tissue massage.

➤ Explain how trigger point massage is most effectively used.

➤ Explain now myofascial release can be used to restore normal functional movement patterns.

➤ Explain how strain–counterstrain, positional release, and active release techniques can be used to treat myofascial trigger points.

➤ Contrast special massage techniques including Rolfing and Trager.

PHYSIOLOGIC EFFECTS OF MASSAGE

Massage is a mechanical stimulation of the tissues by means of rhythmically applied pressure and stretching.[1] Over the years many claims have been made relative to the therapeutic benefits of massage in the patient population, although few are based on well-controlled and well-designed studies.[2–11] Patients have used massage to increase flexibility and coordination as well as to increase pain threshold; decrease neuromuscular excitability in the muscle being massaged; stimulate circulation, thus improving energy transport to the muscle; facilitate healing and restore joint mobility; and remove lactic acid, thus alleviating muscle cramps.[3,6,12–16,112,114] Conclusive evidence of the efficacy of massage as an ergogenic aid in the physically active population is lacking, however.[17]

How these effects may be accomplished is determined by the specific approaches used and how massage techniques are applied. Generally, the effects of massage may be either *reflexive* or *mechanical*.[18] The effect of massage on the nervous system differs greatly according to the method employed, pressure exerted, and duration of applications. Through the reflex mechanism, sedation is induced. Slow, gentle, rhythmical, and superficial effleurage may relieve tension and soothe, rendering the muscles more relaxed. This indicates an effect on sensory and motor nerves locally and some central nervous system response. The mechanical approach seeks to make mechanical or histologic changes in myofascial structures through direct force applied superficially.[18]

Reflexive Effects

The first approach in massage therapy involves a reflexive mechanism. The reflexive approach attempts to exert effects through the skin and superficial connective tissues. Mobilization of soft tissue stimulates sensory receptors in the skin and superficial fascia.[18] If hands are passed lightly over the skin, a series of responses occur as a result of the sensory stimulus of cutaneous receptors. This reflex mechanism is believed to be an autonomic nervous system phenomenon.[19] The reflex stimulus can occur alone (unaccompanied by the mechanical mechanism). Mennell calls this the "reflex effect."[20] In itself, it is not an effect but the cause of an effect (that is, it causes sedation, relieves tension, and increases blood flow).

Effects on Pain

The effect of massage on pain is probably regulated by both the gate control theory and through the release of endogenous opiates (see Chapter 4). In gate control, cutaneous stimulation of large-diameter afferent nerve fibers effectively blocks transmission of pain information carried in small-diameter nerve fibers. Stimulation of painful areas in the skin or myofascia can facilitate the release of β-endorphins and enkephalin, which essentially effect the transmission of pain-associated information in descending spinal tracts.

Effects on Circulation The effect of massage on the circulation of the blood, according to Pemberton, takes place through a reflex influence on blood vessels from a sympathetic division in the nervous system.[21] He believes that vessels in the muscular system are emptied during massage, not only by being squeezed but also by this reflex action. Very light massage (effleurage) produces an almost instantaneous reaction through transient dilation of lymphatics and small capillaries. Heavier pressure brings about a more lasting dilation. If capillary dilation occurs, blood volume and blood flow increase, producing an increase in temperature in the area being massaged.[22]

Massage increases lymphatic flow.[22,104] In the lymphatic system, movement of fluid depends on forces outside of the system. Such factors as gravity, muscle contraction, movement, and massage can affect the flow of lymph. Increased lymphatic flow assists in the removal of edema.[23] When administering massage to an edematous part, elevation also helps to increase lymph flow.

It has been proposed that massage can promote lactate clearance following exercise. However, evidence suggests that increases in blood flow that occur from massage have little or no effect on lactate metabolism and its subsequent clearance from blood and tissues.[24,25,105,113]

Effects on Metabolism

Massage does not alter general metabolism appreciably.[21] There is no change in the acid–base equilibrium of blood. Massage does not appear to have any significant effects on the cardiovascular system.[26] Massage metabolically augments a chemical balance. The increased circulation means increased dispersion of waste products and an increase of fresh blood and oxygen. The mechanical movements assist in the removal and hasten the resynthesis of lactic acid.

Mechanical Effects

The second approach to massage is mechanical in nature. Techniques that stretch a muscle, elongate fascia, or mobilize soft-tissue adhesions or restrictions are all mechanical techniques. The mechanical effects are always accompanied by some reflex effects. As the mechanical stimulus becomes more effective, the reflex stimulus becomes less effective. Mechanical techniques should be performed after reflexive techniques. This is not to imply that mechanical techniques are more aggressive forms of massage. However, mechanical techniques are most often directed at deeper tissues, such as adhesions or restrictions in muscle, tendons, and fascia.

Effects on Muscle

The basic goal of massage on muscle tissue is to "maintain the muscle in the best possible state of nutrition, flexibility, and vitality so that after recovery from trauma or disease the muscle can function at its maximum."[1] Muscle massage is done either for mechanical stretching of the intramuscular connective tissue or to relieve pain and discomfort associated with myofascial trigger points. Massage has been shown to increase blood flow to skeletal muscle, and thus to increase venous return.[27–29] It has also been shown to retard muscle atrophy following injury.[16] Massage has also been shown to increase the range of motion in hamstring muscles owing to the combined decrease in neuromuscular excitability and stretching of muscle and scar tissue.[30,106] Massage does not increase strength or bulk of muscle, nor does it increase muscle tone.

Effect on Skin

Effects of massage on the skin include an increase in skin temperature, possibly as a result of direct mechanical effects, and indirect vasomotor action. It has also been found that increased sweating and decreased skin resistance to galvanic current result from massage.

If skin becomes adherent to underlying tissues and scar tissue is formed, **friction massage** usually can be used to mechanically loosen the adhesions and soften the scar. Massage toughens yet softens the skin. It acts directly on the surface of the skin to remove dead cells that result from prolonged casting of 6–8 weeks. The effect of massage on scar tissue is that it stretches and breaks down the fibrous tissue. It can break down adhesions between skin and subcutaneous tissue and stretch contracted or adhered tissue.[31]

PSYCHOLOGICAL EFFECTS OF MASSAGE

The psychological effects of massage can be as beneficial to some patients as the physiologic effects. The "hands-on" effect helps patients feel as if someone is helping them. A general sedative effect can be most beneficial for the patient. Massage has been shown to lower psychoemotional and somatic arousal such as tension and anxiety.[32] The clinician's approach should inspire a feeling of confidence in the patient, and the patient should respond with a feeling of well-being—a feeling of being helped.

MASSAGE TREATMENT CONSIDERATIONS AND GUIDELINES

The clinician must have a basic essential knowledge of anatomy and of the particular area being treated. The physiology of the area to be treated and the total function of the patient must be considered, and the existing pathology and the process by which repair occurs must be understood. The clinician needs a thorough knowledge of massage principles and skillful techniques, as well as manual dexterity, coordination, and concentration in the use of massage techniques. The clinician also needs to exhibit such traits as patience, a sense of caring for the patient's welfare, and courteousness both in speech and manner.

Perhaps the most important tools in massage therapy are the hands of the clinician. They must be clean, warm, dry, and soft. The nails must be short and smooth. Hands must be washed before and after treatment for sanitary reasons. If the clinician's hands are cold, they should be placed in warm water for a short period. Rubbing them together briskly helps to warm them, too.

Positioning is also important for the clinician. Correct positioning will allow relaxation, prevent fatigue, and permit free movement of arms, hands, and the body. Good posture will

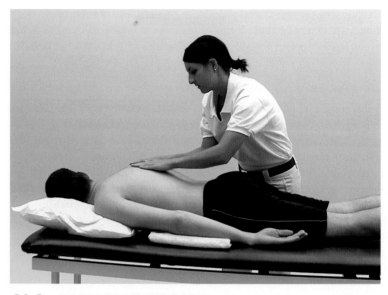

Figure 16–1. Position of clinician for stroking.

also help prevent fatigue and backache. The weight should rest evenly on both feet with the body in good postural alignment. When massaging a large area, the weight should shift from one foot to the other. You must be able to fit your hands to the contour of the area being treated. A good position is required to allow the correct application of pressure and rhythmic strokes during the procedure (Figure 16–1).

The following points are important to consider when administering massage:[33–35,102,103,111]

1. Pressure regulation should be determined by the type and amount of tissue present. It must also be governed by the patient's condition and which tissues are to be affected. The pressure must be delivered from the body, through the soft parts of the hands, and it must be adjusted to contours of the patient's body parts.

2. Rhythm must be steady and even. The time for each stroke and time between successive strokes should be equal.

3. Duration depends on the pathology, size of the area being treated, speed of motion, age, size, and condition of the patient. One also should observe the response of the patient to determine duration of the procedure. Massage of the back or the neck area might take 15–30 minutes. Massage of a large joint (such as a hip or shoulder) may require less than 10 minutes.

4. If swelling is present in an extremity, treatment should begin with the proximal part to help facilitate the lymphatic flow proximally. The subsequent effects of distal massage in removing fluid or edema will be more efficient since the proximal resistance to lymphatic flow will be reduced. This technique has been referred to as the "uncorking effect."

5. Massage should never be painful, except possibly for friction massage, nor should it be given with such force that it causes ecchymosis (discoloration of the skin resulting from contusion).

6. In general, the direction of forces should be applied in the direction of the muscle fibers (Figure 16–2).

7. During a session, one should begin with effleurage, then use maneuvers that increase progressively to the greatest energy possible, follow with maneuvers that decrease energy, and end with effleurage.

8. The clinician must consider the position in which massage can best be given and be sure the patient is warm and in a comfortable, relaxed position.

9. The body part may be elevated if this is necessary and possible.

10. The clinician should be in a position in which the whole body, as well as hands and arms, can be relaxed and the procedure accomplished without strain (see Figure 16–1).

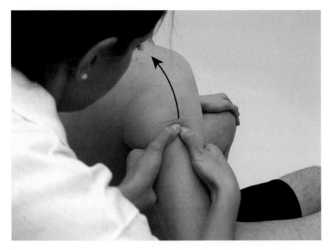

Figure 16–2. In the application of massage, forces should be applied in the direction of muscle fibers.

11. Sufficient lubricant should be used so that the clinician's hands will move smoothly along the skin surface (except in friction). The use of too much lubricant should be guarded against.
12. Massage should begin with superficial stroking; this stroke is used to spread the lubricant over the part being treated.
13. Each stroke should start at the joint or just below the joint (unless massage over joints is contraindicated) and finish above the joint so that strokes will overlap.
14. The pressure should be in line with venous flow followed by a return stroke without pressure. The pressure should be in the centripetal direction (Figure 16–3).
15. Care should be used over body areas. Hands should be relaxed and pressure adjusted to fit the contour of the area being treated.
16. Bony prominences and painful joints should be avoided if possible.
17. All strokes should be rhythmic. The pressure strokes should end with a swing off, in a small half circle, in order that the rhythm will not be broken by an abrupt reversal.

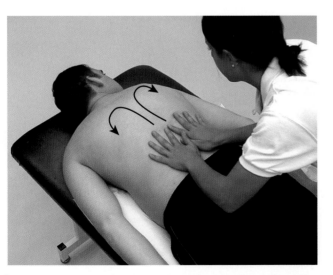

Figure 16–3. Massage pressure should be in line of venous flow followed by a return stroke without pressure. The hands should maintqin contact with the body surface.

Equipment

Table

A firm table, easily accessible from both sides, is most desirable. The height of the table should be reasonably comfortable for the clinician; leaning over or reaching up to perform the required movements should not be necessary. An adjustable table is almost a must in this situation. To facilitate cleaning and disinfecting, a washable plastic surface is much preferred. There should be a storage area close by for linens and lubricant. If the table is not padded, a mattress or foam pad should be used for the comfort of the patient.

Linens and Pillows

The patient should be draped with a sheet or a towel, so only that part to be massaged is uncovered (Figure 16–4). Towels should be handy for removing the lubricant. A cotton sheet between the plastic surface of the table and the patient is required to absorb perspiration and for patient comfort. The surface of the plastic material is generally too cool for comfort. Pillows should be available to support the patient.

Lubricant

Some type of lubricant should be used in almost all massage movements to overcome friction and avoid irritations by ensuring smooth contact of hands and skin. If the patient's skin is too oily, it may be desirable to wash the skin first.

The lubricant should be of a type that is absorbed slightly by the skin but does not make it so slippery that the clinician finds it difficult to perform the required strokes. A light oil is recommended for lubrication. One that works well is a combination of one part beeswax to three parts coconut oil. These ingredients should be melted together and allowed to cool. It is best to use oil in situations in which (1) the clinician's or patient's skin is too dry, (2) a cast has recently been removed, (3) scar tissue is present, or (4) there is excess hair. Some types of oil that may be used are olive oil, mineral oil, cocoa butter, and hydrolanolin. The "warm creams" or analgesic creams are skin irritants and if used in conjunction with massage may cause a burn, depending on the skin type of the patient. They are also thought to cause blood to come to the surface of the skin, moving away from the muscles, which is exactly the opposite of what the trainer trying to accomplish through the massage techniques.

Alcohol may be used to remove the lubricant after massage. It is suggested that alcohol be placed in the clinician's hands before application to avoid the dramatic temperature drop that occurs when alcohol is applied directly to the patient.

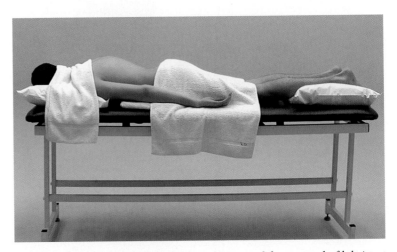

Figure 16–4. Draping of prone patient. Towels are used for removal of lubricants, sheets are used for draping, and pillows are placed under hips and ankles for patient comfort.

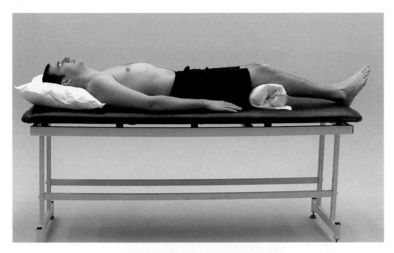

Figure 16–5. Patient supine with pillow under head and knees.

Sometimes unscented powder should be used if the clinician's hands tend to perspire or to prevent skin irritation.

Lubricant is not desired, nor should it be used, when applying friction movements, since a firm contact between the skin and hands of clinician must take place.

Preparation of the Patient

The position of the patient is probably the most important aspect of ensuring a beneficial relaxation of the muscles from massage. The patient should be in a relaxed, comfortable position. Lying down, when possible, is most beneficial to the patient. This position also permits gravity to assist in the venous flow of the blood.

The part involved in the treatment must be adequately supported. It may be elevated, depending on the pathology. When the patient is being treated in the prone position, for massage of the neck, shoulders, back, buttocks, or back of the legs, a pillow or a roll should be placed under the abdomen. Another pillow should be placed under the ankles so that the knees are slightly flexed (see Figure 16–4). If the patient is in the supine position, small pillows should be placed under the head and under the knees (Figure 16–5).

Sometimes the prone position will be too painful for a patient to assume for massaging a shoulder, upper back, or neck. A position that may be more comfortable is sitting in a chair, facing the table while leaning forward and supported by pillows on the table. Forearms and hands are on the table for additional support (Figure 16–6). The clinician can administer the massage while standing behind the patient.

The body areas not being treated should be covered to prevent the patient from being chilled. Clothing should be removed from the part being treated. Towels should cover any clothes near the area being treated to protect them from the lubricant (see Figure 16–4).

MASSAGE TREATMENT TECHNIQUES

Hoffa Massage

Albert Hoffa's Technik der Massage, published in 1900, provides the basis for the various massage techniques that have developed over the years.[36] Hoffa massage is essentially the classical massage technique that uses a variety of superficial strokes, including **effleurage**, **petrissage**, **tapotement**, and **vibration**. Although some clinicians consider this technique to be mechanical, the strokes may be lighter and more superficial, thus making them more reflexive in nature. This technique opens the door for more mechanical techniques that are directed toward underlying tissues.

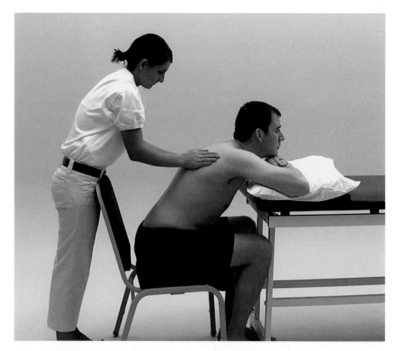

Figure 16–6. Patient resting in a chair facing table and leaning forward is supported by pillows on the table with forearms and hands on the table for support. The clinician stands behind the patient.

Effleurage

This massage maneuver glides over the skin lightly without attempting to move the deep muscle masses. The main physiologic effect occurs when stroking is begun at the peripheral areas and moves toward the heart. This process probably helps the return flow of the venous and lymphatic systems. Circulation to the skin surface also is increased by stroking; the success is traced to the increased rate of metabolic exchange in the peripheral areas.

Treatment Protocols: Massage (Hoffa Massage)

1. After applying lubricant, effleurage is applied with a stroking motion from distal to proximal with light to moderate pressure; the deeper tissue is not moved. The initial strokes serve to distribute the lubricant over the treatment area.
2. Petrissage is a kneading type motion, in which the muscles are lifted and rolled.
3. Tapotement is a series of percussion movements with the tips of the fingers, the ulnar border of the hands, the heel of the hands, or cupped hands.
4. Vibration is a rapid oscillation or tremor of the hands when they are in firm contact with the skin.

The primary purpose of effleurage is to accustom the patient to the physical contact of the clinician. Initially effleurage serves to evenly distribute the lubricant. It also allows sensitive fingers to search for areas of muscle spasm or soreness and to locate trigger points and pressure points that can help in determining the type of procedures to be used during the massage.

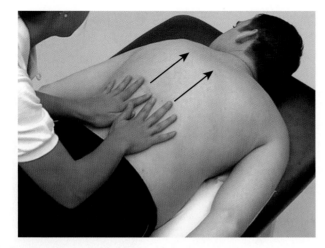

Figure 16–7. The effleurage stroke is performed with the heel of the hand, fingers slightly bent and thumbs spread.

At the start of the massage, the stroke should be performed with a light pressure, coming from the flat of the hand with fingers slightly bent and thumbs spread (Figure 16–7). Once the unidirectional flow is established, going either centripetally or centrifugally, it should be continued throughout the treatment. Movement of the stroke should be toward the heart, and contact should be maintained with the patient at all times to enhance relaxation (Figure 16–8).

Deep stroking massage is also a form of effleurage, except it is given with more pressure to produce a mechanical effect, as well as a reflexing effect (Figure 16–9).[37]

Every massage begins and ends with effleurage. Stroking should also be used between other techniques. Stroking relaxes, decreases the defensive tension against harder massage techniques, and has a generally mentally soothing effect.

Petrissage

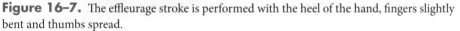

Petrissage consists of kneading manipulations that press and roll the muscles under the fingers or hands. There is no gliding over the skin except between progressions from one area to another. The muscles are gently squeezed, lifted, and relaxed. The hands may remain stationary or may travel slowly along the length of the muscle or limb. The purpose of petrissage is to increase venous and lymphatic return and to press metabolic waste products out of affected areas through intensive, vigorous action. This form of massage can also break up adhesions

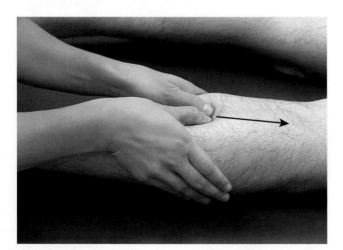

Figure 16–8. The kneading stroke is directed toward the heart, and contact should be maintained with the patient.

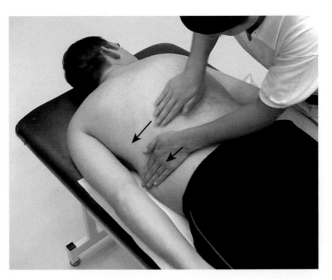

Figure 16–9. Deep stroking massage.

between the skin and underlying tissue, loosen adherent fibrous tissue, and increase skin elasticity.

Petrissage can be described as a kneading technique. It is the repeated grasping, application of pressure, releasing in a lifting or rolling motion, then moving an adjacent area (Figure 16–10). Smaller muscles may be kneaded with one hand (Figure 16–11). Larger muscles, such as the hamstrings or back muscles, will require the use of both hands. When kneading, the hands should move from the distal to the proximal point of the muscle insertion grasping parallel to or at right angles to the muscle fibers.

Tapotement or Percussion

Percussion movements are a series of brisk blows, administered with relaxed hands and following each other in rapid alternating movements. This technique has a penetrating effect that is used to stimulate subcutaneous structures. Percussion is often used to increase circulation or to get a more active flow of blood. Peripheral nerve endings are stimulated so that they convey impulses more strongly with the use of percussion techniques.

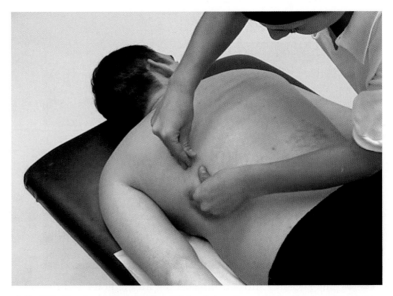

Figure 16–10. Petrissage kneading with both hands on the back.

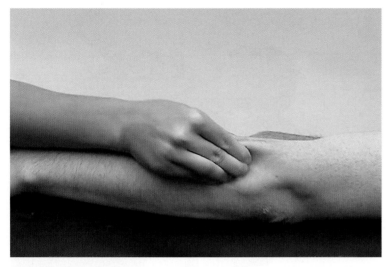

Figure 16–11. Petrissage Kneading with one hand

Types of percussion techniques are hacking, the alternate striking of the patient with the ulnar border of the hand (Figure 16–12); alternate slapping with the fingers (Figure 16–13); beating with the half-closed fist using the hypothenar eminence of the hand (Figure 16–14); tapping with the tips of the fingers (Figure 16–15); and clapping or cupping using fingers, thumb, and palm together to form a concave surface (Figure 16–16). Clapping or cupping is used primarily in postural drainage.

Clinical Decision-Making *Exercise 16-1*

A patient comes into the clinic complaining about a "knot" that is palpable in the gastrocnemius. She explains that several months earlier she had suffered a muscle strain in that same muscle and she now feels that she can not stretch out the muscle and that "it is always tight." What can the clinician do to get rid of the knot?

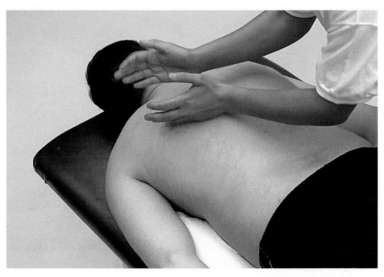

Figure 16–12. Percussion stroke striking with the ulnar border of the hand.

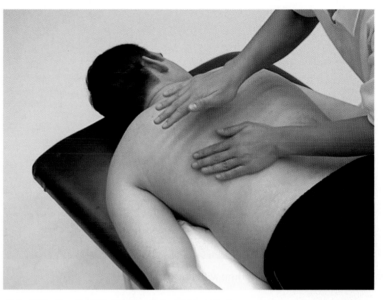

Figure 16–13. Percussion stroke of slapping with fingers.

Vibration

Vibration technique is a fine tremulous movement, made by the hand or fingers placed firmly against a part; this causes the part to vibrate. The hands should remain in contact with the patient and a rhythmic trembling movement will come from the whole forearm, through the elbow (Figure 16–17). The vibration technique is commonly used by clinicians working with patients who require postural drainage, such as individuals who have cystic fibrosis.

Routine

The following is an example of a massage progression or routine.

1. Superficial stroking
2. Deep stroking
3. Kneading

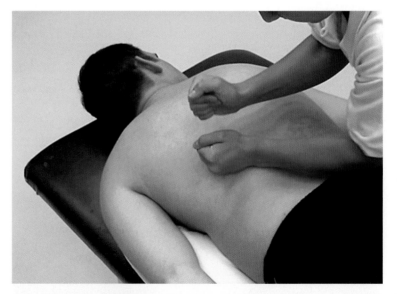

Figure 16–14. Percussion stroke of beating using a half-closed fist using hypothenar eminence.

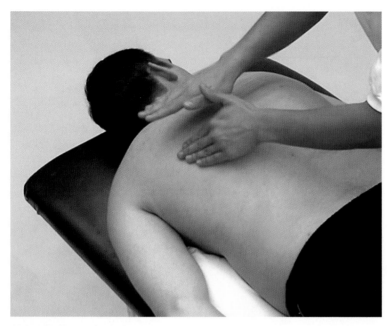

Figure 16–15. Percussion stroke using tips of fingers.

4. Optional friction or tapotement
5. Deep stroking
6. Superficial stroking

The various individual classic massage techniques alone, however, do not make for a good massage. A proper program, intensity, tempo, and rhythm, as well as the proper starting, climax, and closing of the massage, are all important, too. The form of the massage depends on the individual requirements of the patient.

Friction Massage

James Cyriax and Gillean Russell have used a technique called deep friction massage to affect musculoskeletal structures of ligament, tendon, and muscle to provide therapeutic movement

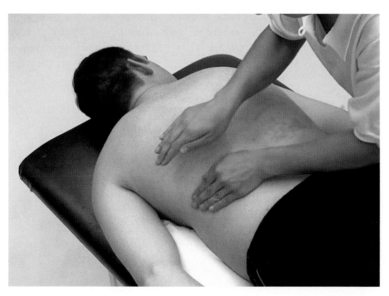

Figure 16–16. Percussion stroke of cupping using fingers, thumb, and palm together.

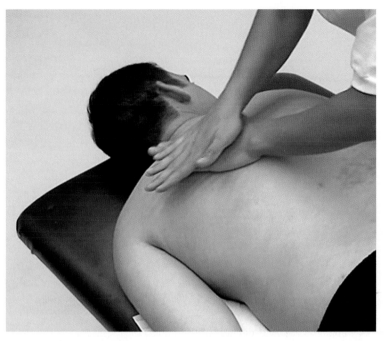

Figure 16–17. Vibration stroke.

over a small area.[38] The purposes for friction movements are to loosen adherent fibrous tissue (scar), aid in the absorption of local edema or effusions, and reduce local muscular spasm. Inflammation around joints is softened and more readily broken down so that the formation of adhesions is prevented. Another purpose is to provide deep pressure over trigger points to produce reflex effects. This technique is performed by the tips of the fingers, the thumb, or the heel of the hand, according to the area to be covered, making small circular movements (Figure 16–18). The superficial tissues are moved over the underlying structures by keeping the hand or fingers in firm contact with the skin (Figure 16–19).

Transverse Friction Massage

Transverse friction massage is a technique for treating chronic tendon inflammations.[38–40] Inflammation is an important part of the healing process. It must occur before the healing process can advance to the fibroblastic stage. In chronic inflammations, however, the inflammatory process "gets stuck" and never really accomplishes what it is supposed to. The purpose of transverse friction massage is to try to increase the inflammation to a point where the inflammatory process is complete and the injury can progress to the later stages of

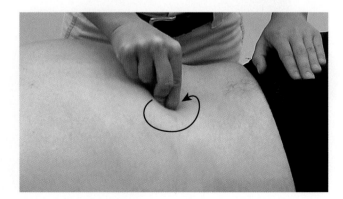

Figure 16–18. Thumb movement in a circle on an trigger point.

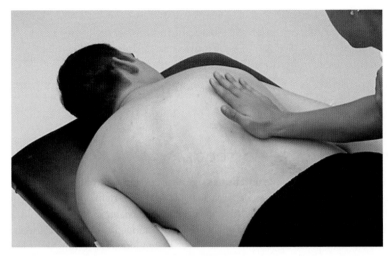

Figure 16–19. Superficial friction applied to the back by using the heel of the hand.

the healing process. This technique is used most often in chronic overuse problems such as lateral or medial humeral epicondylitis, "jumper's knee," and rotator cuff tendinitis.

The technique involves placing the tendon on a slight stretch. Massage is done using the thumb or index finger to exert intense pressure in a direction perpendicular to the direction of the fibers being massaged (Figure 16–20). The massage should last for 7–10 minutes and should be done every other day. Transverse friction massage is a painful technique, and this should be explained to the patient before beginning the massage. Because transverse friction massage is painful, it may help to apply ice to the treatment area prior to massage for analgesic purposes.

Treatment Protocols: Massage (Transverse Friction Massage)

1. No lubricant is used.
2. The tendon or ligament is placed on a slight stretch.

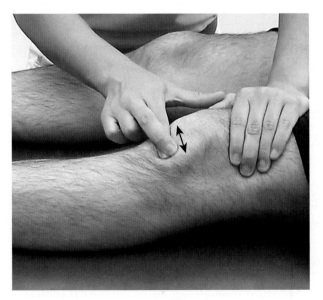

Figure 16–20. Transverse tendon friction massage on the patellar tendon.

3. Using deep pressure, such that the skin and thumb or finger move together over the deeper tissue, apply a back-and-forth motion perpendicular to the fibers of the tendon or ligament.

4. The duration of the massage should be up to 10 minutes, or as tolerated by the patient.

Connective Tissue Massage

Connective tissue massage (**Bindegewebsmassage**) was developed by Elizabeth Dicke, a German physical therapist who suffered from decreased circulation in her right lower extremity for which amputation was advised. In trying to relieve her lower back pain, she massaged the area with pulling strokes (Figure 16–21). She found that with the continued stroking the muscular tension relaxed and she felt a prickling warmth in the area. She continued the technique on herself, and after 3 months, she had no low back pain and she had restored circulation to her right leg.

Connective tissue massage is a stroking technique carried out in the layers of connective tissue on the body surface.[41] This stimulates the nerve endings of the autonomic nervous system.[42] Afferent impulses travel to the spinal cord and the brain, which causes a change in reaction susceptibility.[20]

Connective tissue is an organ of metabolism; therefore, abnormal tension in one part of the tissue is reflected in other parts.[43] All pathologic changes involve an inflammatory reaction in the affected part. One of the changes caused by inflammatory reaction is accumulation of fluid in the affected area. The area where these changes can most readily be detected is on the body surface. These changes are often seen as flattened areas or depressed bands that may be surrounded by elevated areas. The flat areas are the areas of main response and the connective tissue is tight, resisting pulling in any direction with movement.

The technique of connective tissue massage is not used as much in the United States as it is in European countries, especially Germany. As more results are seen, especially in the treatment of diseases associated with the pathology of circulation, this technique should become more widely accepted and used in this country.

General Principles of Connective Tissue Massage

Position of the patient. The patient is usually in the sitting position for a connective tissue massage. Occasionally a patient may be treated in a sidelying or prone position when he or she cannot be treated in a sitting position.

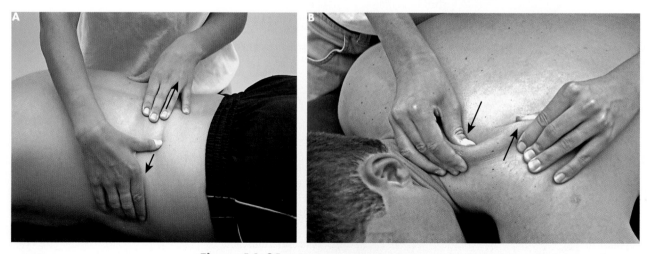

Figure 16–21. Connective tissue massage involves strokes that pull on layers of connective tissue. (a) Pulling technique, (b) Pinching technique.

Position of the clinician. The clinician should be in a position, seated or standing, that provides good body mechanics, is comfortable, and avoids fatigue.

Application technique. The basic stroke of pulling is performed with the tips, or pads, of the middle and ring fingers of either hand. Fingernails must be very short. The stroking technique is characterized by a tangential pull on the skin and subcutaneous tissues away from the fascia with the fingers. This technique should cause a sharp pain in the tissue. The stroke is a pull, not a push of the tissue. No lubricant is used. All treatments are started by the basic strokes from the coccyx to the first lumbar vertebra. Treatments last about 15–25 minutes. After 15 treatments, which are carried out two to three times per week, there should be a rest period of at least 4 weeks.

Treatment Protocols: Massage (Connective Tissue Massage)

1. No lubricant is used.
2. Using the tips of the third and fourth digits, the skin and subcutaneous tissues are pulled away from the fascia.
3. The massage extends from the coccyx to the upper lumbar area, and each pulling stroke should produce a transient, sharp pain.
4. Duration of treatment should be 15–25 minutes or as tolerated by the patient.

Other considerations. Before any logical plan for treatment can be made, it is important to determine where any alterations in the optimum function of connective tissue have taken place, where the changes started, and, if possible, the cause of the alteration.

Evaluation is a most important part of an effective connective tissue massage program. The technique of stroking with two fingers of one hand along each side of the vertebral column will give much information about the sensory changes that are caused by alterations in the tension of surface tissues.

Indications and contraindications. Numerous arterial and venous disorders may respond to connective tissue massage. Specific disabilities include (1) scars on the skin; (2) fractures and arthritis in the bones and joints; (3) lower back pain and torticollis in the muscles; (4) varicose symptoms, thrombophlebitis (subacute), hemorrhoids, and edema in the blood and lymph; and (5) Raynaud's disease, intermittent claudication, frostbite, and trophic changes in the circulatory system. Connective tissue massage can also be used for myocardial dysfunctions, respiratory disturbances, intestinal disorders, ulcers, hepatitis, infections of the ovaries and uterus (subacute), amenorrhea, dysmenorrhea, genital infantilism, multiple sclerosis, Parkinson's disease, headaches, migraines, and allergies. Connective tissue massage is recommended to help in the process of revascularization following orthopedic complications such as fractures, dislocations, and sprains.

Contraindications to connective tissue massage include tuberculosis, tumors, and mental illnesses that result from psychologic dependence.

Connective tissue massage must be learned and performed initially under the direct supervision of someone who has been taught these highly specialized techniques. More detailed information about connective tissue massage can be found listed in the references.[44-46]

Trigger Point Massage

Myofascial Trigger Points

A **myofascial trigger point** is a hyperirritable locus within a taut band of skeletal muscle, in tendons, myofascia, ligaments and capsules surrounding joints, periosteum, or the skin.[47] Trigger points may activate and become painful because of some trauma to the muscle occurring either from direct trauma or from overuse that results in some inflammatory response.[48] Like acupuncture points, pain is usually referred to areas that follow a specific pattern associated with a particular point. Stimulation of these points has also been demonstrated to result in the relief of pain.[49] Trigger points are classified as being latent or active depending on their clinical characteristics.[50] A latent trigger point does not cause spontaneous pain but may restrict movement or cause muscle weakness.[50] The patient presenting with muscle restrictions or weakness may become aware of pain originating from a latent trigger point only when pressure is applied directly over the point. An active trigger point causes pain at rest. It is tender to palpation with a referred pain pattern that is similar to the patient's pain complaint. This referred pain is felt not at the site of the trigger-point origin, but remote from it. The pain is often described as spreading or radiating. Referred pain is an important characteristic of a trigger point. It differentiates a trigger point from a tender point, which is associated with pain at the site of palpation only. Trigger points are palpable within muscles as cord-like bands within a sharply circumscribed area of extreme tenderness. They are found most commonly in muscles involved in postural support.[51] Acute trauma or repetitive microtrauma may lead to the development of stress on muscle fibers and the formation of trigger points.[52]

Treatment Protocols: Massage (Myofascial Trigger Point Massage)

1. No lubricant is used.
2. Technique is similar to transverse friction massage, but is applied to a trigger or acupuncture point (found using a chart or by palpation). Trigger points usually are nodular-like lumps in a muscle, and often feel gritty.
3. Using the tip of any digit, or even the olecranon process, the skin is moved on the trigger point; no motion should take place between the therapist and the patient's skin. The motion is circular, and is confined to the point.
4. Pressure will be painful, and as hard as the patient can tolerate. The pressure may produce pain radiating to distant areas.
5. Duration of the massage is between 1 and 5 minutes per point.

Accurate identification of true, active trigger points is essential for satisfactory outcomes. Look for these clinical characteristics:

- Patients may have regional, persistent pain resulting in a decreased range of motion in the affected muscles. These include muscles used to maintain body posture, such as those in the neck, shoulders, and pelvic girdle.
- Palpation of a hypersensitive bundle or nodule of muscle fiber of harder than normal consistency is the physical finding typically associated with a trigger point. Palpation of the trigger point will elicit pain directly over the affected area and/or cause radiation of pain toward a zone of reference and a local twitch response.[51]
- Contracting the muscle against fixed resistance significantly increases pain.
- Firm pressure applied over the point usually elicits a "jump sign," with the patient crying out, wincing, or withdrawing from the stimulus.[48]
- One or several fasciculations, called the local twitch response, may be observed when firm pressure is applied over the point.

Trigger point massage has been related to **acupressure**, a technique that is based on massage of acupuncture points.[53–55,109] Acupuncture and trigger points are not necessarily one and the same. However, a study by Melzack, Fox, and Stillwell attempted to develop a correlation coefficient between acupuncture and trigger points on the basis of two criteria: spatial distribution and associated pain patterns.[56] They found a remarkably high correlation coefficient of 0.84, which suggested that acupuncture and trigger points used for pain relief, although discovered independently, labeled by totally different methods, and derived from such histori-cally different concepts of medicine, represent a similar phenomenon and may be explained by the same underlying neural mechanisms.[56,57,109]

Physiologic explanations of the effectiveness of trigger point massage may likely be attributed to some interaction of the various mechanisms of pain modulation discussed in Chapter 4.[2] There is considerable evidence that intense, low-frequency stimulation of these points triggers the release of β -endorphin.[46,58,59]

Trigger Point Massage Techniques

Perhaps the easiest method to locate a trigger point is simply to palpate the area until either a small fibrous nodule or a strip of tense muscle tissue that is tender to the touch is felt.[60–62] Once the point is located, massage is begun using the index or middle fingers, the thumb, or per-haps the elbow. Small friction-like circular motions are used on the point (see Figure 16–18). The amount of pressure applied to these acupressure points should be determined by patient tolerance; however, it must be intense and will likely be painful to the patient. Generally, the more pressure the patient can tolerate, the more effective the treatment.

Effective treatment times range from 1 to 5 minutes at a single point per treatment. It may be necessary to massage several points during the treatment to obtain the greatest effects. If this is the case, it is best to work distal points first and to move proximally.

Clinical Decision-Making *Exercise 16-2*

A female athlete is complaining of painful menstrual cramps during practice. She is in such discomfort that she is incapable of continuing with the practice session. Is there anything that the clinician can do to immediately relieve her cramps?

During the massage, the patient will report a dulling or numbing effect and will fre-quently indicate that the pain diminishes or subsides totally during the massage. The lingering effects of acupressure massage vary tremendously from patient to patient. The effects may last for only a few minutes in some but may persist in others for several hours.

CASE STUDY 16–1
MASSAGE

Background: A 30-year-old stockbroker complains of chronic cervical myalgia ("My neck hurts."). There was no prior history of trauma and his family physician reported that his x-rays were within normal limits without evidence of degenerative changes or loss of disk space height. The patient reports no radiation of pain into the shoulders or upper extremities, but did complain of restriction in rotating his head to the left. The patient stated that he spends many hours each day at work cra-dling a telephone with his right side.

Impression: "Occupational Neck": Right Upper Trapezius and Sternocleidomastoid Muscle Spasm.

Treatment Plan: The patient was placed in a forward seated position with the head and neck supported by pillows on the treatment plinth. The arms were likewise supported by

a pillow in the lap. A small amount of pre-warmed massage lotion was applied to the right upper quarter region and a Hoffa massage commenced with light effleurage stroking begun to the SCM and upper trapezius muscles. The light effleurage stroking was followed by several minutes of deep effleurage strokes, which identified several "trigger point" areas in each muscle. Petrissage was directed at each trigger point area for approximately 30 seconds, then the massage concluded with several more minutes of deep, then superfi-cial effleurage strokes. At the completion of the massage, ex-cess lotion was removed, then the patient was instructed in cervical and upper quarter active range-of-motion exercise. The patient was encouraged to perform his home range of motion exercises each a.m. and p.m.

(continued)

CASE STUDY 16–1   (*continued*)
MASSAGE

Response: The patient reported immediate relief of his symptoms following the initial session of massage. He reported the ability to fully turn and bend his head and neck. The patient returned for two additional sessions of massage treatment and was educated as to postural habits that triggered his condition. He continued his range of motion exercises twice a day, added isometric strengthening exercises to his daily regimen, and monitored his postural habits at work. His employer subsequently added once weekly visits by a massage therapist as an employee benefit.

The rehabilitation professional employs therapeutic agent modalities to create an optimum environment for tissue healing while minimizing the symptoms associated with the trauma or condition.

Discussion Questions

- What tissues were injured or affected?
- What symptoms were present?
- What phase of the injury-healing continuum did the patient present for care in?
- What are the therapeutic agent modality's biophysical effects (direct, indirect, depth, and tissue affinity)?
- What are the therapeutic agent modality's indications and contraindications?
- What are the parameters of the therapeutic agent modality's application, dosage, duration, and frequency in this case study?
- What other therapeutic agent modalities could be utilized to treat this injury or condition? Why? How?

Strain–Counterstrain

Strain–counterstrain is an approach to decreasing muscle tension and guarding that may be used to normalize muscle function. It is a passive technique that places the body in a position of greatest comfort, thereby relieving pain.[35,63,64,107,111]

In this technique, the clinician locates a trigger point on the patient's body that corresponds to areas of dysfunction in specific joints or muscles that are in need of treatment. These tender points are not located in or just beneath the skin as are many acupuncture points, but deeper in muscle, tendon, ligament, or fascia. They are characterized by tense, tender, edematous sports on the body; they are 1 cm or less in diameter, with the most acute point 3 mm in diameter, although they may be a few centimeters long within a muscle; there may be multiple points for one specific joint dysfunction; they may be arranged in a chain; and points are often found in a painless area opposite the site of pain and/or weakness.[35,63,64]

The clinician monitors the tension and level of pain elicited by the tender point as he or she moves the patient into a position of ease or comfort. This is accomplished by markedly shortening the muscle. When this position of ease is found, the tender point is no longer tense or tender. When this position is maintained for a minimum of 90 seconds, the tension in the tender point and in the corresponding joint or muscle is reduced or cleared. By slowly returning to a neutral position, the tender point and the corresponding joint or muscle remain pain free with normal tension. For example, with neck pain and/or tension headaches, the tender points may be found on either the front or back of the patient's neck and shoulders.[24] The clinician will have the patient lay on his or her back and will gently and slowly bend the patient's neck until that tender point is no longer tender (Figure 16–22). After holding that position for 90 seconds, the clinician gently and slowly returns the patient's neck to its resting position. Upon pressing that tender point again, the patient should notice a significant decrease in pain at that tender point.[24,65]

Clinical Decision-Making   *Exercise 16–3*

A patient is complaining of pain in the middle of the upper back between the "shoulder blades" that seems to radiate to the left shoulder. What is causing this pain, and what techniques can the clinician use to eliminate this problem?

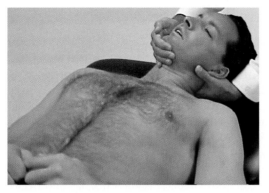

Figure 16–22. Strain–counterstrain technique. The body part is placed in a position of comfort for 90 seconds and then slowly moved back to a neutral position.

The physiologic rationale for the effectiveness of the strain–counterstrain technique can be explained by the stretch reflex. When a muscle is placed in a stretched position, impulses from the muscle spindles create a reflex contraction of the muscle in response to stretch. With strain–counterstrain, the joint or muscle is not placed in a position of stretch but rather a slack position. Thus muscle spindle input is reduced and the muscle is relaxed, allowing for a decrease in tension and pain.[24]

Positional Release Therapy

Positional release therapy (PRT) is based on the strain–counterstrain technique. The primary difference between the two is the use of a facilitating force (compression) to enhance the effect of the positioning.[66-69] Like strain–counterstrain, PRT is an osteopathic mobilization technique in which the body is brought into a position of greatest relaxation.[70] The clinician finds the position of greatest comfort and muscle relaxation for each joint with the help of movement tests and diagnostic tender points. Once located, the tender point is maintained with the palpating finger at a subthreshold pressure. The patient is then passively placed in a position that reduces the tension under the palpating finger and causes a subjective reduction in tenderness as reported by the patient. This specific position is adjusted throughout the 90-second treatment period. It has been suggested that maintaining contact with the tender point during the treatment period exerts a therapeutic effect.[67-69] This technique is one of the most effective and most gentle methods for the treatment of acute and chronic musculoskeletal dysfunction (Figure 16–23).

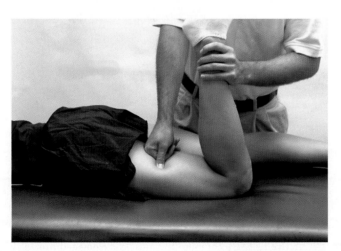

Figure 16–23. The positional release technique places the muscle in a position of comfort with the figure or thumb exerting submaximal pressure on a tender point.

Active Release Technique®

Active release technique® (ART) is a relatively new type of manual therapy that has been developed to correct soft-tissue problems in muscle, tendon, and fascia caused by formation of fibrotic adhesions as a result of acute injury, repetitive or overuse injuries, or constant pressure or tension injuries.[42,71–73,108] When a muscle, tendon, fascia, or ligament is torn (strained or sprained) or a nerve is damaged, the tissues heal with adhesions or scar tissue formation rather than the formation of brand new tissue. Scar tissue is weaker, less elastic, less pliable, and more pain sensitive than healthy tissue. These fibrotic adhesions disrupt the normal muscle function, which in turn affects the bio-mechanics of the joint complex, and can lead to pain and dysfunction. Active release technique® provides a way to diagnose and treat the underlying causes of cumulative trauma disorders that, left uncorrected, can lead to inflammation, adhesions/fibrosis, muscle imbalances resulting in weak and tense tissues, decreased circulation, hypoxia, and symptoms of peripheral nerve entrapment including numbness, tingling, burning, and aching.[72–74]

Active release technique® is a deep tissue technique used for breaking down scar tissue/adhesions and restoring function and movement. In the Active release technique®, the clinician should first, through palpation, locate those adhesions in the muscle, tendon, or fascia that are causing the problem. Once located the clinician then traps the affected muscle by applying pressure or tension with the thumb or finger over these lesions in the direction of the fibers (Figure 16–24). Then the patient is asked to actively move the body part such that the musculature is elongated from a shortened position while the clinician continues to apply tension to the lesion. This should be repeated three to five times per treatment session. By breaking up the adhesions, the patient's condition will steadily improve by softening and stretching the scar tissue, resulting in increased range of motion, increased strength, and improved circulation, which optimizes healing. Treatments tend to be uncomfortable during the movement phases as the scar tissue or adhesions tear apart. This is temporary and subsides almost immediately after the treatment. An important part of active release technique is for the patient to heed the clinician's recommendations regarding activity modification, stretching, and exercise.[42,71–73,75,76]

Myofascial Release

Myofascial release is a term that refers to a group of techniques used for the purpose of relieving soft tissue from the abnormal grip of tight fascia.[77,78] It is essentially a form of stretching

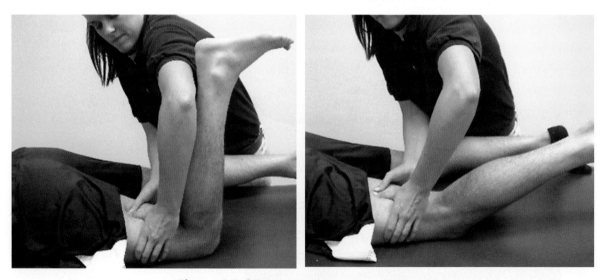

Figure 16–24. Active release technique. The muscle is elongated from a shortened position while static pressure is applied to the tender point.

that has been reported to have significant impact in treating a variety of conditions.[47] Some specialized training is necessary for the clinician to understand specific techniques of myofascial release, in addition to an in-depth understanding of the fascial system.[78,79]

Fascia is a type of connective tissue that surrounds muscles, tendons, nerves, bones, and organs. It is essentially continuous from head to toe and is interconnected in various sheaths or planes. Fascia is composed primarily of collagen along with some elastic fibers. During movement the fascia must stretch and move freely. If there is damage to the fascia owing to injury, disease, or inflammation, it will not only affect local adjacent structures but may also affect areas far removed from the site of the injury.[47] Thus it may be necessary to release tightness in both the area of injury as well as in distant areas.[77,80] It will tend to soften and release in response to gentle pressure over a relatively long period of time.[77,81]

Myofascial release has also been referred to as soft-tissue mobilization, although technically all forms of massage involve mobilization of soft tissue.[20,82] Soft-tissue mobilization should not be confused with joint mobilization, although it must be emphasized that the two are closely related. Joint mobilization is used to restore normal joint arthrokinematics, and specific rules exist regarding direction of movement and joint position based on the shape of the articulating surfaces. Myofascial restrictions are considerably more unpredictable and may occur in many different planes and directions.[83]

Myofascial treatment is based on localizing the restriction and moving into the direction of the restriction regardless of whether that follows the arthrokinematics of a nearby joint.[18] (Figure 16–25) Thus, myofascial manipulation is considerably more subjective and relies heavily on the experience of the clinician.[84]

Clinical Decision-Making   *Exercise 16–4*

A basketball player has a chronic case of patellar tendinitis. The clinician has taken usual anti-inflammatory measures (i.e., rest. medications, etc.) in treating the problem but it has not improved. Suggest an alternative treatment for chronic inflammation.

Myofascial manipulation focuses on large treatment areas, whereas joint mobilization focuses on a specific joint. Releasing myofascial restrictions over a large treatment area can have significant impact on joint mobility.[85] Once a myofascial restriction is located, the massage should be directly through the restriction. The progression of the technique is from superficial to deep. Once more superficial restrictions are released, the deep restrictions can be located and released without causing any damage to superficial tissues. Joint mobilization should follow myofascial release and will likely be more effective once soft-tissue restrictions are eliminated.[86]

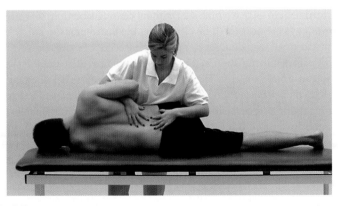

Figure 16–25. Myofascial release is a mild combination of pressure and stretch used to free soft-tissue restrictions.

As the extensibility is improved in the myofascia, elongation and stretching of the musculotendinous unit should be incorporated.[87] In addition, strengthening exercises are recommended to enhance neuromuscular reeducation, which helps promote new, more efficient movement patterns. As freedom of movement improves, postural reeducation may help to ensure the maintenance of the less restricted movement patterns.[79,86]

Generally, acute cases tend to resolve in just a few treatments. The longer a condition has been present, the longer it will take to resolve. Occasionally dramatic results will occur immediately after treatment. It is usually recommended that treatment should be performed at least three times per week.[30]

Treatment Considerations

Protecting the hands. The hands are the primary treatment modality in all forms of massage. Certainly, in myofascial release they are constantly subjected to stress and strain and consideration must be given to protection of the clinician's hands. It is essential to avoid constant hyperextension or hyperflexion of any joints, which may lead to hypermobility. If it is necessary to work in deeper tissues where more force is necessary, then the fist or elbow may be substituted for the thumb and fingers.[18] It bears repeating that hands are the most important tool in massage.

Use of lubricant. It is necessary to use a small amount of lubricant, particularly if large areas are to be treated using long stroking movements. Enough lubricant should be used to allow for traction while reducing painful friction without allowing the hands to slip on the skin.[18]

Positioning of the patient. As with the other forms of massage, it is critical to appropriately position the patient such that the effects of the treatment may be maximized. Pillows or towel rolls may be a great aid in establishing an effective treatment position even before the hands contact the patient (see Figure 16–5). The clinician should make certain that good body mechanics and positioning are considered to protect the clinician as well as the patient.

Graston Technique®

The Graston Technique® is an instrument-assisted soft-tissue mobilization that enables clinicians to effectively break down scar tissue and fascial restrictions as well as to stretch connective tissue and muscle fibers[74,88] (Figure 16–26). The technique utilizes six hand-held specially designed stainless steel instruments, shaped to fit the contour of the body, to scan an area, locate, and then treat the injured tissue that is causing pain and restricting motion.[89] A clinician normally will palpate a painful area looking for unusual nodules, restrictive barriers, or tissue tensions. The instruments help to magnify existing restrictions, which the clinician can feel through the instruments.[88] Then, the clinician can utilize the instruments to supply precise pressure to break up scar tissue, which relieves the discomfort and helps restore normal function. The instruments, with a narrow surface area at the edge, have the ability to separate fibers.

A specially designed lubricant is applied to the skin prior to utilizing the instrument, allowing the instrument to glide over the skin without causing irritation. Using a cross-friction massage in multiple directions, which involves using the instruments to stroke or rub against the grain of the scar tissue, the clinician creates small amounts of trauma to the affected area.[17] This temporarily causes inflammation in the area, which in turn increases the rate and amount of blood flow in and around the area. The theory is that this process helps initiate and promote the healing process of the affected soft tissues. It is common for the patient to experience some discomfort during the procedure and possibly some bruising. Ice application following the treatment may ease the discomfort. It is recommended that an exercise, stretching, and strengthening program be used in conjunction with the technique to help the injured tissues heal.

Rolfing

Rolfing, also referred to as *structural integration*, is a system Ida Rolf devised to correct inefficient structure or to "integrate structure."[90–94] The goal of this technique is to balance the body

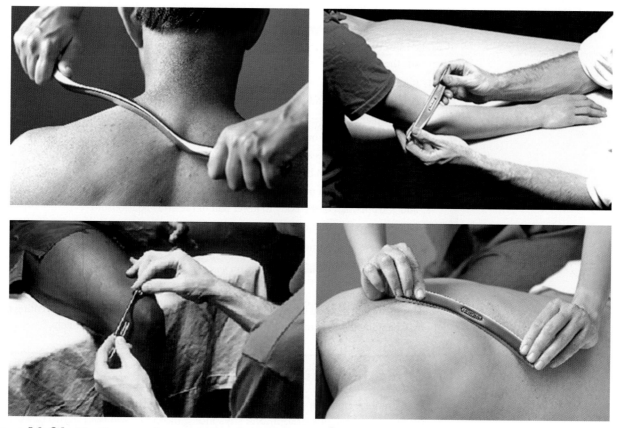

Figure 16–26. The Graston technique uses handheld stainless steel instruments to locate and then separate existing restrictions within muscle.

within a gravitational field through a technique involving manual soft-tissue manipulation.[18] The basic principle of treatment is that if balanced movement is essential at a particular joint yet nearby tissue is restrained, both the tissue and the joint will relocate to a position that accomplishes a more appropriate equilibrium (Figure 16–27).[95,96] It works on the connective tissue to realign the body structurally, harmonizing its fundamental movement patterns in relation to gravity. Rolfing is said to enhance posture and freedom of movement.

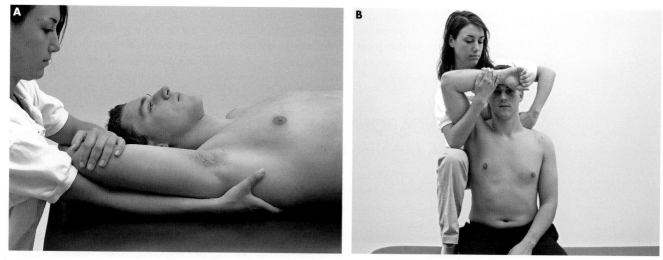

Figure 16–27. Rolfing techniques.

Rolfing is a standardized approach that is administered without regard to symptoms or specific pathologies. The technique involves 10 hour-long sessions, each of which emphasizes some aspect of posture with the massage directed toward the myofascia.[93] The 10 sessions include the following.

1. Respiration.
2. Balance under the body (legs and feet).
3. Sagittal plane balance: lateral line from front to back.
4. Balance left to right: base of body to midline.
5. Pelvic balance: rectus abdominis and psoas.
6. Weight transfer from head to feet: sacrum.
7. Relationship of head to rest of body: occiput and atlas.
8. and 9. Upper half of the body to lower half of the body relationship.
10. Balance throughout the system.

Once these 10 treatments are completed, advanced sessions may be performed in addition to periodic "tune-up" sessions.

A major aspect of this treatment approach is to integrate the structural with the psychologic. An emotional state may be seen as the projection of structural imbalances. The easiest and most efficient method for changing the physical body is through direct intervention in the body. Changing the structural imbalances can alter the psychologic component.[96]

Clinical Decision-Making   Exercise 16–5

A swimmer wants the clinician to give her a full body massage after a particularly difficult workout. She says that a massage will help her to get rid of the lactic acid in her muscles. How should the clinician respond to this request?

Trager

Developed by Milton Trager, **Trager** combines mechanical soft-tissue mobilization and neurophysiologic reeducation.[97-99] Unlike Rolfing, Trager has no standardized protocols or procedures. The Trager system uses gentle, passive, rocking oscillations of a body part. This is essentially a mobilization technique emphasizing traction and rotation as a relaxation technique to encourage the patient to relinquish control. This relaxation technique is followed by a series of active movements designed to alter the patient's neurophysiologic control of movement, thus providing a basis for maintaining these changes. This technique does not attempt to make mechanical changes in the soft tissues but rather to establish neuromuscular control, so that more normal movement patterns can be routinely performed. Essentially it uses the nervous system to make changes rather than making mechanical changes in the tissues themselves.[99]

INDICATIONS AND CONTRAINDICATIONS FOR MASSAGE

The conditions that most often motivate patients to get treatment involve muscle, tendon, and joint problems. Adhesions, muscle spasm, myositis, bursitis, fibrositis, tendinitis or tenosynovitis, and postural strain of the back all generally fall into this category.[100]

Areas of concern that indicate a patient should not be treated with massage include arteriosclerosis, thrombosis or embolism, severe varicose veins, acute phlebitis, cellulitis, synovitis, abscesses, skin infections, cancers, and pregnancy. Acute inflammatory conditions of the skin, soft tissues, or joints are also contraindications.[101] Table 16–1 summarizes indications and contraindications for massage.

Table 16–1 Indications and Contraindications for Therapeutic Massage

INDICATIONS	CONTRAINDICATIONS
Increase coordination	Arteriosclerosis
Decrease pain	Thrombosis
Decrease neuromuscular	Embolism
Excitibility	Severe varicose veins
Stimulate circulation	Acute phlebitis
Facilitate healing	Cellulitis
Restore joint mobility	Synovitis
Remove lactic acid	Abscesses
Alleviate muscle cramps	Skin infections
Increase blood flow	Cancers
Increase venous return	Acute inflammatory conditions
Retard muscle atrophy	
Increase range of motion	
Edema	
Myofascial trigger points	
Stretching scar tissue	
Adhesions	
Muscle spasm	
Myositis	
Bursitis	
Fibrositis	
Tendinitis	
Revascularization	
Raynaud's disease	
Intermittent claudication	
Dysmenorrhea	
Headaches	
Migraines	

SUMMARY

1. Massage is the mechanical stimulation of tissue by means of rhythmically applied pressure and stretching. It allows the clinician, as a health care provider, to assist a patient to overcome pain and to relax through the application of the therapeutic massage techniques.

2. Massage has effects on the circulation, the lymphatic system, the nervous system, the muscles, myofascia, the skin, scar tissue, psychologic responses, relaxation feelings, and pain.

3. Hoffa massage is the classic form of massage and uses strokes that include effleurage, petrissage, percussion or tapotement, and vibration.

4. Friction massage is used to increase the inflammatory response, particularly in cases of chronic tendinitis or tenosynovitis.

5. Massage of acupuncture and trigger points is used to reduce pain and irritation in anatomic areas known to be associated with specific points.

6. Connective tissue massage is a reflex zone massage. It is a relatively new form of treatment in this country and has its best effects on circulatory pathologies.

7. Myofascial release is a massage technique used for the purpose of relieving soft tissue from the abnormal grip of tight fascia.

8. Rolfing is a system devised to correct inefficient structure by balancing the body within a gravitational field through a technique involving manual soft-tissue manipulation.

9. Trager attempts to establish neuromuscular control so that more normal movement patterns can be routinely performed.

REVIEW QUESTIONS

1. What are the physiologic effects of massage?
2. What are the reflexive effects of massage on pain, circulation, and metabolism?
3. What are the mechanical effects of massage on muscle and skin?
4. What psychologic benefits can come with massage?
5. What are the various considerations for setting up equipment and preparing a patient for massage?
6. What are the various stroking techniques used in traditional Hoffa massage?
7. What are the clinical applications for using friction massage?
8. What is connective tissue massage most often used for?
9. What is the difference between acupuncture points and myofascial trigger points?
10. How can myofascial release be used to restore normal functional movement patterns?

SELF-TEST QUESTIONS

True or False

1. Massage will increase blood and lymphatic flow.
2. The "uncorking effect" states massage on a limb with edema should begin distally.
3. The direction of stroking usually follows muscle fibers.

Multiple Choice

4. Which type of massage "kneads" tissue by lifting, rolling, or pressing intermittently?
   a. Effleurage
   b. Petrissage
   c. Tapotement
   d. Vibration

5. Pain relief is one of the reflexive effects of massage. What are the other two effects?
   a. Increased muscle elasticity and decreased adhesions.
   b. Increased muscle elasticity and elongated fascia.
   c. Decreased circulation and metabolism.
   d. Increased circulation and metabolism.

6. Which type of massage does NOT require lubricant?
   a. Petrissage
   b. Effleurage
   d. Hoffa
   d. Friction

7. Acupressure massage technique requires the therapist to identify trigger points and then apply
   a. Pressure
   b. Bindegewebsmassage
   c. Friction
   d. Lubricant
8. Which of the following massage techniques is designed to balance the body by manipulating soft tissue?
   a. Hoffa
   b. Trager
   c. Rolfing
   d. Acupuncture
9. Which of the following is a contraindication to massage?
   a. Acute inflammatory conditions
   b. Edema
   c. Raynaud's disease
   d. Tendinitis
10. Superficial stroking may be utilized at the
    a. Beginning of the massage
    b. End of the massage
    c. Both a and b
    d. Neither a nor b

SOLUTIONS TO CLINICAL DECISION-MAKING EXERCISES

16–1
The clinician may choose to use a petrissage technique, which involves a deep kneading technique. Petrissage is often used to break up adhesions in the underlying muscle and also to assist the lymphatic system in removing waste from the area.

16–2
Acupressure massage to several acupuncture points may help eliminate her cramps in a few minutes by massaging one or several points. The tender points are located 2 inches to the right of T12, 2 inches bilateral to T10, and bilaterally over the first sacral openings. Using a circular massage of these points can potentially eliminate the cramps for several hours.

16–3
It is likely that the patient has a myofascial trigger point in the rhomboids. The clinician could try several different techniques that have proven to be effective, including circular pressure massage, a spray-and-stretch technique (Chapter 4), or a combination of ultrasound and electrical stimulation (Chapter 5).

16–4
A transverse friction massage may help to "jump start" the inflammatory process, thus allowing the healing process to progress to the latter stages. It should be explained that the treatment will be somewhat painful and that the problem should actually get worse before it gets better.

16–5
The clinician should point out that massage post-exercise has not been demonstrated to effectively remove lactic acid. The clinician should also inform the patient that if she has a specific problem that can be helped by incorporating massage, then he or she will be glad to use the technique. However, the policy is generally not to provide full body massage for relaxation purposes.

REFERENCES

1. Wood E, Becker P. *Beard's Massage.* Philadelphia, PA: W.B. Saunders; 1981.
2. Archer PA. *Massage for Sports Health Care Professionals.* Champaign, IL: Human Kinetics; 1999.
3. Archer PA. Three clinical sports massage approaches for treating injured patients, *Athl Ther Today.* 2001;6(3):14–20,36–37,60.
4. Bell GW. Aquatic sports massage therapy. *Clin Sports Med.* 1999;18(2):427–435.
5. Birukov A. Training massage during contemporary sports loads. *Soviet Sports Rev.* 1987;22:42–44.
6. Gazzillo L, Middlemas D. Therapeutic massage techniques for three common injuries. *Athl Ther Today.* 2001;6(3):5–9.
7. Lewis J, Johnson B. The clinical effectiveness of therapeutic massage for musculoskeletal pain: a systematic review. *Physiotherapy.* 2006;92:146–158.
8. Robello N. Therapeutic Massage. *Athl Ther Today.* 2007;12(3):27.
9. Stone JA. Massage as a therapeutic modality—technique. *Athl Ther Today.* 1999;4(5):51–52.
10. Stone JA. Prevention and rehabilitation. Myofascial techniques: trigger-point therapy. *Athl Ther Today.* 2000;5(3):54–55.
11. Vaughn B, Miller K, Fink D. *Massage for Sports Health Care.* Champaign, IL: Human Kinetics; 1998.
12. Hungerford M, Bornstein R. *Sports Massage. Sports Med Guide.* 1985;4:4–6.
13. Kopysov V. Use of vibrational massage in regulating the pre-competition condition of weight lifters. *Soviet Sports Rev.* 1979;14:82–84.
14. Kuprian W. Massage. In: Kuprian W, ed. *Physical Therapy for Sports.* Philadelphia, PA: WB Saunders; 1995.
15. Morelli M, Seaborne PT, Sullivan SJ. Changes in H-reflex amplitude during massage of triceps surae in healthy subjects. *J Orthop Sports Phys Ther.* 1990;12(2):55–59.
16. Sullivan S. Effects of massage on alpha motorneuron excitability. *Phys Ther.* 1991;71:555.
17. Hammer W. Treatment of a case of subacute lumbar compartment syndrome using the Graston technique. *J Manipulative Physiol Ther.* 2005;28(3):199–204.
18. Cantu R, Grodin A. *Myofascial Manipulation:Theory and Clinical Applications.* Gaithersburg, MD: Aspen; 2001.
19. Barr J, Taslitz N. Influence of back massage on autonomic functions. *Phys Ther.* 1970;50:1679–1691.
20. Mennell J. *Physical Treatment,* 5th ed.. Philadelphia, PA: Blakiston; 1968.
21. Pemberton R. The physiologic influence of massage. In: Mock HE, Pemberton R, Coulter JS, eds. *Principles and Practices of Physical Therapy.* Vol. I. Hagerstown, MD: WF Prior; 1939.
22. Ebel A, Wisham L. Effect of massage on muscle temperature and radiosodium clearance. *Arch Phys Med.* 1952;33:399–405.
23. Cafarelli E. Vibratory massage and short-term recovery from muscular fatigue. *Int J Sports Med.* 1990;11:474.
24. Hemmings B, Smith M, Graydon J, Dyson R. Effects of massage on physiological restoration, perceived recovery, and repeated sports performance. *Br J Sports Med.* 2000;34(2):109–114.
25. Martin NA, Zoeller RF, Robertson RJ. The comparative effect of sports massage, active recovery, and rest on promoting blood lactate clearing after supramaximal leg exercise. *J Athl Train.* 1998;33(1):30–35.
26. Boone T, Cooper R, Thompson W. A physiologic evaluation of the sports massage. *Athl Train.* 1991;26(1):51–54.
27. Dubrovsky V. Changes in muscle and venous blood flow after massage. *Soviet Sports Rev.* 1983;18:164–165.
28. Wyper D, McNiven D. Effects of some physiotherapeutic agents on skeletal muscle blood flow. *Phys Ther.* 1976;62:83–85.
29. Zainuddin Z, Newton M, Sacco P. Effects of massage on delayed-onset muscle soreness, swelling, and recovery of muscle function. *J Athl Train.* 2005;40(3):174–180.
30. Crosman L, Chateauvert S, Weisberg J. The effects of massage to the hamstring muscle group on range of motion. *J Orthop Sport Phys Ther.* 1984;6:168.
31. Patino O, Novick C, Merlo A, Benaim F. Massage in hypertrophic scars, *J Burn Care Rehabil.* 1999;20(3):268–271.
32. Longworth J. Psychophysiological effects of slow stroke back massage in normotensive females. *Adv Nurs Sci.* 1982;10:44–61.
33. Moraska A. Sports massage: a comprehensive review. *J Sports Med Phys Fitness.* 2005;45(3):370–380.
34. Tessier D, Draper D. Therapeutic modalities. Sports massage: an overview. *Athletic Therapy Today.* 2005;10(5):67–69.
35. Wheeler L. Advanced strain counterstrain. *Massage Therapy Journal.* 2005;43(4):84–95.
36. Hoffa A. *Technik der massage,* 14th ed. Stuttgart: Ferdinand Enke; 1900.
37. Hart J, Swanik C, Tierney R. Effects of sport massage on limb girth and discomfort associated with eccentric exercise. *J Athl Train.* 2005;40(3):181–185.
38. Cyriax J, Russell G. *Textbook of Orthopedic Medicine.* Baltimore, MD: Williams & Wilkins; 1982.
39. Longhmani M, Avin K, Burr D. Instrument-assisted cross-fiber massage accelerates knee ligament healing. *J Orthop Sports Phys Ther.* 2006;36(1):A7.
40. Trivette K, Boyce D, Brosky J. Cross-friction massage: a review of the evidence (abstract). *J Orthop Sports Phys Ther.* 2004;34(1):A56.
41. Latz J. Key elements of connective tissue massage. *J Massage Ther.* 2003;41(4):44–45,46–50,52–53.
42. George J. The effects of active release technique on hamstring flexibility: a pilot study. *J Manipulative Physiol Ther.* 2006;29(3):224–227.

43. Holey EA. Connective tissue massage: a bridge between complementary and orthodox approaches. *Bodyw Mov Ther.* 2000;4(1):72–80.

44. Ebner M. *Ebner's Connective Tissue Manipulation for Bodyworkers.* Malibar, FL: R.E. Krieger; 1995.

45. Licht S. *Massage, Manipulation and Traction.* New Haven, CT: Elizabeth Licht; 1976.

46. Tappan F, Benjamin P. *Healing massage techniques: holistic, classic, and emerging methods.* Upper Saddle River, NJ: Prentice Hall; 2004.

47. Stone JA. Myofascial release. Athl Ther Today. 2000;5(4): 34–35.

48. Travell J, Simons D. *Myofascial Pain and Dysfunction: The Trigger Point Manual.* Baltimore, MD: Lippincott, Williams & Wilkins; 1998.

49. Fox E, Melzack R. Transcutaneous electrical stimulation and acupuncture: comparison of treatment for low back pain. *Pain.* 1976;2:357–373.

50. Simons DG. Understanding effective treatments of myofascial trigger points. *J Bodyw Mov Ther.* 2002;6(2): 81–88.

51. Hou C. Immediate effects of various physical therapeutic modalities on cervical myofascial pain and trigger-point sensitivity. *Arch Phys Med Rehab.* 2002;83(10):1406–1414.

52. Sefton J. Myofascial release for clinicians, part 2: guidelines and techniques. *Athl Ther Today.* 2004;9(2):52.

53. Man P, Chen C. Acupuncture aesthesia—a new theory and clinical study. *Curr Ther Res.* 1972;14:390–394.

54. Manaka Y. On certain electrical phenomena for the interpretation of chi in Chinese literature. *Am J Chin Med.* 1975;3: 71–74.

55. Mann F. *Acupuncture: The Ancient Chinese Art of Healing and How it Works Scientifically.* New York: Random House; 1973.

56. Melzack R, Stillwell D, Fox E. Trigger points and acupuncture points for pain: correlations and implications. *Pain.* 1977;3:3–23.

57. Wei L. Scientific advances in Chinese medicine. *Am J Chin Med.* 1979;7:53–75.

58. Prentice W. The use of electroacutherapy in the treatment of inversion ankle sprains. *J Nat Athl Train Assoc.* 1982; 17(1):15–21.

59. Sjolund B, Eriksson M. Electroacupuncture and endogenous morphines. *Lancet.* 1976;2:1085.

60. Brickey R, Yao J. *Acupuncture and Transcutaneous Electrical Stimulation Techniques: Course Manual in Acutherapy Post Graduate Seminars.* Raleigh, NC; 1978.

61. Castel J. *Pain Management with Acupuncture and Transcutaneous Electrical Nerve Stimulation Techniques and Photo Stimulation (Laser), Course Manual;* 1982.

62. Cheng R, Pomerantz B. Electroacupuncture analgesia could be mediated by at least two pain relieving mechanisms: endorphin and non-endorphin systems. *Life Sci.* 1979;25:1957–1962.

63. Jones L. *Strain-Counterstrain.* Boise, ID: Jones; 1995.

64. Meseguer A, Fernández-de-las-Peñas C. Immediate effects of the strain/counterstrain technique in local pain evoked by tender points in the upper trapezius muscle. *Clin Chiropr.* 2006;9(3):112–118.

65. Alexander KM. Use of strain-counterstrain as an adjunct for treatment of chronic lower abdominal pain. *Phys Ther Case Rep.* 1999;2(5):205–208.

66. Birmingham, T. Effect of a positional release therapy technique on hamstring flexibility. *Physiother Can.* 2004; 56(3):165–170.

67. Chaitlow L. *Positional Release Techniques (Advanced Soft Tissue Techniques).* Philadelphia, PA: Churchill Livingstone; 2007.

68. Chaitow L. Positional release techniques in the treatment of muscle and joint dysfunction. *Clin Bull Myofascial Ther.* 1998;3(1):25–35.

69. Speicher T, Draper D. Therapeutic modalities: top 10 positional-release therapy techniques to break the chain of pain, parts 1 & 2. *Athl Ther Today.* 2006;11(6):56–58,60–62.

70. D'Ambrogio K, Roth G. *Positional Release Therapy: Assessment and Treatment of Musculoskeletal Dysfunction.* St. Louis, MO: Mosby-Yearbook; 1997.

71. Drover J. Influence of active release technique on quadriceps inhibition and strength: a pilot study. *J Manipulative Physiol Ther.* 2004;27(6):408–413.

72. Leahy M. *Active Release Techniques Soft Tissue Management System Manual.* Colorado Springs, CO: Active Release Techniques, LLP; 1996.

73. Leahy M. Improved treatments for carpal tunnel and related syndromes. *Chiropr Sports Med.* 1995;9(1):6–9.

74. Howitt S, Wong J. The conservative treatment of trigger thumb using Graston techniques and active release techniques. *J Can Chiropr Assoc.* 2006;50(4):249–254.

75. Buchberger D. Use of active release techniques in the post operative shoulder. *J Sports Chiropr Rehab.* 1999;2(6):60–65.

76. Wenban A. Influence of active release technique on quadriceps inhibition and strength: a pilot study. *J Manipulative Physiol Ther.* 2005;28(1):73.

77. Juett T. Myofascial release—an introduction for the patient. *Phys Ther Forum.* 1988;7(41):7–8.

78. Manheim C. *The Myofascial Release Manual.* Thorofare, NJ: Slack Inc.; 2008.

79. Barnes J. Five years of myofascial release. *Phys Ther Forum.* 1987;6(37):12–14.

80. Thomas B. Alleviating atypical tender points through the use of myofascial release of scar tissue. *AAO Journal.* 2007; 17(2):19–24.

81. Luchau T. Myofascial techniques. Working with the cervical core. *Massage Bodyw.* 2009;24(2):122–125,127.

82. Arroyo-Morales M, Olea N. Effects of myofascial release after high-intensity exercise: a randomized clinical trial. *J Manipulative Physiol Ther.* 2008;31(3):217–223.

83. Paolini J, Hubbard T. Review of myofascial release as an effective massage therapy technique. *Athl Ther Today.* 2009;14(5):30–34.

84. Remvig L. Myofascial release: an evidence-based treatment concept? *J Bodyw Mov Ther*. 2008;12(4):385–386.

85. Gordon P. *Myofascial Reorganization*. Brookline, MA: The Gordon Group; 1988.

86. Kierns M. *Myofascial Release in Sports Medicine*. Champaign, Il: Human Kinetics; 2000.

87. Mock LE. Myofascial release treatment of specific muscles of the upper extremity (levels 3 and 4): part 4. *Clin Bull Myofascial Ther*. 1998;3(1):71–93.

88. DeLuccio J. Instrument assisted soft tissue mobilization utilizing Graston Technique: a physical therapist's perspective. *Orthop Phys Ther Pract*. 2006;18(3):32–34.

89. Larkins P, Kass J. Graston technique. *Podiatry Manage*. 2008; 27(1):37–38.

90. Bernau-Eigen M. Rolfing: a somatic approach to the integration of human structures. *Nurse Pract Forum*. 1998;9(4): 235–242.

91. el-Rif J. Rolfing: transformative method of structural integration. *Posit Health*. 2005(117):48–51.

92. James H, Castaneda L. Rolfing structural integration treatment of cervical spine dysfunction. *J Bodyw Mov Ther*. 2009;13(3):229–238.

93. Jones T. Rolfing, Physical Medicine and Rehabilitation. *Clin North Am*. 2004;(4):799–809.

94. Smith H. Rolfing: experience rolfing. *Massage Today*. 2005; 5(7):1,14.

95. Kallen B. Deep impact: rolfing is deeper than the deepest massage—and sometimes more painful. Some patients swear by it anyway. *Men's Fit*. 2000;16(7):96–99.

96. Rolf I. *Rolfing and Physical Reality*. Rochester, VT: Healing Arts Press; 1990.

97. Dalford H, Kingston J. The Trager Approach: what is Trager®? *Posit Health*. 2008;18(3):32–34.

98. Tolle R. The Trager Approach. *Massage Ther J*, 44(1):60-7, 2005.

99. Trager M. Trager psychophysical integration and mentastics. *Trager J.*, 1982;5:10.

100. Horowitz S. Evidence-based indications for therapeutic massage. *Altern Complement Ther*. 2007;13(1):30–35.

101. Batavia M. Contraindications for therapeutic massage: do sources agree? *J Bodyw Mov Ther*.2004;8(1):48–57.

102. Beck M. *Theory and Practice of Therapeutic Massage*, 4th ed. Clifton Park, NJ: Delmar Learning; 2005.

103. Braverman DL, Schulman RA. Massage techniques in rehabilitation medicine. *Phys Med Rehab Clin North Am*. 1999; 10(3):631–649.

104. Elkins E. Effects of various procedures on flow of lymph. *Arch Phys Med*. 1953;34:31–39.

105. Ernst E. Does post-exercise massage treatment reduce delayed onset muscle soreness? A systematic review. *Br J Sports Med*. 1998;32(3):212–214.

106. Harmer P. The effect of preperformance massage on stride frequency in sprinters. *Athl Train*. 1991;26(1):55–59.

107. Heller M. Low-force manual adjusting: "strain-counterstrain." *Dyn Chiropr*. 2003;221(12):16,18.

108. Howitt S. Lateral epicondylosis: a case study of conservative care utilizing ART and rehabilitation. *J Can Chiropr Assoc*. 2006;50(3):182–189.

109. *Hwang Ti Nei Ching* (translation), Berkeley, CA: University of California Press; 1973.

110. King R. *Performance Massage*. Champaign, IL: Human Kinetics; 1993.

111. Lewis C. The use of strain-counterstrain in the treatment of patients with low back pain. *J Man Manip Ther*. 2001;9(2):92–98.

112. Marshall L. Back to basics. *Altern Med Mag*. 2006;92: 70–74.

113. Hart J., Swanik B, Tierney, R. Effects of sport massage on limb girth and discomfort associated with eccentric exercise. *Journal of Athletic Training*. 2005;40(3): 181–185.

114. Stone JA. Prevention and rehabilitation. The rationale for therapeutic massage. *Athl Ther Today*. 1999;4(4):26.

SUGGESTED READINGS

Barnes M, Personius W, Gronlund R. An efficacy study on the effect on myofascial release treatment technique on obtaining pelvic symmetry. *Phys Ther*. 1994;19(1):56.

Basmajian J. *Manipulation, Traction and Massage*. Baltimore, MD: Williams & Wilkins;1985.

Bean B, Henderson H, Martinsen M. Massage: how to do it and what it can do for you. *Scholast Coach*. 1982;52(5):10–11.

Beard G. A history of massage technique. *Phys Ther Rev*. 1952; 32:613–624.

Beck M. *Theory and Practice of Therapeutic Massage*. Clifton Park, NY: ThomsonDelmar Learning; 2006.

Breakey B. An overlooked therapy you can use ad lib. *RN*. 1982;45:7.

Cambron J, Dexheimer J. Changes in blood pressure after various forms of therapeutic massage: a preliminary study. *J Altern Complement Med*. 2006;12(1):65–70.

Chamberlain G. Cyriax's friction massage: a review. *J Orthop Sports Phys Ther*. 1982;4(1):16–22.

Chiropractic approach to pain relief, rehabilitative care. *J Am Chiropr Assoc*. 2009;46(6):16–17.

Cyriax J. *Textbook of Orthopedic Medicine*. 8th ed. Vol I. New York: Macmillan; 1982.

Day J, Mason P, Chesrow S. Effect of massage on serom level of β-endorphin and β-lipotrophin in healthy adults. *Phys Ther*. 1987;67:926–930.

Domenico G. Beards Massage Principles and Practice of Soft Tissue Manipulation. Philadelphia: W.B. Saunders; 2007.

Draper D. The deep muscle stimulator's effects on tissue stiffness in trigger-point therapy. *Athl Ther Today.* 2005;10(6):52.

Ebner M. Connective tissue massage. *Physiotherapy.* 1978;64: 208–210.

Ehrett S. Craniosacral therapy and myofascial release in entry-level physical therapy curricula. *Phys Ther.* 1988;68(4): 534–540.

Ernst E, Matra A, Magyarosy I. Massages cause changes in blood fluidity. *Physiotherapy.* 1987;73:43–45.

Fritz S. Fundamentals of Therapeutic Massage. St. Louis, MO: Mosby; 1995.

Furlan A, Brosseau L, Imamura M. Massage for low-back pain: a systematic review within the framework of the Cochrane Collaboration Back Review Group. *J Orthop Sports Phys Ther.* 2003;33(4):213–214.

Gemmell H, Allen A. Relative immediate effect of ischaemic compression and activator trigger point therapy on active upper trapezius trigger points: a randomised trial. *Clin Chiroprc.* 2008;11(4):175–181.

Goats G. Massage: the scientific basis of an ancient art: part 1, the techniques. *Br J Sports Med.* 1994;28(3):149–152.

Goldberg J, Seaborne D, Sullivan S. The effect of therapeutic massage on H-reflex amplitude in persons with a spinal cord injury. *Phys Ther.* 1994;74(8):728–737.

Gordon C, Emiliozzi C, Zartarian M. Use of a mechanical massage technique in the treatment of fibromyalgia: a preliminary study. *Arch Phys Med Rehabil.* 2006;87(1):145–147.

Hall D. A practical guide to the art of massage. *Runner's World.* 1979;14(10):58–59.

Hammer W. The use of transverse friction massage in the management of chronic bursitis of the hip or shoulder. *J Man Physiol Ther.* 1993;16(2):107–111.

Hanten W, Chandler S. Effects of myofascial release leg pull and sagittal plane isometric contract-relax techniques on passive straight-leg raise angle. *J Orthop Sports Phys Ther.* 1994;20(3):138–144.

Hilbert JE. The effects of massage on delayed onset muscle soreness. *Br J Sports Med.* 2003;37(1):72–75.

Hollis M. *Massage for Physical Therapists.* Oxford, England: Blackwell Scientific; 1987.

Horowitz S. Evidence-based indications for therapeutic massage. *Altern Complement Ther.* 2007;13(1):30–35.

Hovind H, Neilson S. Effect of massage on blood flow in skeletal muscle. *Scand J Rehabil Med.* 1974;6:74–77.

Kewley M. What you should know about massage. *Int Swim.* 1982;September:29–30.

Kirshbaum M. Using massage in the relief of lymphoedema. *Prof Nurse.* 1996;11(4):230–232.

Lewis M, Johnson M. The clinical effectiveness of therapeutic massage for musculoskeletal pain: a systematic review. *Physiotherapy.* 2006;92(3):146–158.

Malkin K. Use of massage in clinical practice. *Br J Nurs.* 1994; 3(6):292–294.

Mancinelli C, Aboulhosn L, Eisenhofer J. The effects of postexercise massage on physical performance and muscle soreness in female collegiate volleyball players. *J Orthop Sports Phys Ther.* 2003;33(2):A-60.

Manheim C. *The Myofascial Release Manual.* Thorofare, NJ: Slack; 2008.

Martin D. Massage. *Jogger.* 1978;10(5):8–15.

McConnell A. Practical massage. *Nurs Times.* 1995;91(36): S2–S14.

McGillicuddy M. Sports massage: three key principles of sports massage. *Massage Today.* 2003;3(5):10.

McKeechie AA. Anxiety states; a preliminary report on the value of connective tissue massage. *J Psychosomat Res.* 1983; 27(2):125–129.

Meagher J, Boughton P. *Sportsmassage.* New York: Doubleday; 1995.

Morelli M, Seaborne D, Sullivan S. H-reflex modulation during manual muscle massage of human triceps surae. *Arch Phys Med Rehabil.* 1991;72(11):915–999.

Morelli M, Seaborne PT, Sullivan SJ. H-reflex modulation during massage of triceps surae in healthy subjects. *Arch Phys Med Rehabil.* 1991;72:915.

Newman T, Martin D, Wilson L. Massage effects on muscular endurance. *J Athl Train.* 1996;(Suppl.)31:S-18.

Paterson C, Allen J. A pilot study of therapeutic massage for people with Parkinson's disease: the added value of user involvement. *Complement Ther Clin Pract.* 2005;11(3): 161–171.

Pellecchia G, Hamel H, Behnke P. Treatment of infrapatellar tendinitis: a combination of modalities and transverse friction massage versus iontophoresis. *J Sport Rehabil.* 1994; 3(2):135–145.

Phaigh R, Perry P. *Athletic Massage.* New York: Simon & Schuster; 1986.

Pope M, Phillips R, Haugh L. A prospective randomized three-week trial of spinal manipulation, transcutaneous muscle stimulation, massage and corset in the treatment of subacute low back pain. *Spine.* 1994;19(22):2571–2577.

Ryan J. The neglected art of massage. *Phys Sports Med.* 1980; 18(12):25.

Smith L, Keating M, Holbert D. The effects of athletic massage on delayed onset muscle soreness, creatine kinase, and neutrophil count: a preliminary report. *J Orthop Sports Phys Ther.* 1994;19(2):93–99.

Stamford B. Massage for patients. *Phys Sports Med.* 1985; 13(10):178.

Steward B, Woodman R, Hurlburt D. Fabricating a splint for deep friction massage. *J Orthop Sports Phys Ther.* 1995;21(3): 172–175.

Stone JA. Prevention and rehabilitation. Strain–counterstrain. *Athl Ther Today.*2000;5(6):30–31.

Sucher B. Myofascial manipulative release of carpal tunnel syndrome: documentation with magnetic resonance imaging. *Journal of the American Osteopathic Association.* 1993;93(12):1273–1278.

Sucher B. Myofascial release of carpal tunnel syndrome. *Journal of the American Osteopathic Association.* 1993;93(1): 92–94,100–101.

Suskind M, Hajek N, Hinds H. Effects of massage on denervated muscle. *Arch Phys Med .* 1946;27:133–135.

Tappan F. *Healing Massage Techniques: A Study of Eastern and Western Methods.* Reston, VA: Reston Publishing; 1980.

Tiidus P, Shoemaker J. Effleurage massage, muscle blood flow and long-term post-exercise strength recovery. *Int J Sports Med.* 1995;16(7):478–483.

Trevelyan J. Massage. *Nurs Times.* 1993;89(19):45–47.

van Schie T. Connective tissue massage for reflex sympathetic dystrophy: a case study. *NZ J Physiother.* 1993;21(2):26.

Wakim KG, Martin GM, Terrier JC. The effects of massage in normal and paralyzed extremities. *Arch Phys Med.* 1949;30:135–144.

Weber M, Servedio F, Woodall W. The effects of three modalities on delayed onset muscle soreness. *J Orthop Sports Phys Ther.* 1994;20(5):236–242.

Whitehill W. Massage and skin conditions: indications and contraindications. *Athl Ther Today.* 2002;7(3):24–28.

Wiktorrson-Moeller M, Oberg B, Ekstrand J. Effects of warming up, massage and stretching on range of motion and muscle strength in the lower extremity. *Am J Sports Med.* 1983;11:249–251.

Yates J. *Physiological Effects of Therapeutic Massage and Their Application to Treatment.* British Columbia: Massage Athletic Trainers Association; 1989.

GLOSSARY

acupressure   The technique of using finger pressure over acupuncture points to decrease pain.

bindegewebsmassage   Reflex zone massage; uses a pulling stroke across connective tissue to effect change.

effleurage   To stroke; any stroke that glides over the skin without attempting to move the deep muscle masses. The hand is molded to the part, stroking with more or less constant pressure, usually upward. Any degree of pressure may be applied, varying from the lightest possible touch to very deep pressure.

friction massage   A technique performed by small circular movements that penetrate into the depth of a muscle, not by moving the fingers on the skin, but by moving the tissues under the skin.

massage   The act of rubbing, kneading, or stroking the superficial parts of the body with the hand or with an instrument for the purpose of modifying nutrition, restoring power of movement, or breaking up adhesions.

myofascial release   A group of techniques used for the purpose of relieving soft tissue from the abnormal grip of tight fascia.

petrissage   Massage technique that is a kneading manipulation. Consists of repeatedly grasping and releasing the tissue with one or both hands or parts thereof, in a lifting, rolling, or pressing movement. The outside characteristic of this movement as contrasted to stroking movements is that the pressure is applied intermittently.

rolfing   A system devised to correct inefficient structure by balancing the body within a gravitational field through a technique involving manual soft tissue manipulation.

tapotement   A percussion massage; any series of brisk blows following each other in a rapid alternating fashion: hacking, cupping, slapping, beating, tapping, and pinchment. It is used when stimulation is the objective.

trager   A technique that attempts to establish neuromuscular control so that more normal movement patterns can be routinely performed.

vibration   A shaking massage technique; a fine tremulous movement made by the hand or fingers placed firmly against a part that will cause the part to vibrate. Often used for a soothing effect; may be stimulating when more energy is applied.

LAB ACTIVITY

Massage

DESCRIPTION

Massage is most likely the oldest form of mechanical therapy for injury. Even very small children know that rubbing an injured area tends to diminish the pain. As with essentially all physical agents, the massage itself does not produce healing, but the therapeutic effects can assist during the healing process.

There are many types of massage, each with proponents and detractors. The different types of massage have different proposed physiologic and therapeutic effects, although there is a great deal of overlap. In essence, all forms of massage involve the application of mechanical force to various tissues of the body, usually with the therapist's hands. Massage may exert an influence on the injured or dysfunctional tissue via either via a direct mechanical action or neurologic reflexes.

PHYSIOLOGIC EFFECTS

- Increase in large-diameter afferent neural input
- Increase in venous outflow
- Increase in lymph outflow

THERAPEUTIC EFFECTS

- Decreased pain
- Decreased soft tissue swelling and congestion
- Remodeling of collagen

INDICATIONS

The indications for massage vary depending on the type of massage used. In general, pain, swelling, and connective tissue contracture are the indications for massage.

CONTRAINDICATIONS

There are probably no absolute contraindications to massage. Obviously, precautions should be used in the case of fractures, open wounds, and severe pain. The amount of pressure applied can be regulated based on the irritability of the tissue and the desired effect.

MASSAGE			
PROCEDURE	EVALUATION		
	1	2	3
1. Check supplies.			
a. Obtain sheet or towels for draping.			
b. Obtain lubricant as indicated.			
2. Question patient.			
a. Verify identity of patient (if not already verified).			
b. Verify the absence of contraindications.			
c. Ask about previous massage treatments, check treatment notes.			
3. Position patient.			
a. Place patient in a well-supported, comfortable position. Positioning is particularly crucial for massage.			
b. Expose body part to be treated.			
c. Drape patient to preserve patient's modesty, protect clothing, but allow access to body part.			

4. Inspect body part to be treated.			
a. Check light touch perception.			
b. Check circulatory status (pulses, capillary refill).			
c. Verify that there are no open wounds or rashes.			
d. Assess function of body part (e.g., ROM, irritability).			
5a. Apply Hoffa massage			
a. After applying lubricant, effleurage is applied with a stroking motion from distal to proximal with light to moderate pressure; the deeper tissue is not moved. The initial strokes serve to distribute the lubricant over the treatment area.			
b. Petrissage is a kneading type motion, where the muscles are lifted and rolled.			
c. Tapotement is a series of percussion movements with the tips of the fingers, the ulnar border of the hands, the heel of the hands, or cupped hands.			
d. Vibration is a rapid oscillation or tremor of the hands when they are in firm contact with the skin.			
5b. Apply transverse friction massage.			
a. No lubricant is used.			
b. The tendon or ligament is placed on a slight stretch.			
c. Using deep pressure, such that the skin and thumb or finger, move together over the deeper tissue, apply a back-and-forth motion perpendicular to the fibers of the tendon or ligament.			
d. The duration of the massage should be up to 10 minutes, or as tolerated by the patient.			
5c. Apply connective tissue massage (Bindegewebsmassage).			
a. No lubricant is used.			
b. Using the tips of the third and fourth digits, the skin and subcutaneous tissues are pulled away from the fascia.			
c. The massage extends from the coccyx to the upper lumbar area, and each pulling stroke should produce a transient, sharp pain.			
d. Duration of treatment should be 15–25 minutes or as tolerated by the patient.			
5d. Acupressure/Trigger Point Massage.			
a. No lubricant is used.			
b. Technique is similar to transverse friction massage, but is applied to a trigger or acupuncture point (found using a chart, or by palpation). Trigger points usually are nodular-like lumps in a muscle, and often feel gritty.			
c. Using the tip of any digit, or even the olecranon process, the skin is moved on the trigger point; no motion should take place between the therapist and the patient's skin. The motion is circular, and is confined to the point.			